ENGLISH
FOR NUTRITIONISTS

ENGLISH
FOR NUTRITIONISTS

IRENA BAUMRUKOVÁ

ISBN:	Softcover	978-1-5144-9381-6
	eBook	978-1-5144-9382-3

Print information available on the last page.

Rev. date: 05/10/2016

To order additional copies of this book, contact:
Xlibris
800-056-3182
www.Xlibrispublishing.co.uk
Orders@Xlibrispublishing.co.uk
737268

Contents

PREFACE

The **first part** of the textbook, **Practical part**, is designed for **students, assistants, professionals in healthy life style and exercises, and nutritional specialists** who have to communicate in English or who wish to work in English speaking countries.

The level is lower intermediate to **intermediate,** but some of the texts can be used by **well motivated self-study beginners** as well. The language is easy and **vocabularies** give a very good selection of important words and they also indicate how the terms are **pronounced**. The students of various nationalities are supposed to **find out the meanings** by themselves and that is why the book can be used also in multilingual classes. Some learners will find it useful to **keep a notebook** containing the meanings of the new words.

Theoretical part of the textbook is designed for **medical students, physicians, nurses, nutritionists and nutritional scientists** whose first language is not English. This part is very good help to those who want to learn **professional journals** and textbooks, or to **take part in conferences** conducted in English. Exercises in each unit can be used as a basis for discussions.

The level of this part is intermediate to upper-intermediate. The book is a valuable resource for both individual and group study. You may choose to **work through the book from beginning to end or** you may find it more useful to **select chapters** according to your **interests and needs.** The book uses medical terms derived from Greek and Latin.

Knowledge of medicine is not essential for teachers using this book, and the students' professional knowledge may be a valuable learning combination. Teachers can use this book to **supplement more general course books** as well. The texts are English based and are therefore suitable for both **classroom use and for self-study.**

PRACTICAL PART

Chapter I
Healthy living

Unit 1 - Fit for life. Walking for fitness.

Exercise is for everyone

Whether you are young or old, male or female, your health will benefit from some form of regular exercise. **Exercise two or three times every week for 20 minute periods** to keep yourself fit for life. Regular exercise will make your heart and lungs more efficient and your muscles stronger. As well as improving your figure and posture and enhancing your overall sense of well-being.

Setting realistic targets

Set yourself **targets that are suitable for your level of fitness** and keep a daily record to monitor your progress. If you are out of shape, start slowly and gradually build up your exercise routine, increasing the length of time and the amount of effort you put in as your fitness improves. A stopwatch is a useful tool for monitoring progress.

Getting started

Choose a form of exercise that you enjoy, that your fitness level permits, and fits easily into your lifestyle. Otherwise you are unlikely to stick at it. Use stairs rather than lifts, and walk or cycle on short trips instead of taking your car. If you are elderly, obese, or have a medical disorder, **visit your doctor for a routine check-up before starting an exercise regime.**

- Health drive: when playing a competitive game like golf, be sure to compete against your own performance rather than your opponent.
- Don't jump in at the deep end: A gentle swim is an ideal way to begin a fitness programme. Swim at

your own pace for twenty minutes, three times a week.

Safety first

While some sports injuries are clearly unavoidable accidents, many can be prevented by taking simple precautions before starting exercise or by paying more attention to the appropriate safety guidelines.

- Do not exercise while you are still **aching from a previous session**.
- Do not take strenuous exercise if you have a condition such as **high blood pressure or heart disease**.
- Never exercise while you are under the influence of **drugs or alcohol**
- Since many sports injuries result from faulty technique, it is wise to seek basic **professional coaching**.

Clothing and equipment

Always wear the right protective equipment. Find out what you need and buy the appropriate model for your requirements.

- Always wear the equipment that is the **correct size**. This applies to rackets and bats, not just pads and helmets.
- Take off your **jewellery** before you participate in sport.
- Even good swimmers should wear **a life jacket** for water sports such as sailing or water-skiing
- Protective **eye wear**: choose goggle lenses made of shatter-proof plastic
- Good quality protective **helmets** carry an authorized safety standard kite mark.
- **Training shoes** should be comfortable and shock absorbent to avoid injury.

Stretch yourself

Prepare yourself for strenuous activity with a routine of stretching exercises. This will help you avoid damaging your muscles or joints. **Warm up** wisely. Although lotions and liniments may feel good and relieve some pain and stiffness incurred during strenuous exercise, never employ them as a substitute for your regular warm-up routine; lotions cannot help prevent injuries to muscles.

- Regular stretching enhances your **body's flexibility**. Always wear comfortable loose-fitting clothing when warming up.
- Stretch to the point where you feel a pull, **never bounce or jerk**.
- **Repeat your stretch routine when you finish** exercising to minimize the resulting aches and pains.
- Begin your stretching routine with a **gentle, aerobic activity**, start a brisk walk, to increase the flow of blood to your muscles.

- Swing your **arms**: stretch your arms out straight over your head and make large circling movements. Rotate your arms forwards five times, then back five times.
- **Shoulder** stretch: raise your arms away from your back. Clasp your hands behind you, then slowly raise your arms up. Hold the pull for a count of five seconds. Repeat this stretch five times.
- **Calf** stretch: Keep your back straight. With one leg in front of the other, gradually lean your weight onto your front leg. Hold for a count of five. Repeat five times. Feel a gentle pull on your calf muscle.
- **Leg** raises: Feel your hamstring stretch. Stand on one leg and raise your other leg up to your chest. Hold your leg against your chest for a count of five. Repeat five times.
- **Squats**: Lower yourself gently into a squat. Stand up again slowly, without using your hands to help you. Repeat this movement five times. Feel a gentle stretch in your thigh muscles.

Exercise 1a
Match the column A with the column B. Try to learn the expressions and/ or sentences by heart.

A

1. Regular exercise will
2. Do not exercise while
3. Do not take strenuous exercise
4. Never exercise
5. Take off your jewellery
6. Even good swimmers
7. Prepare yourself for strenuous activity
8. Always wear comfortable loose-fitting clothing
9. Repeat your stretch routine
10. Set yourself targets
11. If you are elderly, obese, or have a medical disorder

B

a) before you participate in sport.
b) if you have a condition such as high blood pressure or heart disease.
c) make your heart and lungs more efficient and your muscles stronger.
d) should wear a life jacket.
e) that are suitable for your level of fitness.
f) visit your doctor for a routine check-up before starting an exercise regime.
g) when warming up.
h) when you finish exercising to minimize the resulting aches and pains.
i) while you are under the influence of drugs or alcohol.

j) with a routine of stretching exercises.

k) you are still aching from a previous session.

Walking for fitness

Take regular walks to improve your health, whatever your age or level of fitness. Aim to walk about 3 km, at least three times a week. Start at a slow pace and gradually build up speed and distance. Walk fast enough to become a little tired, but never leave yourself exhausted.

Aerobic exercise

Walking, jogging, swimming, and rowing are all aerobic exercises because they can be performed for at least 12 minutes without a break. **Aerobic exercises**, which increase the efficiency of your heart and lungs **are an essential part of a fitness routine**

- Skip to health: **skipping is a convenient aerobic activity**, once the technique is mastered. Alternate this exercise with jogging on the spot. Do not jump higher than 10 cm.

How fit is your heart?

Age	**20 – 29 years**	**30 – 39 years**	**40 – 49 years**	**50+ years**
Fitness level				
Men				
excellent	under 60	under 64	under 66	under 68
good	60 - 69	64 - 71	66 - 73	68 -75
fair	70 -85	72- 87	74 - 89	76 - 91
poor	over 85	over 87	over 89	over 91
Women				
excellent	under 70	under 72	under 74	under 76
good	70 - 77	72 - 79	74 - 81	76 - 83
fair	78 - 94	86 - 96	82 - 98	84 - 100
poor	over 94	over 96	over 98	over 100

Heart beat

A resting pulse over 100 beats per minute may indicate a heart problem. You should therefore consult your doctor. The table above shows you how **resting pulse rate can indicate your overall level of fitness**. To find your resting pulse take your pulse **when you first wake up** – count your pulse for 15 seconds, then multiply by four to get a heart rate per minute. Then compare your pulse against the chart according to your age and sex. **How soon your pulse returns to normal after exercise also indicates the fitness of your heart**.

- Take your own pulse: the easiest place to locate and record your pulse is on the front of your wrist at the base of your thumb.
- Pulse recovery: step up and down a stair, moving one foot after another. Take your pulse rate after completing a step-up routine or similar strenuous exercise. **Your pulse rate should return to normal after four or five minutes.**

Exercise for strength

Any exercise that improves the condition of your muscles

will make day-to-day tasks like housework and shopping easier. It is a good idea **to join a gym where you can use apparatus under the supervision of a qualified instructor.** However, you do not need weights to improve muscle tone. Exercises can be performed by working against gravity.

- Abdominal exercise: bend your knees, sit-ups strengthen your abdominal muscles and lessen the risk of back injuries.

Exercise for the elderly

Regular exercise is the best preventive medicine available. It helps to maintain the normal functioning of joints, bones and muscles well into old age. If you are not used to exercise, **go to your doctor for a check up before you start**.

- Yoga provides a gentle form of exercise.

Exercise at home

A home exercise routine will help you build up the confidence to take part in other sports. **A wide variety of exercise machines** are now available for home use. **Exercise bikes and rowing machines** are the most popular devices. Don't buy costly exercise equipment that you are likely to discard after a few weeks.

On your bike:

- press-ups strengthen the upper arms and the pectorals across the front of your chest
- legs raises and sit-ups strengthen your abdominals. Remember always bend your knees when performing sit-ups.
- Use your stairs for step-ups to tone your thighs and calves.

Leg raises:

- lie on your back with your legs bent and draw your knees up one at a time towards your chin. Keep your leg bent during the exercise.

Press-ups:

- place your palms flat on the floor, shoulder-width apart, and bend your arms until your chin touches the floor.
- do not allow your back to arc
- keep your legs straight

Food and exercise

A healthy balanced diet is vital to provide the energy needed for activity. However, eating less than an hour before exercising may make you feel nauseous. When exercising, you must **drink plenty of water** to replace fluid lost due to perspiration

Don't overstretch yourself

Exercising can do more harm than good if you do not take time to **rest between sessions**. Never attempt any strenuous activity while your muscles are still aching from your last workout.

- **Allow 48 hours for your muscles to recover** after they have been worked to maximum capacity
- **It is normal to feel a little stiff after exercise**, but see a doctor if symptoms persist after about 5 days.
- **Signs of over training:** warning signs such as **recurrent infections or minor injuries** can soon appear if you exercise too frequently. Other symptoms are loss of appetite, insomnia, feelings of exhaustion or listlessness, and the loss of desire to keep fit.

Exercise 1b
Match the column A with the column B. Try to learn the expressions and/ or sentences by heart.

A

1. Start walking at a slow pace
2. Walking, jogging, swimming, and rowing
3. Skipping is a convenient aerobic activity,
4. A resting pulse over 100 beats per minute
5. The easiest place to locate and record your pulse
6. Your pulse rate should
7. Abdominal exercises
8. Regular exercise
9. Eating less than an hour before exercising
10. When exercising,
11. Signs of over training

B

a) *and gradually build up speed and distance.*
b) *are all aerobic exercises because they can be performed for at least 12 minutes without a break.*
c) *can soon appear if you exercise too frequently.*
d) *helps to maintain the normal functioning of joints, bones and muscles well into old age.*
e) *is on the front of your wrist at the base of your thumb.*
f) *may indicate a heart problem.*
g) *may make you feel nauseous.*
h) *once the technique is mastered.*
i) *return to normal after four or five minutes.*
j) *strengthen your abdominal muscles and lessen the risk of back injuries.*
k) *you must drink plenty of water to replace fluid lost due to perspiration.*

Exercise 2
Translate the expressions. Try to explain their meanings in English.

Efficient enhancing, accident, precautions, session, strenuous, coaching, racket, bat, protective equipment, participate, life jacket, lotions and liniments, stiffness, strenuous exercise, stretch out, clasp hands, keep straight, hold, squat, stick at, stopwatch, medical disorder, check-up, competitive game, at your own pace, speed and distance, exhausted, jogging, rowing, efficiency skipping, convenient, resting pulse, overall, multiply, chart, wrist, thumb, weights, gravity, abdominal, knees, back injuries, joints, bones and muscles, build up the confidence, discard, arms, pectorals, chest, knees, thighs, calves, leg, chin, palms, shoulder, arms nauseous, perspiration, persist, loss of appetite, insomnia, exhaustion, listlessness.

Exercise 3
Answer the following questions. Prepare short talks and/or dialogues on these topics.

1. What are the benefits of regular exercise?
2. Describe the appropriate safety guidelines.
3. Speak about suitable clothing and equipment.
4. Why are stretching exercises important?
5. Explain the importance of walking for fitness.
6. What do we understand by aerobic exercises?
7. How can resting pulse rate indicate your overall level of fitness?
8. Why is it a good idea to join a gym?
9. How can you exercise at home?
10. What are the symptoms of over stretching?

Vocabulary 1

Fill in the meanings in your mother language:

abdominal /æb'dɒm.ɪ.nəl/
absorbent /əb'sɔːbənt/
accident /'æksɪdənt/
ache /eɪk/
aim /eɪm/
allow /ə'laʊ/
alternate /'ɒl.tə.neɪt/
apart /ə'pɑːt/
apparatus /'æpəˌreɪtəs/
appear /ə'pɪər/
appropriate /ə'prəʊ.pri.ət/
arc /ɑːk/
arm /ɑːm/
attempt /ə'tempt/
attention /ə'ten.ʃən/
authorized /'ɔː.θər.aɪzd/
back /bæk/
balanced /'bæl.ənt.st/
bat /bæt/
be out of shape /ʃeɪp/
bend /bend/ **(bent, bent)**
bike /baɪk/
blood /blʌd/ **pressure** /'preʃ.ər/
bounce /'baʊnt .s/
break /breɪk/
brisk /brɪsk/
calf /kɑːf/ pl **calves** /kævz/
chart /tʃɑːt/
check /tʃek/ **-up** /ˌʌp/
chest /tʃest/
circle /'sɜː.kl̩/
clasp /klɑːsp/
coach /kəʊtʃ/
compare /kəm'peər/
compete /kəm'piːt/
competitive /kəm'pɛt. ɪ.tɪv/
complete /kəm'pliːt/

condition /kən'dɪʃən/
confidence /'kɒn.fɪ.dəns/
convenient /kən'viː.ni.ənt/
costly /'kɒstlɪ/
count /kaʊnt/
desire /dɪ'zaɪər/
device /dɪ'vaɪs/
discard /dɪ'skɑːd/
disease /dɪ'ziːz/
disorder /dɪ'sɔː.dər/
distance /'dɪs.tənt s/
draw /drɔː/
drive /draɪv/
efficiency /ɪ'fɪʃ.ən.si/
efficient /ɪ'fɪʃ.ənt/
effort /'ef.ət/
elderly /'el.dəl.i/
enhance /ɪn'hɑːns/
equipment /ɪ'kwɪp.mənt/
essential /ɪ'sen.t ʃəl/
excellent /'ek.səl.ənt/
exhausted /ɪg'zɔː.stɪd/
exhaustion /ɪg'zɔːs.tʃən/
eyewear /'aɪweər/
faulty /'fɒl.ti/
feel /fiːl/
figure /fɪgjər/
fitness /'fɪt.nəs/
flexibility /ˌflek.sɪ'bɪl.ə.ti/
flow /fləʊ/
gentle /'dʒen.tlˌ/
goggle /'gɒgəl/
gradually /'grædʒ.ʊ.li/
gravity /'græv.ɪ.tɪ/
guideline /'gaɪd.laɪn/
gym /dʒɪm/
hamstring /'hæmˌstrɪŋ/
heart /hɑːt/ **rate** /reɪt/
helmet /'hel.mət/
hold /həʊld/
housework /'haʊsˌwɜːk/
improve /ɪm'pruːv/
incurred /ɪn'kɜːrd/
influence /'ɪn.flʊ.əns/
injury /'ɪn.dʒər.i/
insomnia /ɪn'sɒm.ni.ə/
jerk /dʒɜːk/
jewellery /'dʒuː.əl.ri/
joint /dʒɔɪnt/
kitemark /'kaɪt.mɑːk/
lean /liːn/
leg /leg/
length /leŋk θ/
lense /lenz/
lie /laɪ/
life /laɪf/ **jacket** /'dʒæk.ɪt/
liniment /'lɪn.ɪ.mənt/
listlessness /'lɪst.lɪs.nɪs/
loose /luːs/**-fitting** /fɪt.ɪŋ/
lotion /'ləʊ.ʃən/
master /'mɑː.stər/
minor /'maɪ.nə/
movement /'muːv.mənt/
multiply /'mʌltɪplaɪ/
muscle /'mʌs.əl/
nauseous /'nɔː.zi.əs/
obese /əʊ'biːs/
opponent /ə'pəʊ.nənt/
overall /ˌəʊ.və'rɔːl/
overstretch /ˌəʊvə'stretʃ/
overtraining / 'əʊvə.treɪn.ɪŋ/
pace /peɪs/
pad /pæd/
pain /peɪn/
palm /pɑːm/
participate /pɑː'tɪs.ɪ.peɪt/
pectoral /'pek.tər.əl/
permit /pə'mɪt/
perspiration /ˌpɜː.spər'eɪ.ʃən/
posture /'pɒs.tʃər/
precaution /prɪ'kɔː.ʃən/
press-up /pres.ʌp/
prevent /prɪ'vent/
previous /'priː.vi.əs/
progress /'prəʊ.gres/
protective /prə'tek.tɪv/
pull /pʊl/
qualified /'kwɒlɪˌfaɪd/
racket /'ræk.ɪt/
raise /reɪz/

record /'rekɔːd/
recover /rɪ'kʌv.ər/
recovery /rɪ'kʌv.ər.i/
recurrent /rɪ'kʌr.ənt/
relieve /rɪ'liːv/
repeat /rɪ'piːt/
requirement /rɪ'kwaɪə.mənt/
rest /rest/
resting /'rest.ɪŋ/ **pulse** /pʌls/
rotate /rəʊ'teɪt/
routine /ruː'tiːn/
rowing /'rəʊ.ɪŋ/
safety /'seɪftɪ/
sailing /'seɪlɪŋ/
seek /siːk/ **(sought, sought)**
session /'seʃ.ən/
setting /'setɪŋ/
shatter /'ʃæt.ər/ **-proof** /pruːf/
shoulder /'ʃəʊl.dər/
sit-up /sɪt.ʌp/
skip /skɪp/
spot /spɒt/
squat /skwɒt/
stick at /stɪk/
stiffness /'stɪf.nəs/
stopwatch /'stɒpˌwɒt/
straight /streɪt/
strength /streŋθ/
strenuous /'stren.ju.əs/
stretch /stretʃ/
substitute /'sʌb.stɪ.tjuːt/
suitable /'sj uː.tə.blˌ/
supervision /ˌsuː.pə'vɪʒ.ən/
swing /swɪŋ/
target /'tɑː.gɪt/
thigh /θaɪ/
thumb /θʌm/
tired /'taɪəd/
tool /tuːl/
training /'treɪ.nɪŋ/
unavoidable /ˌʌn.ə'vɔɪ.də.bl̩/
unlikely /ʌn'laɪ.kli/
upper /'ʌp.ər/
warm /ˌwɔːm/ **up** /ʌp/
water-skiing /'wɔː.tər.skiː.ɪŋ/
weight /weɪt/
well-being /ˌwel'biː.ɪŋ/
width /wɪtθ/
wise /waɪz/
workout /'wɜː.kaʊt/
wrist /rɪst/

Solution to Exercise 1a
1c, 2k, 3b, 4i, 5a, 6d, 7j,
8g, 9h, 10e, 11f

Solution to Exercise 1b
1a, 2b, 3h, 4f, 5e, 6i, 7j,
8d, 9g, 10k, 11c

Unit 2 - Weight watching. Learning to relax.

Apart from excess fat, other signs of weight problems include frequent breathlessness and aching joints in the lower back, hips, and knees.

- **Skin fold test**: to assess approximately how much body fat you are carrying, try pinching a fold of skin between your thumb and index finger. Take care not to include any muscle tissue in the pinch. If you find that you are able to pinch more than one inch of fat, then you would benefit from losing some weight by changing your eating and exercise habits.

Causes of weight gain

Most people put on weight simply because they eat more food than their body requires. However, it is not the amount eaten, but rather the type of food, that causes weight problems.

- **Sweet snacks**: many soft drinks have added sugar and should not be part of a healthy diet.
- **Fatty foods**: eating calorie-rich foods high in fat will cause weight gain.
- Avoid **fried foods.**

Dangers of obesity

Fat should account for about 15 to 20% of body weight in healthy young adult men and 20 to 25% in healthy young adult women. A person who is more than 40% over the desirable weight for his or her age and height runs twice the **risk of early death from coronary heart disease**. Obese people may suffer from **back pain**. This is because the upper part of the body is heavy, putting pressure on the lower spine.

Hazards of long-term obesity:

- **Strokes** are twice as likely to occur in obese people because they often have **a high level of blood cholesterol or high blood pressure**.
- Obesity can cause **breathlessness** during exertion and in the most severe cases even when the obese person is at rest.
- The increase in mortality among people who are obese is due mainly to circulatory diseases, such as **coronary heart disease**
- Obese people are vulnerable to skin chafing and **fungal infections** in areas where folds of skin rub together, for example in the groin.
- Extra weight places **strain on the joints in the legs**. Joint swelling and pain associated with **osteoarthritis** may be made worse by obesity.

How to stop overeating

If you are overweight, **eating frequent small meals** – rather than bingeing on large infrequent meals with unhealthy snacks in between – is the best way to control your weight. The foods you eat **should be nutritious** and must not add up to an excessive number of calories.

Dieting do's and don'ts

Popular diets are often unpalatable and monotonous. At worst such regimes may even be detrimental to your health, causing indigestion, wind, or aggravating any existing metabolic disorders. It is generally best to opt for **a balanced, calorie-controlled diet, rich in fibre and low in fat and refined carbohydrates**, which can be maintained when you have reached your ideal weight.

- **See your doctor before you start any type of diet** if you are very overweight or if you are suffering from a medical disorder such as diabetes or heart disease.

- **Join a slimming organization** if you think this will help to keep you motivated.
- It is important to **eat your food slowly** – not only will your meal last longer and seem more substantial, you will also decrease the risk of indigestion. If you eat fast, by the time you feel that you have eaten enough you will actually have eaten too much.
- **Don't miss meals: if you miss meals, your body will receive warning signals telling it** to try to conserve energy (so burning fewer calories) in response to the temporary absence of food. By eating three healthy meals each day you will find that you are less tempted to snack on high-calorie fast foods.
- If your calorie intake is greater than your energy and body maintenance requirements, then you will gain weight.

Exercises to lose weight

Never use the fact that you are overweight as an excuse for avoiding exercise. **Regular physical activity** will help you lose weight by burning up calories. It also raises your basal metabolic rate, thereby increasing the number of calories your body will burn up when you are at rest.

- Walking: **brisk walking** can help you to lose weight and gives your heart and lungs a workout at the same time.
- Beat the bulge: try this **exercise to strengthen your abdominal muscles.** Lie on your back with your knees bent and curl your knees and your head towards each other.
- Gentle exercise: many overweight people are too embarrassed to participate in sport. **Stretching exercises** and other physical activities can be done in your own home.

Exercise 1a
Match the column A with the column B. Try to learn the expressions and/ or sentences by heart.

A

1. Signs of weight problems include
2. Most people put on weight
3. Many soft drinks
4. Eating calorie-rich foods high in fat
5. Strokes are twice as likely to occur in obese people
6. Obesity can cause
7. Joint swelling and pain associated with osteoarthritis
8. Eating frequent small meals
9. Popular diets
10. It is generally best
11. If you eat fast,

12. If you miss meals,
13. Regular physical activity

B

a) *because they eat more food than their body requires.*
b) *because they often have a high level of blood cholesterol or high blood pressure.*
c) *breathlessness during exertion and in the most severe cases even when the obese person is at rest.*
d) *by the time you feel that you have eaten enough you will actually have eaten too much.*
e) *frequent breathlessness and aching joints in the lower back, hips, and knees.*
f) *have added sugar and should not be part of a healthy diet.*
g) *is the best way to control your weight.*
h) *may be made worse by obesity.*
i) *may even be detrimental to your health, causing indigestion, wind, or aggravating any existing metabolic disorders.*
j) *raises your basal metabolic rate, thereby increasing the number of calories your body will burn up when you are at rest.*
k) *to opt for a balanced, calorie-controlled diet, rich in fibre and low in fat and refined carbohydrates.*
l) *will cause weight gain.*
m) *your body will receive warning signals telling it to try to conserve energy (so burning fewer calories).*

Learning to relax

Organize your life so as not to cause yourself too much stress and learn relaxation exercises to combat the stress you cannot control. A positive self-image and a **healthy attitude to life** will help you to cope with stressful situations both at home and in your place of work.

Fight or flight

Human bodies are designed to respond physically, rather than mentally, to a stressful situation. This **instinctive reaction** is known as the 'fight or flight' response. If the body is aroused without any accompanying physical response, then stress is likely to be harmful. Such situations demand self-control. Natural response to a stressful situation triggers the 'fight or flight' response in humans and animals.

Stress-related illnesses

Although is is not possible to avoid all **stressful situations,** a prolonged period of severe stress or several sources of minor stress, can lead to **physical or mental illness**. Excessive stress puts your body into a state of emotional turmoil. This agitation may affect **a variety of organs and systems within the body** and can eventually produce many different types of diseases.

Mental problems may be brought on by stress. Long-term stress can lead to **mental disorders**. Some **asthmatics** find their condition is aggravated by emotional upset. Stress is known to cause or aggravate many diseases of the **digestive tract**.

Prolonged stress can weaken the immune system, making you more susceptible to **minor infections**. Skin disorders such as **eczema** may flare up during periods of abnormal stress. Stress can **increase blood pressure**, which in turn increases the risk of a **heart attack**. Many people develop an **irritable bladder** as a direct response to stressful events. In men, stress is the most common cause of **impotence** and premature ejaculation. In women, stress can lead to **menstrual disorders.**

Are you stressed?

Recognizing that you are stressed is the first step to regaining control of your emotional health. Some common **symptoms of stress** are listed here:

- Being **indecisive or lacking concentration**
- Finding it **difficult to fall asleep or relax.**
- Constantly **feeling tired and lethargic**.
- Becoming **irritable and impatient.**
- Suffering from **recurrent headaches**.
- **Eating** when you are not hungry.
- Suffering from **nervous ticks**.
- **Smoking or drinking** more.
- Often **wanting to cry**.

What is causing your stress?

Identifying the cause of your stress is the first step towards reducing it. The cause may be obvious to you – **the death of a family member** or a close friend, for example can lead to serious depression. **Marriage and divorce** are also extremely stressful events, as is **pregnancy**. Any major career change can also be stressful: beginning **a new job**, **being fired** or made redundant. Sometimes the cause of your stress may not be so obvious. It may be caused by a change in your **eating habits**, or a change in social activities. Your stress may be caused by a combination of many problems.

Beating PMS

Some women suffer acute depression due to **premenstrual syndrome**, which may occur at any time in the two weeks prior to a period. Try the following measures:

- **Avoid salt, caffeine, and chocolate** in the two weeks before your period begins.
- **Exercise aerobically** - swimming is ideal.
- Visit your doctor – **hormone therapy** may be beneficial. Oral contraceptives may be prescribed to regulate hormone levels.
- Capsules of oil of evening primrose or vitamin B_6

taken for ten days before your period may help.

Reducing stress at work

Having too much to do is a common cause of stress. Stress at work may be due to interpersonal problems such as **hostility** from colleagues or **sexual harassment**. If you cannot solve the problem yourself, make a formal complaint.

- Don't accept **unrealistic demands**.
- Learn to **delegate tasks** if possible.
- Always set yourself **realistic goals**.
- Accept any **changes** optimistically.
- **Learning to say 'no'** to excessive demands is a skill that must be learned to avoid stress at work.
- **Working long hours, taking work home, cancelling holidays** due to pressure at work, are all signs that you are working too hard.

Exercise 1b
Match the column A with the column B. Try to learn the expressions and/ or sentences by heart.

A

1. A positive self-image and a healthy attitude to life
2. A stressful situation
3. A prolonged period of severe stress or several sources of minor stress
4. Prolonged stress can weaken the immune system,
5. Recognizing that you are stressed
6. Some women suffer acute depression
7. Stress at work may be due to

B

a) *can lead to physical or mental illness.*
b) *due to premenstrual syndrome, which may occur at any time in the two weeks prior to a period.*
c) *interpersonal problems such as hostility from colleagues or sexual harassment.*
d) *is the first step to regaining control of your emotional health.*
e) *making you more susceptible to minor infections.*
f) *triggers the 'fight or flight' response in humans and animals.*
g) *will help you to cope with stressful situations.*

Exercise 2
Translate the expressions. Try to explain their meanings in English.

Aching joints, hips, approximately, index finger, put on weight, soft drinks, weight gain, desirable weight, suffer from, back pain, high level, breathlessness, exertion, at rest, mortality, vulnerable to, groin, strain on the joints, swelling and pain, overweight, excessive, unpalatable, detrimental, indigestion, aggravating, medical disorder, substantial, snack, basal metabolic rate, embarrassed, combat, cope with, aroused, harmful, triggers, 'fight or flight' response, turmoil, agitation, aggravated, emotional upset, susceptible, flare up, recognizing, indecisive, fall asleep, impatient, recurrent, obvious, redundant, beneficial, contraceptives, formal complaint.

Exercise 3
Answer the following questions. Prepare short talks and/or dialogues on these topics.

1. Why do people put on weight?
2. What are the dangers of obesity?
3. How to stop overeating?
4. Dieting do's and don'ts.
5. Explain the term 'fight or flight' response.
6. Speak about different types of diseases brought on by stress (mental disorders, increased blood pressure, heart attack, digestive tract disorders).
7. Describe some common symptoms of stress: lacking concentration, feeling tired, becoming irritable, having recurrent headaches, smoking or drinking more.
8. What can cause your stress?
9. How would you reduce stress at work?

Vocabulary 2

Fill in the meanings in your mother language:

accept /ək'sept/
accompany /ə'kʌm.pə.ni/
aching /eɪk.ɪŋ/
added /'æd.ɪd/
aggravate /'æg.rə.veɪt/
agitation /ˌædʒ.ɪ'teɪ.ʃən/
approximately /ə'prɒk.sɪ.mət.lɪ/
arouse /ə'raʊz/
assess /ə'ses/
associated /ə'səʊ.si.eɪ.tɪd/
attitude /'æt.ɪ.tjuːd/
avoid /ə'vɔɪd/
be tempted to /'temptɪd/
beneficial /ˌben.ɪ'fɪʃ.əl/
binge /bɪndʒ/
bladder /'blæd.ər/
breathlessness /'breθ.ləs.nəs/
bulge /bʌldʒ/
burning /'bɜː.nɪŋ/
caffeine /'kæf.iːn/
calorie /'kælərɪ/
cancel /'kæn.səl/
capsule /'kæp.sjuːl/
carbohydrate /ˌkɑː.bəʊ 'haɪ.dreɪt/
career /kə'rɪə/
cause /kɔːz/
chafe /tʃeɪf/
combat /'kɒm.bæt/
common /'kɒm.ən/
complaint /kəm'pleɪnt/
conserve /kən'sɜːv/
constantly /'kɒnt .stənt.li/
contraceptive /ˌkɒn.trə'sep.tɪv/
cope /kəʊp/
coronary /'kɒr.ən.ər.i/ **heart** / hɑːt/ **disease** /dɪ'ziːz/
cry /kraɪ/
curl /kɜːl /
danger /'deɪn.dʒər/
delegate /'delɪˌgeɪt/
demand /dɪ'mɑːnd/

desirable /dɪˈzaɪə.rə.bl̩/
detrimental /ˌdet.rɪˈmen.təl/
diabetes /ˌdaɪəˈbiː.tiːz/
mellitus /məˈlaɪ.təs/
digestive /da ɪˈdʒes.tɪv/
divorce /dɪˈvɔːs/
eczema /ˈek.sɪ .mə/
ejaculation /ɪˌdʒækjʊˈleɪʃən/
embarrassed /ɪmˈbær.əst/
evening /ˈiːv.nɪŋ/ **primrose** / ˈprɪm.rəʊz/
event /ɪˈvent/
excessive /ekˈses.ɪv/
excuse /ɪkˈskjuːz/
exertion /ɪɡˈzɜː.ʃən/
extremely /ɪkˈstriːm.li/
fall /ˈfɔːl/ **asleep** /əˈsliːp/
fast food /fɑːst.fuːd/
fat /fæt/
fibre /ˈfaɪ.bər/
fight or flight /ˌfaɪt.ɔː.ˈflaɪt/
finding /ˈfaɪn.dɪŋ/
fire /faɪə/
flare /fleər/ **up** /ʌp/
fold /fəʊld/
food /fuːd/
fried /fraɪd/
fungal /ˈfʌŋ.gəl/
groin /ɡrɔɪn/
habits /ˈhæb.ɪts/
harassment /ˈhær.əs.mənt/
harmful /ˈhɑːm.fəl/
hazard /ˈhæz.əd/
heart /hɑːt/ **disease** /dɪˈziːz/
hip /hɪp/
human /hjuːmən/
illness /ˈɪl.nəs/
impatient /ɪmˈpeɪ.ʃənt/
impotence /ˈɪm.pə.təns/
inch /ɪntʃ/
indecisive /ˌɪndɪˈsaɪ.sɪv/
index /ˈɪn.deks/ **finger** /ˈfɪŋ.gər/
indigestion /ˌɪn.dɪ.dʒes.tʃən/
infrequent /ɪnˈfriː.kwənt/
instinctive/ɪnˈstɪŋk.tɪv/
irritable /ˈɪr.ɪ.tə.bl̩/
lack /læk/
lethargic /ləˈθɑː.dʒɪk/
lose /luːz/
lung /lʌŋ/
maintenance /ˈmeɪn.tɪ.nəns/
marriage /ˈmær.ɪdʒ/
measure /ˈmeʒ.ər/
menstrual /ˈmen.strəl/
period /ˈpɪə.ri.əd/
mental /ˈmen.təl/
mentally /ˈmen.təl.i/
miss /mɪs/
monotonous /məˈnɒtənəs/
mortality /mɔːˈtæl.ə.ti/
natural /ˈnætʃ.ər.əl/
nutritious /njuːˈtrɪʃəs/
obesity /əʊ ˈbiː.sɪ.ti/
obvious /ˈɒb.vi.əs/
opt /ɒpt/
osteoarthritis /ˌɒs.ti.əʊ.ɑːˈθraɪ.tɪs/
overeating /ˌəʊvərˈiːtɪŋ/
overweight /ˌəʊ.vəˈweɪt/
period /ˈpɪə.ri.əd/
physically /ˈfɪz.ɪ.kəl.i/
pinching /pɪntʃ.ɪŋ/
pregnancy /ˈpreg.nən.si/
premature /ˈprem.ə.tʃər/
premenstrual /priːˈmens.trʊ.əl/
prescribe /prɪˈskraɪb/
prior /praɪər/
prolonged /prəˈlɒŋd/
receive /rɪˈsiːv/
recognize /ˈrek.əg.naɪz/
reduce /rɪˈdjuːs/
redundant /rɪˈdʌn.dənt/
refined /rɪˈfaɪnd/
regain /rɪˈgeɪn/
relax /rɪˈlæks/
response /rɪˈspɒns/
rub /rʌb/
self-control /ˌself.kənˈtrəʊl/
self-image /ˌself.ˈɪm.ɪdʒ/
severe /sɪˈvɪər/
skill /skɪl/

skin /skɪn/
slim /slɪm/
snack /snæk/
soft /sɒft/ **drink** /drɪŋk/
solve /sɒlv/
spine /spaɪn/
strain /streɪn/
stressful /ˈstres.fəl/
stroke /strəʊk/
substantial /səbˈstæn.ʃəl/
suffer /ˈsʌf.ər/
susceptible /səˈsep.tɪ.bl̩/
swelling /ˈswel.ɪŋ/
syndrome /ˈsɪn.drəʊm/
temporary /ˈtem.pər.ər.i/
tick /tɪk/
tissue /ˈtɪʃ.uː/
trigger /ˈtrɪg.ər/
turmoil /ˈtɜː.mɔɪl/
unpalatable /ʌnˈpæl.ət.əb.əl/
upset /ʌpˈset/
vulnerable /ˈvʌl.nər.ə.bl̩/
warning /ˈwɔː.nɪŋ/
watching /ˌwɒtʃ.ɪŋ/
weaken /ˈwiː.kən/
weight /weɪt/ **gain** /geɪn/
wind /wɪnd/

Solution to Exercise 1a
1e, 2a, 3f, 4m, 5b, 6c, 7h, 8g, 9i, 10l, 11d, 12n, 13j

Solution to Exercise 1b
1g, 2f, 3a, 4e, 5d, 6b, 7c

Unit 3 - Coping with stress. Yoga.

Time management

Reduce your stress levels by learning to manage your time effectively.

- Prioritize your **tasks for each working day**.
- **Prepare a list of tasks** every day.
- Concentrate on **difficult jobs first**.
- Transfer all uncompleted tasks to the following day's prioritized list.
- Divide any large projects into smaller, more manageable, portions.
- **Don't put things off** unnecessarily.
- Try to view unwelcome projects as a challenge, and reward yourself for all work completed successfully.

Take a break

Regular breaks should be taken at intervals during the working day to help to relieve pressure and refresh your mind after a session of concentrated mental or physical effort, or if you find yourself becoming frustrated with a particular project.

- Take **regular holidays** or weekend breaks.
- Take **regular exercise**. Physical activity reduces tension, helps you to sleep better, releases pent-up emotions, and helps to take your mind off your problems.

Stress for dinner

Unhealthy eating habits have been blamed for aggravating symptoms of stress. The presence of caffeine, and a host of additives, in many of the snack foods that we purchase has been connected with insomnia and other stress-related conditions.

- Certain common **food additives**, are blamed for causing hyperactivity.
- **Too much salt** with your food can aggravate high blood pressure. **Soy sauce** and other condiments are also frequently high in sodium content.
- Too much **coffee** may cause some unpleasant side effects – **difficulty sleeping, irritability, and tremors.**

Exercises to ease tension

1. **Slow your breathing**
2. Shut your eyes and **imagine a beautiful scene.** For five minutes, explore the sights and sounds, savouring every detail.
3. Close your eyes. **Count backwards from 20,** whispering each number every time you breathe out
4. **Lie down** in a quiet, dimly lit room. **Relax your hands** with your **palms facing upwards.** Keep your **legs straight but relaxed,** and let your feet flop outwards. Close your eyes and **breathe gently and deeply** at your own resting rhythm.
5. Next, **screw up your face muscles tightly** for about 10 seconds, **then allow them to relax.**
6. **Lift up your head slowly** off the floor, and **let it fall back.** Relax your jaw and neck so that you can feel your throat opening.
7. **Keep your legs straight** but relaxed. **Press your shoulders against the floor** for 10 seconds and then relax them again.
8. Keep your head back on the floor. **Stretch out your arms and fingers. Hold them rigid** for 10 seconds before relaxing.
9. **Feel your spine stretch, then relax.** Lift your buttocks up off the floor and then relax gently and let them fall back down.
10. Keep your **breathing gentle and rhythmical.** Keeping your heels together, **stretch your legs and toes outwards; then relax completely.**

Exercise 1a
Match the column A with the column B. Try to learn the expressions and/ or sentences by heart.

A

1. Reduce your stress levels
2. Regular breaks should be taken
3. Physical activity
4. The presence of caffeine, and a host of additives
5. Too much coffee

B

a) by learning to manage your time effectively.
b) during the working day to help to relieve pressure and refresh your mind
c) has been connected with insomnia and other stress-related conditions.
d) may cause some unpleasant side effects – difficulty sleeping, irritability, and tremors.
e) reduces tension, helps you to sleep better, releases pent-up emotions, and helps to take your mind off your problems.

Yoga

Yoga is an ancient discipline and teaches **coordinated movement and postures, relaxation, breathing control, and meditation techniques**. Correctly practised, yoga is a useful method of relaxation, which helps maintain body flexibility, and **can increase both muscle stress and endurance**. Yoga exercises both sides of the body equally.

- **Side way stretch**: to achieve a healthy balance, it is crucial to keep all parts of the body strong and supple. Keep your legs straight. Stretch to the same extent on each side.
- **Spinal twist**: the spinal twist is an excellent position for improving flexibility in the spine and relieving back pain.
- **Head to knee**: lean forwards from your hips. Draw your chest as close to your knees as possible. Hold this pose for 30 seconds. Keep your spine as straight as possible. Don't force your head down.
- **Stretching back**: from a standing position, stretch your arms back over your head. Keep your arms parallel to your ears. Arch your chest and hips, and keep your feet together. Keep your knees straight.
- **Double leg raise**: lie with your feet together and your hands flat on the floor. Breathe in, and raise both legs. Repeat five times

Meditation

Regular meditation is useful for reducing stress and for **relieving many stress-related disorders**. Begin by sitting in a comfortable position, with your back straight and your eyes closed. Choose a word that has no emotional significance for you and repeat it silently to yourself. **Prevent your mind from wandering by concentrating on your breathing.**

- Keep your back straight
- If possible, sit in a cross-legged position

Thinking positively

A positive self-image and healthy attitude to life **will increase your resistance to stress**. If you feel a loss of confidence and self-esteem, try making a list of your positive characteristics and think positively about those things that you have succeeded in doing in the past.

Massage

Giving or receiving a relaxing massage is a useful way to reduce stress. **Stroking, rubbing, kneading and pummelling** different areas of the body can **increase blood flow, reduce pain, relax muscles, and make the skin more supple**. When giving a massage, use firm pressure on large muscles; on smaller areas, apply gentle pressure with your fingertips.

- **Hand massage:** You will be able to massage many areas of your body yourself. Hands are hard-working parts of the body, so it is good to pamper them for a change.
- **Treat your feet**: A foot massage not only keeps your feet flexible and healthy, but also helps to relax and refresh your whole body.
- **Back massage**: A soothing back rub can cure tension and muscular pain in the back. It can also impart a feeling of peace and relaxation, so aiding restful sleep.

Techniques for massage

When giving a massage, it is crucial to use **a warm, dimly lit room** where you won't be disturbed. Give the massage on **a firm, padded surface**, such as thick blankets placed on the floor. Remove all jewellery and use **carrier oils to prevent friction.**

- **Cover the body with towels**; only expose those areas of the body that are being massaged.
- **Keep one of your hands in contact** with the body all the time, and use rhythmic motions.
- During the massage, **concentrate on the movements**, do not chatter.

Need for sleep

Make sure that you get sufficient sleep to rest and restore your body. The brain and the body's metabolic processes require **regular periods of rest to recover**. Growth hormone is released during sleep, renewing tissues and producing new bone and red blood cells. Sleeping poorly at night will soon begin to affect your health.

- Losing sleep: try to stop worrying about not sleeping – just resting in bed will do you some good.

Avoid taking tranquillizers

Although **tranquillizers can prove helpful in cases of extreme stress**, such as bereavement, they are not a long-term solution.

Tranquillizers should only be taken when all other measures have failed. Only take tranquillizers for the shortest possible time to **avoid the risk of becoming dependent on them**. This will also give you the chance to build up your own ability to live with and fight against pressures you are under.

Exercise 1b
Match the column A with the column B. Try to learn the expressions and/or sentences by heart.

A

1. Yoga is a useful method of relaxation,
2. The spinal twist is an excellent position
3. Regular meditation
4. Prevent your mind from wandering
5. A positive self-image and healthy attitude to life
6. A foot massage
7. When giving a massage,
8. Make sure that you get sufficient sleep
9. Only take tranquillizers for the shortest possible time

B

a) by concentrating on your breathing.
b) for improving flexibility in the spine and relieving back pain.
c) is useful for reducing stress and for relieving many stress-related disorders.
d) it is crucial to use a warm, dimly lit room where you won't be disturbed.
e) not only keeps your feet flexible and healthy, but also helps to relax and refresh your whole body.
f) to avoid the risk of becoming dependent on them.
g) to rest and restore your body.
h) which helps maintain body flexibility, and can increase both muscle stress and endurance.
i) will increase your resistance to stress.

Exercise 2
Translate the expressions. Try to explain their meanings in English.

Prioritize, challenge, reward, session, tension, blamed, aggravating, caffeine, additives, condiments, insomnia, irritability, tremors, explore, savouring, whisper, flop outwards, screw up, allow to relax, lift up, let it fall back, keep straight, press against the floor, stretch out, hold rigid, spine stretch, ancient, flexibility, endurance, equally, crucial, extent, spinal twist, relieving, arch, raise, repeat, significance, wandering, cross-legged position, self-esteem, impart, stroking, rubbing, kneading and pummelling, supple, pamper, soothing, cure, friction, expose, motions, chatter, growth hormone, tranquillizers, bereavement.

Exercise 3
Answer the following questions. Prepare short talks and/or dialogues on these topics.

1. What do you understand by time management at work?
2. Speak about unhealthy eating habits.
3. Describe some exercises to ease tension.
4. Speak about yoga and meditation as useful methods of relaxation.
5. Why is thinking positively so important?
6. What can you say about giving and receiving massage?
7. Why do we need to get sufficient sleep?

Vocabulary 3

Fill in the meanings in your mother language:

ability /əˈbɪl.ɪ.ti/
additive /ˈæd.ɪ.tɪv/
affect /əˈfekt/
ancient /ˈeɪn.tʃənt/
bereavement /bɪˈriːv.mənt/
blame /bleɪm/
blanket /ˈblæŋ.kɪt/
break /breɪk/
buttock /ˈbʌt.ək/
carrier /ˈkærɪ.ə/ **oil** /ɔɪl/
chatter /ˈtʃæt.ər/
challenge /ˈtʃæl.ɪndʒ/
condiment /ˈkɒn.dɪ.mənt/
content /kənˈtent/
correctly /kəˈrekt.li/
cross /krɒs/ **-legged** /ˈlegd/
crucial /ˈkruː.ʃəl/
cure /kjʊər/
dependent /dɪˈpen.dənt/
dimly /ˈdɪmlɪ/
discipline /ˈdɪsɪplɪn/
disturb /dɪˈstɜːb/
double /ˈdʌb.l̩/
ease /iːz/
emotion /ɪˈməʊ.ʃən/
endurance /ɪnˈdjʊə.rənt s/
explore /ɪkˈsplɔːr/
extent /ɪkˈstent/
face /feɪs/
fall /ˈfɔːl/ **back** /bæk/
fingertip /ˈfɪŋ.gə.tɪp/
firm /fɜːm/
flat /flæt/
flop /flɒp/
force /fɔːs/
friction /ˈfrɪk.ʃən/
frustrated /frʌˈstreɪtɪd/
Growth /grəʊθ/ **Hormone** /ˈhɔː.məʊn/
heel /hiːl/
host /həʊst/
hyperactivity /ˌhaɪ.pərˈækˈtɪv.ɪ.ti/
impart /ɪmˈpɑːt/
incomplete /ˌɪn.kəmˈpliːt/
interval /ˈɪn.tə.vəl/
irritability /ˌɪr.ɪ.təˈbɪl.ɪ.ti/
jaw /dʒɔː/
keep /kiːp/
knead /niːd/
lift /lɪft/ **up** /ʌp/
list /lɪst/
lit /lɪt/
maintain /meɪnˈteɪn/
manageable /mænɪdʒəbəl/
management /ˈmæn.ɪdʒ.mənt/
massage /ˈmæs.ɑːʒ/
meditation /ˌmedɪˈteɪ.ʃən/
mind /maɪnd/
motion /ˈməʊ.ʃən/
padded /ˈpæd.ɪd/
pamper /ˈpæm.pə/
parallel /ˈpær.ə.lel/
pent-up /pent.ʌp/
pose /pəʊz/

practised /'præktɪst/
pressure /'preʃ.ə/
prioritize /praɪ'ɒrɪˌtaɪz/
prove /pruːv/
pummel /'pʌməl/
purchase /'pɜːtʃ.ɪs/
put /pʊt/ **off** /ɒf/
red /red/ **blood** /blʌd/ **cell** /sel/
refresh /rɪ'freʃ/
relaxation /ˌriː.læk'seɪ.ʃən/
renew /rɪ'njuː/
resistance /rɪ'zɪs.tənts/
restful /'restfʊl/
resting /'rest.ɪŋ/
reward /rɪ'wɔːd/
rhythm /'rɪðəm/
rigid /'rɪdʒ.ɪd/
savour /'seɪ.və/
screw /skruː/ **up** /ʌp/
side /saɪd/ **effect** /ɪ'fekt/
sideways /saɪdˌweɪz/
sodium /'səʊ.di.əm/
soothing /'suː.ðɪŋ/
soy /sɔɪ/ **sauce** /sɔːs/
stand /stænd/
stroke /strəʊk/
succeed /sək'siːd/
supple /sʌpəl/
task /tɑːsk/
throat /θrəʊt/
tightly /'taɪt.li/
toe /təʊ/
tranquillizer /'træŋ.kwɪ.laɪ.zər/
treat /triːt/
tremor /'trem.ər/
twist /twɪst/
wander /'wɒn.dər/
whisper /'wɪspə/
yoga /'jəʊgə/

Solution to Exercise 1a
1a, 2b, 3e, 4c, 5d

Solution to Exercise 1b
1h, 2b, 3c, 4a, 5i, 6e, 7d, 8g, 9f

Unit 4 - Nutritional know-how

Fuel for your body

Good nutrition is vital for good health. Food provides the body with the energy needed to sustain life. It is the **raw material for growth, repair, and maintenance of vital organs and tissues**. The substances in food that fulfil these functions are known as **nutrients**. Carbohydrates, fats, proteins, fibre, vitamins, and minerals are six vital elements that can be extracted from a varied, well balanced diet.

Carbohydrates

Carbohydrates, which can be divided into two main types – **sugars and starches**, are the body's principal **source of energy**. Starch, which can be found in pasta, bread, potatoes, and the majority of fruits, is the optimum source of energy and should always be eaten in preference of sugars, which are found in foods like ice cream. Even if slimming, starch should play a major role in your diet. Experts believe that **carbohydrates,** which are found in fruit and vegetables, should make up **about 55% of a healthy diet**.

Brown or white?

You should always choose to eat **unrefined carbohydrates** and cut down on all refined foods, especially those that have added sugar. To make a refined carbohydrate, such as white sugar, or white rice, the manufacturer employs a process that actually removes a large percentage of the food's fibre and other nutrients such as vitamins and minerals. Unrefined carbohydrates, such as **brown pasta and wholemeal bread** have a higher nutrient value than refined carbohydrates such as white sugar or white rice.

Fat facts

Fats should constitute **up to 30% of a healthy diet**. They are a highly concentrated energy source and are vital to the process of cell growth and repair. There are two types of fats: **saturated, found in animal and dairy products**, and **unsaturated, found in vegetables.**

Chose unsaturated fats instead of saturated fats to lessen the risk of heart disease. Excess fat is stored under the skin causing weight gain.

- **Unsaturated fats**: many types of food have high levels of unsaturated fats. The fat in poultry, fish, soft margarine, and certain fruits, such as avocados, is largely unsaturated. The main source of unsaturated fat, however, is **vegetable oil.**

Controlling cholesterol

Cells throughout the body **use cholesterol to produce many important hormones** required for growth and reproduction. **Excess cholesterol** remains in the blood stream and clings to the artery walls as fatty deposits that obstruct the flow of blood. To lower your blood cholesterol level you must eat fewer fatty foods. People with high cholesterol levels risk suffering from **heart attacks, angina, or circulation disorders.**

- **Cholesterol-producing food**: the main source of cholesterol are those foods that are high in saturated fats (sausage, eggs, cheese, shellfish).

Proteins

A regular intake of protein in your diet provides your body cells with an adequate **supply of amino acids**, which are used as building blocks in the **formation of new cells**. They also assist in the growth, repair, and replacement of body tissues, such as **bones, muscles, connective tissues, and the walls of hollow organs**. Meat, fish, and eggs are rich sources of protein.

- **Red meat** provides all the essential amino acids you need, but it is also high in saturated fats.
- **Sources of protein:** meat, poultry, fish, and dairy products are good sources of protein. Plant sources include potatoes, rice, bread, and pasta.

Proteinaceous plants

Foods from plant sources, such as nuts, beans, and the grain in cereals and bread, are known as **partially complete proteins because they are deficient in** one or more **essential**

amino acids. (A complete protein is one that contains all the essential amino acids). But the **amino acids missing in one plant food are often present in another**. In order to obtain a complete protein from these foods, they must be **eaten in combination** with one another: legumes and wheat, legumes and rice, nuts and rice.

Exercise 1a
Match the column A with the column B. Try to learn the expressions and/ or sentences by heart.

A

1. Carbohydrates, fats, proteins, fibre, vitamins, and minerals
2. Carbohydrates, which can be divided into two main types – sugars and starches,
3. Starch, which can be found in pasta, bread, potatoes, and the majority of fruits,
4. Unrefined carbohydrates,
5. There are two types of fats:
6. The main source of unsaturated fat
7. Excess cholesterol
8. People with high cholesterol levels
9. A regular intake of protein in your diet
10. Proteins
11. A complete protein
12. In order to obtain a complete protein

B

a) *are six vital elements that can be extracted from a varied, well balanced diet.*
b) *are the body's principal source of energy.*
c) *assist in the growth, repair, and replacement of body tissues, such as bones, muscles, connective tissues, and the walls of hollow organs.*
d) *foods must be eaten in combination with one another.*
e) *is one that contains all the essential amino acids.*
f) *is the optimum source of energy and should always be eaten in preference of sugars.*
g) *is vegetable oil.*
h) *provides your body cells with an adequate supply of amino acids, which are used as building blocks in the formation of new cells.*
i) *remains in the blood stream and clings to the artery walls as fatty deposits that obstruct the flow of blood.*
j) *risk suffering from heart attacks, angina, or circulation disorders.*
k) *saturated, found in animal and dairy products, and unsaturated, found in vegetables.*
l) *such as brown pasta and wholemeal bread have a higher nutrient value than*

refined carbohydrates such as white sugar or white rice.

The importance of fibre

Every adult should eat about 25 grams of fibre a day. Fibre has a crucial role to play in maintaining a healthy body. By increasing the bulk of the faeces, it encourages the efficient **passage of waste products through the intestine**. By reducing the absorption of digested fats, fibre **lowers cholesterol levels**, thereby reducing the risk of heart disease.

Fibre-rich foods

Fibre comes from fruit, grain, husks, and vegetables. **High-fibre foods are filling, but low in calories, so that they can help you lose weight**.

- **Eat the skins of fruit and vegetables** (but wash them thoroughly first).
- Choose **wholemeal bread, whole grain cereals, and brown rice,** rather than highly refined alternatives.
- **Introduce** fibre-rich food products **gradually**, or you may suffer from stomach cramps and flatulence.

Vitamins are vital

A balanced, varied diet will contain all the vitamins you need, so supplements are needed only by those people who are in poor health or do not eat well. Vitamins stimulate energy production and control the growth and repair of tissues.

- **Vitamin A**: forms **bones and teeth**. Keeps **skin and hair** healthy. **Protects** lining of **respiratory, urinary, and digestive tracts**.
- **Vitamin B_1 (Thiamine):** promotes the production of energy, which is needed for the healthy **functioning of the nerves, muscles, and heart.**
- **Vitamin B_2 (Riboflavin)**: helps stimulate the release of energy from nutrients. Helps maintain a **healthy mouth, tongue and skin**. Promotes hormone production.
- **Niacin:** aids energy production. Assists the functioning of the **nervous and digestive systems**. Promotes the production of **sex hormones**.
- **Vitamin B_6 (Pyridoxine)**: helps **form red blood cells and antibodies**. Assists **digestive and nervous systems**. Helps maintain **healthy skin**.
- **Vitamin B_{12}**: keeps **nervous system healthy**. Aids production of genetic matter inside cells – essential for the **formation of new cells.**
- **Vitamin C**: maintains **gums, teeth, bones, and blood vessels**. Improves iron absorption. Aids the **immune system**. Enhances **wound healing.**
- **Vitamin D:** aids absorption from food. **Forms strong**

teeth and bones. Maintains healthy **blood clotting, muscles, and nerves**.

- **Folic acid:** helps maintain a healthy **nervous system**. Aids the production of genetic material inside cells – **needed for cell growth**.
- **Vitamin E:** assists in the **formation of red blood cells**. Protects cell lining in the lungs and other tissues. May slow down cell ageing.

Minerals for the metabolism

At least 20 different minerals play a role in controlling the body's metabolism. Some minerals, like **magnesium and sodium, are needed in fairly large amounts**. Others, like **iron and fluoride**, are only required **in tiny quantities.** A balanced diet usually supplies all the necessary minerals, but deficiencies of iron and calcium are not uncommon.

- **Sodium**: controls body's **water balance**. Maintains normal **heart rhythm.** Helps in **generation of nerve impulses**.
- **Potassium**: controls body's **water balance**. Maintains normal **heart rhythm**. Helps in **generation of nerve impulses**.
- **Calcium**: forms and maintains **teeth and bones**. Controls transmission of **nerve impulses**. Aids efficiency of **muscle contraction**.
- **Magnesium**: Forms and maintains **healthy teeth and bones**. Activates energy-producing chemical reactions inside cells.
- **Iron**: helps **form haemoglobin,** which carries oxygen in the red blood cells. Aids **enzyme production** that stimulates metabolism.
- **Zinc:** assists **wound healing**. Maintains **skin and hair**. Enables **growth and sexual development** to occur normally.
- **Copper:** controls enzyme activity that stimulates the formation of **connective tissues and pigments** that protect the skin.
- **Fluoride**: **hardens tooth enamel,** which helps the **prevention of dental decay**. Helps to strengthen bones.
- **Selenium: protects cells against damage from oxidizing substances** in the blood. May reduce the risk of developing some cancers.

When to take supplements

Only take vitamin and mineral supplements **on medical advice**, which may be based on blood tests that show a deficiency. Women who have heavy periods may lack iron, for example. People on low-calorie diets may also need supplements. Generally, however, **a varied, balanced diet will provide all the nutrients** you need.

- **Overdose**: taking too much of a vitamin or mineral can be dangerous -high doses of vitamin A can be fatal.

Exercise 1b
Match the column A with the column B. Try to learn the expressions and/ or sentences by heart.

A

1. Every adult
2. Fibre comes from
3. Choose wholemeal bread, whole grain cereals, and brown rice,
4. Supplements are needed only by those people
5. Vitamin A
6. Vitamin B_2 (Riboflavin)
7. Vitamin B_6 (Pyridoxine)
8. Vitamin C
9. Vitamin D
10. Sodium
11. Calcium
12. Iron
13. Zinc
14. Fluoride
15. Selenium
16. Taking too much of a vitamin or mineral

B

a) *assists wound healing.*
b) *can be dangerous - high doses of vitamin A can be fatal.*
c) *controls body's water balance, maintains normal heart rhythm and helps in generation of nerve impulses.*
d) *forms and maintains teeth and bones.*
e) *forms bones and teeth; keeps skin and hair healthy and protects lining of respiratory, urinary, and digestive tracts.*
f) *forms strong teeth and bones and maintains healthy blood clotting, muscles, and nerves.*
g) *fruit, grain, husks, and vegetables.*
h) *hardens tooth enamel, which helps the prevention of dental decay.*
i) *helps form haemoglobin, which carries oxygen in the red blood cells.*
j) *helps maintain a healthy mouth, tongue and skin.*
k) *helps maintain healthy skin.*
l) *maintains gums, teeth, bones, and blood vessels.*
m) *protects cells against damage from oxidizing substances in the blood.*
n) *rather than highly refined alternatives.*
o) *should eat about 25 grams of fibre a day.*
p) *who are in poor health or do not eat well.*

Exercise 2
Translate the expressions. Try to explain their meanings in English.

Sustain life, repair, maintenance, carbohydrates, fats, proteins, fibre, vitamins, and minerals, starches, preference, slimming, wholemeal bread, unsaturated fats, excess, cling, fatty deposits, obstruct, suffering from, building blocks, grain, complete, crucial role, maintaining, bulk, passage, grain, husks, filling foods, wholemeal bread, whole grain cereals, cramps and flatulence, supplements, lining, promote, release, genetic matter, enhances wound healing, blood clotting, cell lining, ageing, deficiencies, not uncommon, generation of nerve impulses, potassium, calcium, magnesium, copper, transmission, maintain, connective tissues, harden, enamel, dental decay, medical advice, supplements, overdose, fatal.

Exercise 3
Answer the following questions. Prepare short talks and/or dialogues on these topics.

1. Why is good nutrition important?
2. Speak about carbohydrates.
3. Speak about saturated and unsaturated fats.
4. Why is excess cholesterol dangerous?
5. What is the function of proteins in the body?
6. What are proteinaceous plants?
7. Explain the importance of fibre.
8. Why are vitamins vital? Describe the function of each vitamin in the body.
9. Why are minerals vital? Describe the function of each mineral in the body.

Vocabulary 4

Fill in the meanings in your mother language:

absorption /əbˈzɔːp.ʃən/
activate /ˈæk.tɪ.veɪt/
advice /ədˈvaɪs/
ageing /ˈeɪ.dʒɪŋ/
Acquired /əˌkwaɪ.əd/ **Immune** /ɪˈmjuːn/ **Deficiency** /dɪˈfɪʃ.ən.si/ **Syndrome** /ˈsɪn.drəʊm/ **AIDS**
alternative /ɒlˈtɜː.nə.tɪv/
angina /ænˌdʒaɪ.nə/
antibody /ˈæn.tiˌbɒd.i/
artery /ˈɑːtərɪ/
assist /əˈsɪst/
avocado /ˌævəˈkɑːdəʊ/
bean /biːn/
blood /blʌd/ **stream** /striːm/
blood /blʌd/ **vessel** /ˈves.əl/
bone /bəʊn/
building /ˈbɪl.dɪŋ/ **block** /blɒk/
bulk /bʌlk/
calcium /ˈkæl.si.əm/
carry /ˈkær.i/
cereal /ˈsɪə.ri.əl/
cholesterol /kəˈles.tər.ɒl/
circulation /ˌsɜː.kjʊˈleɪ.ʃən/
cling /klɪŋ/
clotting /ˈklɑt̬.ɪŋ/
connective /kəˌnek.tɪv/
constitute /ˈkɒn.stɪ.tjuːt/
contraction /kənˈtrækʃən/
copper /ˈkɒp.ər/
cramp /kræmp/
cut /kʌt/ **down** /daʊn/
dairy /ˈdeə.ri/
decay /dɪˈkeɪ/
deficiency /dɪˈfɪʃ.ənt.si/
deficient /dɪˈfɪʃ.ənt/
deposit /dɪˈpɒz.ɪt/
development /dɪˈvel.əp.mənt/
element /ˈel.ɪ.mənt/
employ /ɪmˈplɔɪ/
enable /ɪˈneɪ.bl̩/

enamel /ɪ'næm.əl/
encourage /ɪn'kʌr.ɪ.dʒ/
enzyme /'en.zaɪm/
excess /ek'ses/
extract /ɪk'strækt/
faeces /'fiː.siːz/
fatal /'feɪ.təl/
filling /'fɪl.ɪŋ/
flatulence /'flæt.jʊ.lənts/
fluoride /'flʊə.raɪd/
folic acid /ˌfəʊ.lɪk'æs.ɪd/
fuel /fjʊəl/
fulfil /fʊl'fɪl/
generation /ˌdʒen.ə'reɪ.ʃən/
genetic /dʒə'net.ɪk/
grain /greɪn/
haemoglobin /ˌhiː.mə'gləʊ.bɪn/
harden /'hɑː.dən/
healing /hiːlɪŋ/
husk /hʌsk/
importance /ɪm'pɔː.tənts/
inside /ɪn'saɪd/
intestine /ɪn'tes.tɪn/
introduce /ˌɪn.trə'djuːs/
iron /aɪən/
legume /'leg.juːm/
lessen /'les.ən/
lining /'laɪn.ɪŋ/
magnesium /mæg'niː.zi.əm/
major /'meɪ.dʒər/
majority /mə'dʒɒrɪtɪ/
manufacturer /ˌmæn.jʊ'fæk.tʃər.ər/
margarine /ˌmɑː.dʒə'riːn/
matter /'mæt.ər/
metabolism /mə'tæb.əl.ɪ.zəm/
missing /'mɪs.ɪŋ/
nervous /'nɜː.vəs/
niacin /'naɪə.sɪn/
nutrient /'njuː.tri.ənt/
obstruct /əb'strʌkt/
optimum /'ɒp.tɪ.məm/
overdose /'əʊ.və.dəʊs/
oxygen /'ɒk.sɪ.dʒən/
partially /'pɑː.ʃəl.i/
passage /'pæs.ɪdʒ/
pasta /'pæstə/
percentage /pə'sen.tɪdʒ/
pigment /'pɪg.mənt/
plant /plɑːnt/
potassium /pə'tæs.i.əm/
preference /'pref.ər.ənt s/
prevention /prɪ'ven.ʃən/
principal /'prɪnt.sɪ.pəl/
protein /'prəʊ.tiːn/
proteinaceous /'prəʊ.tiːneɪ.ʃəs/
provide /prə'vaɪd/
pyridoxine /ˌpɪrɪ'dɒksiːn/
raw /rɔː/ **material** /mə'tɪərɪəl/
release /rə'liːs/
remove /rɪ'muːv/
repair /rɪ'peə/
replacement /rɪ'pleɪs.mənt/
reproduction /ˌriː.prə'dʌk.ʃən/
respiratory /rɪ'spɪr.ə.tər.i/
riboflavin /ˌraɪ.bəʊ'fleɪ.vɪn/
sausage /'sɒs.ɪdʒ/
selenium /sə'liː.ni.əm/
shellfish /'ʃelˌfɪʃ/
source /sɔːs/
starch /stɑːtʃ/
stomach /'stʌm.ək/
store /stɔːr/
substance /'sʌb.stəns/
sustain /sə'steɪn/
thiamine /'θaɪ.ə.miːn/
throughout /θruː'aʊt/
tiny /'taɪ.ni/
tongue /tʌŋ/
transmission /trænz'mɪʃ.ən/
uncommon /ʌn'kɒm.ən/
unrefined /ˌʌn.rɪ'faɪnd/
urinary /'jʊə.rɪ.nər.i/
value /'væl.juː/
varied /'veə.rɪd/
vital /'vaɪ.təl/
wheat /wiːt/
wholemeal /'həʊlˌmiːl/

Solution to Exercise 1a
1a, 2b, 3f, 4l, 5k, 6g, 7i, 8j, 9h, 10c, 11e, 12d

Solution to Exercise 1b
1o, 2g, 3n, 4p, 5e, 6j, 7k, 8l, 9f, 10c, 11d, 12i, 13a, 13h, 14h, 15m, 16b

Unit 5 - Nutrient deficiencies. The health-conscious cook.

Many symptoms and minor skin problems are due to deficiencies in one, or several nutrients, caused by eating a lot of processed foods or a highly restricted diet. Such deficiencies should be confirmed by your doctor before any treatment is started.

- Women need greater quantities of **iron, folic acid, calcium,** and other nutrients **in pregnancy or while breastfeeding**.
- Older people may risk incurring deficiencies through changes in the digestive system due to **ageing process**.

Nutrient	Symptom	People at risk
Iron	Tiredness, pale skin, sore mouth, and nail changes	Those who eat a poor diet, women with heavy periods
Calcium	Increased risk of fractures in later life due to osteoporosis	Needed during growth spurts, pregnancy, and breast-feeding
Potassium	Weakness and palpitations	People with chronic diarrhoea or taking diuretics
Zinc	Loss of appetite and delayed wound healing	Those who eat a poor diet or a lot of processed foods
Vitamin B_2 riboflavin	Chapped lips and sore tongue	Those who eat a poor diet or a lot of overcooked food
Folic acid	Reduced resistance to infection and fatigue	Pregnant women or anyone with a prolonged illness

Eating for health
Your health in the balance

Satisfy your nutritional needs by eating a range of food every day from five separate categories – bread, cereals and other grain products; fruit; vegetables; meat, poultry, fish, eggs, and plant protein sources such as dried beans and dairy produce.

- For a healthy diet, eat **fresh fruit and vegetables** at least twice a day.
- The recommended intake of **meat is 100 – 150 g a day**. Have at least one meat-free day a week.
- Drink **plenty of water** to keep your digestive system working.
- Start the day with a **hearty breakfast**. High-fibre cereals are a good choice.
- Drink **orange juice** rather than coffee.
- A glass of **milk** provides an excellent source of protein, and also contains valuable carbohydrates.
- Eat only four **eggs** a week. They are very high in cholesterol. Avoid fried breakfasts.

- Eat plenty of **vegetables** and salad at lunchtime. Choose lean meats.
- **Fish** is healthier and lower in calories than red meat.
- Finish your meal with **fruit** rather than rich desserts that are high in calories.
- Although alcohol is extremely harmful in excess, a glass of **wine** with your meal will aid digestion.

The importance of water

Drink **at least eight glasses of water a day**. Many bodily processes need water in order to function normally.

- If you do not drink enough water you are likely to become constipated.
- Try to **avoid drinking** too much **carbonated water**. It introduces gas into the digestive tract.

Meals in moderation

It is better to **eat three moderate-size meals a day** rather than one large feast. Your metabolism works more efficiently with a regular supply of nutrients. If you eat too many large meals, or one big meal a day, you are more likely to become obese, or suffer from indigestion and ulcers.

Choosing healthier snacks

Snacks can be healthy and nutritious, as well as tasty. Sweets, biscuits, potatoes crisps, chocolate, and cakes are high in calories, refined sugar, and saturated fats.

- Choose a piece of **fresh fruit, a raw vegetable, or a yoghurt** to provide you with essential vitamins, minerals, and fibre.
- Fruit is a healthy option, and choose wholemeal pizza or sandwiches rather than burgers or hot dogs.
- Drink **fruit juice** as a nutritious **alternative to soft drinks with added sugar.**

Cutting down on caffeine

Reduce your caffeine intake by drinking water, diluted fruit juices, or decaffeinated products. **Caffeine** is a stimulant that **reduces fatigue and improves your concentration.** However, just three or four cups of tea a day may be enough to produce **adverse side effects, such as tremors, irritability, insomnia, and diarrhoea.**

Shopping wisdom

While you are shopping, always **check food and drink labels**.

- Buy **fresh food** rather than processed alternatives.
- Choose **low-calorie soft drinks**.
- Select **low-fat dairy products** like skimmed milk and low-fat cheese.
- Buy tinned foods that **do not have added salt or sugar**.

Exercise 1a
Match the column A with the column B. Try to learn the expressions and/ or sentences by heart.

A

1. Women need greater quantities of iron, folic acid, calcium, and other nutrients
2. Older people may risk incurring deficiencies
3. For a healthy diet
4. The recommended intake of meat
5. Drink plenty of water
6. Finish your meal with fruit
7. If you do not drink enough water
8. If you eat too many large meals, or one big meal a day,
9. Sweets, biscuits, potatoes crisps, chocolate, and cakes
10. Choose a piece of fresh fruit, a raw vegetable, or a yoghurt
11. Just three or four cups of tea a day
12. Buy tinned foods

B

a) are high in calories, refined sugar, and saturated fats.
b) eat fresh fruit and vegetables at least twice a day.
c) in pregnancy or while breastfeeding.
d) is 100 – 150 g a day.
e) may be enough to produce adverse side effects, such as tremors, irritability, insomnia, and diarrhoea.
f) rather than rich desserts that are high in calories.
g) that do not have added salt or sugar.
h) through changes in the digestive system due to ageing process.
i) to keep your digestive system working.
j) to provide you with essential vitamins, minerals, and fibre.
k) you are likely to become constipated.
l) you are more likely to become obese, or suffer from indigestion and ulcers.

The health-conscious cook

In the kitchen, trim excess fat from meat and remove chicken skin. **Bake, boil, grill, steam, or stir-fry** your food **rather than frying** it. If you do fry food, **use olive oil** or polyunsaturated vegetable oil rather than butter or lard. Add little, if any salt to your cooking. Try to avoid overcooking your food and use fresh ingredients when possible.

- **Try not to fry. Bake or grill** your food to minimize the fat content. To help preserve vitamins, cook fruits and vegetables in their skins.
- **Trimming red meat**: be sure to trim all visible fat off meat. Try to use alternative sources of protein to red meat when possible, such as poultry or fish.
- **Skimming off the fat**: cook stews and soups

slowly, skimming off fat at regular intervals. Make your own salt-free stock.

Meatless meals

Vegetarian food is healthy and nutritious. The vegetarian food is normally **low in fat** because it does not contain fatty cuts of meat. It is also **richer in fibre** from beans, pulses, and grains, which helps the bowels to function normally.

Food for a healthy heart

Heart disease accounts for about one third of all adult deaths, but dietary changes could help:

- **Eat more fibre**. It reduces the amount of cholesterol you absorb while digesting fatty food.
- **Cut down on fatty foods**. Eat more fish and poultry, and switch to low-fat dairy produce.
- **Reduce your salt intake**. It may raise your blood pressure, which increases your risk of developing coronary heart disease.

Food for healthy bones

Every bone is a living tissue, which needs **a variety of nutrients** from your diet **to maintain its strength and resilience**. Eat lots of **calcium-rich foods**. Milk and most dairy products, fish with edible bones (sardines and tinned salmon), green leafy vegetables, citrus fruit, nuts, and dried peas and beans are all good sources of calcium. Skimmed milk has as much calcium as whole milk, but less saturated fat. Cut down on **alcohol and caffeine**: they can **weaken your bones.**

Food for healthy teeth

To develop strong, healthy teeth, your diet must provide adequate amounts of **six essential nutrients**: **calcium, phosphorus, magnesium, vitamins C and D, and fluoride.** If you eat a balanced diet, you will be taking more than enough of the first five nutrients. Fluoride, which strengthens the enamel, is found in seafood and in some drinking water. Apples can freshen up your mouth, and cheese can neutralize acids that attack your teeth after you eat.

Reducing the risk of cancer

Cancer specialists have published dietary recommendations based on the results of their studies:

- **Fat should account for no more than 30%** of your daily **calorie intake**.
- Increase your **fibre intake** to between **20 and 30 grams** a day.
- **Alcoholic drinks** should only be consumed **in moderation**.
- **Body weight** should be kept within **normal limits**.
- **Smoked, nitrate-cured, and salted foods** should **not be eaten regularly**.
- **Vitamin A curbs cancer** by a direct action on cells.

- **Vitamin C** may help **prevent cancer of the oesophagus**.
- **Vitamin E** is thought to help **prevent cancer**.
- **Selenium** is thought to **prevent cancers** caused by oxidizing substances.
- **Cruciferous vegetables**, such as cabbage, may **reduce the risk of digestive cancers.**

Avoid food poisoning

Always **wash your hands** before touching any food and after handling raw meat. This will help prevent food poisoning due to eating food that is contaminated.

- **High risk** foods include **poultry, seafood, and undercooked meat**.
- **Store raw meat away** from all other food. Eat it as soon as it is cooked.
- Never use food from a **container that is leaking, bulging, or damaged**.
- Always **thaw frozen meat** or poultry completely before cooking.
- **Reheat** meat **thoroughly**.

Exercise 1b

Match the column A with the column B. Try to learn the expressions and/or sentences by heart.

A

1. If you fry food,
2. Try to avoid overcooking your food -
3. To help preserve vitamins,
4. Cook stews and soups slowly,
5. The vegetarian food is
6. Cut down on fatty foods -
7. Reduce your salt intake because
8. Milk and dairy products, fish, green leafy vegetables, citrus fruit, nuts, and dried peas and beans
9. To develop strong, healthy teeth,
10. Fat should account for
11. Increase your fibre intake
12. Smoked, nitrate-cured, and salted foods
13. Avoid food poisoning –
14. Store raw meat
15. Always thaw

B

a) use fresh ingredients when possible.
b) are all good sources of calcium.
c) away from all other food.
d) cook fruits and vegetables in their skins.
e) eat more fish and poultry.
f) frozen meat or poultry completely before cooking.
g) high risk foods include poultry, seafood, and undercooked meat.
h) it may raise your blood pressure.
i) no more than 30% of your daily calorie intake.
j) to between 20 and 30 grams a day.

k) *richer in fibre from beans, pulses, and grains, which helps the bowels to function normally.*
l) *should not be eaten regularly.*
m) *skimming off fat at regular intervals.*
n) *use olive oil or polyunsaturated vegetable oil rather than butter or lard.*
o) *your diet must provide adequate amounts of six essential nutrients: calcium, phosphorus, magnesium, vitamins C and D, and fluoride.*

Exercise 2
Translate the expressions. Try to explain their meanings in English.

Processed foods, restricted diet, confirmed, breastfeeding, fatigue, tiredness, pale skin, sore tongue, growth spurts, weakness, palpitations, diarrhoea, diuretics, chapped lips, valuable, lean meats, harmful, become constipated, moderate-size, feast, indigestion, ulcers, snacks, alternative, caffeine, option, diluted, adverse side effects, tremors, irritability, insomnia, wisdom, skimmed milk, tinned foods, trim, bake, boil, steam, stir-fry, lard, overcooking, ingredients, skin, skimming off, stews, cut down on, switch to, coronary heart disease, edible, tinned, weaken, strengthen, drinking water, freshen up, recommendations, account for, salted, in moderation, curb, oesophagus, cabbage, poisoning, handling, raw meat, thaw, container, leaking.

Exercise 3
Answer the following questions. Prepare short talks and/or dialogues on these topics.

1. What are the symptoms of iron (calcium, potassium, zinc, vitamin B_2, folic acid) deficiencies? Who are the people at risk?
2. How to satisfy nutritional needs (fruit, vegetables, meat, water, eggs, milk)?
3. Speak about the importance of a regular supply of nutrients. Give examples of healthy snacks.
4. Which are the adverse side effects of caffeine?
5. Give some tips on health-conscious cook.
6. Give advice on food for a healthy heart (food for healthy bones, food for healthy teeth)
7. Talk about reducing the risk of cancer.
8. What should you do to avoid food poisoning?

Vocabulary 5

Fill in the meanings in your mother language:

account /əˈkaʊnt/ **for** /fə/
acid /ˈæs.ɪd/
adverse /ˈæd.vɜːs/
appetite /ˈæp.ɪ.taɪt/
attack /əˈtæk/

bake /beɪk/
bodily /ˈbɒd.ɪ.li/
boil /bɔɪl/
breastfeed /ˈbrest.fiːd/
burger /ˈbɜːgə/
cabbage /ˈkæb.ɪdʒ/
carbonated /ˈkɑr.bəˌneɪ.t̬ ɪd/
chapped /ˈtʃæpt/
check /tʃek/
confirmed /kənˈfɜːmd/
conscious /ˈkɒn.tʃəs/
constipated /ˈkɒn.stɪ.peɪt.ɪd/
consume /kənˈsjuːm/
contaminated /kənˈtæm.ɪ.neɪ.tɪd/
cruciferous /kruːˈsɪfərəs/
dessert /dɪˈzɜːt/
develop /dɪˈvel.əp/
diarrhoea /ˌdaɪ.əˈriː.ə/
dilute /daɪˈluːt/
diuretic /ˌdaɪ.jʊə ˈret.ɪk/
edible /ˈed.ɪ.bl̩/
feast /fiːst/
fracture /ˈfræk.tʃə/
freshen /ˈfreʃ.ən/
frozen /ˈfrəʊ.zən/
fry /fraɪ/
handling /ˈhænd.lɪŋ/
hearty /ˈhɑːtɪ/
hot /hɒt/ **dog** /ɒg/
in order to /ˈɔː.dər/
incur /ɪnˈkɜː/
ingredient /ɪnˈgriː.di.ənt/
intake /ˈɪn.teɪk/
label /ˈleɪ.bəl/
lard /lɑːd/
leafy /ˈliː.fi/
leak /liːk/
lip /lɪp/
living /ˈlɪv.ɪŋ/
loss /lɒs/
moderate /ˈmɒd.ər.ət/
nail /neɪl/
neutralize /ˈnjuː.trə.laɪz/
nitrate /ˈnaɪ.treɪt/
nitrate /ˈnaɪtreɪt/ **-cured** /kjʊəd/
oesophagus /ɪˈsɒf.ə.gəs/
option /ˈɒp.ʃən/
osteoporosis /ˌɒs.ti.əʊ.pəˈrəʊ.sɪs/
overcook /ˌəʊ.vəˈkʊk/
oxidize /ˈɒk.sɪ.daɪz/
pale /peɪl/
palpitations /ˌpæl.pɪˈteɪ.ʃənz/
phosphorus /ˈfɒs.fər.əs/
poisoning /ˈpɔɪ.zən.ɪŋ/
process /ˈprəʊ.ses/
pulse /pʌls/
raw /rɔː/
reheat /ˌriːˈhiːt/
resilience /rɪˈzɪl.i.əns/
restrict /rɪˈstrɪkt/
salmon /ˈsæm.ən/
salted /ˈsɒl.tɪd/
satisfy /ˈsæt.ɪs.faɪ/
separate /ˈsep.ər.ət/
skim /skɪm/
smoked /sməʊkt/
sore /sɔːr/
spurt /spɜːt/
steam /stiːm/
stew /stjuː/
stir-fry /ˈstɜː.fraɪ/
stock /stɑːk/
strengthen /ˈstreŋ.θən/
supply /səˈplaɪ/
sweet /swiːt/
switch /swɪtʃ/
tasty /ˈteɪ.sti/
thaw /θɔː/
thoroughly /ˈθʌr.ə.li/
thought /θɔːt/
tinned /tɪnd/
tiredness /ˈtaɪəd.nəs/
touch /tʌtʃ/
treatment /ˈtriːt.mənt/
ulcer /ˈʌl.sər/
weaken /ˈwiː.kən/
weakness /ˈwiːk.nəs/
wisdom /ˈwɪz.dəm/

Solution to Exercise 1a
1c, 2h, 3b, 4d, 5i, 6f, 7k, 8l, 9a, 10j, 11e, 12g

Solution to Exercise 1b
1n, 2a, 3d, 4m, 5k, 6e, 7h, 8b, 9o, 10i, 11j, 12l, 13g, 14c, 15f

Unit 6 - The dangers of addiction. Hygiene and health care.

Unhealthy habits

The most widely abused drugs are not illegal substances like cocaine but the readily available, usually legal, drugs: alcohol, tobacco, and caffeine. Smokers often cannot kick the habit even though they know that cigarettes increase their risk of dying prematurely. **Any drug abuse is likely to lead to various physical, psychological, social, and financial problems**. Even taking tranquillizers for more than two weeks can cause dependence.

Know your limits

Although alcohol is socially acceptable, it is important to remember that it is still potentially an addictive drug. **Monitor your weekly intake of alcohol and keep it below a maximum of 21 units for men and 14 units for women**. Half a pint of beer, one glass of table wine, and one single measure of spirits each contains one unit of alcohol. Be sure to have at least two alcohol-free days a week.

The dangers of alcohol

Drink alcohol in moderation. **Regular consumption of substantial amounts of alcohol will inevitably damage the liver, the heart, and the brain.** Alcohol abuse can also cause a number of different cancers.

- Even a little alcohol will **impair your judgement and concentration**, so do not drink if you are driving.
- Heavy drinking while pregnant may cause **foetal alcohol syndrome**, where a baby is born retarded.
- Abuse of alcohol leads to destruction of brain cells, causing **depression and memory loss.**
- Alcohol increases the risk of **cancers in the mouth, throat, and oesophagus**.
- People who drink heavily are likely to suffer from **high blood pressure, a heart attack, or a stroke.**
- Heavy drinking may cause **cirrhosis, hepatitis, or liver cancer**.
- Excessive drinking can result in severe abdominal pain, caused by **gastritis, pancreatitis, or ulcers.**
- Because alcohol is rich in calories, **obesity** is a common problem among heavy drinkers.
- In men, excess alcohol can lead to **impotence**. In women it commonly causes **menstrual problems**.

- **Skin problems**: alcoholics often have a persistent flush which is due to damage to blood vessels under the surface of the skin.

How to control your intake

- **Learn to say no** to friends who urge you to have just one more.
- Buy your own drinks so that you are able to drink at your pace.
- When you go out, **start with a soft drink** to quench you first.
- Choose low-alcohol or non-alcoholic drinks. Many taste just as good as their alcoholic equivalents.
- **Dilute your drinks** to slow down your alcohol intake by adding a mixer like tonic or soda water.

The dangers of smoking

As soon as you do stop smoking, you lower your risk of dying from smoking-related diseases. Although most people are fully aware of the increased cancer risk from smoking, there are numerous other smoking-related diseases that are less known.

- **White or red patches in your mouth** may be the result of early cancerous changes due to smoking.
- Smoking impairs lung capacity and can result in difficulty in breathing or **chronic bronchitis**.
- **Smoker's cough:** a persistent cough in a smoker may be due to chronic bronchitis, or occasionally lung cancer.
- Smoking is a major risk factor in **coronary heart disease**. Coughing up blood is also a symptom of **lung cancer**.
- **Gastritis and peptic ulcers** can be caused or aggravated by smoking.
- The appearance of blood in your urine may be a symptom of **bladder or kidney cancer**, both of which are more likely to develop in smokers.
- Unless you stop smoking, **leg ulcers and gangrene** may develop, requiring major surgery.
- Smoking in pregnancy: **miscarriage, still birth, and premature or low birth weight babies** are more common among women who smoke during pregnancy.
- **Passive smoking**: non-smokers who are regularly exposed to tobacco smoke increase their risk of cancer by 10 to 30%.

How to stop smoking

You must really want to stop. It is harder for those who started before the age of 20 to give up smoking than for those who took up the habit when they were older.

- Throw away cigarettes and avoid places where you are tempted to smoke.
- Cut down on red meat, tea, coffee, and alcohol: they can make you crave a cigarette.
- **Stop altogether, not gradually.**

Beating drug abuse

If you become dependent on drugs, consult your doctor who can refer you to a rehabilitation centre.

- **Reduce your dosage** over several weeks, **under medical supervision**, to minimize **withdrawal symptoms.**
- Moving to a new environment away from drug-taking friends may reduce the risk of re-addiction.
- **Psychotherapy** may be advised to help discover the root causes of your dependency.
- **Heroin addiction** is sometimes treated by abrupt abstinence and the use of **methadone**, a painkiller, to relieve the withdrawal symptoms.
- **Self-help groups** can help provide and maintain the motivation to stay off drugs.
- **Prescribed drugs**: tranquillizers are often prescribed by doctors to treat anxiety and insomnia, but there is a danger that they **can be abused** for their relaxing effects.

Exercise 1a
Match the column A with the column B. Try to learn the expressions and/ or sentences by heart.

A

1. The most widely abused drugs are
2. Smokers often cannot kick the habit even though
3. Half a pint of beer, one glass of table wine, and one single measure of spirits
4. Even a little alcohol
5. Heavy drinking while pregnant
6. Abuse of alcohol
7. Alcohol increases the risk
8. Heavy drinking may cause
9. Excessive drinking can result in
10. As soon as you do stop smoking,
11. Smoker's cough:
12. Gastritis and peptic ulcers
13. The appearance of blood in your urine
14. Miscarriage, still birth, and premature or low birth weight babies
15. If you become dependent on drugs,
16. Reduce your dosage over several weeks, under medical supervision,

B

a) *a persistent cough in a smoker may be due to chronic bronchitis, or occasionally lung cancer.*

b) *are more common among women who smoke during pregnancy.*

c) *can be caused or aggravated by smoking.*

d) *causes depression and memory loss.*

e) *cirrhosis, hepatitis, or liver cancer.*

f) *consult your doctor who can refer you to a rehabilitation centre.*

g) *each contains one unit of alcohol.*

h) *may be a symptom of bladder or kidney cancer.*

i) *may cause foetal alcohol syndrome, where a baby is born retarded.*

j) *of cancers in the mouth, throat, and oesophagus.*

k) *severe abdominal pain, caused by gastritis, pancreatitis, or ulcers.*

l) *the readily available, usually legal, drugs: alcohol, tobacco, and caffeine.*

m) *they know that cigarettes increase their risk of dying prematurely.*

n) *to minimize withdrawal symptoms.*

o) *will impair your judgement and concentration.*

p) *you lower your risk of dying from smoking-related diseases.*

Hygiene and health care
The importance of hygiene

Good personal hygiene is essential. It will help prevent the spread of bacteria, which can lead to infections. Wash every day with a mild soap. Taking a shower is the best option – too many long baths tend to dry out the skin. Although sweating is a natural part of your body's cooling system, perspiration drying on the skin may make it sore and can smell unpleasant. The **condition of your skin, hair, and nails** is a good indication of the overall state of your health.

- Clean cut: if you cut yourself, keep the wound spotlessly clean to prevent infection from germs found in dirt.
- Cleanliness around the home is vital, bur never more so than when you have a baby.

Caring for your skin

- **Clean your skin** with water and a mild soap to remove excess oil and help prevent spots.
- **Sunbathe sensibly.** If you are fair-skinned you should only sunbathe for 15 minutes when the sun is strong. Use a high-factor sunscreen.
- Remove all the **make-up** every night.

- Remove dead skin on your feet with a **pumice stone**. Always dry between your toes thoroughly.
- **Do not squeeze spots** – this will spread the infection and can cause permanent scarring.
- Old and blunt **razors** can cause cuts and spots to become infected.
- Examine your skin often to check for changes that may indicate health problems.

Healthy hair

Shampoo and condition your hair regularly to remove oil and dirt. **Comb**, rather than brush, your hair when it is wet. If you blow dry your hair, hold the **hair dryer** at least 15 cm away from your hair to avoid heat damage, such as split ends. Leave your hair slightly damp.

Healthy nails

There are many practical steps you can take to keep your nails strong and healthy.

- **Keep nails short** to stop them from splitting.
- **File** your fingernails using an emery board. File from the sides inwards towards the centre.
- **Trim** your nails after a hot bath – that is when they are at their softest. Always cut your toenails in a straight line to avoid ingrowing nails.

Looking after your eyes

Always treat your eyes gently and respect how delicate they are.

- Wear **protective goggles** when using dangerous chemicals, high speed machinery, and when you are swimming in chlorinated water.
- Try to **avoid rubbing** your eyes – this can easily spread infection.
- Do not stare at TV or computer screens for too long – you may strain the muscles in your eyes.
- **Have your eyes tested** regularly – every two years if you are over the age of 40.
- Consult your doctor if you have any eye pain or **irritation, blurred vision, or see haloes** around lights.

How to avoid ear trouble

If you think that you are not hearing as well as you should be, ask your doctor to test your ears.

- Do not use **cotton buds** to clean your ears, you **may damage your ear drum** or cause an **infection.**
- Wear **protective ear muffs** if you are constantly exposed to loud noise in your work.
- Do not play your personal stereo system too loudly.

How to keep your teeth healthy

Brush your teeth every morning and evening and after each meal, to prevent the build up of **plaque**, stop bad breath, and **keep your teeth and gums healthy**. Cut down on sugary foods. Finish your meals with cheese to help neutralize the acids that attack your teeth. Floss every day, but be careful not to pull up the floss too hard, or you may damage your gums.

- **Brushing technique**: brush your teeth with a fluoride toothpaste using small circular strokes.
- **Dental floss:** floss every day to remove plaque and food particles from between your teeth.
- Buying a brush: choose a **brush with soft bristles. A small-headed brush** will enable you to reach awkward areas.

Exercise 1b
Match the column A with the column B. Try to learn the expressions and/or sentences by heart.

A

1. Good personal hygiene
2. The condition of your skin, hair, and nails
3. If you are fair-skinned
4. Do not squeeze spots
5. Shampoo and condition your hair regularly
6. Keep nails short
7. Wear protective goggles
8. Consult your doctor if you have any
9. Do not use cotton buds to clean your ears,
10. Brush your teeth every morning and evening and after each meal,
11. Brush your teeth with a fluoride toothpaste
12. A small-headed brush with soft bristles

B

a) *– this will spread the infection and can cause permanent scarring.*
b) *eye pain or irritation, blurred vision, or see haloes around lights.*
c) *is a good indication of the overall state of your health.*
d) *to prevent the build up of plaque, stop bad breath, and keep your teeth and gums healthy.*
e) *to remove oil and dirt.*
f) *to stop them from splitting.*
g) *using small circular strokes.*
h) *when using dangerous chemicals, high speed machinery, and when you are swimming in chlorinated water.*
i) *will enable you to reach awkward areas.*
j) *will help prevent the spread of bacteria, which can lead to infections.*
k) *you may damage your ear drum or cause an infection.*

l) you should only sunbathe for 15 minutes when the sun is strong.

Exercise 2
Translate the expressions. Try to explain their meanings in English.

Available, kick the habit, prematurely, tranquillizers, dependence, addictive, spirits, consumption, substantial, inevitably, impair judgement, retarded, destruction, memory loss, stroke, cirrhosis, hepatitis, gastritis, pancreatitis, ulcers, persistent, flush, urge, at your pace, quench, dilute, aware, patches, coughing up, aggravated, appearance, urine, bladder, miscarriage, still birth, premature, exposed to, habit, tempted, crave, dependent, dosage, withdrawal symptoms, addiction, abrupt, painkiller, tranquillizers, anxiety, abused, mild soap, option, tend to, sweating, perspiration, indication, overall state, spotlessly, sunbathe sensibly, fair-skinned, sunscreen, squeeze, scarring, blow dry, hair dryer, damp, splitting, file, delicate, goggles, rubbing, stare at, strain the muscles, blurred vision, cotton buds, ear drum, ear muffs, brush, plaque, pull up the floss, circular strokes, soft bristles, a small-headed brush.

Exercise 3
Prepare short talks and/or dialogues on these topics.

1. The dangers of addiction; beating drug abuse
2. The dangers of alcohol; how to control your intake.
3. The dangers of smoking; how to stop smoking.
4. The importance of good personal hygiene
5. Caring for your skin, nails and healthy hair
6. Looking after your eyes
7. How to avoid ear trouble.
8. How to keep your teeth healthy.

Vocabulary 6

Fill in the meanings in your mother language:

abrupt /ə'brʌpt/
abuse /ə'bjuːz/
acceptable /ək'sept.ə.bl̩/
addiction /ə'dɪk.ʃən/
addictive /ə'dɪk.tɪv/
altogether /ˌɔːl.tə'geð.ər/
anxiety /æŋ'zaɪ.ə.ti/
available /ə'veɪ.lə.bl̩/
aware /ə'weər/
awkward /'ɔː.kwəd/
bacteria /bæk'tɪə.ri.ə/
bath /bɑːθ/
beat /biːt/
birth /'bɜːθ/
blunt / blʌnt/
blurred /blɜːd/
brain /breɪn/
bristle /'brɪs.l̩/
bronchitis /brɒŋ'kaɪ.tɪs/
brush /brʌʃ/
build up, buildup /'bɪld.ʌp/
cancer /'kænt .sər/
chlorinated /'klɔː.rɪ.neɪ.tɪd/
cirrhosis /sɪ'rəʊ.sɪs/
cocaine /kəʊ 'keɪn/
comb /kəʊm/
cooling /'kuː.lɪŋ/
cotton /'kɒt.ən/ **bud** /bʌd/
cough /kɒf/

crave /kreɪv/
cut /kʌt/
damp /dæmp/
delicate /ˈdel.ɪ.kət/
dependence /dɪˈpen.dənt s/
dependency /dɪˈpen.dənt .si/
destruction /dɪˈstrʌk.ʃən/
discover /dɪˈskʌv.ər/
dosage /ˈdəʊ.sɪdʒ/
ear muffs /ˈɪə.mʌfs/
effect /ɪˈfekt/
emery /ˈem.ər.i/ **board** /bɔːd/
environment /ɪnˈvaɪə .rən .mənt/
equivalent /ɪˈkwɪv.əl.ənt/
examine /ɪgˈzæm.ɪn/
exposed /ɪkˈspəʊzd/
fair-skinned /ˌfeəˈskɪnd/
file /faɪl/
floss /flɒs/
flush /flʌʃ/
foetal /ˈfiː.təl/ **alcohol** /ˈæl.kə.hɒl/ **syndrome** /ˈsɪn.drəʊm/
gangrene /ˈgæŋ.griːn/
gastritis /gæsˈtraɪ.tɪs/
germ /dʒɜːm/
give /gɪv/ **up** /ʌp/
habit /ˈhæb.ɪt/
halo /ˈheɪ.ləʊ/
hearing /ˈhɪə.rɪŋ/
heart /hɑːt/ **attack** /əˈtæk/
heavily /ˈhev.ɪ.li/
hepatitis /ˌhep.əˈtaɪ.tɪs/
heroin /ˈherəʊɪn/
high /haɪ/ **-speed** /spiːd/
hygiene /ˈhaɪ.dʒiːn/
illegal /ɪˈliː.gəl/
impair /ɪmˈpeər/
indication /ˌɪn.dɪˈkeɪ.ʃən/
inevitably /ɪˈnev.ɪ.tə.bli/
ingrowing /ˈɪŋˌgrəʊ.ɪŋ/ **nail** /neɪl/
inwards /ˈɪn.wədz/
irritation /ˌɪr.ɪˈteɪ.ʃən/
judgement /ˈdʒʌdʒ.mənt/
kick /kɪk/ **the habit** /ˈhæbɪt/
kidney /ˈkɪd.ni/
liver /ˈlɪv.ər/
look /lʊk/ **after** /ˈɑːf.tər/
machinery /məˈʃiː.nə.ri/
memory /ˈmem.ər.i/
methadone /ˈmeθ.ə.dəʊn/
miscarriage /ˈmɪsˌkær.ɪdʒ/
mixer /ˈmɪksə/
occasionally /əˈkeɪ.ʒən.əl.i/
painkiller /ˈpeɪnˌkɪlə/
pancreatitis /ˌpæŋ.krɪ.əˈtaɪ.tɪs/
particle /ˈpɑː.tɪ.kl̩/
patch /pætʃ/
peptic /ˈpep.tɪk/ **ulcer** /ˈʌl.sər/
persistent /pəˈsɪs.tənt/
pint /paɪnt/
plaque /plɑːk/
potentially /pəˈten.ʃəl.i/
pregnant /ˈpregnənt/
prematurely /ˌpri.məˈtʃʊr.li/
pull /pʊl/ **up** /ʌp/
pumice stone /ˈpʌm.ɪsˌstəʊn/
quench /kwentʃ/
razor /ˈreɪ.zər/
readily /ˈred.ɪ.li/
refer /rɪˈfɜːr/ **to** /tʊ/
retarded /rɪˈtɑːd.ɪd/
root /ruːt/
scarring /skɑːr.ɪŋ/
sensibly /ˈsen.sɪ.bli/
slow /sləʊ/ **down** /daʊn/
small-headed /smɔːlˈhed.ɪd/
spirit /ˈspɪr.ɪt/
split /splɪt/
spotlessly /ˈspɒt.ləs.li/
spread /spred/
squeeze /skwiːz/
still /stɪl/ **birth** /bɜːθ/
sunbathe /ˈsʌn.beɪð/
sunscreen /ˈsʌn.skriːn/
surface /ˈsɜː.fɪs/
surgery /ˈsɜː.dʒər.i/
tempted /ˈtemptɪd/
throw /θrəʊ/ **(threw, thrown)**
trouble /ˈtrʌb.l̩/
unhealthy /ʌnˈhelθɪ/
urge /ɜːdʒ/
urine /ˈjʊə.rɪn/

vision /ˈvɪʒ.ən/
withdrawal /wɪðˈdrɔː.əl/

Solution to Exercise 1a
1l, 2m, 3g, 4o, 5i, 6d, 7j, 8e, 9k, 10p, 11a, 12c, 13h, 14b, 15f, 16n

Solution to Exercise 1b
1j, 2c, 3l, 4a, 5e, 6f, 7h, 8b, 9k, 10d, 11g, 12i

Chapter II
Understanding food and nutrition

Unit 1 - How your body uses food. Turning food into nutrients. Energy.

Everything that goes into your stomach is mixed with enzymes, chemicals that broke food down, into its **basic components (nutrients).** The mixture then passes from your **stomach** into your **intestines**, where the nutrients are absorbed into your **blood stream**. Your blood transports the nutrients around your body to the cells where they are used or stored. Food components that are not absorbed are excreted.

Your gastrointestinal tract

Your gastrointestinal tract is a tube around seven metres long, which begins at your mouth and ends at your anus. Each section of the tube has its role to play in digestion.

The mouth

Digestion begins as soon as you start **chewing** food. **Saliva** excreted by glands in your mouth, is mixed with the food to make it easier to swallow. Saliva contains an enzyme called **amylase**, which breaks down starch carbohydrate foods into **simpler sugars** that can be absorbed into your body. Amylase can work only in an alkaline environment, such as in the mouth.

The stomach

Once food is **swallowed**, it travels down your **oesophagus** (gullet) to your **stomach**. At its entrance and exit, your stomach has rings of muscle called **sphincters**, which act as valves. When food arrives at your stomach, the top sphincter opens so that food can enter. The top sphincter then closes, keeping the food and **digestive juices** inside your stomach. If this sphincter leaks, you experience heartburn.

Digestive juices contain chemicals that break down food. Two of the chemicals are the enzyme **protease and hydrochloric acid**. Protease breaks down proteins. Hydrochloric acid destroys most of the bacteria present in food and provides the acid conditions in which protease works. Alcohol is not subject to these digestive processes: alcohol is absorbed into your bloodstream directly from your stomach.

Semi-liquid food remains in your stomach for two to four hours before being released in small amounts, through the lower sphincter, into your small intestine.

The small intestine

The small intestine is five to six metres long. It is narrow, only two to four centimetres in diameter. Your small intestine has three distinct parts: **the duodenum, the jejunum, and the ileum**. When food enters your duodenum, it is still acid from the stomach juices. **Alkaline digestive juices** are now added to neutralise it. They are produced in the **pancreas**, and they contain enzymes that continue to digest food. **Bile** is also added to the mixture. This green, watery fluid, which is **produced in your liver** and stored in your **gallbladder**, helps to keep fatty material in solution. The major food components are broken down into their constituents:

- **proteins** into **amino acids**
- **carbohydrates** into **glucose** and other **simple sugars**
- **fat** into **fatty acids** and **glycerol**

The jejunum and ileum

In your jejunum and ileum, the end-products of digestion are absorbed through the intestinal wall into your bloodstream. Food is passed along your intestine by contractions of muscles in the intestinal wall; this is called **peristalsis.**

The intestinal wall consists of millions of tiny finger-like protrusions called **villi**. Water-soluble vitamins and minerals are also absorbed at this stage of digestion. Once the **nutrients** have been **absorbed**, the remaining **undigested food** passes into your **large intestine**. Your body can store some nutrients, such as those providing energy and some vitamins and minerals. Excess of nutrients are lost in **faeces**.

The large intestine

Your large intestine consists of your **colon, rectum and anus**. It **reabsorbs the water** that is used in digestion and **eliminates undigested food and fibre**. Bacteria in the colon break down fibre residues, and release fatty acids, which are important for the nutrition of the colon itself. Once water has been reabsorbed in your colon, the faeces, which are now drier and more solid, are passed along your **rectum** by peristalsis and are finally **expelled** through your **anus**. When faeces reach your rectum, they trigger the desire to defecate, owing to reflex contractions of your rectum and the relaxation of your anal sphincter muscles. It usually takes between one and three days for food to pass from your mouth to your anus.

The importance of fibre

Fibre or non-starch polysaccharides (NSPs) are derived from plant material. **Insoluble fibre** cannot be broken down by digestive enzymes, so it passes through your gastrointestinal tract without being absorbed. As it adds bulk to your diet, fibre makes you feel full and also **regulates your bowel movements**.

Constipation

If you eat a high-fibre diet with plenty of fluids, your faeces will be bulky and pass through more quickly and easily. This prevents constipation. Changing to a **high-fibre diet and drinking more fluids** can ease constipation in most people. Laxatives should be used only on medical advice, as their abuse can lead to loss of muscle tone in the bowel.

Diverticular disease

A high-fibre diet also helps prevent a common disorder called **diverticular disease**. Most sufferers have a history of constipation, which leads to increased pressure in the colon. Straining to pass hard faeces can stretch the wall of the large intestine, encouraging the formation of small pouches, called diverticula, which are pushed outwards from the bowel wall. **Inflammation and bacterial overgrowth** in these **pouches** may cause pain and diarrhoea.

Bowel cancer

Fibre in the diet is also important in connection with bowel cancer, the third most common type of cancer. If detected early enough, it has a very good prognosis. It has been shown that a diet that is low in fibre increases the risk of developing bowel cancer. Recent research has suggested that eating lots of **red meat** (for example, beef, pork and lamb) and **processed meat** (for example, salami, bacon and some sausages) may also increase the risk of bowel cancer. Try alternating meat in your main meals with fish, cheese or other vegetarian options. Swap processed meats for alternatives such as spicy chicken.

Key points

- **Food is broken down** into its building blocks **by enzymes in your mouth, stomach and small intestine.**
- **Nutrients are absorbed** into your **bloodstream from your intestine**.
- Some **excess nutrients can be stored** in your body, but **others are excreted**.
- **Fibre** is essential for the normal movement of food along your bowel and **has a key role in food digestion and absorption.**

Exercise 1a
Match the column A with the column B. Try to learn the expressions and/ or sentences by heart.

A

1. Food is broken down
2. Saliva contains an enzyme called amylase,
3. Everything that goes into your stomach
4. Your blood transports the nutrients

5. Food components
6. Once food is swallowed,
7. Digestive juices contain chemicals (the enzyme protease and hydrochloric acid)
8. Semi-liquid food remains in your stomach
9. When food enters your duodenum,
10. Bile which is produced in your liver and stored in your gallbladder,
11. Food is passed along your intestine
12. The intestinal wall consists of
13. Nutrients are absorbed
14. Once the nutrients have been absorbed,
15. Some excess nutrients can be stored,
16. Once water has been reabsorbed in your colon,
17. Fibre
18. Insoluble fibre
19. Changing to a high-fibre diet and drinking more fluids
20. A high-fibre diet
21. Small pouches, called diverticula,
22. Eating lots of red meat (for example, beef, pork and lamb) and processed meat (for example, salami, bacon and some sausages)

B

a) *alkaline digestive juices, produced in the pancreas, are added to neutralise it.*

b) *are pushed outwards from the bowel wall and inflammation may cause pain and diarrhoea.*

c) *around your body to the cells where they are used or stored.*

d) *by contractions of muscles in the intestinal wall; this is called peristalsis.*

e) *by enzymes in your mouth, stomach and small intestine.*

f) *can ease constipation in most people.*

g) *for two to four hours before being released in small amounts, through the lower sphincter, into your small intestine.*

h) *has a key role in food digestion and absorption.*

i) *helps prevent a common disorder called diverticular disease.*

j) *helps to keep fatty material in solution.*

k) *into your bloodstream from your intestine.*

l) *is mixed with enzymes, chemicals that broke food down, into its basic components (nutrients).*

m) *it travels down your oesophagus (gullet) to your stomach.*

n) *may increase the risk of bowel cancer.*

o) *millions of tiny finger-like protrusions called villi.*

p) *others are excreted.*

q) passes through your gastrointestinal tract without being absorbed.
r) that are not absorbed are excreted.
s) that break down food.
t) the faeces are passed along your rectum by peristalsis and are finally expelled through your anus.
u) the remaining undigested food passes into your large intestine.
v) which breaks down starch carbohydrate foods into simpler sugars that can be absorbed into your body.

Energy
Calories

Your body's primary need, apart from water, is for energy. Calories are often used as a negative term, with people worrying about taking in too many. In contrast, people talk positively about having lots of energy, meaning that they feel healthy. **In nutritional terms**, however, **calories and energy are the same thing**.

Why you need energy

Your body needs energy for life, voluntary activities (such as movement) and special purposes such as pregnancy, breast feeding and growth. You need it to breathe, digest and absorb food and maintain your body temperature. **The rate at which you use energy is known as your metabolic rate**. Your **resting metabolic rate (RMR)** is the number of kilocalories or kilojoules that **you use** just by existing **(breathing, pumping blood around your body, etc.)** and represents about **70 per cent** of your total energy **expenditure**.

How much energy do you need?

If your level of activity increases, either at work or because you start to take more exercise, your total energy requirement will increase too. Your **energy requirements change** at different stages of your life, for example growth requires a lot of energy. A child uses up less energy than an adult. However, if you compare energy requirements per kilogram of body weight, **a child** actually needs a higher proportion of energy per body weight than an adult. After maturity, the **adult** energy requirement is fairly constant, but shows a slight, and continuing decline from the age of 30.

Energy requirements increase during **pregnancy** to meet the needs of the uterus, placenta and foetus. A pregnant woman's blood volume increases and she lays down extra fatty tissue. The increase in **estimated average requirement** (EAR) for pregnancy in the last trimester, from around week 26, is 191 kcal per day. A woman who is **breast-feeding** exclusively needs, on average, an extra 335 kcal per day to maintain a good supply of milk.

When men need more energy than women

Your body weight is determined by two components: fat and fat-free mass (FFM). **Fat-free mass** consists of your body's lean tissues, including **muscle, bone, blood and internal organs**. These structures are responsible for most of your energy consumption. Men have a higher proportion of FFM than women and therefore **burn more calories**. This means that a man needs more calories per day than a woman of the same age and weight.

Gaining and losing weight

If you eat the same amount of calories as you use, your weight will remain constant. If you eat more calories than you need, your weight will increase. To lose weight, you need to use more calories than you take in. **Over a long period, any excess energy is stored as fat**. If you continue to eat more than you need, you will continue to gain weight. To lose weight, you must eat fewer calories. As you lose weight, you lose FFM and lower your energy requirements. This means that you will need to take in even less energy if you are to continue losing weight. When you reach your target weight, you can **consume the amount of calories that will balance your energy intake with your energy expenditure** and you will then stabilise at your new weight.

Where does energy come from?

Energy in your diet is provided by **carbohydrate, fat, protein and alcohol.** Almost all the weight of a food is made up of these components **plus water**. Some foods, such as many **fruit and vegetables, contain a lot of water**, which has no calorific value, and **have less protein, fat or carbohydrate** for a given weight and are therefore **low in calories**. A fatty food, such as butter, which contains relatively little water, is rich in calories.

The following foods all contain approximately **100 kcal**

- 150 ml (half a mug) whole milk
- 290 ml (one mug) skimmed milk
- 290 ml (approx. half a pint) lager
- 2 slices wholemeal bread
- 25 g Cheddar cheese
- 20 g chocolate
- 95 g potato baked in jacket
- 1 kg cooked cauliflower
- a third (approx.) of a Mars bar
- 50 g bag of crisps

Alcohol

Alcohol is a source of energy but contains no other nutrients. It is **rapidly absorbed from your stomach** and **slowly** broken down (**metabolised**) by your **liver**. The rate at which this occurs determines how quickly you become intoxicated. Generally, smaller people metabolise alcohol more slowly than large people, and women more slowly than men. Drinking alcohol with food slows down the rate at which the alcohol is absorbed from your stomach, so that it has a less intoxicating effect.

The maximum recommended intake of alcohol is **three units a day for men** and **two units a day for women**. A **unit provides about eight grams of alcohol** and is equivalent to one small glass of wine, half a pint of beer or one pub measure of spirits. Recent studies have shown a relationship between **moderate intakes** of alcohol and a **decrease in the rate of coronary heart disease**. It is thought that alcohol probably has a beneficial effect on certain types of fat in the bloodstream that help to stop the arteries becoming clogged.

Key points

- Your body needs **energy to survive**
- **Children have higher energy requirements** than adults in relation to their body weight; **older people have lower energy requirements**
- **Fat is your body's main energy store** and is used when you don't eat enough food
- **People put on weight** when their **energy intake exceeds** their **energy requirements**

Exercise 1b
Match the column A with the column B. Try to learn the expressions and/or sentences by heart.

A

1. Your body needs energy
2. The rate at which you use energy
3. If your level of activity increases,
4. A child
5. Energy requirements increase during pregnancy
6. Fat-free mass consists of
7. Men have a higher proportion
8. If you eat the same amount of calories as you use,
9. Over a long period,
10. Energy in your diet
11. Alcohol is
12. Recent studies have shown a relationship
13. Fat is your body's main energy store

B

a) and is used when you don't eat enough food.
b) any excess energy is stored as fat.
c) between moderate intakes of alcohol and a decrease in the rate of coronary heart disease.
d) is known as your metabolic rate.
e) is provided by carbohydrate, fat, protein and alcohol.
f) needs a higher proportion of energy per body weight than an adult.
g) of fat-free mass than women and therefore burn more calories.
h) rapidly absorbed from your stomach and slowly broken down (metabolised) by your liver.

i) *to breathe, digest and absorb food and maintain your body temperature.*
j) *to meet the needs of the uterus, placenta and foetus.*
k) *your body's lean tissues, including muscle, bone, blood and internal organs.*
l) *your total energy requirement will increase too.*
m) *your weight will remain constant.*

Exercise 2
Translate the expressions. Try to explain their meanings in English.

Components, mixture, intestines, stored, digestion, chewing, saliva, alkaline, swallowed, oesophagus, valves, sphincter, heartburn, released, diameter, pancreas, liver, gallbladder, solution, jejunum, ileum, contractions, protrusions, villi, colon, rectum, residues, derived, plant material, insoluble fibre, bowel movements, bulky, constipation, laxatives, medical advice, muscle tone, straining, stretch, diverticula, pushed outwards, overgrowth, detected, alternating, options, bloodstream, voluntary activities, resting metabolic rate, expenditure, requirements, compare, proportion, maturity, decline, uterus, estimated, average, consumption, gain weight, lose weight, target, calorific value, mug, whole milk, skimmed milk, lager, slices, wholemeal bread, cauliflower, crisps, become intoxicated, relationship, clogged, survive, exceed.

Exercise 3
Answer the following questions. Prepare short talks and/or dialogues on these topics.

1. Describe the gastrointestinal tract.
2. Describe the causes of disorders and diseases of the gastrointestinal tract.
3. Why do you need energy and how much energy do you need?
4. Gaining and losing weigh; where does energy come from?
5. Alcohol as a source of energy but no nutrients.

Vocabulary 1

Fill in the meanings in your mother language:

abuse /ə'bjuːz/
added /'æd.ɪd/
advice /əd'vaɪs/
alkaline /'æl.kəl.aɪn/
alternate /'ɒl.tə.neɪ.t/
amino acid /əˌmiː.nəʊ'æs.ɪd/
amylase /'æm.ɪ.leɪz/
anus /'eɪ.nəs/
apart /ə'pɑːt/
approximately /ə'prɒksɪmɪtlɪ/
arrive /ə'raɪv/
average /'æv.ər.ɪdʒ/
bacon /'beɪ.kən/
bake /beɪk/
balance /'bæləns/
bar /bɑː/
beef /biːf/
beneficial /ˌben.ɪ'fɪʃ.əl/
bile /baɪl/
bloodstream /'blʌd.striːm/

bowel /ˈbaʊ.əl/
break /breɪk/ **down** /daʊn/
breast-feed /ˈbrest.fiːd/
breathe /briːð/
building /ˈbɪl.dɪŋ/
bulk /bʌlk/
carbohydrate /ˌkɑː.bəʊ ˈhaɪ.dreɪt/
cauliflower /ˈkɒl.ɪˌflaʊ.ər/
chew /tʃuː/
clogged /klɒgd/
colon /ˈkəʊ.lɒn/
compare /kəmˈpeər/
component /kəmˈpəʊ.nənt/
condition /kənˈdɪʃən/
constant /ˈkɒn.stənt/
constipation /ˌkɒnt.stɪˈpeɪ.ʃən/
constituent /kənˈstɪt.ju.ənt/
consumption /kənˈsʌmp.ʃən/
contain /kənˈteɪn/
continue /kənˈtɪn.juː/
contraction /kənˈtrækʃən/
coronary /ˈkɒr.ən.ər.i/
crisp /krɪsp/
decline /dɪˈklaɪn/
defecate /ˈdef.ə.keɪt/
derive /dɪˈraɪv/
desire /dɪˈzaɪər/
destroy /dɪˈstrɔɪ/
detect /dɪˈtekt/
determine /dɪˈtɜː.mɪn/
diameter /daɪˈæm.ɪ.tər/
diarrhoea /ˌdaɪ.əˈriː.ə/
digest /daɪˈdʒest/
digestive /daɪˈdʒes.tɪv/
distinct /dɪˈstɪŋkt/
diverticular /ˌdaɪ.vəˌtɪk.
jʊˈlər/ **disease** /dɪˈziːz/
diverticulum /ˈdaɪ.vəːˌtɪk.
juˈləm/ pl **diverticula**
duodenum /ˌdjuː.əˈdiː.nəm/
eliminate /ɪˈlɪm.ɪ.neɪt/
encourage /ɪnˈkʌr.ɪ.dʒ/
environment /ɪnˈvaɪə.rən.mənt/
equivalent /ɪˈkwɪv.əl.ənt/
estimated /ˈes.tɪ.meɪt.ɪd/
excess /ekˈses/
exclusively /ɪkˈskluː.sɪv.li/
excrete /ɪkˈskriːt/
expel /ɪkˈspel/
expenditure /ɪkˈspendɪtʃə/
experience /ɪkˈspɪə.ri.ənt s/
faeces /ˈfiː.siːz/
fairly /ˈfeə.lɪ/
fetus, foetus /ˈfiː.təs/
fibre /ˈfaɪ.bər/
fluid /ˈfluː.ɪd/
gallbladder /ˈgɔːlˈblæd.ər/
gland /glænd/
glucose /ˈgluː.kəʊs/
glycerol /ˈglɪs.ə.rɒl/
growth /grəʊθ/
gullet /gʌlɪt/
heart /hɑːt/ **disease** /dɪˈziːz/
heartburn /ˈhɑːt.bɜːn/
hydrochloric acid /ˌhaɪd.
rə.klɒr.ɪkˈæs.ɪd/
ileum /ˈɪl.i.əm/ pl **ilea**
importance /ɪmˈpɔː.tənts/
inflammation /ˌɪn.fləˈmeɪ.ʃən/
insoluble /ɪnˈsɒl.jʊ.blˌ/
internal /ɪnˈtɜː.nəl/
intoxicated /ɪnˈtɒk.sɪ.keɪ.tɪd/
jacket /ˈdʒækɪt/
jejunum /dʒɪˈdʒu nəm/
juices /dʒuːs.ɪz/
lager /ˈlɑːgə/
lamb /læm/
large /lɑːdʒ/ **intestine** /ɪnˈtes.tɪn/
laxative /ˈlæk.sə.tɪv/
lay /leɪ/ **down** /daʊn/
leak /liːk/
lean /liːn/ **tissue** /ˈtɪʃuː/
maturity /məˈtjʊə.rɪ.ti/
metabolic /ˌmet.əˈbɒl.ɪk/ **rate** /reɪt/
metabolise /mɪˈtæbəˌlaɪz/
mixture /mɪks.tʃər/
moderate /ˈmɒd.ər.ət/
movement /ˈmuːv.mənt/
mug /mʌg/
muscle /ˈmʌsəl/ **tone** /təʊn/
occur /əˈkɜːr/
oesophagus /ɪˈsɒf.ə.gəs/

option /'ɒp.ʃən/
overgrowth /ˌəʊ.və.grəʊθ/
owing /'əʊɪŋ/
pancreas /'pæŋ.kri.əs/
pass /pɑːs/
peristalsis /ˌpɛrɪ'stælsɪs/
placenta /plə'sen.tə/
polysaccharide /ˌpɒlɪ'sækəˌraɪd/
pork /pɔːk/
pouch /paʊtʃ/
pregnancy /'preg.nən.si/
primary /'praɪ.mə.ri/
process /'prəʊ.ses/
prognosis /prɒg'nəʊ.sɪs/
protease /'prəʊ.tiː.eɪz/
protein /'prəʊ.tiːn/
protrusion /prə'tru.ʒən/
pump /pʌmp/
purpose /'pɜː.pəs/
push /pʊʃ/
put /pʊt/ **on weight** /weɪt/
reabsorbs /riːæb'sɔrb/
reach /riːtʃ/
recent /'riː.sənt/
recommend /ˌrekə'mend/
rectum /'rek.təm/ pl **recta**
relation /rɪ'leɪ.ʃən/
relationship /rɪ'leɪ.ʃən.ʃɪp/
remain /rɪ'meɪn/
requirement /rɪ'kwaɪə.mənt/
residue /'rez.ɪ.djuː/
responsible /rɪ'spɒnt.sɪ.bl̩/
resting /'rest.ɪŋ/
ring /rɪŋ/
salami /sə'lɑːmɪ/
sausage /'sɒsɪdʒ/
semi /ˌsem.i/ **-liquid** /'lɪk.wɪd/
skim /skɪm/
slight /slaɪt/
slow /sləʊ/ **down** /daʊn/
small /smɔːl/ **intestine** /ɪn'tes.tɪn/
solid /'sɒl.ɪd/
soluble /'sɒljʊbəl/
solution /sə'luː.ʃən/
sphincter /'sfɪŋktə/
spicy /'spaɪsɪ/
spirit /'spɪr.ɪt/
stabilise /'steɪbɪˌlaɪz/
stage /steɪdʒ/
starch /stɑːtʃ/
store /stɔːr/
straining /streɪn.ɪŋ/
stretch /stretʃ/
sufferer /'sʌf.ər.ər/
suggest /sə'dʒest/
supply /sə'plaɪ/
survive /sə'vaɪv/
swallow /'swɒl.əʊ/
swap /swɒp/
target /'tɑː.gɪt/
temperature /'tem.prə.tʃər/
third /θɜːd]/
tiny /'taɪ.ni/
trigger /'trɪg.ər/
turn /tɜːn/
uterus /'juː.tər.əs/ pl **uteri**
valve /vælv/
villus /'vɪlə/ **villi** /'vɪlaɪ/
volume /'vɒl.juːm/
voluntary /'vɒl.ən.tər.i/
watery /'wɔː.təri/
whole /həʊl/ **milk** /mɪlk/
wholemeal /'həʊlˌmiːl/

Solution to Exercise 1a
1e, 2v, 3l, 4c, 5r, 6m, 7s, 8g, 9a, 10j, 11d, 12o, 13k, 14u, 15p, 16t, 17h, 18q, 19f, 20i, 21b, 22n

Solutions to Exercise 1b
1i, 2d, 3l, 4f, 5j, 6k, 7g, 8m, 9b, 10e, 11h, 12c, 13a

Unit 2 - Proteins. Fats.

Proteins in your body

Proteins are the building blocks of your body. Without them, you would not be able to replace or repair your body cells.

Why you need protein

Protein has many important uses in your body. It is a major component of structural tissues such as **skin and collagen**, which is found **in connective tissue** such as **tendons and ligaments. Blood** requires protein for **red blood cells, white blood cells** and numerous compounds in **plasma**. Your body's immunity is also dependent on protein, which is needed for the **formation of antibodies** and white blood cells that fight disease. **Enzymes** and some **hormones** (for example, **insulin**) are also proteins.

If your diet doesn't provide enough energy, your body will eventually use functional body proteins (proteins incorporated into the essential structure of your body). Your body can **adapt to a lack of protein in the short term**. However, conditions such as **injury, infection, cancer**, uncontrolled **diabetes and starvation** can cause substantial **protein losses**. The body starts to lose muscle in order to generate enough energy. If left unchecked, this can become life threatening.

What are proteins?

Proteins are large **compounds of** smaller units called **amino acids**. Amino acids contain **carbon, hydrogen, oxygen, nitrogen and occasionally sulphur**. All amino acids have an **acid group** and an **amino group** attached to different **carbon atoms. Amino** is the chemical name for the combination of **nitrogen** and **hydrogen** in these compounds. When **more than two amino acids** join together, a **polypeptide** is formed. A typical **protein** may contain **500 or more amino acids** joined together. The size and shape of each polypeptide determine what protein it is and its function.

How your body uses proteins

Proteins are **broken down** into amino acids and small peptides by **enzymes (proteases) in your gut**. The small peptides and **amino acids** are **taken via your bloodstream to your liver**, where they are **used or transported** to your body's cells. Your liver is the most important site of amino acid and protein metabolism. Amino acids are chemically changed so that they can be **used for energy, or converted** into other amino acids or proteins, or into **urea** (the form in which they are **excreted**). Some proteins, such as collagen in connective tissue or tendons, are very resistant to digestion and pass through your gut unchanged.

All the proteins that your body needs can be made from 20 different amino acids. You can make some of these from other amino acids, but **there are seven that can't** be made by your body **and must be supplied by your diet.** These are called **essential amino acids**. Children need two further amino acids for growth.

Where is protein found?

Protein can be found in animal produce such as **meat, fish, eggs, milk and milk products, and in plant foods such a cereals, beans**

and pulses. It is important **to eat a mixture of protein sources** to ensure that you have an adequate supply of all essential amino acids. If the diet contains a lot of „empty calories", such as sugar or alcohol, which provide energy but little protein the diet will be deficient in protein.

Special needs

Children

Children need **extra protein** so that they can **grow properly**. The mixture of essential amino acids should be in the correct proportions. There are extra essential amino acids that children need for growth. **Vegan or macrobiotic diets** are not suitable for small children. They **are unlikely to provide all the essential amino acids**. As they contain large amounts of **bulky fibrous foods**, these diets are **unlikely to supply sufficient energy** as fat or carbohydrate and, therefore, protein may be used to make up the deficit.

Vegetarians and vegans

Provided that you follow guidelines on what constitutes a balanced diet, you can get all the essential amino acids and other nutrients that you need without eating meat or fish. However, you should **mix your sources of protein**. **An ova-lacto-vegetarian** eats animal proteins such as **eggs, milk and milk products,** especially cheese. **A vegan** who consumes **only vegetable sources of protein** may find it harder to ensure that they get all the necessary nutrients, but it certainly isn't impossible.

If you are bringing up your **child as a vegetarian,** it is important to make sure that his or her energy needs are met. **Weaning foods such as pulses, cereals, bananas and avocado pears** should be given frequently. The timing of **introduction of some foods** should follow **current guidelines**, for example wheat should not be introduced before six months of age. Aim to include different plant sources of protein at each meal because this will provide a better balance of amino acids. It will be necessary to **supplement** your child's **diet with vitamins and minerals.**

Pregnant and breast feeding women

A pregnant woman needs an **extra six grams of pure protein daily** to allow her baby to grow and develop properly. This will also meet her own needs, which increase as **she develops extra body tissues. Breast-feeding** is very demanding in terms of both energy and protein. To maintain an adequate milk supply, which is a rich source of protein, it is estimated that the mother requires **an extra 11 grams of protein per day from birth until her baby is six months old.** After this she needs eight grams extra per day. Most babies start eating some solids around this age. If you are on a **strict vegan or macrobiotic diet**, you may need **iron and vitamin supplements** while pregnant or breast feeding. Babies should not routinely be given **soya milk** because it is not supplemented with the necessary vitamins and minerals.

Key points

- **Proteins** are made **of amino acids.**
- **Essential amino acids cannot be made in your body** and therefore need to be obtained from food.
- **Vegetarian diets** can be suitable **for all age groups**, but **vegan diets** are **not suitable for children**, especially those under school age.

Exercise 1a
Match the column A with the column B. Try to learn the expressions and/ or sentences by heart.

A

1. Protein
2. Blood requires protein
3. Protein is needed
4. Injury, infection, cancer, uncontrolled diabetes and starvation
5. Proteins are large compounds
6. Amino acids contain
7. All amino acids have an acid group and an amino group
8. A typical protein
9. Proteins are broken down
10. Your liver is the most important site
11. Amino acids are chemically changed
12. There are seven amino acids (called essential amino acids)
13. Protein can be found in
14. There are extra essential amino acids
15. An ova-lacto-vegetarian
16. A vegan
17. A pregnant woman needs
18. To maintain an adequate milk supply,
19. If you are on a strict vegan or macrobiotic diet,
20. Vegetarian diets

B

a) an extra six grams of pure protein daily to allow her baby to grow and develop properly.
b) attached to different carbon atoms.
c) can be suitable for all age groups, but vegan diets are not suitable for children, especially those under school age.
d) can cause substantial protein losses.
e) carbon, hydrogen, oxygen, nitrogen and occasionally sulphur.
f) consumes only vegetable sources of protein.
g) eats animal proteins such as eggs, milk and milk products.
h) for red blood cells, white blood cells and numerous compounds in plasma.
i) for the formation of antibodies and white blood cells that fight disease.

j) *into amino acids and small peptides by enzymes (proteases) in your gut.*
k) *is a major component of structural tissues such as skin and collagen.*
l) *may contain 500 or more amino acids joined together.*
m) *meat, fish, eggs, milk and milk products, and in plant foods such a cereals, beans and pulses.*
n) *of amino acid and protein metabolism.*
o) *so that they can be used for energy, or converted into other amino acids or proteins, or into urea.*
p) *of smaller units called amino acids.*
q) *that can't be made by your body and must be supplied by your diet.*
r) *that children need for growth.*
s) *the mother requires an extra 11 grams of protein per day from birth until her baby is six months old.*
t) *you may need iron and vitamin supplements while pregnant or breast feeding.*

Fats

Visible and invisible fats

Fats (or **lipids**) in your diet are often divided into two types: visible and invisible. **Visible fats** are those that **are obvious**, such as butter, margarine and other spreads, cooking oils and fat on meat. **Invisible (hidden) fats** are **incorporated** during **cooking** (for example, in cakes and biscuits) or during food **preparation** (as in sausages). **Emulsions of fats** are used extensively in products such as mayonnaise. Such foods such as eggs are also rich in fat.

Why do you need fat?

A great deal has been written about the harmful effects of fat, but fat is an essential part of your diet for three important reasons.

- **Taste**: Fat makes many foods taste better. It's no use a food being nutritious if people don't like it and therefore won't eat it.
- **Energy:** Fats are concentrated sources of energy, providing 9 kcal per gram (38 kJ per gram).
- **Essential nutrients:** Fat in your diet provides **fat-soluble vitamins** and **essential fatty acids.**

What are fats?

The basic building blocks of fat are **fatty acids** and **glycerol**. A fatty acid is made up of a chain of carbon atoms with an acid group at one end and methyl group at the other. A methyl group consists of one carbon atom and three hydrogens. **Three different fatty acids combine with glycerol** to form a **triglyceride**. The **fat in your food** is made up of a **mixture of triglycerides**.

Saturated and unsaturated fats

The amount and type of the fatty acids that you eat influence the way in which your body handles them and therefore their role in diseases such as coronary heart disease. Each carbon atom in a fatty acid chain is attached to one or two hydrogen atoms. **If the fatty acid has all the hydrogen atoms that it can hold, it is said to be saturated.**

If, however, **some hydrogen atoms are missing**, the fatty acid is said to be **unsaturated**. In unsaturated fats, the missing hydrogen atoms are replaced by a double bond between the carbon atoms.

All fats contain both saturated and unsaturated fatty acids, and the relative proportion of saturated and unsaturated gives each fat its predominant **characteristics** (for example, **oil or solid**). **The level of saturation** of a fat is also referred to as **hydrogenation**. It is possible to **alter this level** of saturation (or hydrogenation) in the **manufacture of fats and oils.** Generally, fats from **animal sources**, such as butter, have a **high level of saturation**. Saturated fats are more solid at room temperature than unsaturated fats. **The less saturated the fat molecule, the more liquid it will be.** Food **manufacturers** have developed ways of producing unsaturated solid fats by using **stabilisers and emulsifiers**.

Essential fatty acids

Most fatty acids can be made in your body. However, linoleic acid and linolenic acid must be supplied by your diet. These are known as essential fatty acids (EFAs). Some others can be produced to a limited extent from these two essential fatty acids.

Essential fatty acids keep cell walls in good condition and working properly. They are also **important in the transport, breakdown and excretion of cholesterol.** They are used to manufacture other chemicals in your body such as prostaglandins. Most vegetable oils and oily fish are good sources of EFAs.

Omega 3 fatty acids

These fatty acids are found in **oily fish and fish oils**, and some **seeds**, for example flaxseed. An increase in their consumption has health benefits such as **reducing the risk of heart disease.**

Fats known as "trans" fats

"Trans" fats are produced industrially by **modifying the natural structure of a fatty acid.** There is evidence linking **trans fatty acids** with increased risk of **atherosclerosis** and some **cancers**. Some countries have banned trans fatty acids in food production.

How do you use fats?

Fats are **insoluble in water**. They have to be **emulsified by bile** to make them accessible to digestive enzymes. This occurs to a limited extent in your **stomach**, but is completed in your

small intestine. The presence of undigested fat in your stomach delays the rate of emptying.

Fat is broken down by the enzymes **into** smaller compounds such as **fatty acids and glycerols**. These compounds form small particles called **micelles**, which are **small enough to be absorbed** through your gut wall. In your intestinal wall, the micelles are reassembled into larger compounds which are transported to your liver.

Your **liver** then produces **lipoproteins**, such as high-density lipoprotein (HDL), very-low-density lipoprotein (VLDL) and low-density lipoprotein (LDL). The amount and type of fat in your diet influence the ratio in which these lipoproteins are produced.

The recommended dietary intake of EFAs for adults is one to two per cent of the total energy intake and one per cent for children and babies. For adults this means two to five grams per day.

Cholesterol

Cholesterol is used by your body to make **steroid hormones** and **bile salts** and to **maintain the structure of cell membranes**. However, **raised** blood cholesterol **levels** are associated with an **increased risk of coronary heart disease** (CHD). This is because cholesterol can be deposited in **arteries**, making them **narrower**.

One or more **blood vessels** can become totally **blocked**, preventing blood from reaching the tissues served by a vessel. If the blood supply is stopped, the tissue dies. If the blocked vessel is one of the **coronary arteries** supplying blood to the heart, the result is a **heart attack.**

Diet and cholesterol levels

Although some foods are rich in cholesterol, **most cholesterol (95 per cent) is made in your body.** Your body makes cholesterol from saturated fat. **The more saturated fat in your diet, the higher your blood cholesterol levels**. Eating more **high-fibre food,** especially soluble fibre, which is found in foods such as oats and beans, also helps to **reduce your cholesterol levels. Soluble fibre binds cholesterol in bile**, **preventing its re-absorption** by your body and increasing its excretion.

Low levels of cholesterol have been linked to an increased risk of cancer. However, **any disadvantages of a low cholesterol diet are outweighed by its benefits** in reducing the risk of coronary heart disease.

Key points

- **Fat** is an **essential** part of your diet
- **Cutting down on your total fat intake**, especially of saturated fat, is better than trying to substitute one kind of fat for another
- **Fat should provide a maximum of 35 per cent** of your total daily **calories**

Exercise 1b
Match the column A with the column B. Try to learn the expressions and/or sentences by heart.

A

1. Visible fats are those
2. Invisible (hidden) fats
3. Fat in your diet provides
4. The basic building blocks of fat
5. If the fatty acid has all the hydrogen atoms
6. If some hydrogen atoms are missing,
7. Fats from animal sources, such as butter,
8. Food manufacturers
9. Essential fatty acids
10. "Trans" fats are produced industrially
11. Fats are insoluble in water and
12. Fat is broken down by the enzymes
13. Small particles called micelles,
14. In your intestinal wall, the micelles are reassembled
15. Your liver produces lipoproteins;
16. Cholesterol is used by your body
17. Raised blood cholesterol levels are associated
18. Cholesterol can be deposited in arteries,
19. The more saturated fat in your diet,
20. Eating more high-fibre food,
21. Soluble fibre

B

a) *are absorbed through your gut wall.*
b) *are fatty acids and glycerol.*
c) *are important in the transport, breakdown and excretion of cholesterol.*
d) *are incorporated during cooking or during food preparation.*
e) *binds cholesterol in bile, preventing its re-absorption by your body and increasing its excretion.*
f) *by modifying the natural structure of a fatty acid.*
g) *fat-soluble vitamins and essential fatty acids.*
h) *have a high level of saturation.*
i) *have developed ways of producing unsaturated solid fats by using stabilisers and emulsifiers.*
j) *helps to reduce your cholesterol levels.*
k) *into larger compounds which are transported to your liver.*
l) *into smaller compounds such as fatty acids and glycerols.*
m) *making them narrower.*
n) *that are obvious, such as butter, margarine and other spreads, cooking oils and fat on meat.*
o) *that it can hold, it is said to be saturated.*
p) *the amount and type of fat in your diet influence the ratio in which these lipoproteins are produced.*

q) *the fatty acid is said to be unsaturated.*
r) *the higher your blood cholesterol levels.*
s) *they have to be emulsified by bile to make them accessible to digestive enzymes.*
t) *to make steroid hormones and bile salts and to maintain the structure of cell membranes.*
u) *with an increased risk of coronary heart disease.*

Exercise 2
Translate the expressions. Try to explain their meanings in English.

Replace, repair, connective tissue, tendons, ligaments, provide, incorporated, essential, adapt, starvation, generate, carbon, hydrogen, oxygen, nitrogen, sulphur, acid group, amino group, polypeptide, gut, converted, urea, excreted, resistant, pulses, deficient, sufficient, make up, ova-lacto-vegetarian, bringing up, emulsions, harmful, fat-soluble vitamins, methyl group, handle, attached, hold, saturated, double bond, proportion, predominant, solid, referred to, alter, manufacture, stabiliser, emulsifier, condition, properly, prostaglandins, trans fats, banned, accessible, digestive enzymes, emptying, compounds, gut wall, reassembled, high-density, lipoprotein, ratio, bile salts, maintain, raised, increased, deposited, blood supply, soluble fibre, bind, bile, preventing, re-absorption, excretion, disadvantage, outweighed, cutting down, substitute.

Exercise 3
Answer the following questions. Prepare short talks and/or dialogues on these topics.

1. What are proteins? Where are they found?
2. Why do you need protein? How does your body use protein?
3. Special needs (children, pregnant and breast feeding women).
4. What are fats? Why do you need fat? How do you use fats?
5. Characterize saturated and unsaturated fats.
6. Explain the term: Essential fatty acids.
7. What are "trans" fats?
8. Diet and cholesterol levels.

Vocabulary 2

Fill in the meanings in your mother language:

accessible /ək'ses.ə.bl̩/
adapt /ə'dæpt/
aim /eɪm/ **at** /ət/
allow /ə'laʊ/
amino /ə'maɪnəʊ/
amount /ə'maʊnt/
antibody /'æn.ti.bɒd.i/
artery /'ɑ:tərɪ/
atherosclerosis /ˌæθ.ə.rəʊ.sklə'rəʊ.sɪs/
atom /'ætəm/
attached /ə'tætʃt/
banned /'bænd/
bile /baɪl/ **salts** /sɒlts/

bind /baɪnd/
blood /blʌd/ **cell** /sel/
blood /blʌd/ **vessel** /ˈves.əl/
bond /bɒnd/
bring /brɪŋ/ **up** /ʌp/
bulky /ˈbʌl.ki/
carbon /ˈkɑː.bən/
chain /tʃeɪn/
cholesterol /kəˈles.tər.ɒl/
collagen /ˈkɒl.ə.dʒən/
combination /ˌkɒm.bɪˈneɪ.ʃən/
complete /kəmˈpliːt/
compound /ˈkɒm.paʊnd/
connective tissue /kəˌnek.tɪvˈtɪʃ.uː/
constitute /ˈkɒn.stɪ.tjuːt/
convert /kənˈvɜːt/
current /ˈkʌr.ənt/
cut /kʌt/ **down** /daʊn/
deal /dɪəl/
deficient /dɪˈfɪʃ.ənt/
delay /dɪˈleɪ/
demanding /dɪˈmɑːn.dɪŋ/
density /dent.sɪ.ti/
dependent /dɪˈpen.dənt/
deposit /dɪˈpɒz.ɪt/
disadvantage /ˌdɪs.ədˈvɑːn.tɪdʒ/
divide /dɪˈvaɪd/
double /ˈdʌb.lˌ/
empty /ˈemp.ti/
emulsifier /ɪˈmʌlsɪˌfaɪə/
emulsion /ɪˈmʌl.ʃən/
ensure /ɪnˈʃɔːr/
essential /ɪˈsen.tʃəl/
eventually /ɪˈven.tju.əl.i/
evidence /ˈev.ɪ.dəns/
excretion /ɪkˈskriː.ʃən/
extensively /ɪkˈsten.sɪv.li/
extent /ɪkˈstent/
fat /fæt/ **-soluble** /ˈsɒl.jʊ.blˌ/
fibrous /ˈfaɪ.brəs/
fight /faɪt/
flaxseed /ˈflæksˌsiːd/
functional /ˈfʌŋk.ʃən.əl/
generate /ˈdʒen.ər.eɪt/
glycerol /ˈglɪsəˌrɒl/
guidelines /ˈgaɪdˌlaɪnz/
gut /gʌt/
handle /ˈhæn.dlˌ/
harmful /ˈhɑːm.fəl/
hidden /ˈhɪd.ən/
hold /həʊld/
hydrogen /ˈhaɪ.drɪ.dʒən/
hydrogenation /ˌhaɪ.drɪ.dʒəˈneɪ.ʃən/
immunity /ɪˈmjuː.nɪ.ti/
incorporate /ɪnˈkɔː.pər.eɪt/
industrially /ɪnˈdʌstrɪəlɪ/
influence /ˈɪn.flʊ.əns/
intestinal /ˌin.ˈtes.tin.əl/
introduction /ˌɪn.trəˈdʌk.ʃən/
invisible /ɪnˈvɪzəbəl/
iron /aɪən/
lack /læk/
life-threatening /ˈlaɪfˌθret.ən.ɪŋ/
ligament /ˈlɪgəmən/
linoleic /lɪˈnoʊ li ɪk/ **acid** /ˈæsɪd/
linolenic /ˈlæ noʊ lɪ nɪk/ **acid** /ˈæsɪd/
lipid /ˈlɪp.ɪd/
lipoprotein /ˌlɪp.ə .ˈprəʊ.tiːn/
macrobiotics /ˌmækrəʊbaɪˈɒtɪks/
manufacture /ˌmæn.jʊˈfæk.tʃər/
manufacturer /ˌmæn.jʊˈfæk.tʃər.ər/
meet /miːt/ **the needs** /niːdz/
membrane /ˈmem.breɪn/
methyl /ˈmɛθ əl/
modify /ˈmɒd.ɪ.faɪ/
molecule /ˈmɒl.ɪ.kjuːl/
natural /ˈnætʃ.ər.əl/
nitrogen /ˈnaɪ.trə.dʒən/
oats /əʊts/
obtain /əbˈteɪn/
obvious /ˈɒb.vi.əs/
oily /ˈɔɪlɪ/
ova /ˈoʊ və/**-lacto** /ˌlæk toʊ/-
vegetarian /ˌvɛdʒ ɪˈtɛər i ən/
oxygen /ˈɒk.sɪ.dʒən/
particle /ˈpɑː.tɪ.kl̩/
pass /pɑːs/ **through** /θruː/
pear /peə/
peptide /ˈpep.taɪd/
per /pər/ **day** /deɪ/
plasma /ˈplæz.mə/

polypeptide /ˌpɒl.ɪˈpep.taɪd/
predominant /prɪˈdɒmɪnənt/
prevent /prɪˈvent/
properly /ˈprɒp.əl.i/
prostaglandin /ˌprɒstəˈglændɪn/
protease /ˈprəʊ.tiː.eɪz/
provide /prəˈvaɪd/
pure /pjʊər/
ratio /ˈreɪ.ʃi.əʊ/
reabsorption /riː.əbˈzɔːp.ʃən/
reassemble /ˌriːəˈsɛmbəl/
relative /ˈrel.ə.tɪv/
repair /rɪˈpeə/
replace /rɪˈpleɪs/
resistant /rɪˈzɪs.tənt/
saturated /ˈsæt.jʊ.reɪ.tɪd/
seed /siːd/
spread /spred/
stabilizer /ˈsteɪbɪˌlaɪzə/
starvation /stɑːˈveɪ.ʃən/
steroid /ˈstɪərɔɪd/
hormone /ˈhɔːməʊn/
strict /strɪkt/
substitute /ˈsʌb.stɪ.tjuːt/
suitable /ˈsj uː.tə.bl̩/
sulphur /ˈsʌl.fər/
supplement /ˈsʌp.lɪ.mənt/
tendon /ˈten.dən/ pl **tendines**
timing /ˈtaɪ.mɪŋ/
trans fats /ˈtrænz.fæts/
triglyceride /traɪ.glɪs.ə.raɪd/
unchecked /ʌnˈtʃekt/
uncontrolled /ˌʌn.kənˈtrəʊld/
unlikely /ʌnˈlaɪ.kli/
unsaturated /ʌnˈsætʃ.ər.eɪ.tɪd/
urea /jʊəˈriː.ə/
vegan /ˈviːgən/
via /ˈvaɪə/
visible /ˈvɪz.ɪ.bl̩/
weaning /wiːnɪŋ/
wheat /wiːt/

Solution to Exercise 1a
1k, 2h, 3i, 4d, 5p, 6e, 7b, 8l, 9j, 10n, 11o, 12q, 13m, 14r, 15g, 16f, 17a, 18s, 19t, 20c

Solution to Exercise 1b
1n, 2d, 3g, 4b, 5o, 6q, 7h, 8i, 9c, 10f, 11s, 12l, 13a, 14k, 15p, 16t, 17u, 18m, 19r, 20j, 21e

Unit 3 - Carbohydrates. Starches.

Sugars, starches and fibre

Carbohydrates are your main source of energy. When carbohydrates are combined with oxygen (oxidised) in cells, carbon dioxide and water are formed and energy is released.
Glucose + Oxygen = Energy + Carbon dioxide + Water

Nutritionists classify carbohydrates into **sugars, starches and fibre**. The **basic chemical structure** of carbohydrates is a compound called a **saccharide**. Sugars are formed either from a single saccharide, called a **monosaccharide**, or form two saccharides joined together, forming a **disaccharide**. Many saccharides joined together make a **polysaccharide**.

How your body uses sugars

Sugars are important sources of dietary energy. **Glucose** is used as **fuel** by your body's **cells**, and your brain is almost entirely dependent on it for all its functions, including thinking. Disaccharides are broken down by digestive enzymes in your intestine, and absorbed as monosaccharides. **Excess sugars** are **stored in your liver as glycogen**. If the stores are full, sugars are **converted into fa**t and stored in

adipose tissue. Your body is able to **regulate the levels of glucose** in your blood. If you eat a lot of carbohydrate, your **pancreas produces more of the hormone insulin**, which encourages the conversion of sugars into glycogen. This returns your blood glucose levels to normal. When you exercise, you use more glucose and need less insulin.

Where is sugar found?

Sugars are found in a variety of foods. Those occurring **naturally** in the structure of foods are called **intrinsic sugars**. **Those added** in the production process are called **extrinsic sugars**.

Glucose is found in small amounts in fruit and vegetables, such as grapes and onions, and, with **fructose**, it is one of the main constituents of honey. Free glucose is not a common natural sugar, but is produced commercially from starch. Fructose is found in fruit, vegetables and honey. **Galactose**, combined with glucose is found in milk. **Sucrose** is the most commonly used disaccharide, and is extracted commercially from sugar beet or sugar cane. It is present in fruit and vegetables, but table sugar, which is 99 per cent pure sucrose, is the major source in the diet. **Maltose** is produced commercially by breaking down starch. It is present in malted wheat and barley, which are used to produce malted foods and in the brewing industry to make beer. **Lactose** is found naturally only in milk and milk products. It consists of glucose and galactose.

Commercial sugar comes in many forms, including white, granulated, caster, icing, demerara, cane, soft brown, dark brown, treacle, golden syrup, molasses and cubes. The stage and type of processing determine the colour and form of the sugar. None of these sugars contains substantial amounts of any other nutrients. Sugar alcohols, such as **sorbitol**, are compounds that are sweet but have the same chemical structure as alcohol. Sorbitol is found naturally in some fruits, such as cherries, but it is also made commercially from glucose. The intake of refined or added sugars may contribute to the development of obesity. Sugars contribute energy but no other nutrients to diet and are therefore often called empty calories.

Sugars and dental disease

Sugars in the diet have been linked to dental disease. **Dental plaque** is the white layer that builds up on teeth between brushings. Plaque is made of **bacteria, water, polysaccharides** and sometimes **dead cells** from your mouth. It collects in areas that are difficult to clean, which are often called food traps. **Sugars** from food pass into the plaque and **are changed into acid by bacteria**. The acid starts to **dissolve the hard enamel** coating of your teeth, causing **tooth decay** or dental caries. When the acid is neutralised, your tooth can heal, but a frequent intake of sugars maintains the **acid environment, stopping the healing process.**

People who eat large amounts of refined sugars, such as sucrose, have the most dental decay. The more frequent the intake of refined sugars, the greater the number of cavities found. **There is no evidence to suggest that intrinsic sugars**, such as fructose in fruit and lactose in milk and milk products, **have any adverse effects on teeth**. However, the use of fruit juices in comforters (dummies), which maintain prolonged periods of contact with teeth, can contribute to decay. There is strong evidence to suggest that **extrinsic sugars,** such as sucrose, **are involved in the development of dental decay**.

Exercise 1a

Match the column A with the column B. Try to learn the expressions and/or sentences by heart.

A

1. When carbohydrates are combined with oxygen (oxidised) in cells,
2. Nutritionists classify carbohydrates
3. The basic chemical structure of carbohydrates
4. Glucose
5. Excess sugars
6. Sugars are converted
7. If you eat a lot of carbohydrate,
8. Glucose is found
9. Fructose
10. Galactose,
11. Sucrose is extracted
12. Maltose is
13. Lactose
14. Sorbitol
15. Sugars in the diet
16. Plaque is made of
17. Sugars
18. The acid starts
19. Fruit juices in comforters (dummies),

B

a) are changed into acid by bacteria.
b) are stored in your liver as glycogen.
c) bacteria, water, polysaccharides and sometimes dead cells from your mouth.
d) can contribute to decay.
e) carbon dioxide and water are formed and energy is released.
f) combined with glucose is found in milk.
g) commercially from sugar beet or sugar cane.
h) has the same chemical structure as alcohol.
i) have been linked to dental disease.
j) in fruit and vegetables.
k) into fat and stored in adipose tissue.
l) into sugars, starches and fibre.
m) is a compound called a saccharide.
n) is found in fruit, vegetables and honey.

o) is found naturally only in milk and milk products.
p) is used as fuel by your body's cells, and your brain is almost entirely dependent on it.
q) to dissolve the hard enamel coating of your teeth, causing tooth decay.
r) used in the brewing industry to make beer.
s) your pancreas produces more of the hormone insulin, which returns your blood glucose levels to normal.

Starches

Starchy foods are an important part of your diet. Starch is a large, complex compound (a polysaccharide) made up of many glucose molecules. **The glucose can combine in many different ways or patterns**, and this affects the rate at which you digest and absorb starch. Raw starch is very difficult to digest. **Processing**, such as cooking, can change the patterns of glucose molecules, **making the starch more digestible**. Heating starch in water causes it to swell and thicken, and then the digestive enzyme amylase can break it down into glucose, which can be absorbed into your body. The major **source of starches** in the diet are staple foods such as **potatoes, cereal grains** (wheat, barley, maize, oats and rye) and **rice**. A healthy diet should provide an average of **37 per cent of energ**y from starches, intrinsic sugars and milk sugars. The best nourishment for babies is breast milk, which does not contain starch.

Diabetes

Rapidly absorbed carbohydrates, such as sucrose, result in **high glucose levels in the blood. Healthy people** are able to cope with this by **adjusting their insulin production** accordingly. Insulin is a hormone, secreted by the pancreas, that helps to move glucose from the blood into the body's cells. If you have diabetes, this mechanism doesn't work. **People with diabetes either do not produce insulin and need to inject it (type 1** diabetes mellitus) **or produce insulin but are resistant to its action (type 2** diabetes mellitus); they are usually treated by diet and/or tablets but may need insulin. High levels of glucose in the blood result in the **acute symptoms** of diabetes, such as **thirst and increased urination** and, in the **long term,** in complications such as **eye, nerve and circulatory disorders. Starches are important** to people with diabetes because they **do not cause rapid changes in blood glucose levels**, yet provide **energy and fibre**. Sorbitol is often used in products manufactured for people with diabetes. It has less effect on blood glucose than sucrose. However, **sorbitol** has **more calories** per gram and too much of it can give you diarrhoea.

Fibre or non-starch polysaccharides

Fibre was originally called roughage and is now referred to as non-starch polysaccharides (NSPs).

What is fibre and what does it do?

Fibre is the major **component of plant cell walls** and is resistant to enzymes that digest food. Most of the fibre in diet comes from **fruit, vegetables and cereals.** In wheat, maize and rice, the fibre is mainly insoluble, whereas, in oats, barley and rye, it is mainly soluble. **In fruit and vegetables, the ratio of insoluble to soluble fibre is variable.** Each kind of fibre plays a different role in digestion. Insoluble fibre increases the bulk and wetness of faeces and prevents and relieves constipation by holding water in your bowel. The increased bulk speeds up the transit time of faeces and reduces the pressure in your bowel.

Soluble and insoluble fibre sources

Insoluble fibre passes through the intestine unchanged whereas soluble fibre is partly broken down by bacteria in the intestine. The following foods are examples of each type:

Soluble fibre

- Beans, for example baked beans
- Lentils
- Peas
- Oats
- Oranges
- Apples

Insoluble fibre

- Wholemeal bread
- Wholemeal breakfast cereals
- Wholemeal biscuits and crisp breads
- Brown rice
- Wheat bran
- Oats

Soluble fibre has little effect on stool bulk. However, it binds bile acids, which are rich in cholesterol. The cholesterol found in bile is usually reabsorbed into your body. Soluble fibre prevents its re absorption, so **more cholesterol is lost in the faeces and less is taken back into your bloodstream**. This can be **important in the prevention of coronary heart disease. The digestion and absorption of carbohydrates are slower** if there is a good supply of fibre in your diet. This results in a **more gradual release of glucose into your blood**, which is especially important for people with diabetes. **Fibre makes you feel full** because, once it has absorbed water, it has a larger bulk. Generally, foods rich in fibre have more bulk, are less energy dense and are more likely to reduce hunger than fibre-free foods. This suggests that they can **play a useful role in weight-reducing diets.**

Glycaemic index

The glycaemic index (GI) is a way of **ranking foods**, depending on the type of carbohydrate that they contain and **the effect that**

they have on blood sugar levels. Low GI foods are slowly absorbed. Quickly absorbed foods have a high GI. Low GI foods can help even cut blood glucose levels in people with diabetes and may help people on a weight-reducing diet. Diets with high GI may increase the risk of heart disease. **The way in which foods are manufactured and cooked will affect their GI.**

How the glycaemic index works

The glycaemic index **runs from 0 to 100** and usually uses **glucose – which has a GI value of 100 – as the reference.** The effect that other foods have on blood sugar levels is then compared with this. The GI tells us whether **a food raises blood sugar levels dramatically** (high GI value), **moderately** (medium GI value) or **a little bit** (low GI level)

Low GI	**Medium GI**	**High GI**
Apples	Pitta bread	White or wholemeal bread
Beans	Weetabix	Cooked brown or white rice
Porridge	Boiled white basmati rice	Jacket potato
Sweet corn	New potatoes – peeled and boiled	Mashed potato
Sweet potato	Couscous	Glucose
Durum wheat pasta	Honey	Cornflakes

Glycaemic load

The glycaemic load of a food considers the combined **effect of the amount of a food and its glycaemic index on blood sugar levels**. A healthy diet should have a low glycaemic load.

Key points

- **Carbohydrate** is an important **source of energy** in your diet
- Try to eat more carbohydrate foods and **reduce the fat content** of your diet
- **Complex carbohydrates** (starches and fibre) **make you feel full**

Exercise 1b
Match the column A with the column B. Try to learn the expressions and/ or sentences by heart.

A

1. The glucose can combine in many different ways or patterns,
2. Processing, such as cooking,
3. The major source of starches in the diet
4. Insulin is a hormone, secreted by the pancreas,
5. People with diabetes
6. Acute symptoms of diabetes are
7. Long term complications of diabetes
8. Starches are important to people with diabetes
9. In wheat, maize and rice, the fibre is mainly insoluble,
10. Insoluble fibre increases the bulk and wetness of faeces

11. Insoluble fibre passes through the intestine unchanged
12. Soluble fibre
13. Foods rich in fibre
14. Low GI foods are slowly absorbed;
15. The way in which foods are manufactured and cooked
16. The GI tells us whether a food raises blood sugar levels
17. The glycaemic load of a food considers

B

a) *and prevents and relieves constipation.*
b) *and this affects the rate at which you digest and absorb starch.*
c) *are eye, nerve and circulatory disorders.*
d) *are staple foods such as potatoes, cereal grains (wheat, barley, maize, oats and rye) and rice.*
e) *because they do not cause rapid changes in blood glucose levels, yet provide energy and fibre.*
f) *can change the patterns of glucose molecules, making the starch more digestible.*
g) *can play a useful role in weight-reducing diets.*
h) *dramatically (high GI value), moderately (medium GI value) or a little bit (low GI level).*
i) *either do not produce insulin or produce insulin but are resistant to its action.*
j) *binds bile acids, which are rich in cholesterol, so more cholesterol is lost in the faeces and less is taken back into your bloodstream.*
k) *quickly absorbed foods have a high GI.*
l) *that helps to move glucose from the blood into the body's cells.*
m) *the combined effect of the amount of a food and its glycaemic index on blood sugar levels.*
n) *thirst and increased urination.*
o) *whereas soluble fibre is partly broken down by bacteria in the intestine.*
p) *whereas, in oats, barley and rye, it is mainly soluble.*
q) *will affect their GI.*

Exercise 2
Translate the expressions. Try to explain their meanings in English.

Entirely, dependent, converted, adipose tissue, encourage, occur, naturally, added, grapes, onion, commercially, sugar beet, sugar cane, pure, malted wheat, barley, brewing industry, caster, icing, demerara, treacle, molasses, cube, processing, substantial, cherries, dental plaque, dissolve, enamel, coating, decay, heal, cavities, adverse effects, comforter, patterns, raw starch, processing, digestible, thicken, staple foods, grains, wheat, barley, maize, oats, rye, nourishment, breast milk, cope with, adjusting, resistant, urination, long term, diarrhoea, component, oats, barley, rye, ratio, bulk, wetness, relieve, constipation, speeds up, beans, lentils, peas, wholemeal, wheat bran, bile acids, reabsorb, take back, gradual release, fibre-free, weight reducing, glycaemic index, reference, compared, moderately, pasta, cornflakes, couscous, peeled, mashed potato, jacket potato, porridge.

Exercise 3
Answer the following questions. Prepare short talks and/or dialogues on these topics

1. Explain how your body uses sugars. Where is sugar found?
2. Forms of commercial sugar. Sugars and dental disease
3. Why are starchy foods an important part of your diet?
4. How are healthy people able to cope with high glucose levels in the blood?
5. What are acute symptoms and long term complications of diabetes?
6. What is fibre and what does it do? Soluble and insoluble fibre sources.
7. Glycaemic index. How does the glycaemic index work?

Vocabulary 3

Fill in the meanings in your mother language:

accordingly /ə'kɔː.dɪŋ.li/
action /'æk.ʃən/
adipose /'æd.ɪ.pəʊz/
adjust /ə'dʒʌst/
adverse /'æd.vɜːs/
affect /ə'fekt/
barley /'bɑː.li/
beet /biːt/
bile /baɪl/ **acid** /'æs.ɪd/
brain /breɪn/
bran /bræn/
breast /brest/ **milk** /mɪlk/
brew /bruː/
brush /brʌʃ/
build up, buildup /'bɪld.ʌp/
cane /keɪn/
carbon /'kɑː.bən/ **dioxide** / daɪ'ɒk.saɪd/
caries /'keəriːz/
caster /kɑːstə/ **sugar** /'ʃʊgə/
cavity /'kæv.ə.ti/
cherry /'tʃer.i/
coating /'kəʊtɪŋ/
collect /kə'lekt/
comforter /'kʌmfətə/
commercially /kə'mɜː.ʃəl.i/
contribute /kən'trɪb.juːt/
conversion /kən'vɜː.ʃən/
cope /kəʊp/ **with** /wɪð/
corn /kɔːn/
cornflakes /'kɔːnˌfleɪks/
couscous /'kuːskuːs/
cube /kjuːb/
dead /ded/
decay /dɪ'keɪ/
demerara /ˌdɛmə'rɛərə/
dental /'den.təl/ **disease** /dɪ'ziːz/
digestible /daɪ'dʒes.tə.bl̩/
disaccharide /daɪ'sækəˌraɪd/
disorder /dɪ'sɔː.dər/
dissolve /dɪ'zɒlv/
dramatically /drə'mætɪkəli /
dummy /'dʌm.i/
durum /'djʊərəm/ **wheat** /wiːt/
entirely /ɪn'taɪə.li/
extract /ɪk'strækt/
extrinsic /ek'strɪnt.sɪk/
faeces /'fiː.siːz/
fructose /'frʌktəʊs/
fuel /fjʊəl/

galactose /gəˈlæktəʊz/
glycaemic /glaɪˈsi mik/ **index** /ˈɪndɛks/
glycogen /ˈglaɪ.kəʊ.dʒən/
gradual /ˈgræd.jʊ.əl/
grain /greɪn/
granulate /ˈgrænjʊˌleɪt/
grape /greɪp/
heal /hiːl/
heating /ˈhiː.tɪŋ/
icing /ˈaɪsɪŋ/
inject /ɪnˈdʒekt/
intrinsic /ɪnˈtrɪn.sɪk/
layer /ˈleɪ.ə/
lentil /ˈlɛntɪl/
likely /ˈlaɪ.kli/
link /lɪŋk/
load /ləʊd/
maize /meɪz/
major /ˈmeɪ.dʒər/
malted /mɔːltid/
maltose /ˈmɔːltəʊz/
mashed /mæʃt/
moderately /ˈmɒd.ər.ət.li/
molasses /məˈlæsɪz/
monosaccharide /ˌmɒnəʊˈsækəˌraɪd/
nourishment /ˈnʌr.ɪʃ.mənt/
onion /ˈʌn.jən/
oxidise /ˈɒksɪˌdaɪz/
pattern /ˈpæt.ən/
pea /piː/
peel /piːl/
pitta /ˈpɪtə/ bread /bred/
plaque /plɑːk/
porridge /ˈpɒrɪdʒ/
processing /ˈprəʊ.ses.ɪŋ/
produce /prəˈdjuːs/
rank /ræŋk/
reference /ˈref.ər.ənt s/
release /rəˈliːs/
relieve /rɪˈliːv/
roughage /ˈrʌfɪdʒ/
rye /raɪ/
saccharide /ˈsækəˌraɪd/
sorbitol /ˈsɔːbɪˌtɒl/
speed /spiːd/ **up** /ʌp/
staple /ˈsteɪpəl/
stool /stuːl/
sucrose /ˈsuː.krəʊz/
syrup /ˈsɪr.əp/
thicken /ˈθɪk.ən/
transit /ˈtrænsɪt/
trap /træp/
treacle /ˈtriːkəl/
treat /triːt/
unchanged /ʌnˈtʃeɪndʒd/
urination /ˌjʊə.rɪˈneɪ.ʃən/
variable /ˈveə.ri.ə.bl̩/
Weetabix /wit.ə.bəks/
wetness /wɛtnəs/
whereas /weərˈæz/
wholemeal /ˈhəʊlˌmiːl/ **bread** /bred/

Solution to Exercise 1a
1e, 2l, 3m, 4p, 5b, 6k, 7s, 8j, 9n, 10f, 11g, 12r, 13o, 14h, 15i, 16c, 17a, 18q, 19d

Solution to Exercise 1b
1b, 2f, 3d, 4l, 5i, 6n, 7c, 8e, 9p, 10a, 11o, 12j, 13g, 14k, 15q, 16h, 17m

Unit 4 - Vitamins

Micro-nutrients

Vitamins and minerals are an essential part of a balanced diet. A lack of vitamins or minerals can lead to ill-health and cause deficiency diseases. Vitamins can also play a part in preventing diseases such as cancer.

What are vitamins?

Vitamins are complex **chemical substances**. Most can't be made in your body, so you have to **obtain them from food**. Vitamin D can be made in your skin on exposure to sunlight. Bacteria, which aren't part of your body but live inside your gut, can also make some vitamins. Vitamins can be split into two groups: water soluble and fat soluble. **Water-soluble vitamins** can be dissolved in water and, therefore, are found in non-fatty, water-rich foods such as fruit and vegetables. **Fat-soluble vitamins** are found in fatty foods, as their chemical structures allow them to be dissolved in fat. **The fresher the foods**, and the less they are cooked, the better the supplies of vitamins available. Vitamin C is destroyed by heat, and vitamin B_1 (thiamine) is sensitive to light. **Frozen vegetables** are often better sources of vitamins because they are frozen very soon after harvest and the vitamins are preserved.

How much do you need?

Only small amounts of each vitamin are required each day. There are **recommended daily allowances** (Rd As) for several vitamins. The RDA varies between different groups of people; **infants, children, elderly people, adults and pregnant and breast-feeding women** all require different amounts.

Water-soluble vitamins

Vitamin C (ascorbic acid)

Vitamin C helps to maintain your **skin and connective tissue** and helps **iron to be absorbed** from your gut. People who don't get enough vitamin C develop a condition called **scurvy**, which causes fatigue, bleeding and poor wound healing. Vitamin C **deficiency** can affect people with illnesses such as **cancer, malabsorption syndromes and alcoholism**, or those who are being fed intravenously. Vitamin C is found in **citrus fruit, tomatoes, spinach, potatoes and broccoli.** Foods rich in vitamin C should be stored in a cool, dark place.

Taking **high doses** of vitamin C has been claimed to reduce your chances of catching the common cold. Taking too much can be harmful, causing diarrhoea and kidney stones. As vitamin C increases iron uptake, taking too much can also lead to iron overload.

Vitamin B_1 (thiamine)

Thiamine helps to **break down carbohydrate, fat and alcohol**. People who have thiamine **deficiency** (known as **beri-beri**) cannot process carbohydrates or fat properly and develop a range of symptoms including cardiac and neurological problems. The condition mainly affects people with **chronic disease, malabsorption or problems with anorexia**. Chronic binge-drinking **alcoholics** can also develop thiamine deficiency. Major sources are **fortified cereals and bread, offal, pork, nuts and legumes** (peas and beans).

Large doses of thiamine, in excess of 3 grams per day, may cause headaches, insomnia, weakness and skin problems.

Vitamin B_2 (riboflavin)

Your body needs vitamin B_2 to **extract energy from fat,**

protein and carbohydrate in food. The main sources are **dairy products, meat, fish, asparagus, broccoli, poultry and spinach**. Some cereals are fortified with riboflavin. Riboflavin is **sensitive to ultraviolet light**. Riboflavin **deficiency** can cause **skin disorders**, especially in and around the mouth.

Vitamin B_6 (pyridoxine)

Pyridoxine is essential for the **metabolism of proteins and haemoglobin** (the oxygen-carrying red pigment in your blood), and so the quantity that you need depends on how much protein you eat. Pyridoxine **deficiency** causes **skin problems** in and around the mouth and **neurological problems**. Bacteria in your gut make pyridoxine, some of which is absorbed through your intestinal wall. **Poultry, fish, pork, eggs and offal** are rich **sources** of pyridoxine, as are **oats, peanuts and soy-beans. High doses** of pyridoxine over a period of time have been associated with nerve damage.

Vitamin B_{12} (cyanocobalamin)

Cyanocobalamin is involved in the **production of red blood cells. Foods derived from animals** are a good source of **vitamin** B_{12}. Strict vegetarians and vegans may need to take supplements to make up for any deficiency in their diets. **People who have a stomach disorder** preventing them from making enough intrinsic factor **cannot absorb vitamin** B_{12} properly; they develop **pernicious anaemia.**

Exercise 1a
Match the column A with the column B. Try to learn the expressions and/ or sentences by heart.

A

1. A lack of vitamins or minerals
2. Most vitamins can't be made in your body,
3. Vitamin D can be
4. Water-soluble vitamins
5. Fat-soluble vitamins
6. Vitamin C is destroyed by heat,
7. Infants, children, elderly people, adults and pregnant and breast-feeding women
8. Vitamin C helps
9. Scurvy causes
10. Vitamin C is found
11. Taking high doses of vitamin C
12. Thiamine helps to
13. People who have thiamine deficiency (known as beri-beri)
14. Major sources of vitamin B_1 (thiamine)
15. Your body needs vitamin B_2 (riboflavin)
16. The main sources of riboflavin are
17. Vitamin B_6 (pyridoxine)
18. Poultry, fish, pork, eggs and offal are rich sources of pyridoxine,
19. Vitamin B_{12} (cyanocobalamin)
20. Foods derived from animals

B

a) all require different amounts of each vitamin.
b) and vitamin B1 (thiamine) is sensitive to light.
c) are a good source of vitamin B12.
d) are fortified cereals and bread, offal, pork, nuts and legumes (peas and beans).
e) are found in fatty foods.
f) are found in fruit and vegetables.
g) as are oats, peanuts and soy-beans.
h) break down carbohydrate, fat and alcohol.
i) can lead to ill-health and cause deficiency diseases.
j) cannot process carbohydrates or fat properly and develop a range of symptoms including cardiac and neurological problems.
k) dairy products, meat, fish, asparagus, broccoli, poultry and spinach.
l) fatigue, bleeding and poor wound healing.
m) has been claimed to reduce your chances of catching the common cold.
n) in citrus fruit, tomatoes, spinach, potatoes and broccoli.
o) is essential for the metabolism of proteins and haemoglobin.
p) is involved in the production of red blood cells.
q) made in your skin on exposure to sunlight.
r) so you have to obtain them from food.
s) to extract energy from fat, protein and carbohydrate in food.
t) to maintain your skin and connective tissue and helps iron to be absorbed from your gut.

Folate

Folate (folic acid) is essential for the normal **formation of red blood cells**. People with folic acid **deficiency** may develop a condition called **megaloblastic anaemia** in which the red blood cells are enlarged. **Sources** of folates include **liver, yeast extract and green, leafy vegetables**. A good supply is particularly important for women who are planning to conceive and those who are in the **first 12 weeks of pregnancy**, when the recommended intake is 400 micrograms per day. Folate has been shown to reduce the risk of having a baby with a neural tube defect such as spina bifida. **High intakes** of folate may affect the absorption of zinc and interfere with tests used to diagnose vitamin B12 deficiency.

Niacin

Niacin is involved in **fat metabolism** and is necessary to maintain the condition of your skin. Niacin **deficiency** is rare in developed countries, but in Asia and Africa it results in a condition called **pellagra**, which can be fatal if untreated. **Meat** is a good **source** of niacin and cereals provide moderate amounts. Niacin can also be made in your body from the amino acid tryptophan. Excess niacin is excreted in your urine, although very large doses can cause liver problems.

Pantothenic acid and biotin

Pantothenic acid and biotin are involved in fat and carbohydrate metabolism and are found in foods derived from animal sources and in cereals and pulses.

Fat soluble vitamins

Vitamin A (retinol)

Vitamin A can be **made in your body** from substances called **beta-carotenes**, which are found in **dark-green, orange and yellow vegetables** such as spinach and carrots. Retinol is obtained from animal **sources**, such as **meat and dairy products,** and is added to margarine. **Deficiency** is a major cause of **blindness** in children in some developing countries. Retinol is **toxic in large doses**, but most damage is done by **accumulation**. Toxicity can lead to **liver and bone damage** and cause **birth defects.** You shouldn't take supplements or eat large quantities of liver just before or during pregnancy.

Vitamin D (calciferol)

Vitamin D is important in the **growth and maintenance of bone** because it **controls the absorption of calcium and phosphorus**, which are essential in bone metabolism. Children who don't get enough vitamin D develop **rickets** and adults develop **osteomalacia,** which is a condition with **weak, soft bones**. **Sources** of vitamin D include **fatty fish**, such as pilchards, sardines, mackerel and tuna, **eggs and fortified foods** such as margarine and some breakfast cereals. Vitamin D can be made in your skin by **ultraviolet rays** in sunlight. **Deficiency** is rare. It is more common in people who have little vitamin D in their diet and whose skins are rarely exposed to sunlight. **Large doses** can lead to high blood levels of calcium, especially in children, and may result in bone malformations, although this is extremely rare.

Vitamin E (tocopherol)

Tocopherol acts as an **antioxidant**, which means that it stops your body's cells being attacked by chemicals called oxygen-generated free radicals. Vitamin E is important in maintaining the structure of lipids (fats) in your body and any structures, such as membranes surrounding cells, that are rich in lipids. Dietary **sources** include **vegetable oils, nuts, vegetables and cereals.**

Vitamin K (phylloquinone, menaquinone and menadione)

Vitamin K is involved in **blood clotting** and a deficiency will lead to bruising and excessive bleeding. Deficiency is rare except in newborn babies and people who have diseases affecting vitamin absorption or metabolism. **Dark green leafy**

vegetables are the major sources in the diet, although **bacteria in your gut** can make vitamin K, which is absorbed into your blood.

Exercise 1b
Match the column A with the column B. Try to learn the expressions and/ or sentences by heart.

A

1. Folate (folic acid) is essential
2. Sources of folates
3. Folate has been shown to reduce
4. Niacin is involved in
5. Meat is a good source of niacin
6. Pantothenic acid and biotin are involved in fat and carbohydrate metabolism
7. Vitamin A can be made in your body
8. Retinol is toxic in large doses,
9. Vitamin D is important in the growth and maintenance of bone
10. Children who don't get enough vitamin D
11. Sources of vitamin D include
12. Dietary sources of vitamin E (tocopherol)
13. Vitamin K is involved in
14. Dark green leafy vegetables are the major sources in the diet,

B

a) *although bacteria in your gut can make vitamin K, which is absorbed into your blood.*
b) *and are found in foods derived from animal sources and in cereals and pulses.*
c) *and cereals provide moderate amounts.*
d) *because it controls the absorption of calcium and phosphorus.*
e) *blood clotting and a deficiency will lead to bruising and excessive bleeding.*
f) *but most damage is done by accumulation.*
g) *develop rickets and osteomalacia.*
h) *fat metabolism and is necessary to maintain the condition of your skin.*
i) *fatty fish, eggs and fortified foods such as margarine and some breakfast cereals.*
j) *for the normal formation of red blood cells.*
k) *from substances called beta-carotenes, which are found in dark-green, orange and yellow vegetables.*
l) *include liver, yeast extract and green, leafy vegetables.*
m) *include vegetable oils, nuts, vegetables and cereals.*
n) *the risk of having a baby with spina bifida.*

Exercise 2
Translate the expressions. Try to explain their meanings in English.

Essential, deficiency, complex substances, obtain, exposure, split, dissolved, therefore, the supplies of, sensitive, frozen, harvest, preserved, required, elderly, connective tissue, scurvy, fatigue, healing, fed, stored, claimed, catching cold, harmful, uptake, overload, beri-beri, a range of, condition, binge-drinking, offal, fortified cereals, in excess of, insomnia, weakness, asparagus, broccoli, poultry, spinach, pork, peanuts, derived, to make up for, pernicious anaemia, yeast extract, conceive, spina bifida, interfere with, pellagra, blindness, maintenance, rickets, osteomalacia, malformations, oxygen-generated free radicals, blood clotting, bruising, excessive bleeding.

Exercise 3
Answer the following questions. Prepare short talks and/or dialogues on these topics

1. What are vitamins?
2. What do you know about vitamin C?
3. What do you know about vitamin B_1, B_2, B_6 and B_{12}?
4. Why is a good supply of folate particularly important in pregnancy?
5. What is the cause of a condition called pellagra?
6. What are the sources of vitamin A?
7. Why is vitamin D particularly important for young children?
8. What is the cause of a condition called rickets?
9. Dietary sources of vitamin E.
10. The importance of vitamin K.

Vocabulary 4

Fill in the meanings in your mother language:

accumulation /əˌkjuː.mjʊˈleɪ.ʃən/
allowance /əˈlaʊəns/
asparagus /əˈspær.ə.gəs/
associated /əˈsəʊ.si.eɪ.tɪd/
available /əˈveɪ.lə.bl̩/
beriberi /ˌber.ɪˈber.i/
beta /ˈbiː.tə/-**carotene** /ˈkærəˌtiːn/
binge /bɪndʒ/ **drinking** /ˈdrɪŋ.kɪŋ/
biotin /baɪˈɒt.iːn/
blindness /ˈblaɪnd.nəs/
broccoli /ˈbrɒk.əl.i/
bruising /ˈbruː.zɪŋ/
calciferol /kælˈsɪfərɒl/
catch /kætʃ/ a **cold** /kəʊld/
claim /kleɪm/
clotting /ˈklɑt̬.ɪŋ/
complex /ˈkɒm.pleks/
conceive /kənˈsiːv/
cyanocobalamin /ˌsaɪənəʊkəʊˈbæləmɪn/
dairy /ˈdeə.ri/
excessive /ekˈses.ɪv/
exposure /ɪkˈspəʊ.ʒər/
fatal /ˈfeɪ.təl/
fatigue /fəˈtiːg/
folate /ˈfoʊ leɪt/
fortified /ˈfɔː.tɪˌfaɪd/
frozen /ˈfrəʊ.zən/
haemoglobin /ˌhiː.məˈgləʊ.bɪn/
harvest /ˈhɑː.vɪst/
infant /ˈɪn.fənt/

inside /ɪnˈsaɪd/
insomnia /ɪnˈsɒm.ni.ə/
interfere /ˌɪn.təˈfɪər/
intravenously /ˌɪn.trəˈviː.nəs.li/
kidney /ˈkɪd.ni/ **stones** /stəʊnz/
leafy /ˈliː.fi/
mackerel /ˈmæk.rəl/
make /meɪk/ **up** /ʌp/ **for** /fɔːr/
malabsorption /ˌmæləbˈsɔːpʃən/
malformation /ˌmæl.fəˈmeɪ.ʃən/
margarine /ˌmɑː.dʒəˈriːn/
megaloblastic /ˌmɛgələʊˈblæstɪk/
anaemia /əˈniːmɪə/
menadione /ˌmɛnəˈdaɪəʊn/
menaquinone /ˌmɛnəkwɪˈnəʊn/
micronutrient /ˌmaɪkrəʊˈnjuːtrɪənt/
neural /ˈnjʊə.rəl/ **tube** /tjuːb/
newborn /ˈnjuː.bɔːn/
offal /ˈɒfəl/
osteomalacia /ˌɒstɪəʊməˈleɪʃɪə/
overload /ˌəʊ.vəˈləʊd/
pantothenic /ˌpæntəˈθɛnɪk/
acid /ˈæsɪd/
part /pɑːt/
particularly /pəˈtɪk.jʊ.lə.li/
peanut /ˈpiː.nʌt/
pellagra /pəˈleɪgrə/
pernicious /pəˈnɪʃəs/
anaemia /əˈniːmɪə/
phosphorus /ˈfɒs.fər.əs/
phylloquinone /ˌfɪləʊkwɪˈnəʊn/
pilchard /ˈpɪltʃəd/
pork /pɔːk/
poultry /ˈpəʊl.tri/
pyridoxine /ˌpɪrɪˈdɒksiːn/
quantity /ˈkwɒn.tɪ.ti/
range /reɪndʒ/
rare /reər/
ray /reɪ/
retinol /ˈrɛtɪˌnɒl/
rickets /ˈrɪk.ɪts/
sardine /sɑːˈdiːn/
scurvy /ˈskɜː.vi/
sensitive /ˈsent.sɪ.tɪv/
soybean /ˈsɔɪˌbiːn/
spina bifida /ˌspaɪ.nəˈbɪf.ɪ.də/
spinach /ˈspɪn.ɪtʃ/
split /splɪt/
sunlight /ˈsʌn.laɪt/
thiamine /ˈθaɪ.ə.miːn/
tocopherol /tɒˈkɒfəˌrɒl/
tryptophan /ˈtrɪptəˌfæn/
tuna /ˈtjuː.nə/
ultraviolet /ˌʌltrəˈvaɪəlɪt/
untreated /ʌnˈtriː.tɪd/
uptake /ˈʌp.teɪk/
urine /ˈjʊə.rɪn/
weakness /ˈwiːk.nəs/
yeast /jiːst/

Solution to Exercise 1a
1i, 2r, 3q, 4f, 5e, 6b, 7a, 8t, 9l, 10n, 11m, 12h, 13j, 14d, 15s, 16k, 17o, 18g, 19p, 20c

Solution to Exercise 1b
1j, 2l, 3n, 4h, 5c, 6b, 7k, 8f, 9d, 10g, 11i, 12m, 13e, 14a

Unit 5 - Minerals. Healthy eating.

Minerals are **single chemical elements** that are involved in various processes in your body. If you eat a varied diet, you should obtain all the minerals that you need. Unlike vitamins, **minerals do not deteriorate during storage or cooking, so mineral deficiency is rare**, except in people being fed intravenously or who have certain diseases. One exception is **iron deficiency**, which is often the result of **blood loss** or may develop in people who are **strict vegetarians or vegans**. Taking mineral supplements may cause problems: **overloading** with one mineral may decrease the absorption of another that is absorbed in your body via the same route.

Sodium, potassium and chromium

Sodium, potassium and chromium are also referred to, in solution, as **electrolytes**. They are widely distributed throughout you body and have **many functions**, including maintaining your nerves in proper working order. **Deficiencies and high levels** of these chemicals are usually caused by a **problem with a person's metabolism** – for example, certain diseases or dehydration caused by excessive vomiting. Electrolytes are readily available in animal and vegetable foods.

Other minerals and trace elements

Other minerals and trace elements used by your body include **aluminium, antimony, boron, bromine, cadmium, lithium, nickel, sulphur and strontium.** They are **readily available in your diet** and are only necessary in trace (tiny) quantities.

Antioxidants and disease prevention

Recently, there has been evidence that some vitamins and the mineral selenium may act as defences against certain diseases. **When oxygen is used in chemical reactions** in your body, it produces, as a **by-product, potentially harmful chemicals called free radicals**. These cause **tissue damage** and may lead to some conditions such as **heart disease** and some **cancers. Antioxidants, such as vitamin A, beta-carotene, vitamins C and E, selenium, zinc and lycopene**, are able to **stop the action of these radicals**. Dietary **sources** of antioxidants are **fruit and vegetables, nuts, cereals, and fish** (and their oils). The best way of ensuring that you get enough of the relevant nutrients is to eat five portions of fruit and vegetables a day.

Sources of antioxidants

Antioxidant	Present in:
Vitamin A	Dairy products, oily fish (herring, sardines, tuna) and fish oils
Beta-carotene	Fruit and vegetables
Vitamin C	Fruit and vegetables (spinach, tomato, potato, broccoli, strawberry, orange and citrus)
Vitamin E	Fruit, vegetables, cereals, dairy, nuts, eggs
Selenium	Cereal grains, meat, fish
Zinc	Meat, leafy and root vegetables, whole grains, eggs, nuts
Lycopene	Cooked/processed tomatoes from sauces

Key points

- A **balanced diet** provides all the necessary vitamins and minerals for healthy adults
- The benefits of **large doses** of vitamins (much higher than the recommended daily allowance) are not proven; large doses of fat-soluble vitamins can actually be harmful
- Some people are at **risk of a vitamin or a mineral deficiency** (for example, pregnant women, and

vegetarians), and may benefit from supplements of the correct dosage

- Research has found links between a low vitamin and mineral intake and heart disease and some cancers; it is believed that **five portions of fruit and vegetables per day** can reduce the risk of developing these diseases.
- Taking the **recommended dose of folate supplement** before and for the first 12 weeks of **pregnancy** reduces the risk of having a baby with spina bifida

Exercise 1a
Match the column A with the column B. Try to learn the expressions and/or sentences by heart.

A

1. Unlike vitamins,
2. Iron deficiency
3. Overloading with one mineral
4. Sodium, potassium and chromium
5. Other minerals and trace elements used by your body
6. Some vitamins and the mineral selenium
7. When oxygen is used in chemical reactions in your body, it produces, as a by-product,
8. Antioxidants, such as vitamin A, beta-carotene, vitamins C and E, selenium, zinc and lycopene,
9. A balanced diet provides
10. Some people are at risk of a vitamin or a mineral deficiency
11. Research has found links

B

a) *(for example, pregnant women, and vegetarians), and may benefit from supplements of the correct dosage.*
b) *all the necessary vitamins and minerals for healthy adults.*
c) *are able to stop the action of free radicals.*
d) *are also referred to, in solution, as electrolytes.*
e) *between a low vitamin and mineral intake and heart disease and some cancers.*
f) *include aluminium, antimony, boron, bromine, cadmium, lithium, nickel, sulphur and strontium.*
g) *is often the result of blood loss or may develop in people who are strict vegetarians or vegans.*
h) *may act as defences against certain diseases.*
i) *may decrease the absorption of another that is absorbed in your body via the same route.*
j) *minerals do not deteriorate during storage or cooking, so mineral deficiency is rare.*
k) *potentially harmful chemicals called free radicals.*

Healthy eating

It is important **to view your diet as a whole**. If you deny yourself a particular favourite food, you are more likely to become obsessed with it and crave it all the time. When you do succumb, you're more likely to over-indulge that if you include it in your diet every now and again.

The five food groups

There are five food groups:

- Fruit and vegetables
- Bread, cereals, pasta and potatoes (carbohydrates)
- Meat, fish and alternatives (protein foods)
- Milk and dairy foods
- Foods containing fat or sugar

To achieve a balanced diet, you should **choose a variety of foods from the first four groups**. This will supply you with enough of the various nutrients that your body needs. **Foods in the fifth group** do not always provide a wide variety of nutrients, but can make your diet more enjoyable. They **should be eaten only in moderation**. Aim to have three meals a day with small snacks in between if you want them. **Snacks** don't have to be high in calories or fat – fruit or a couple of wholemeal biscuits is a better bet. **Breakfast** is an important meal and shouldn't be missed. The longer you go between meals or snacks, the more likely you are to overeat when you next get the chance. Foods should be included in your **diet in relative proportions**.

Your eating plan
Fruit and vegetables

Fruit and vegetables provide vitamins, minerals and fibre. Frozen, dried and tinned fruit and vegetables are just as nutritious as fresh foods.

Healthy snacks

Snacks can be healthy and nutritious as well as easy to prepare. Include **foods that are low in sugar, fat and salt, and high in fibre**. The most healthy snack and easiest to prepare is fresh fruit.

- Fresh fruit
- Dried fruit (be careful if watching calories)
- Raw chopped vegetables, for example, carrot or celery sticks
- Plain popcorn
- Plain scone or currant bun
- Low-fat yoghurt or fromage frais
- Bread sticks

What is a portion?

This chart shows examples of the portion sizes of particular foods.

Food	Portion
Apple, banana, orange	1 fruit
Plums	2 fruits
Dried fruit	1 tablespoon
Grapes, cherries	1 cupful
Fruit juice	1 small glass
Vegetables	2 tablespoons
Salad	1 dessert bowlful

Carbohydrates

It is important to eat plenty of carbohydrates, as they are **good sources of energy, fibre, calcium,**

iron and B vitamins. Wholemeal bread and pasta and brown rice are particularly good sources of fibre. As well as **preventing constipation and bowel disease**, eating lots of fibre will make you feel full helping you to **stop overeating**. High-fibre diets can also **lower blood cholesterol**, reducing the risk of coronary heart disease.

Fat

Fat is an essential part of your diet but you don't need very much. It **provides energy, essential fatty acids and vitamins** and makes food easier to eat. However, high levels are associated with coronary heart disease and obesity, so it is important to **cut down your intake**, especially when it comes to **saturated fat**. You can do this by eating **less fat and oil** for cooking and spreading. Food manufacturers offer a wide choice of low-fat products. Some products, such as **cakes or biscuits, contain invisible fats**, so you need to read food labels carefully. Try using products that are high in polyunsaturated fats and low in saturated fats. Eating **oily fish twice a week** can help to prevent heart disease. Oily fish include **salmon, kippers, tuna, sardines, pilchards, mackerel, herring, trout and anchovies**.

Sugary food and drinks

These contain calories and no other nutrients. They are particularly **harmful to your teeth** and are best eaten at the end of meals.

Alcohol

Drinking one or two units of alcohol has been shown to be beneficial to health by reducing the risk of coronary disease. However, drinking **large quantities** of alcohol increases the **risk to your health**, and this applies even if you abstain all week and then binge at weekends.

Salt

There is now evidence to suggest that **sodium, found in salt** is associated with **high blood pressure**. Hypertension can increase the risk of heart disease and stroke. Try to reduce your salt intake by adding less salt to food when cooking and at the table, consuming fewer salted foods and choosing processed foods with low salt or reduced salt options.

Exercise 1b
Match the column A with the column B. Try to learn the expressions and/ or sentences by heart.

A

1. If you deny yourself a particular favourite food,
2. There are five food groups:
3. Snacks don't have to be high in calories or fat
4. Breakfast is an important meal
5. Fruit and vegetables
6. Healthy snacks include
7. It is important to eat plenty of carbohydrates,
8. Eating lots of fibre will make you feel full

9. Fat provides
10. Cut down your intake,
11. Some products, such as cakes or biscuits,
12. Eating oily fish twice a week
13. Sugary food and drinks
14. Large quantities of alcohol increases the risk to your health,
15. Try to reduce your salt intake

B

a) *– fruit or a couple of wholemeal biscuits is a better bet.*
b) *1) fruit and vegetables, 2) bread, cereals, pasta and potatoes, 3) meat, fish and alternatives, 4) milk and dairy foods, 5) foods containing fat or sugar.*
c) *and shouldn't be missed.*
d) *and this applies even if you abstain all week and then binge at weekends.*
e) *are particularly harmful to your teeth.*
f) *as they are good sources of energy, fibre, calcium, iron and B vitamins.*
g) *by adding less salt to food when cooking and at the table, consuming fewer salted foods and choosing processed foods with low salt or reduced salt options.*
h) *can help to prevent heart disease.*
i) *contain invisible fats, so you need to read food labels carefully.*
j) *energy, essential fatty acids and vitamins and makes food easier to eat.*
k) *especially when it comes to saturated fat.*
l) *foods that are low in sugar, fat and salt, and high in fibre.*
m) *helping you to stop overeating.*
n) *provide vitamins, minerals and fibre.*
o) *you are more likely to become obsessed with it and crave it all the time.*

Exercise 2

Translate the expressions. Try to explain their meanings in English.

Deteriorate, storage, fed intravenously, exception, overloading, route, dehydration, vomiting, available, trace elements, aluminium, antimony, boron, bromine, cadmium, lithium, nickel, sulphur, strontium, defences, by-product, harmful, tissue damage, ensuring that, relevant, leafy and root vegetables, whole grains, recommended daily allowance, proven, dosage, research, deny, particular, obsessed, crave, succumb, over-indulge, every now and again, enjoyable, aim to, wholemeal biscuits, proportions, tinned fruit, nutritious, raw, chopped, celery sticks, plain popcorn, scone, currant, bun, fromage frais, bread sticks, dessert bowlful, cupful, tablespoon, cut down, intake, cooking and spreading, salmon, kippers, tuna, sardines, pilchards, mackerel, herring, trout, anchovies, abstain, binge, evidence, heart disease, stroke, options.

Exercise 3
Answer the following questions. Prepare short talks and/or dialogues on these topics

1. What are minerals?
2. Functions of sodium, potassium and chromium.
3. Give the names of other minerals and trace elements.
4. Talk about antioxidants and disease prevention.
5. Sources of vitamin A, beta-carotene, vitamin C, vitamin E, selenium, zinc, lycopene.
6. Risks of a vitamin or a mineral deficiency.
7. Healthy eating and the five food groups.
8. Give examples of healthy snacks.
9. What is a portion?
10. Sources of carbohydrates.
11. Fats and their importance in your diet.
12. Why should you cut down your intake of fats?
13. Dangers of sugary food and drinks; dangers of alcohol.
14. Why should you try to reduce your salt intake?

Vocabulary 5

Fill in the meanings in your mother language:

abstain /æb'steɪn/
aim /eɪm/
aluminium /ˌæl.jə'mɪn.i.əm/
anchovy /'æn.tʃə.vi/ pl **anchovies**
antimony /'æntɪmənɪ/
bet /bet/
binge /bɪndʒ/
boron /'bɔːrɒn/
bowlful /'bəʊlˌfʊl/
bread /bred/ **stick** /stik/
bromine /'brəʊmiːn/
by product /'baɪˌprɒd.ʌkt/
cadmium /'kædmɪəm/
carrot /kærət/
celery /'selərɪ/ **stick** /stɪk/
chop /tʃɒp/
chromium /'krəʊmɪəm/
crave /kreɪv/
cupful /'kʌpˌfʊl/
currant /'kʌrənt/ **bun**/ bʌn/
damage /'dæm.ɪdʒ/
defence /dɪ'fens/
dehydration /ˌdiː.haɪ'dreɪ.ʃən/
deny /dɪ'naɪ/
dessert /dɪ'zɜːt/
deteriorate /dɪ'tɪə.ri.ə.reɪt/
dosage /'dəʊ.sɪdʒ/
dried /draɪd/
electrolyte /ɪ'lek.trə.laɪt/
enjoyable /ɪn'dʒɔɪəbəl/
ensure /ɪn'ʃɔːr/
exception /ɪk'sep.ʃən/
favourite /'feɪvrɪt/
free /friː/ **radical** /'ræd.ɪ.kəl/
fromage frais /'frɒmɑːʒ 'freɪ/
herring /'herɪŋ/
hypertension /ˌhaɪ.pə'ten.t ʃən/
in moderation /ˌmɒd.ər'eɪ.ʃən/
indulge /ɪn'dʌldʒ/
intake /'ɪn.teɪk/
kipper /'kɪpə/
lithium /'lɪθ.i.əm/
lycopene /'laɪkəˌpiːn/
nickel /'nɪkəl/
nutritious /njuː'trɪʃəs/
obsessed /əb'sest/
overeating /ˌəʊvər'iːtɪŋ/
particular /pə'tɪk.jʊ.lər/

plain /pleɪn/
plum /plʌm/
popcorn /ˈpɒpˌkɔːn/
potassium /pəˈtæs.i.əm/
potentially /pəˈten.ʃəl.i/
processed /prəˈsest/
proportion /prəˈpɔː.ʃən/
proven /ˈpruː.vən/
raw /rɔː/
refer /rɪˈfɜːr/ **to** /tʊ/
research /rɪˈsɜːtʃ/
root /ruːt/ **vegetable** /ˈvedʒ.tə.bl̩/
route /ruːt/
salmon /ˈsæmən/
scone /skɒn/
selenium /səˈliː.ni.əm/
solution /səˈluː.ʃən/
spoon /spuːn/
stable /ˈsteɪ.bl̩/
strawberry /ˈstrɔːbərɪ/
stroke /strəʊk/
strontium /ˈstrɒntɪəm/
succumb /səˈkʌm/
tinned /tɪnd/
trace /treɪs/ **element** /ˈɛlɪmənt/
trout /traʊt/
unlike /ʌnˈlaɪk/
vomit /ˈvɒm.ɪt/
whole /həʊl/

Solution to Exercise 1a
1j, 2g, 3i, 4d, 5f, 6h, 7k, 8c, 9b, 10a, 11e

Solution to Exercise 1b
1o, 2b, 3a, 4c, 5n, 6l, 7f, 8m, 9j, 10k, 11i, 12h, 13e, 14d, 15g

Unit 6 - A healthy weight. Food labelling.

The right weight for you

People in the correct weight have a **body mass index (BMI)** of between **18.5 and 24.9.** To calculate your BMI divide your weight in kilograms by your height in metres squared. If your BMI is 25 to 29.9, you are a bit overweight. If your BMI is above 30, you are overweight and should consider losing weight otherwise your health will suffer. **At BMI values greater than 30**, there is an **increased risk of many diseases.** These include coronary heart disease (CHD), high blood pressure (a risk factor for CHD), some cancers, diabetes mellitus, musculoskeletal problems, reproductive disorders and gallbladder disease.

Losing weight wisely

To lose weight you should eat a **high-fibre, low-fat diet** that follows the given guidelines but has **smaller portions. Exercise** is an important part of weight maintenance. It does not have to be strenuous but just enough to make you feel slightly out of breath – a brisk walk, for example. Aim to exercise for **20 to 30 minutes two or three times a week**. The recommended rate of **weight loss is 450 g per week.** If you lose weight too quickly, your body may lose body tissues that are not associated with the excess weight (that is, fat-free mass). This will make it harder for you to maintain your new weight. You'll **lose more weight when you first start to diet** because your body uses up its stores of glycogen from your liver and muscle. How much weight you lose in this initial stage will depend on the energy and carbohydrate content of your diet before you started. **The distribution of fat** in the body is also important. People with relatively **large waists** (apple shaped) are more at risk of health problems than those with relatively large hips (pear shaped). Men should try to keep their waist at or below 94 centimetres and women at or below 80 centimetres.

Feeding children

Up to the **age of six months, breast of formula milk** provides all the nutrients that a baby needs. You can begin to **introduce solids** around this time, starting with **puréed fruit and vegetables.** Over the following weeks and months, you can gradually increase the amount and texture, so that, at **12 months** your child is eating a varied diet of **three meals and two or three snacks** a day. Gradually introducing different textures will encourage your child to chew. Whether you opt for bought or home made food is a matter of personal choice. **Preparing baby and toddler meals** doesn't have to be time-consuming and fiddly, and is certainly less expensive. For example, you can make extra of a particular dish, such as fruit and vegetables, portions can be **puréed and frozen**. Remember, however, **not to add salt** or sugar for yourself until your child's portion has been put into a separate dish. Keep the portions small when you first start – **ice cube trays** make ideal containers for freezing foods. That way, not much is wasted if your baby doesn't like a particular food. An **older toddler** can be served with the rest of your family and his or her **food simply mashed** in the serving bowl. Although children under two years should **not eat too much fat**, there is no need for them to be on a low-fat diet. They need a lot of energy to grow, some of which can be provided by fat.

Fussy eaters

Some children won't eat a variety of foods or at times **appear to eat very little.** Although it is very frustrating and upsetting for you as a parent, the best approach is to stay calm as you can and not give your child too much attention. If you allow eating to become an issue you will simply make the problem worse. You may be able to avoid this situation if you give your child a wide variety of foods and try to make mealtimes a relaxing and enjoyable experience. If you are concerned about your child's diet, **a referral from your GP to a paediatric dietitian** may be helpful. She will be able to assess your child's diet and, with the doctor, his or her growth and development. Most fussy children are actually growing well and require little or no intervention from health professionals.

Key points

- Have **three meals** a day and don't **skip breakfast**
- There is no reason to avoid snacks
- Eat **more fibre and carbohydrate and reduce fat**
- Eat **five portions of fruit and vegetables** per day

- Food should be a pleasure, not another thing to worry about

Exercise 1a
Match the column A with the column B. Try to learn the expressions and/or sentences by heart.

A

1. To calculate your BMI
2. If your BMI is above 30, you are overweight and
3. To lose weight you should
4. Exercise does not have to be strenuous
5. You'll lose more weight when you first start to diet
6. People with relatively large waists (apple shaped)
7. Up to the age of six months,
8. You can begin to introduce solids,
9. At 12 months your child
10. Remember,
11. Although children under two years should not eat too much fat,
12. If you allow eating to become an issue
13. If you are concerned about your child's diet,

B

a) a referral from your GP to a paediatric dietitian may be helpful.
b) are more at risk of health problems than those with relatively large hips (pear shaped).
c) because your body uses up its stores of glycogen from your liver and muscle.
d) breast of formula milk provides all the nutrients that a baby needs.
e) but just enough to make you feel slightly out of breath – a brisk walk, for example.
f) divide your weight in kilograms by your height in metres squared.
g) eat a high-fibre, low-fat diet that follows the given guidelines but has smaller portions.
h) is eating a varied diet of three meals and two or three snacks a day.
i) not to add salt or sugar for yourself until your child's portion has been put into a separate dish.
j) should consider losing weight otherwise your health will suffer.
k) starting with puréed fruit and vegetables.
l) there is no need for them to be on a low-fat diet.
m) you will simply make the problem worse.

Food labelling
How do you choose healthy foods?

You can choose from a wide selection of imported fresh foods with a long shelf-life. This is partly the result of improved storage methods such as refrigeration and freezing. Other ways to extend shelf-life are the addition of chemicals and the use of irradiation to delay spoiling.

Extending the shelf-life of foods

Food-preserving techniques prevent the contamination and deterioration of food. They act by **inhibiting bacterial activity** and the action of enzymes in the foods that break down cells.

Refrigeration

Reducing the storage temperature to 3 to 5 ℃ reduces the deterioration of fats (rancidity) and slows down microbial growth.

Freezing

Reducing the storage temperature to -18 to -20 ℃ stops the growth of microbes but does not kill them. Microbes will still be present, and will resume growth once the food is defrosted. The deterioration of fats is slowed even further by freezing than by refrigeration, but will not stop if the food is defrosted. This is why food should not be refrozen after thawing.

Chemicals

Altering the chemical composition of food reduces the impact of microbe contamination and oxidation.

Irradiation

High doses of radiation sterilise food. Low doses can be used to delay ripening of fruit.

The information on a food label

- **Name** As well as the name of food, all labels should list:
- **ingredients** – substances that may cause allergies or intolerances must be included and emphasised, for example in bold letters
- **date** by which the food should be eaten
- **storage** instructions to prevent spoilage
- **preparation** instructions if necessary
- **additives**, with E numbers
- **nutritional information**
- **genetically modified** ingredients
- **country** of origin
- **manufacturer** details and batch number

Names

Some foods have **trade names**, whereas others have a **descriptive name** such as gravy browning. Names such as wholemeal are defined by law. The name must be precise enough to **distinguish the food** from other products. There are **exceptions** for some food, including whole, unpeeled fresh fruit and vegetables, flavourings, cheese and butter. Names **must not be misleading**, for example, cherry cheesecake must have its flavour coming mainly from real cherries, as must a product with fresh cherries pictured on the packet. Cherry flavour, on the other hand, means that the product's flavour is derived mainly from artificial flavourings.

Ingredients

Most foods must have the **ingredients listed in descending order of weight.** Water is not always included, unless it falls within the constraints of legislation, because it is often considered an integral part of food. If added water takes up five per cent or more of the finished product, it must be listed with the other ingredients. There has been a recent trend towards **listing water as aqua.**

Additives and E numbers

Ingredients that fall into this category are usually added in small quantities and therefore appear towards the end of the list. The approved name or E number may be used. An **E number** indicates that **the additive is permitted under European Union legislation.** Additives are used for **flavouring, sweetening or colouring**, to enhance the **preservation** of food or to affect its **consistency or texture**.

Date mark

Foods that have a **shelf-life greater than three months** must show a **month and year** by which they should be eaten. Foods with a **shelf-life of less than three months** must show **the day and month** by which they should be used. Products with a sell-by date rather than a best before date should tell you within how many days the food should be eaten from this sell-by date. Retailers can be prosecuted for displaying products for sale after these dates.

Storage

Following storage instructions **prevents food spoilage**, reduces the risk of food poisoning and ensures that foods are eaten at their best. Star symbols are frequently shown to indicate a food's **suitability for refrigeration or freezing.**

Preparation

For foods that need heating, labels provide suitable information on **temperature and timing** for both conventional and microwave cookers, to ensure that food tastes at its best. Following cooking instructions ensures that food is thoroughly heated, reducing the risk of food poisoning.

Exercise 1b

Match the column A with the column B. Try to learn the expressions and/or sentences by heart.

A

1. Food-preserving techniques
2. Reducing the storage temperature to 3 to 5 ℃
3. Reducing the storage temperature to -18 to -20 ℃
4. The deterioration of fats is slowed even further
5. Altering the chemical composition of food
6. High doses of radiation sterilise food;
7. All labels should list:

8. The name must be precise enough
9. Most foods must have the ingredients
10. If added water takes up five per cent or more of the finished product,
11. An E number indicates
12. Additives are used for
13. Foods that have a shelf-life greater than three months
14. Foods with a shelf-life of less than three months
15. Following storage instructions
16. For foods that need heating,

B

a) by freezing than by refrigeration, but will not stop if the food is defrosted.
b) flavouring, sweetening or colouring, to enhance the preservation of food or to affect its consistency or texture.
c) ingredients, date by which the food should be eaten, storage and preparation instructions, additives, nutritional information, genetically modified ingredients, country of origin and manufacturer details.
d) it must be listed with the other ingredients.
e) labels provide suitable information on temperature and timing for both conventional and microwave cookers, to ensure that food tastes at its best.
f) listed in descending order of weight.
g) low doses can be used to delay ripening of fruit.
h) must show a month and year by which they should be eaten.
i) must show the day and month by which they should be used.
j) prevent the contamination and deterioration of food.
k) prevents food spoilage, reduces the risk of food poisoning and ensures that foods are eaten at their best.
l) reduces the deterioration of fats (rancidity) and slows down microbial growth.
m) reduces the impact of microbe contamination and oxidation.
n) stops the growth of microbes but does not kill them.
o) that the additive is permitted under European Union legislation.
p) to distinguish the food from other products.

Exercise 2

Translate the expressions. Try to explain their meanings in English.

Calculate, divide, metres squared, overweight, consider, suffer, values, skip, musculoskeletal problems, reproductive disorders, gallbladder disease, wisely, guidelines, maintenance, strenuous, brisk walk, associated, mass, initial stage, content, waist, formula milk, introduce solids, puréed, gradually, texture, fussy, encourage, chew, opt for, toddler, time-consuming, fiddly, add salt, containers, wasted, mashed, bowl, upsetting, approach, attention, referral, intervention, labelling, shelf-life, refrigeration, freezing, irradiation, spoiling, extending, inhibiting, rancidity, resume, defrosted, thawing, altering, impact, ripening, ingredients, emphasised, bold letters, spoilage, additives, batch number, trade names, precise, distinguish, exceptions, unpeeled, flavourings, misleading, artificial, descending order, constraints, integral, additives, approved, permitted, preservation, consistency, texture, retailers, prosecuted, food poisoning, suitability, timing, cookers.

Exercise 3
Answer the following questions. Prepare short talks and/or dialogues on these topics

1. How would you calculate your BMI?
2. Losing weight wisely.
3. Talk about feeding children.
4. How do you choose healthy foods?
5. Food-preserving techniques (refrigeration, freezing, chemicals, irradiation)
6. The information on a food label (name, ingredients, date, storage instructions, preparation instructions, additives, nutritional information, genetically modified ingredients, country of origin, manufacturer details)

Vocabulary 6

Fill in the meanings in your mother language:

addition /əˈdɪʃ.ən/
additive /ˈæd.ɪ.tɪv/
approved /əˈpruːvd/
aqua /ˈækwə/
artificial /ˌɑː.tɪˈfɪʃ.əl/
attention /əˈten.ʃən/
batch /bætʃ/
bold /bəʊld/ **letter** /ˈletə/
brisk /brɪsk/
calculate /ˈkælk.jʊˌleɪt/
cheesecake /ˈtʃiːzˌkeɪk/
concerned /kənˈsɜːnd/
consider /kənˈsɪd.ər/
consistency /kənˈsɪs.tənt .si/
constraint /kənˈstreɪnt/
container /kənˈteɪ.nər/
contamination /kənˌtæm.ɪˈneɪ.ʃən/
conventional /kənˈvent .ʃən.əl/
cooker /ˈkʊkə/
defrost /diːˈfrɒst/
derive /dɪˈraɪv/
descending /dɪˈsend.ɪŋ/
descriptive /dɪˈskrɪp.tɪv/
deterioration /dɪˌtɪə.ri.əˈreɪ.ʃən/
dish /dɪʃ/
display /dɪˈspleɪ/
distinguish /dɪˈstɪŋ.gwɪʃ/
emphasise /ˈemfəˌsaɪz/
extend /ɪkˈstend/
fiddly /ˈfɪdlɪ/
flavour /ˈfleɪ.vər/
flavouring /ˈfleɪ.vər.ɪŋ/
formula /ˈfɔːmjʊlə/
freezing /ˈfriː.zɪŋ/
fussy /ˈfʌsɪ/

general /ˈdʒen.ər.əl/ **practitioner** /prækˈtɪʃ.ən.ər/, **GP**
genetically /dʒəˈnet.ɪk.əl.i/
gradually /ˈgrædʒ.ʊ.li/
gravy /ˈgreɪvɪ/ **browning** /ˈbraʊ nɪŋ/
hip /hɪp/
ice /aɪs/ **cube** /kjuːb/
impact /ˈɪm.pækt/
inhibit /ɪnˈhɪb.ɪt/
initial /ɪˈnɪʃ.əl/
integral /ˈɪn tɪ grəl/
intervention /ˌɪn.təˈven.ʃən/
intolerance /ɪnˈtɒl.ər.əns/
irradiation /iˌrei.diˈei.ʃən/
issue /ˈɪʃ.uː/
label /ˈleɪ.bəl/
legislation /ˌledʒɪsˈleɪʃən/
list /lɪst/
maintenance /ˈmeɪn.tɪ.nəns/
mark /mɑːk/
microbe /ˈmaɪ.krəʊb/
microwave /ˈmaɪ.krə.weɪv/
misleading /ˌmɪsˈliː.dɪŋ/
musculoskeletal /ˌmʌs. kjə.ləʊˈskel.ɪ.təl/
opt /ɒpt/
order /ˈɔː.dər/
origin /ˈɒr.ɪ.dʒɪn/
overweight /ˌəʊvəˈweɪt/
packet /ˈpæk.ɪt/
permit /pəˈmɪt/
poisoning /ˈpɔɪ.zən.ɪŋ/
precise /prɪˈsaɪs/
preserve /prɪˈzɜːv/
prosecute /ˈprɒsɪˌkjuːt/
purée /ˈpjʊəreɪ/
radiation /ˌreɪ.diˈeɪ.ʃən/
rancid /ˈrænsɪd/
referral /rɪˈfɜː.rəl/
refrigeration /rɪˌfrɪdʒ.əˈreɪ.ʃən/
reproductive /ˌriː.prəˈdʌk.tɪv/
resume /rɪˈzjuːm/
retailer /ˈriːteɪlə/
ripen /ˈraɪpən/
selection /sɪˈlek.ʃən/
sell-by /baɪ/ **date** /deɪt/
shelf /ʃelf/ **life** /laɪf/
skip /skɪp/
spoil /spɔɪl/
spoilage /ˈspɔɪlɪdʒ/
square /skwɛə/
sterilise /sterɪˌlaɪz/
strenuous /ˈstren.ju.əs/
suffer /ˈsʌf.ər/
suitability /ˌsuːtəˈbɪlɪtɪ/
texture /ˈteks.tʃər/
thaw /θɔː/
thoroughly /ˈθʌr.ə.li/
time-consuming /ˈtaɪm.kənˌsjuː.mɪŋ/
toddler /ˈtɒd.lər/
trade /treɪd/ **name** /ˈneɪm/
tray /treɪ/
unpeeled /ʌnpiːld/
upsetting /ʌpˈset.ɪŋ/
waist /weɪst/
wasted /ˈweɪs.tɪd/
wisely /ˈwaɪzlɪ/

Solution to Exercise 1a
1f, 2j, 3g, 4e, 5c, 6b, 7d, 8k, 9h, 10i, 11l, 12m, 13a

Solution to Exercise 1b
1j, 2l, 3n, 4a, 5m, 6g, 7c, 8p, 9f, 10d, 11o, 12b, 13h, 14i, 15k, 16e

Unit 7 - Nutritional claims. Food additives.

The nutritional claims made by manufacturers:

- **Energy**: Low energy, Energy-reduced, Energy-free
- **Fat**: Low fat, Fat free, Low saturated fat, Saturated fat free, High polyunsaturates, High unsaturated fat
- **Salt** (sodium): Low sodium/ salt, Very low sodium/ salt, Sodium or salt free

- **Fibre**: Source of fibre, High fibre
- **Natural/naturally**: Prefix natural/naturally may be used where food naturally meets the conditions for nutrition claims

Ingredients that may cause allergies

Labels must state clearly if they contain **ingredients** to which **people may be allergic or intolerant**. It must be clear if any of these ingredients are present. For example, it is not enough to state glazer; the label must state glaze made from eggs.

Nutritional claims

Nutritional values should be expressed **per 100 grams of food**, and **per portion** if the packet contains less than 100 grams. Information should be given about **energy, protein, fat and carbohydrate**, then about **dietary fibre and sodium**, and then about **sugars, vitamins and minerals**. Vitamin and mineral values are given when they are present in amounts greater than one-sixth of the recommended dietary intake. Manufacturers who falsify claims can be prosecuted. However, the terminology used can be confusing.

Genetically modified foods

Any ingredient that has been involved in **gene modification**, either human or animal genes, **must appear on the label.**

Manufacturer and batch numbers

Manufacturers give their **contact details** on product labels, enabling consumers to write or telephone with enquiries or complaints. All foods are marked with an **identity number** to allow both manufacturers and consumers to **identify food batches** easily.

Recommended daily allowance

Nutrition labelling often includes the **recommended daily allowance** (RDA) of **energy, protein, vitamins or minerals**. This is the amount that will **supply the requirements of most people**. There is no RDA for carbohydrate or fat because they are interchangeable sources of energy. A substance can only be listed in this way when more than one-sixth of the RDA is present. **Estimated average requirement** (EAR) is defined for energy, protein and vitamins **for a specified group of people**, for example, a specific age range. About half of this group will need more than the EAR and the other half will need less. **Reference nutrient intake** (RNI) is defined for protein, vitamins and minerals, is the amount that is **enough for about 97 per cent of the population.** These data are included on food labels for information and as a marketing tool. In everyday life, such precise knowledge is not needed.

Traffic light labelling

The government recommends that food manufacturers use this system of labelling to **help consumers compare products** and to **make healthy choices**. Details are shown of the amounts of **total fat, saturated fat, sugars and salt in an average serving**. To make it easier, the traffic light labels give an at-a-glance way of **identifying foods** that have **high (red), medium (amber) and low (green) amounts** in them. A healthy diet will contain a mixture of foods with each colour label. However, there should be fewer foods with red labels that those with amber labels. Include red-labelled foods as an occasional treat. **There should be more foods with green labels** than foods with amber labels.

Guideline daily amounts

Some food manufacturers believe that it is better to give guideline daily amounts (GDAs) on packaging. GDAs summarise recommendations for energy, fat, sugar and salts and are **intended as a guide when comparing products.**

Key points

- **Food labelling** helps you to decide whether to buy food products, now that there is more storage, preserving and processing
- **Laws** determine what **nutritional claims** manufacturers may make
- **The list of ingredients** tells you what ingredients the food contains and in what proportions
- RDA is the **recommended daily allowance** that will supply the requirements of almost everyone
- Following **manufacturers'** guidelines for **food storage and preparation** can reduce the risk of food poisoning

Exercise 1a
Match the column A with the column B. Try to learn the expressions and/ or sentences by heart.

A

1. Labels must state clearly
2. Information should be given about
3. Any ingredient that has been involved in gene modification,
4. Manufacturers give their contact details on product labels,
5. The recommended daily allowance (RDA) of energy, protein, vitamins or minerals
6. Estimated average requirement (EAR) is defined
7. Reference nutrient intake
8. Food manufacturers use the traffic light labelling
9. The traffic light labels
10. Guideline daily amounts (GDAs) summarise recommendations for energy, fat, sugar and salts
11. The list of ingredients
12. RDA is the recommended daily allowance

13. Following manufacturers' guidelines for food storage and preparation

m) to help consumers compare products and to make healthy choices.

B

a) and are intended as a guide when comparing products.
b) can reduce the risk of food poisoning.
c) enabling consumers to write or telephone with enquiries or complaints.
d) energy, protein, fat and carbohydrate, then about dietary fibre and sodium, and then about sugars, vitamins and minerals.
e) must appear on the label.
f) for a specified group of people.
g) is the amount that is enough for about 97 per cent of the population.
h) give an at-a-glance way of identifying foods that have high (red), medium (amber) and low (green) amounts in them.
i) if they contain ingredients to which people may be allergic or intolerant.
j) is the amount that will supply the requirements of most people.
k) tells you what ingredients the food contains and in what proportions
l) that will supply the requirements of almost everyone.

Food additives

The debate over additives

Without additives, the variety of foods available and their shelf-lives should be greatly reduced. However, the use of additives in food is a controversial subject, with claims that they can trigger allergies or are toxic. Some people are **sensitive to certain additives**, especially colourings, and should check food labels carefully to see what additives the food contains.

Why use additives?

Many of the foods that we eat today contain additives. Additives are used in food for many reasons including the following:

- To **keep foods fresh** until eaten, widening food choice
- To enable food to be **conveniently packaged, stored, prepared and used**
- To make the product look **more appealing**
- To extend the food's **shelf-life**
- To **reduce the ingredient cost**
- To add **additional nutrients**

Approximately 3,500 additives are in use today. **All permitted additives** are considered **safe and necessary**, and are **controlled by law**. Food additives must gain approval before their use in food manufacture is permitted. Many additives are natural substances; for example, ascorbic acid (vitamin C) is used as a flour improver to speed up bread production. **Natural additives** must **also undergo testing** and approval before they can be used in food manufacture.

E numbers

E numbers are given to permitted food additives **regarded as safe for use within the European Union**. Some additives have a number but no E prefix, as they are under consideration for licensing by the EU. All food labels must show the additive's **name or E number in the list of ingredients**.

Colourings (E 100-180)

Food is coloured to restore losses that occur in manufacture and storage, to meet consumer expectations and to maintain uniformity of products. An example of this is that oranges have green patches when picked and are coloured orange before sale.

Preservatives (E 200-290)

Food spoils easily: **bacteria** cause the structure to **rot and putrefy**; **enzymes** cause changes such as **browning**; **injury** causes some fruit cells to die, leading to **discolouring** and eventually **rotting**; **fats** become **rancid** as a result of **oxidation. Preservatives stop food going off** in these ways and make a wide range of goods available out of the usual season. **Traditional** preservatives include **salt, vinegar, alcohol and spices. Acetic acid** is the major component of vinegar and may be considered as a natural additive, but it has undergone extensive testing and has an E number (E 260),

Examples of natural and synthetic colourings

Many colours are used for cosmetic reasons. About half are the natural pigments, such as carbon and riboflavin. Artificial colourings such as tartrazine and amaranth are also used.

Natural colours

Name	Colour	E	Typical use
Riboflavin	Yellow	E101	Processed cheese
Chlorophyll	Green	E140	Fats, oils, canned vegetables
Carbon	Black	E153	Jams and jellies
Alpha-carotene	Yellow/orange	E160	Margarine and cakes

Synthetic colours

Tartrazine	Yellow	E102	Soft drinks
Sunset	Yellow	E110	Orange drinks
Amaranth	Red	E123	Blackcurrant products
Erythrosine	Red	E127	Glacé cherries
Indigo Carmine	Blue	E132	Savoury food mixes
Green 5	Green	E142	Tinned peas, mint jelly and sauce

Frequently used preservatives

Name	E number	Food use
Sorbic acid *	E200–E203	Cheese, yoghurt and soft drinks
Acetic acid	E260	Pickles and sauces
Lactic acid	E270	Margarine, confectionery and sauces

Propionic acid *	E280–E283	Bread, cakes and flour confectionery
Benzoic acid *	E210–E219	Soft drinks, pickles, fruit products
Sulphur dioxide	E220	Soft drinks, fruit products, beer, cider, wine
Nitrites	E249, E250	Cured meats, cooked meats and meat products
Nitrates	E251, E252	Bacon, ham and cheese (not Cheddar or Cheshire)

* Includes derivative products

Radiation

Radiation can be used as a preservative because it **destroys bacteria and enzymes that spoil food**. It can also be used to **delay ripening of fruit and sprouting** in vegetables such as potatoes.

Exercise 1b
Match the column A with the column B. Try to learn the expressions and/or sentences by heart.

A

1. Some people are sensitive to certain additives, especially colourings,
2. Additives are used in food
3. Additives are also used in food
4. All permitted additives
5. Natural additives must also undergo testing and approval
6. E numbers are given to permitted food additives
7. All food labels must show
8. Preservatives stop food going off
9. Traditional preservatives include
10. The natural pigments are e.g. carbon and riboflavin;
11. Radiation destroys

B

a) and make a wide range of goods available out of the usual season.
b) and should check food labels carefully to see what additives the food contains.
c) are considered safe and necessary, and are controlled by law.
d) artificial colourings such as tartrazine and amaranth are also used.
e) bacteria and enzymes that spoil food.
f) before they can be used in food manufacture.
g) regarded as safe for use within the European Union.
h) salt, vinegar, alcohol and spices.
i) the additives name or E number in the list of ingredients.
j) to extend the food's shelf-life, to reduce the ingredient cost and to add additional nutrients.
k) to keep foods fresh until eaten and to enable food to be conveniently packaged, stored, prepared and used.

Exercise 2
Translate the expressions. Try to explain their meanings in English.

Claims, contain, ingredients, intolerant, glaze, nutritional values, falsify, intended, prosecuted, confusing, gene modification, batch numbers, enquiries, complaints, allowance, estimated, average, reference, traffic light, occasional treat, guideline, recommendations, trigger, allergies, sensitive, widening, conveniently, appealing, additional, spoil, permitted, approval, ascorbic acid, undergo testing, prefix, expectations, rot, putrefy, rancid, going off, vinegar, spices, acetic acid, canned vegetables, pickles, processed cheese, cured meats, confectionery, ripening, sprouting.

Exercise 3
Answer the following questions. Prepare short talks and/or dialogues on these topics.

1. The nutritional claims made by manufacturers (energy, fat, salt, fibre, ingredients that may cause allergies, genetically modified foods, contact details)
2. What do you understand by the terms recommended daily allowance (estimated average requirement, reference nutrient intake)?
3. How does traffic light labelling help consumers?
4. The use of additives in food.
5. E numbers.
6. Colourings and preservatives.
7. Radiation.

Vocabulary 7

Fill in the meanings in your mother language:

acetic /ə'siːtɪk/ **acid** /'æsɪd/
alpha /'ælfə/ **-carotene** /ˈkærəˌtiːn/
amaranth /'æməˌrænθ/
amber /'æm bər/
appealing /əˈpiːlɪŋ/
appear /əˈpɪər/
approval /əˈpruː.vəl/
at-a-glance /glæns/
benzoic /bɛnˈzəʊɪk/ **acid** /'æsɪd/
blackcurrant /ˌblækˈkʌrənt/
canned /kænd/
carefully /ˈkeə.fəl.i/
check /tʃek/
Cheddar /ˈtʃɛdə/
Cheshire /ˈtʃɛʃə/
chlorophyll /ˈklɔːrəfɪl/
cider /ˈsaɪdə/
colouring /ˈkʌlərɪŋ/
complaint /kəmˈpleɪnt/
confectionery /kənˈfekʃənərɪ/
confusing /kənˈfjuːzɪŋ/
consideration /kənˌsɪd.əˈreɪ.ʃən/
controversial /ˌkɒn.trəˈvɜː.ʃəl/
convenient /kənˈviː.ni.ənt/
cure /kjʊə/
debate /dɪˈbeɪt/
derivative /dɪˈrɪvətɪv/
enable /ɪˈneɪ.bl̩/
enquiry /ɪnˈkwaɪə.ri/
erythrosine /ɪˈrɪθ rə sɪn/
expectation /ˌek.spekˈteɪ.ʃən/
expressed /ɪkˈspresd/
falsify /ˈfɔːlsɪˌfaɪ/
flour /ˈflaʊə/
gene /dʒiːn/
glacé /ˈglæsɪ/

glaze /gleɪz/
go /gəʊ/ **off** /ɒf/
goods /gʊdz/
identify /aɪˈden.tɪ.faɪ/
identity /aɪˈden.tɪ.ti/
improver /ɪmˈpruːv.ə/
indigo /ˈɪndɪˌgəʊ/ **carmine** /ˈkɑːmaɪn/
intended /ɪnˈten.dɪd/
interchangeable /ˌɪn tərˈtʃeɪn dʒə bəl/
lactic /ˈlæk.tɪk/ **acid** /ˈæs.ɪd/
licence /ˈlaɪsəns/
marketing /ˈmɑːkɪtɪŋ/ **tool** /tuːl/
mint /mɪnt/ **jelly** /dʒelɪ/
mint /mɪnt/ **sauce** /sɔːs/
nitrate /ˈnaɪ.treɪt/
occasional / əˈkeɪ.ʒə.nəl/
pickle /ˈpɪkəl/
polyunsaturate /ˌpɒlɪʌnˈsætʃəˌreɪtɪd/
prefix /ˈpriːfɪks/
preservative /prɪˈzɜːvətɪv/
product /ˈprɒdʌkt/
propionic /ˌproʊ piˈɒn ɪk/ **acid** /ˈæsɪd/
putrefy /ˈpjuːtrɪˌfaɪ/
regarded /rɪˈgɑːd.ɪd/
rot /rɒt/
savoury /ˈseɪvərɪ/
serving /ˈsɜːvɪŋ/
soft /sɒft/ **drink** /drɪŋk/
sorbic /ˈsɔːbɪk/ **acid** /ˈæsɪd/
sprout /spraʊt/
state /steɪt/
subject /ˈsʌb.dʒekt/
sulphur /ˈsʌlfə/ **dioxide** /daɪˈɒksaɪd/
summarise /ˈsʌməˌraɪz/
sunset /ˈsʌnˌset/
tartrazine /ˈtɑːtrəˌziːn/
treat /triːt/
vinegar /ˈvɪn.ɪ.gər/
widen /ˈwaɪ.dən/

Solution to Exercise 1a
1i, 2d, 3e, 4c, 5j, 6f, 7g, 8m,
9h, 10a, 11k, 12l, 13b

Solution to Exercise 1b
1b, 2k, 3j, 4c, 5f, 6g, 7i,
8a, 9h, 10d, 11e

Unit 8 - Other preservatives. Food allergy and intolerance.

Benzoic acid and benzoates

These preservatives are found in **many fresh foods** such as **peas, bananas and berries**. Benzoates cause **adverse reactions** in some people.

Sulphur dioxide

Sulphur dioxide is used as a **preservative to destroy yeasts**, which can cause fermentation in food products. Its use is not permitted in foods that are a significant source of the vitamin thiamine, because sulphur dioxide destroys thiamine.

Nitrates and nitrites

These preservatives **kill bacteria that cause botulism,** a potentially lethal form of **food poisoning,** and also preserve the red colour in meat. Nitrites may react with other chemicals in the gut to form **nitrosamines**, which have been shown to cause cancer in experimental animals, although there is no evidence that they do the same in people.

Antioxidants (E 300-322)

Fats and oils become **rancid through oxidation**, which causes an unpleasant taste and smell. The higher the fat content of a product, the faster the food becomes rancid.

This process can be delayed, but not stopped, by low temperatures (for example, refrigeration). **The use of antioxidants prevents oxidation.** The most common antioxidants are **butylated hydroxyanisole (BHA)** and **butylated hydroxytoluene (BHT).**

Permitted antioxidants

Antioxidants prevent or delay the effects of oils and fats turning food rancid. Some antioxidants are **natural substances** such as **vitamins C and E.** Others are **synthetic**, such as **BHA and BHT.**

Name	E	Food use
Ascorbic acid (vitamin C) *	E300-E305	Beer, soft drinks, powdered milk, fruit and meat products
Tocopherols (vitamin E) *	E306-E309	Vegetable oils
Gallates	E310-E320	Vegetable oils and fats, margarine
Butylated hydroxy anisole (BHA)	E320	Margarine and fat in baked products, e.g. pies
Butylated hydroxy toluene (BHT)	E321	Crisps, margarine, vegetable oils and fats, convenience foods

∗ Includes derivative products

Emulsifiers and stabilisers (E 400-495)

These additives are used to increase the shelf-life of foods and affect their **texture and consistency. Emulsifiers** are **fatty compounds** that change the chemical properties of some foods so that they can be **mixed.** An example of this is **vinaigrette,** which will normally separate out with oil floating on the top of the vinegar. If an emulsifier, such as **lecithin**, is added, the oil and vinegar stay mixed together in an emulsion.

Examples of emulsifiers and stabilisers

Emulsifiers are used to prevent the oil and water components of many foods from separating. Stabilisers are added to improve texture and are often made from plant matter such as seaweed.

Name	E	Food use, Category
Lecithins *	E322	Chocolate, margarine and potato snacks, Emulsifier
Citric acid * *	E472a-c	Pickles, dairy and baked products, Emulsifier
Tartaric acid * *	E472d-f	Baking powder, Emulsifier
Alginic acid * *	E400-E401	Ice cream, instant desserts and puddings, Emulsifier
Agar	E406	Tinned ham, ice cream, Emulsifier
Carrageenan	E407	Ice cream, Emulsifier
Gums	E410-E415	Ice cream, soups and confectionery, Emulsifier
Pectin	E440	Preserves and jellies, Stabilizer

∗ May also be used as an antioxidant.
∗ ∗ Includes derivative products.

Stabilisers (for example **pectin**) are usually large **carbohydrates.** They form a structure that is capable of holding the smaller chemicals in foods together, forming a **more stable product**. This is the largest group of additives and many are natural substances – for example, **carrageenan** which is derived from seaweed and is used as a **gelling agent.**

Thickeners are carbohydrates that alter or control the consistency of a product during cooling or heating, or in storage.

Raising agents are used to give a **light spongy texture** to cakes and other baked products, and include **bicarbonate of soda,** tartaric acid and baking powder (a mixture of sodium bicarbonate and pyrophosphoric acid).

Sweeteners

These are divided into two groups. **Caloric sweeteners** add energy to the diet, and include **mannitol, sorbitol, xylitol** and hydrogenated **glucose syrup**. The caloric sweetener **agave syrup/** nectar is also now available. **Non-caloric sweeteners** are synthetic sweeteners, and include **acesulfame K, aspartame, saccharin and thaumatin**. Another non-caloric sweetener approved for use in the EU since 2011 is **stevia.** Sucrose, glucose, fructose and lactose are all classified as foods rather than sweeteners or additives.

Fortifiers

Foods can be fortified to reduce the risk of deficiency diseases within a population. Fortification takes place either when a particular nutrient had been lost during processing, or when the addition of a nutrient(s) is beneficial to health. By law, **flour is fortified with certain B vitamins, calcium and iron**, and **margarine is fortified with vitamins A and D**. Voluntary fortification includes the addition of **B vitamins and iron to breakfast cereals and infant formulas.** Vegan products are sometimes fortified with vitamin B_{12}.

Other additives

Glazing agents are used to give food an appealing shiny appearance, and include egg-based products. **Flour improvers** are used to produce bread with a lighter texture and to slow staling.

Other additives include: **flavour enhancers**, such as **monosodium glutamate** (which intensifies the flavour of food); **anti-foaming agents** (which prevent frothing during processing); and **propellant gases** (which are used, for example, in aerosol cream). **Polyphosphates** enable products to **retain water**, so increasing their weight, and are used in foods such as **frozen poultry and cured meats.**

Key points

- Food **additives** prolong the **shelf-life of foods** and make them more appealing to eat.
- If you are concerned about **the safety of additives, check food labels carefully.**
- Fortified foods **supplement dietary intakes of certain nutrients**.

Exercise 1a
Match the column A with the column B. Try to learn the expressions and/or sentences by heart.

A

1. Benzoates cause
2. Sulphur dioxide is used as a preservative to destroy yeasts,
3. Nitrates and nitrites
4. Fats and oils become rancid through oxidation,
5. Antioxidants prevent or delay
6. Emulsifiers are fatty compounds
7. Stabilisers are added
8. Stabilisers (for example pectin)
9. Thickeners
10. Raising agents are used
11. Caloric sweeteners
12. Non-caloric sweeteners are synthetic
13. Fortification takes place either when a particular nutrient had been lost during processing,
14. Glazing agents
15. Flour improvers
16. Other additives include:
17. Polyphosphates enable products to retain water

B

a) add energy to the diet, and include mannitol, sorbitol, xylitol hydrogenated glucose syrup, and agave syrup/nectar is also now available.

b) adverse reactions in some people.

c) alter or control the consistency of a product during cooling or heating, or in storage.

d) and are used in foods such as frozen poultry and cured meats.

e) are used to give food an appealing shiny appearance, and include egg-based products.

f) are used to produce bread with a lighter texture and to slow staling.

g) flavour enhancers, anti-foaming agents and propellant gases.

h) form a structure that is capable of holding the smaller chemicals in foods together, forming a more stable product.

i) kill bacteria that cause botulism, a potentially lethal form of food poisoning.

j) or when the addition of a nutrient(s) is beneficial to health.

k) sweeteners, and include acesulfame K, aspartame, saccharin, thaumatin and stevia.

l) that change the chemical properties of some foods so that they can be mixed.

m) the effects of oils and fats turning food rancid.

n) to give a light spongy texture to cakes and other baked products, and include bicarbonate of soda, tartaric acid and baking powder.

o) to improve texture and are often made from plant matter such as seaweed.

p) which can cause fermentation in food products.

q) which causes an unpleasant taste and smell.

Food allergy and intolerance

What is a food allergy?

Food allergies and intolerances cause similar symptoms, but involve different mechanisms. **Food allergies** are caused by the **immune system reacting abnormally to food**. Most food could trigger an allergic response, but preparation, cooking and the action of digestive acid and enzymes destroy most of this potential. When your body's **defence system meets** a potentially **harmful substance**, it responds with an **immunological reaction**. This **releases histamine** and other chemicals **into your circulation**, causing itching of the skin and changes in blood vessels. **In serious cases**, the changes in blood vessels can lead to a rapid **fall in blood volume** and a dramatic, and potentially fatal, reaction, known as **anaphylactic shock**, which can interfere with a person's ability to breathe. The **chemicals released** in this reaction also cause **constriction of lung tissues** and are associated with **asthma**.

What is a food intolerance?

Food intolerances do not involve an immunological reaction. Some of the mechanisms involved are not fully understood. Food intolerance reactions include the following:

Non-allergic histamine release

Shellfish and strawberries cause this reaction in some people, who usually develop a rash.

Enzyme defects

People with a lactase deficiency, for example, have a reduced ability to digest **the milk sugar lactose**. The treatment consists of a diet low in milk and milk products.

Pharmacological reactions

These occur in response to food components, such as amines. Amines are found in foods that contain nitrogen (for example amino acids in foods such as **tea, coffee, cola drinks and chocolate**). The effects may be triggered by small amounts of food and include **migraine, tremor, sweating and palpitations**, which can be alarming.

Irritant effects

Foods such as **curry** can irritate the gut. Monosodium **glutamate** can cause a condition known as a **Chinese restaurant syndrome,** which results in **chest pain, palpitations and weakness.**

Lactose intolerance

People with lactase deficiency should **avoid the products** listed below. Several lactose-reduced milks and products are available commercially.

- **Cows', goats', and sheep's milk**
- Milk products, such as **cheese and skimmed milk**
- **Milk derivatives** often used in food manufacture. Remember to read the list of ingredients.
- Foods such as **stock cubes and crisps**, which often contain **whey**
- **Medicines** that use milk products as fillers

Diagnosing an allergy

Anyone suspected of having a food allergy must be diagnosed and treated by a dietitian. Diagnosis often involves eliminating **possible allergens – substances that cause an allergic reaction** – from the diet. An elimination diet is sometimes based on the very few foods that are unlikely to cause allergic reactions, and such a limited diet is difficult to plan and stick to. As each food is gradually reintroduced to the diet, the dietitian can assess which of them is responsible for any symptoms. This process needs **careful monitoring**. It is not safe to try excluding suspect foods from your diet by yourself. It is necessary to use a very **restrictive diet**, there is a risk of nutritional deficiencies developing, unless it is carefully controlled. This is especially **important in children**, who need an **adequate supply of the right nutrients** in order to grow normally and maintain good health. The danger of anaphylaxis, or other severe reactions associated with the diagnosis of food allergy, means that the dietitian works closely with medical colleagues.

Exercise 1b
Match the column A with the column B. Try to learn the expressions and/ or sentences by heart.

A

1. Food allergies and intolerances cause similar symptoms,
2. Food allergies are caused
3. When your body's defence system meets a potentially harmful substance,
4. In serious cases, the changes in blood vessels
5. Anaphylactic shock
6. The chemicals released in anaphylactic shock
7. Food intolerances
8. Shellfish and strawberries cause
9. People with a lactase deficiency,
10. Pharmacological reactions
11. The effects of amino acids in foods such as tea, coffee, cola drinks and chocolate
12. Mono-sodium glutamate can cause
13. People with lactase deficiency should avoid
14. Diagnosis often involves

15. An elimination diet is
16. As each food is gradually reintroduced to the diet,
17. Children need an adequate supply of the right nutrients

B

a) a Chinese restaurant syndrome, which results in chest pain, palpitations and weakness.
b) based on the very few foods that are unlikely to cause allergic reactions.
c) but involve different mechanisms.
d) by the immune system reacting abnormally to food.
e) can interfere with a person's ability to breathe.
f) can lead to a rapid fall in blood volume and anaphylactic shock.
g) cause constriction of lung tissues and are associated with asthma.
h) do not involve an immunological reaction.
i) eliminating possible allergens – substances that cause an allergic reaction – from the diet.
j) have a reduced ability to digest the milk sugar lactose.
k) in order to grow normally and maintain good health.
l) include migraine, tremor, sweating and palpitations.
m) it responds with an immunological reaction.
n) milk, milk derivatives, stock cubes and crisps, which often contain whey and medicines that use milk products as fillers.
o) non-allergic histamine release in some people, who usually develop a rash.
p) occur in response to food components, such as amines.
q) the dietitian can assess which of them is responsible for any symptoms.

Exercise 2
Translate the expressions. Try to explain their meanings in English.

Fermentation, botulism, fat content, powdered milk, texture, convenience, consistency, floating, seaweed, thickeners, raising agents, spongy, baking powder, deficiency, beneficial, infant formulas, appealing, staling, flavour enhancers, anti-foaming agents, propellant gases, cured meats, intolerances, trigger, potential, defence system, harmful substance, release, histamine, itching, blood volume, interfere with, constriction, rash, lactase, deficiency, treatment, amines, nitrogen, migraine, tremor, sweating, irritant, palpitations, mono-sodium glutamate, weakness, skimmed milk, stock cubes, crisps, whey, stick to, gradually, dietitian, assess, responsible, restrictive diet.

Exercise 3
Answer the following questions. Prepare short talks and/or dialogues on these topics

1. Characterize these preservatives: benzoic acid and benzoates, sulphur dioxide, nitrates and nitrites.
2. Where are these antioxidants used: vitamin C, vitamin E, tocopherols, gallates, butylated hydroxyanisole, butylated hydroxytoluene?
3. Talk about emulsifiers and stabilisers: lecithins, citric acid, tartaric acid, alginic acid, agar, carrageenan, gums, pectin.
4. Do you know any other additives?
5. Give the names of artificial sweeteners.
6. When does fortification take place?
7. What is a food allergy? What is a food intolerance?
8. Which products should people with lactase deficiency avoid?
9. Diagnosing an allergy by a dietitian, the possibility of treatment.

Vocabulary 8

Fill in the meanings in your mother language:

ability /ə'bɪl.ɪ.ti/
acesulfame K, /eɪsɪːsʌl.feɪm/
aerosol /'eə.rəʊ .sɒl/ **cream** /kriːm/
agar /'eɪgə/
agave /ə'geɪvɪ/
alarm /ə'lɑːm/
alginic /'ældʒɪn.ɪk/ **acid** /'æsɪd/
allergen /'æl.ə.dʒən/
anaphylactic /ˌæn.ə.fɪ'læk.tɪk/
anti /'æntɪ/ **-foaming** /fəʊm.ɪŋ/ **agent** /'eɪdʒənt/
antioxidant/ˌæn.ti'ɒk.sɪ.dənt/
aspartame /ə'spɑːˌteɪm/
assess /ə'ses/
asthma /'æsmə/
baking /'beɪkɪŋ/ **powder** /'paʊdə/
benzoate /'bɛnzəʊˌeɪt/
bicarbonate of soda / baɪˌkɑː.bən.ət.əv'səʊ.də/
butylated /'bjuːˌtaɪ.leɪtɪd/
hydroxyanisole /haɪ.drəʊ'ænɪˌsəʊl/
capable /'keɪ.pə.bl̩/
carrageenan /ˌkærə'giːnən/
chest /tʃest/ **pain** /peɪn/
citric acid /'sɪtrɪk 'æsɪd/
constriction /kən'strɪk.ʃən/
convenience /kən'viːnɪəns/
cooling /'kuː.lɪŋ/
curry /'kʌrɪ/
dietitian /ˌdaɪɪ'tɪʃən/
fall /'fɔːl/
fermentation /ˌfɜːmɛn'teɪʃən/
filler /'fɪl.ər/
flavour /'fleɪvə/ **enhancer** /ɪn'hɑːnsər/
float /'fləʊ/
fortifier /'fɔːtɪˌfaɪ/
froth /frɒθ/
gallate /'gæl.ət/
gelling /dʒɛl/ **agent** /'eɪdʒənt/
glazing /'gleɪzɪŋ/ **agent** /'eɪdʒənt/
goat /gəʊt/
gum /gʌm/
histamine /'hɪs.tə.miːn/
hydrogenate /'haɪdrədʒɪˌneɪt/
immunological /ˌɪm.jʊ.nəʊ.'lodʒ.ɪ.kəl/
infant /'ɪnfənt/ **formula** /'fɔːmjʊlə/
instant /'ɪn.stənt/
intensify /ɪn'tɛnsɪˌfaɪ/
involve /ɪn'vɒlv/
irritant /'ɪr.ɪ.tənt/
irritate /'ɪr.ɪ.teɪt/
itching /'ɪtʃ.ɪŋ/
lactase /'lækteɪs/
lecithin /'lɛsɪθɪn/

lethal /ˈliːθəl/
mannitol /ˈmænɪˌtɒl/
medical /ˈmed.ɪ.kəl/
migraine /ˈmiːgreɪn/
monosodium /ˌmɒnəʊˈsəʊdɪəm/
glutamate /ˈgluːtəˌmeɪt/
nectar /ˈnektə/ nektar
nitrosamine /ˌnaɪtrəʊsəˈmiːn/
palpitations /ˌpæl.pɪˈteɪ.ʃənz/
pectin /ˈpɛktɪn/ pektin
polyphosphate /ˈpɒlɪˈfɒsfeɪt/
potential /pəˈten.ʃəl/
powdered /ˈpaʊdəd/ **milk** /mɪlk/
propellant /prəˈpɛlənt/ **gas** /gæs/
pyrophosphoric /ˈpaɪrəʊˌfɒsˈfɒrɪk/ **acid** /ˈæsɪd/
raising /ˈreɪzɪŋ/ **agent** /ˈeɪdʒənt/
rash /ræʃ/
reintroduce /riːˌɪntrəˈdjuːs/
restrictive /rɪˈstrɪk.tɪv/
retain /rɪˈteɪn/
saccharin /ˈsækərɪn/
seaweed /ˈsiːˌwiːd/
separate /ˈsep.ər.ət/
sheep /ʃiːp/
shiny /ˈʃaɪ.ni/
skimmed /skɪməd/ **milk** /mɪlk/
smell /smel/
spongy /ˈspʌndʒɪ/
stale /steɪl/
stevia /ˈstɛv i ə/
stick /stɪk/
stock /stɒk/ **cube** /kjuːb/
storage /ˈstɔː.rɪdʒ/
suspected /səˈspek.tɪd/
sweating /swet.ɪŋ/
sweetener /ˈswiːtənə/
tartaric /tɑːˈtærɪk/ **acid** /ˈæsɪd/
taste /teɪst/
thaumatin /ˈtɔːmætɪn/
thickener /ˈθɪkənə/
tremor /ˈtrem.ər/
vinaigrette /ˌvɪneɪˈgrɛt/
whey /weɪ/
xylitol /ˈzaɪlɪˌtɒl/

Solution to Exercise 1a
1b, 2p, 3i, 4q, 5m, 6l, 7o, 9c, 10n, 11a, 12k, 13j, 14e, 15f, 16g, 17d

Solution to Exercise 1b
1c, 2d, 3m, 4f, 5e, 6g, 7h, 8o, 9j, 10p, 11l, 12a, 13n, 14i, 15b, 16q, 17k

Unit 9 - Foods that may cause allergies. Dietary supplements, alternative diets and 'health foods'.

Manufacturers must clearly announce the presence of the following in any product, as they may cause allergies:

- **Celery**
- Cereals containing **gluten**: wheat, rye, oats, barley
- Crustaceans, for example **lobster, crab**
- **Milk**
- **Eggs**
- **Fish**
- **Mustard**
- **Soy-beans**
- **Peanuts**
- **Nuts**: almonds, pistachios, Brazil nuts, walnuts, hazelnuts, cashews, pecans, macadamia nuts
- **Sesame seeds**
- **Sulphur dioxide and sulphites** at levels above 10 milligrams per kilogram or litre

Preventing food allergies

Many people do themselves more harm than good by excluding nutritionally important foods (such as milk), to which they believe they have an allergy. **Get expert advice** before following this course. Some food allergies are **inherited** or may be related to a **child becoming sensitised** while in the womb or in the first months after birth.

Atopic eczema

Atopic eczema affects children with a **family history** of allergies, including **hay fever and asthma**, and has been linked to food allergies. Some people have suggested that **pregnant and breast-feeding women** should **change their diets** to reduce or prevent the risk of their children developing allergies to foods. Mothers of children at risk of developing **atopic eczema** (the kind that runs in families, often together with asthma) should try to **avoid highly allergenic foods** such as **milk products, nuts, eggs and soya beans**. It may also be worth **delaying the introduction** of any of these foods to the children until they are over eight months old. Breast milk appears to give some protection, but no one is sure whether cow's milk plays any role in triggering allergies.

Nut allergy

Peanuts are the most common cause of the serious (and sometimes fatal) allergic reaction known as **anaphylaxis. Immediate medical attention** is usually needed, although some people who are aware of their allergy **carry emergency medication** to counteract their body's response. Not all peanut allergy sufferers have such a dramatic and rapid allergic reaction. Recent studies have shown that peanut allergy is more common that previously realized and **appears to be on increase**. This is probably related to the fact that women often eat larger quantities of peanuts and products containing peanut oil while pregnant or breast-feeding. Peanut products should not be given to children aged less than six months. Whole peanuts should also not be given to children under that age. Peanut or other **nut allergies can be inherited,** and any women with a family history of this type of allergy should avoid these foods during pregnancy and breast-feeding.

Hyperactivity

A link between hyperactive children and food additives was first suggested in the 1970s. Some scientists have found that the behaviour of these children improve when certain foods are eliminated from their diet. These include milk, eggs, wheat, nuts and colourings and additives such as tartrazine and benzoic acid. There is a link between food and hyperactivity in a minority of children, especially those with allergic conditions such as asthma and eczema. However, there is **no conclusive evidence** that any food is responsible for triggering the behaviour of most hyperactive children.

Key points

- **Food allergies** involve **immunological reactions; food intolerances** involve many different **non-immunological mechanisms**
- **Never put your child on a restricted diet**, even if you suspect an allergy, *without getting expert advice first, no matter how mild the symptoms are.*

Exercise 1a
Match the column A with the column B. Try to learn the expressions and/or sentences by heart.

A

1. Manufacturers must clearly announce the presence of
2. Some food allergies are inherited or
3. Atopic eczema affects children
4. Mothers of children at risk of developing atopic eczema
5. Peanuts are the most common cause
6. Peanut or other nut allergies can be inherited, and any women with a family history of this type of allergy
7. Some scientists have found that the behaviour of hyperactive children
8. Food allergies involve immunological reactions;
9. Never put your child on a restricted diet,

B

a) celery, wheat, rye, oats, barley, lobster, crab, milk, eggs, fish, mustard, soy-beans, peanuts, nuts, sesame seeds.
b) food intolerances involve many different non-immunological mechanisms.
c) improve when milk, eggs, wheat, nuts and colourings and additives such as tartrazine and benzoic acid are eliminated from their diet.
d) may be related to a child becoming sensitised while in the womb or in the first months after birth.
e) of the serious (and sometimes fatal) allergic reaction known as anaphylaxis.
f) should avoid these foods during pregnancy and breast-feeding.
g) should try to avoid highly allergenic foods such as milk products, nuts, eggs and soya beans.
h) with a family history of allergies, including hay fever and asthma, and has been linked to food allergies.
i) without getting expert advice first, no matter how mild the symptoms are.

Dietary supplements, alternative diets and 'health foods'
A growing range

The growing interest in diet and health has stimulated an increase in the market for dietary supplements. The **range of supplements** available in health food shops, chemists and supermarkets is growing, with **vitamins, minerals, fish liver oils and evening primrose oil** being the most popular. Dietary **supplements fall between medicines and foods** in terms of legal controls, and it is therefore difficult to regulate the way that they are promoted and sold. Some manufacturers make **misleading claims** about what their products can do and provide little, if any, information on **possible side effects** and the **hazards of overdosing**. No medical claims can legally be made for these products unless they have been thoroughly testes and licensed.

Nutrient supplements

The role of vitamins and minerals is well established. However, the use of large doses is controversial. A **balanced diet** will provide **nutrients in sufficient quantities** to satisfy your body's requirements. The only people who need **supplements** are those who have **medical conditions affecting the absorption or metabolism** of certain nutrients and those who have increased needs. Housebound elderly people may require vitamin D supplements. Their limited exposure to sunlight reduces the amount of vitamin D that they can synthesise.

Folate and iron

The need to supplement the diet of pregnant women with folate and iron is one of the few exceptions. **Folate supplementation before conception and in early pregnancy** has been shown to reduce the incidence of neural tube defects such as spina bifida. The need to take **iron** in pregnancy is not totally accepted by doctors; some argue that the low blood concentrations of iron are due to a normal dilution by the increased blood volume that occurs in pregnancy. The amount of iron normally taken by pregnant women does not, however, appear to cause side effects so, although it may not always do any good, it **does no harm** either.

Pyridoxine

Many other supplements make claims that have little or no scientific justification. Pyridoxine supplements are taken by some women to reduce symptoms associated with **premenstrual syndrome**. There is limited evidence that pyridoxine supplements may be helpful in relieving in premenstrual symptoms but taking **high doses** over a period of time has been associated with **nerve damage.**

Vitamins for children

Children between the ages of six months and five years may be advised to be given **vitamin drops** containing vitamins A, C and D, however, there is no evidence to support the theory that giving children vitamin supplements makes them more intelligent. All children need a balanced diet to function normally and to grow, and any dietary problems will obviously undermine their ability to their school work well.

Legislation

This legislation sets safety and quality standards for supplements. For example, there are **regulations** about the **chemical form** that the vitamins and minerals are in and about the **minimum levels** of vitamins and minerals that a supplement must include. The following must be shown on the **label**:

- details of the **nutrients included**
- the **amount recommended** to be taken daily
- a warning **not to exceed** this dose
- a statement that supplements should **not be used as a substitute for a varied diet**
- a warning to keep the product **out of reach of children**

Exercise 1b
Match the column A with the column B. Try to learn the expressions and/ or sentences by heart.

A

1. The range of supplements
2. Dietary supplements
3. Some manufacturers
4. The only people who need supplements
5. Folate supplementation before conception and in early pregnancy
6. Pyridoxine supplements are taken by some women
7. All children need a balanced diet
8. The following must be shown on the label:

B

a) *are those who have medical conditions affecting the absorption or metabolism of certain nutrients and those who have increased needs.*
b) *fall between medicines and foods in terms of legal controls.*
c) *is growing, with vitamins, minerals, fish liver oils and evening primrose oil being the most popular.*
d) *nutrients included, the amount recommended, a warning not to exceed the dose, a statement that supplements should not be used as a substitute for a varied diet and a warning to keep the product out of reach of children.*
e) *provide little information on possible side effects and the hazards of overdosing.*
f) *reduce the incidence of neural tube defects such as spina bifida.*

g) to function normally and to grow.

h) to reduce symptoms associated with premenstrual syndrome.

Exercise 2

Translate the expressions. Try to explain their meanings in English.

Gluten, sulphur dioxide, sulphites, excluding, sensitised, womb, atopic eczema, hay fever, introduction, aware of, sufferers, increase, link, minority, allergic conditions, conclusive evidence, restricted diet, mild symptoms, promoted, misleading claims, side effects, overdosing, established, satisfy requirements, exposure to sunlight, exception, conception, incidence, argue, dilution, harm, scientific justification, relieving, be advised to, obviously, include, undermine, amount, recommended, not to exceed, statement, substitute.

Exercise 3

Answer the following questions. Prepare short talks and/or dialogues on these topics

1. Which foods may cause allergies?
2. How to prevent food allergies?
3. What do you know about atopic eczema?
4. What do you know about nut allergy?
5. Which are the most popular dietary supplements available?
6. What kind of information should manufacturers provide?
7. When do people need supplements?
8. When do women take folate (iron, pyridoxine) supplements?
9. What information must be shown on the label?

Vocabulary 9

Fill in the meanings in your mother language:

allergenic /ˌæl.əˈdʒen.ɪk/
almond /ˈɑːmənd/
anaphylaxis /ˌæn.ə.fɪˈlæk.sɪs/
argue /ˈɑːg.juː/
atopic /əˈtɒpɪk/ **exzema** /ˈek.sɪ.mə/
aware /əˈweər/
brazil /brəˈzɪl/ **nut** /nʌt/
cashew /kæˈʃuː/
celery /ˈselərɪ/
chemist /ˈkemɪst/
conception /kənˈsep.ʃən/
conclusive /kənˈkluːsɪv/
counteract /ˌkaʊn.tərˈækt/
course /kɔːs/
crab /kræb/
crustacean /krʌˈsteɪʃən/
emergency /ɪˈmɜː.dʒənt .si/
exzema /ˈek.sɪ.mə/
fish /fɪʃ/ **liver** /ˈlɪvə/ **oil** /ɔɪl/
gluten /ˈgluːtən/
hay /heɪ/ **fever** /ˈfiː.vər/
hazard /ˈhæz.əd/
hazelnuts /heɪzəlˌnʌt/
housebound /ˈhaʊsˌbaʊnd/
hyperactive /ˌhaɪ.pərˈæk.tɪv/
improve /ɪmˈpruːv/
inherit /ɪnˈher.ɪt/
justification /ˌdʒʌs.tɪ.fɪˈkeɪ.ʃən/

legal /ˈliː.gəl/
lobster /ˈlɒbstə/
macadamia /ˌmækəˈdeɪmɪə/ **nut** /nʌt/
medication /ˌmed.ɪˈkeɪ.ʃən/
minority /maɪˈnɒr.ɪ.ti/
mustard /ˈmʌs.təd/
out of reach /riːtʃ/
overdose /ˈəʊ.və.dəʊs/
pecan /ˈpiːkən/
pistachio /pɪˈstɑːʃɪˌəʊ/
promote /prəˈməʊt/
realize /ˈrɪə.laɪz/
scientist /ˈsaɪəntɪst/
sesame /ˈsesəmɪ/ **seed** /siːd/
side /saɪd/ **effect** /ɪˈfekt/
statement /ˈsteɪt.mənt/
sulphite /ˈsʌlfaɪt/
synthesise /ˈsɪnθɪˌsaɪz/
undermine /ˌʌndəˈmaɪn/
walnut /ˈwɔːlˌnʌt/
warning /ˈwɔː.nɪŋ/
womb /wuːm/

Solution to Exercise 1a
1a, 2d, 3h, 4g, 5e, 6f, 7c, 8b, 9i

Solution to Exercise 1b
1c, 2b, 3e, 4a, 5f, 6h, 7g, 8d

Unit 10 - High-energy and protein supplements. Alternative diets.

These products are aimed at **exercise enthusiasts** who want to eat more calories as they use up more energy. These people are often trying to **increase their muscle mass** and **require more protein** to do this. Calories are used mainly by lean tissue, of which muscle is a major component. As the muscle mass increases, **more calories are needed** to maintain the more muscular frame. These extra calories and protein can easily be supplied by eating more food. **Elderly convalescents** and their carers may also use these supplements. The products are often based on milk and need to **be mixed with milk** before they are used. Although they may be of some benefit, their **strong flavourings and rich nature** make them unpalatable to some people with poor appetites. It is usually **better to offer convalescents frequent, small snacks** and meals consisting of foods that they like and therefore will eat.

'Health foods'

This term is usually used to describe foods that are not readily available in supermarkets but which are sold in **specialist shops**. The name implies that these foods are particularly healthy. This is misleading, as people who already eat a balanced diet are unlikely to derive any benefit from them. However, there are many useful products sold in health food shops. Wholemeal foods are a good example, although you can normally buy them just as easily in your local supermarket. **Organic foods such as cereals, fruit and vegetables** are becoming more widely available in both specialist shops and supermarkets, but they are invariably more expensive as a result of **higher production costs**. The use of natural farming methods has obvious advantages in reducing the reliance on **pesticides and fertilisers**. However, there is little scientific evidence to support the theory that organic foods are healthier than those produced by modern methods.

Functional foods

Over the last few years a new type of food has lined supermarket and health shop shelves. These foods are known as functional foods and are **fortified with a range of phytochemicals** that suggest that they can treat or prevent certain diseases such as heart disease. Any product should be assessed by its individual merits, but it is important to remember that nothing can replace the benefits of a healthy balanced diet. **Phytoestrogens** are a group of compounds found naturally in plant foods. The best food sources are **soya-bean** and its products such as **textured vegetable protein, tofu, tempeh and soya milk/flour.** Recently, there has been interest in the role of phyto-oestrogens in the relief of **menopausal symptoms**, such as hot flushes. Although phytoestrogens appear to be a natural alternative to HRT, there is only limited research to support this at present.

Foods containing bacteria

In adults the gastrointestinal tract contains about **one kilogram and 500 different types of bacteria.** The **presence and balance of these bacteria are important** and, if this balance is disturbed, the health of the gastrointestinal tract will be affected. Recently, products have become available that help to maintain this balance. **Probiotics** contain live bacteria – for example, **lactobacilli** – which help prevent disease in the gut. There is some evidence to suggest that they reduce the incidence of diarrhoea and may help lactose intolerance. Manufacturers must, however, fulfil strict criteria about their safety, production and storage. Bacteria in the gut require **substances to help them grow** and **prebiotics** – for example, **fructo-oligosaccharides** – are products that do this. They help the beneficial bacteria to grow and may therefore be useful in the treatment of constipation. Prebiotics are found in a range of foods, including dairy and bakery products. Both probiotics and prebiotics are being investigated further to look at their potential benefits.

Health claims

Making health claims about a food is tightly regulated by the EU and any claim must be approved by the EU.

Exercise 1a
Match the column A with the column B. Try to learn the expressions and/ or sentences by heart.

A

1. Exercise enthusiasts are often trying to increase their muscle mass
2. As the muscle mass increases,
3. It is usually better to offer convalescents frequent, small snacks

4. The use of natural farming methods
5. Functional foods
6. Phytoestrogens are a group of compounds
7. The best food sources of phytoestrogens are soya-bean and its products
8. Recently, there has been interest in the role of phyto-oestrogens
9. In adults the gastrointestinal tract
10. Probiotics contain live bacteria
11. Bacteria in the gut require substances to help them grow
12. Making health claims about a food

B

a) – for example, lactobacilli – which help prevent disease in the gut.
b) and meals consisting of foods that they like and therefore will eat.
c) and prebiotics – for example, fructo-oligosaccharides – are products that do this.
d) and require more protein to do this.
e) are fortified with a range of phytochemicals that suggest that they can treat or prevent certain diseases such as heart disease.
f) contains about one kilogram and 500 different types of bacteria.
g) found naturally in plant foods.
h) has obvious advantages in reducing the reliance on pesticides and fertilisers.
i) in the relief of menopausal symptoms, such as hot flushes.
j) is tightly regulated by the EU and any claim must be approved by the EU.
k) more calories are needed to maintain the more muscular frame.
l) such as textured vegetable protein, tofu, tempeh and soya milk/flour.

Alternative diets

In modern society, health is a major concern, and people are always looking to **optimise the benefits from their diet**. At times, this has resulted in an increase in the number of people willing to pay for alternative diets, many of which are expensive with debatable, if any, benefits.

Detoxification diets

These are recommended by various health writers and therapists to **cleanse the body**, and often involve **fasting, bathing and ex-foliating** (removal of dead skin by rubbing and brushing) **to remove toxins**. If your liver and kidneys are functioning properly, your body will clear any waste substances naturally. There is no scientific evidence to support the benefits of these diets. Always **consult your medical practitioner** before trying one of them.

Anti-candida diets

It has been suggested that **overgrowth of yeasts**, particularly *Candida albicans*, can lead to a variety of **debilitating symptoms**. This overgrowth is supposedly triggered by **diets rich in yeasts and sugar** (which is used as food by yeasts), **oral contraceptives** and the use of **broad-spectrum antibiotics**. This is alleged to result in **toxin production,** which **weakens the immune system,** making susceptible people prone to a wide range of illnesses. The **diet** is used to treat this condition involves **avoiding bread, vinegar, alcohol, pickles, cheese, yeast extracts and all products containing sucrose.** There is no **medically controlled evidence** to justify the use of these diets.

Food-combining (Hay) diet

Supporters of diets such as this **claim that the body cannot digest acid and alkaline foods** together. They also claim that **mixing protein and carbohydrate foods** results in many health problems, such as **headaches, allergies and obesity. In reality, the digestive system is fully capable of digesting** a meal containing **a mixture of foods,** using varying acid and alkaline conditions.

Slimming diets

There are many diets that are supposed to make it easy for people to **lose weight.** Many totally eliminate one food group from the diet. It is suggested that these diets **'burn fat' or 'speed up the metabolism'.** Some slimming diets are based on single foods, such as grapefruit. Such claims have **no scientific basis** and, if you succeed in losing weight on these diets, it is because of their restrictive nature. Such diets will not help you change to a healthy eating pattern in the long term. They can also **cause nutritional deficiencies.**

Very-low-calorie diets

Very-low-calorie diets (VLCDs) were very popular in the 1980s and provided **less than 400 kcal per day**. Medical evidence linked these diets to cardiac problems. These diets should not be used for longer that three to four weeks and then **only by obese people under medical supervision**. The energy content and presentation of these diets were then **changed to provide 600 to 800 kcal per day**, incorporating snack bars and prepared meals. Their popularity has greatly declined over recent years.

The Atkins diet

Low-carbohydrate diets, for example, the Atkins diet, were first promoted in the 1960s but have recently become very popular. Reducing your intake of carbohydrate leads to the **mobilisation of fat stores, releasing** chemicals called **ketones**. Ketones are **made from the breakdown of fat** and can be **used by the body,** but not the brain, **as an energy source** for a limited period. These diets succeeded in restricting energy intake, as many people find it difficult to eat large amounts of fat or protein without carbohydrate.

The lack of carbohydrate results in the rapid **use of glycogen energy stores** and this also causes the loss of water, which accounts for the **initial rapid weight loss.** When **carbohydrate is reintroduced** into the diet, **weight gain** occurs.

The healthiest approach

The best approach to losing weight is to adopt a healthy diet. This will make sure that your weight remains as it should be in the long term, as well as providing all the nutrients you need for good health.

Key points

- The use of specialised food **supplements** is **often unnecessary.**
- **Normal foods can be modified** to provide any additional requirements.
- **Lack of appetite** is **an important factor** when trying to persuade someone to eat more.
- Most **healthy people** are **unlikely** to experience any **specific nutrient deficiency.**

Exercise 1b
Match the column A with the column B. Try to learn the expressions and/ or sentences by heart.

A

1. Detoxification diets are recommended to cleanse the body,
2. There is no scientific evidence
3. Overgrowth of yeasts, is supposedly
4. The diet is used to treat this condition
5. Supporters of food-combining diet claim that the body cannot digest acid and alkaline foods together
6. In reality, the digestive system
7. Slimming diets
8. It is suggested that slimming diets 'burn fat' or 'speed up the metabolism',
9. Very-low-calorie diets
10. Low-carbohydrate diets, for example, the Atkins diet,
11. Low-carbohydrate diets succeeded in restricting energy intake,
12. The lack of carbohydrate results in the rapid use of glycogen energy stores

B

a) and mixing protein and carbohydrate foods results in many health problems, such as headaches, allergies and obesity.

b) and often involve fasting, bathing and exfoliating to remove toxins.

c) and this also causes the loss of water, which accounts for the initial rapid weight loss.

d) are supposed to make it easy for people to lose weight.

e) as many people find it difficult to eat large

amounts of fat or protein without carbohydrate.

f) *but such claims have no scientific basis and can even cause nutritional deficiencies.*

g) *involves avoiding bread, vinegar, alcohol, pickles, cheese, yeast extracts and all products containing sucrose.*

h) *is fully capable of digesting a meal containing a mixture of foods.*

i) *should not be used for longer that three to four weeks and then only by obese people under medical supervision.*

j) *to support the benefits of these diets.*

k) *triggered by diets rich in yeasts and sugar, oral contraceptives and the use of broad-spectrum antibiotics.*

l) *were first promoted in the 1960s but have recently become very popular.*

Exercise 2

Translate the expressions. Try to explain their meanings in English.

Aimed at, component, muscle mass, flavourings, unpalatable, convalescent, imply, misleading, derive, wholemeal foods, invariably, reliance, assessed, relief, hot flushes, research, disturbed, affected, incidence, constipation, investigated, optimise, willing, debatable, benefits, fasting, bathing, rubbing and brushing, dead skin, overgrowth of yeasts, debilitating symptoms, oral contraceptives, susceptible, prone to, justify, acid and alkaline, capable of digesting, slimming, eliminate, restrictive nature, nutritional deficiencies, medical supervision, incorporating, declined, promoted, breakdown of fat, succeeded in, restricting intake, accounts for, additional requirements, persuade.

Exercise 3

Answer the following questions. Prepare short talks and/or dialogues on these topics.

1. What is the use of high-energy and protein supplements?
2. Explain the terms organic foods and functional foods.
3. What are the functions of probiotics and prebiotics?
4. Characterise detoxification diets.
5. What do you know about anti-candida diets?
6. What are the rules of food-combining diet?
7. Talk about slimming diets and very-low-calorie diets.
8. Low-carbohydrate diets, and what accounts for the initial rapid weight loss.

Vocabulary 10

Fill in the meanings in your mother language:

adopt /əˈdɒpt/
aimed /eɪmd/ **at** /æt/
alleged /əˈledʒd/
alternative /ɒlˈtɜː.nə.tɪv/
approach /əˈprəʊtʃ/
approved /əˈpruːvd/

bakery /ˈbeɪkərɪ/
broad /brɔ:d/ **-spectrum** /ˈspɛktrəm/
antibiotic /ˌæntɪbaɪˈɒtɪk/
carer /ˈkeərə/
cleanse /klenz/
concern /kənˈsɜ:n/
contraceptive /ˌkɒn.trəˈsep.tɪv/
convalescent /ˌkɒnvəˈlesənt/
criterion /kraɪˈtɪə.ri.ən/ pl **criteria**
debatable /dɪˈbeɪtəbəl/
debilitating /dɪˈbɪl.ɪ.teɪt.ɪŋ/
decline /dɪˈklaɪn/
detoxification /di:ˌtɒk.sɪ.fɪˈkeɪ.ʃən/
disturb /dɪˈstɜ:b/
enthusiast /ɪnˈθju:.zi.æst/
exfoliate /ɛksˈfəʊlɪˌeɪt/
fasting /fɑ:stɪŋ/
fertilizer /ˈfɜ:.tɪ.laɪ.zər/
frame /freɪm/
fructo /ˈfrʌktəʊ **-oligosaccharide** /ˌɒlɪgəʊˈsækəˌraɪd/
fulfil /fʊlˈfɪl/
Hay /heɪ/ **diet** /ˈdaɪət/
hot /hɒt/ **flush** /flʌʃ/
incidence /ˈɪnt .sɪ.dənts/
invariably /ɪnˈveə.ri.ə.bli/
investigate /ɪnˈves.tɪ.geɪt/
justify /ˈdʒʌs.tɪ.faɪ/
ketone /ˈki:.təʊn/
lactobacillus /ˌlæktəʊbəˈsɪləs/
lactobacilli /-laɪ/
live /lɪv/
menopausal /ˌmenəˈpɔ:zəl/
merit /ˈmɛrɪt/
muscle /ˈmʌs.əl/ **mass** /mæs/
nature /ˈneɪ.tʃə/
optimize /ˈɒp.tɪ.maɪz/
organic /ɔ:ˈgænɪk/ **food** /fu:d/
persuade /pəˈsweɪd/
pesticide /ˈpɛstɪˌsaɪd/
phytochemical /ˌfaɪtəʊˈkɛmɪkəl/
phytoestrogen /ˌfaɪtəʊˈi:strədʒən/
practitioner /prækˈtɪ.ʃən.ər/
prebiotic /ˌpri:baɪˈɒtɪk/
probiotic /ˌprəʊbaɪˈɒtɪk/
prone /prəʊn/
reliance /rɪˈlaɪ.əns/
relief /rɪˈli:f/
restrict /rɪˈstrɪkt/
rub /rʌb/
slimming /slɪm.ɪŋ/
succeed /səkˈsi:d/
supervision /ˌsu:.pəˈvɪʒ.ən/
support /səˈpɔ:t/
supposed /səˈpəʊzɪd/
susceptible /səˈsep.tɪ.bl̩/
tempeh /ˈtɛmpeɪ/
tightly /taɪt.li/
tofu /ˈtəʊˌfu:/
unpalatable /ʌnˈpælətəbəl/
vegetable /ˈvedʒ.tə.bl̩/
willing /ˈwɪl.ɪŋ/

Solution to Exercise 1a
1d, 2k, 3b, 4h, 5e, 6g, 7l, 8i, 9f, 10a, 11c, 12j

Solution to Exercise 1b
1b, 2j, 3k, 4g, 5a, 6h, 7d, 8f, 9i, 10l, 12c

Chapter III
Be your own nutritionist

Unit 1 - Modern diets. About digestion.

People throughout the **developed world** are **fatter**, becoming increasingly **diabetic** and suffering near epidemic levels of **cancer**, **heart attacks** and **strokes**. There are so many different ideas of what healthy foods are, how and when to eat them and such a **profusion of different dietary theories** that those who do want to eat healthily are baffled from the outset. We need to develop a new relationship with what we eat, a genuinely healthy diet that is clearly understood and that will sit comfortably within our mainstream culture. There are **five key factors** for dietary health: **climate, gut function, emotion, flavour analysis and food type.**

When it comes to diets for health, nothing quite compares to the **traditional Chinese approach**. This is supported by numerous and extremely detailed anthropological, epidemiological, and nutritional studies. Traditional Chinese nutrition underpins the diet of **the healthiest and longest-living populations** in the world: those of **Japan, Hong Kong and Singapore**. And not only is this approach remarkably healthy, it is also truly versatile. **It can be adapted to all climates** (which have a profound effect on our health and the food we should eat), **seasons, lifestyles, foods and illnesses** in the world.

The Chinese had retained their connection with their dietary past. In much of the developed world, however, we seem to have lost touch with our roots altogether. Yet, there are striking **similarities**. Both:

- use foods **in relation to variations** in **digestibility, climate, season, lifestyle, stage of life, emotion and disease**
- are **diagnostic** in nature and **adaptable** for individual cases
- are extremely **diverse**
- are packed with **vegetables, nuts, seeds and fruit**
- put a special **emphasis** on **rich foods** like fish, animal and plant fats as an adaptation to cold and damp climate, and place these in the context of **aromatic, warm, cooked and hearty dishes** to enhance digestibility
- use **fermented foods**, strongly **flavoured herbs**, **spices** and **condiments** extensively
- rely on regular consumption of **medicinal foods** such as **offal, shellfish, walnuts, chestnuts** and certain herbs and spices to extend life and sustain health.

What went wrong with modern diets

The rise of junk food

The Western diet has infiltrated the nutrition in every layer of society. Even the most health-conscious of us are still **exposed** to **hidden salt** in shop-bought salads, **hidden sugar** and salt in breakfast cereals or **cheap fat** and **additives** in sandwiches, biscuits, ice cream and cakes. It is likely that, if you don't prepare everything yourself from high quality ingredients, you'll always be exposed to some aspect of the Western diet.

It is easy enough to see how the Western diet became ubiquitous. A good starting point is **recent research** that suggests that eating salt, sugar, and cheap fat triggers the same **addictive neurological pathways as heroin** consumption and withdrawal. Some ingredients - the types of ingredients that are invariably found in **ready meals and junk food snacks** – seem to be **truly addictive**; and as consumers, intentionally or not, we are damaging ourselves by eating them.

One of the methods that junk food manufacturers and retailers use to promote and market their products is to **manipulate the language of science**. They take a cheap and healthy product with a low nutritional value, packed with ingredients that create compulsion like salt and sugar, and then cover the boxes, packets and wrappers with scientific terminology that gives the illusion of health and nutrition. As consumers of the Western diet, we compulsively eat nutritionally deficient food, often under the illusion that it is good for us.

Banish the fads

In recent decades many people have turned to diets other that the Western diet in an attempt to undo its harm, and in particular to lose weight. These **alternative diets** – or rather, fad diets ostensibly exist to promote health and weight loss, but **in reality** they **share many of the failings of the Western diet.**

Looking back over **the past half-century**, we have been offered a steady stream of **high-protein, low-protein, high-carb, low-carb, calorie-controlled, eat-what-you-want, blood-type and raw-food diets – all contradicting each other** in scientific-sounding ways, despite seeming to have the same goals of weight loss and health enhancement. Not all of these diets can be right in their stated benefits and it's up to us to work out where the dietary value lies, a process that can be bewilderingly complex.

The extraordinary number of fad diets and slimming companies, combined with the tons of "health foods" that are eaten show that there is a genuine desire to eat healthier foods. And yet we are experiencing more and more food-related illness.

Big business

It isn't difficult to see that this rise in diet-related illness has come about as a result of the machinations of food corporations. They exist to maximise profit for their shareholders – and that means selling more junk food.

Just like any marketplace, a fad diet is as successful as its ability to sell it, through PR, marketing, and celebrity and media connections. That's why there are so many of them around, in book shops, on the web, TV, and other media; lots of people want to cash in on such a big market.

Sometimes, there may be a very genuine motivation behind the selling of a fad diet, because it is worked for its originator. They are passionate about the diet because, they say, it solved a health issue or made them feel healthy and vibrant – at least for a certain time. But it doesn't mean that the same diet would work for everyone else.

Exercise 1a
Match the column A with the column B. Try to learn the expressions and/or sentences by heart.

A

1. There are five key factors for dietary health:
2. Traditional Chinese nutrition is remarkably healthy, it is diverse and adaptable for individual cases,
3. Traditional nutrition is packed with vegetables, nuts, seeds and fruit;
4. Traditional Chinese nutrition also
5. Even the most health-conscious of us
6. The types of ingredients that are invariably found in ready meals and junk food snacks
7. Alternative diets, or rather, fad diets ostensibly exist
8. Not all of the diets can be right in their stated benefits

B

a) *and it's up to us to work out where the dietary value lies.*
b) *and uses foods in relation to variations in digestibility, climate, season, lifestyle, stage of life, emotion and disease.*
c) *are still exposed to hidden salt in shop-bought salads, hidden sugar and salt in breakfast cereals or cheap fat and additives in sandwiches, biscuits, ice cream and cakes.*
d) *climate, gut function, emotion, flavour analysis and food type.*
e) *it puts a special emphasis on rich foods, and uses aromatic, warm, cooked and hearty dishes to enhance digestibility.*
f) *seem to be truly addictive.*
g) *to promote health and weight loss, but in reality they share many of the failings of the Western diet.*
h) *uses fermented foods, strongly flavoured herbs, spices and condiments extensively.*

About digestion

The problem of modern gastroenterological science is the **complexity of the human gut**, and the **nutritional diversity of the food** we put in it. In terms of anatomy an average human adult gut is nine metres long and consists of at least **seven different sections**.

It is serviced by **two major secreting organs**, and **the nerves** that supply it weigh the same as the brain and the spinal cord put together; indeed, these nerves are so **substantial, powerful and significant** that they are classified as a discreet nervous system – the **Enteral nervous system** (ENS). It can **operate** on its own **without requiring signals from the brain** and its **own stimuli** can feed back and **directly alter brain chemistry**.

And the food that we eat is just as complicated. Let's take as an example a common dish like beef stew and dumplings. Such a dish might have upwards of fifteen **ingredients**, with each of those ingredients consisting of **thousands of molecules**, many of which have neither been labelled scientifically, nor had their nutritional roles identified.

In the course of being cooked, eaten and metabolised, these molecules are **combined, heated, chewed, broken down, absorbed and used** within the body's cells. So in the end we're talking about the **transformation, absorption and assimilation** of many tens of thousands of molecule types.

An astonishing number of chemical processes take place as a result of the preparation and consumption of even a relatively simple dish. To date, it has been virtually impossible to fully understand these chemical processes in scientific terms; they are far **too extensive and complex**.

Where dietary science has been very successful is in **linking single nutrients to major diseases**; i.e. where there is a deficiency of the nutrient, the disease arises. Examples of this include **vitamin D and rickets**, **vitamin C and scurvy**, and **vitamin B_1 and beri beri**.

When the link between the nutrient and disease was first identified, it seemed miraculous that such severe illness could be fixed with a simple dietary change. In reality, when it comes to whole food, groups of foods and their interactions with our very complex digestive systems and metabolisms, effective scientific understanding is distinctly lacking.

The traditional diet for health is based on a small number of digestive concepts that are easily applied to climate, lifestyle, individual foods and food combinations. These concepts are symbiosis, secretion and motility.

- **Symbiosis** is all about countless **microbes, that live in our guts,** help us to break down our food and also produce vital nutrients
- **Secretion** is the process by which **the gut produces the chemical substances** that break foods down so that they can be absorbed as they are moved along.
- **Motility** refers to **the movement of the gut**, when it is in harmony or when it is distressed.

The **three digestive processes** are independent and utterly influenced by the foods that we eat, the environment that we live in and the lifestyles that we lead. Together, they provide a comprehensive view of digestive function.

Exercise 1b
Match the column A with the column B. Try to learn the expressions and/ or sentences by heart.

A

1. In terms of anatomy
2. It is serviced by two major secreting organs, and the nerves
3. It can operate on its own without requiring signals from the brain
4. In the course of being cooked, eaten and metabolised,
5. Where dietary science has been very successful
6. The traditional diet for health is based on a small number of digestive concepts;
7. Symbiosis is all about countless microbes,
8. Secretion is the process by which
9. Motility refers

B

a) *an average human adult gut is nine metres long and consists of at least seven different sections.*
b) *and its own stimuli can feed back and directly alter brain chemistry.*
c) *are so substantial, powerful and significant that they are classified as a discreet nervous system – the enteral nervous system.*
d) *is in linking single nutrients to major diseases; i.e. vitamin D and rickets, vitamin C and scurvy, and vitamin B1 and beri beri.*
e) *that live in our guts, help us to break down our food and also produce vital nutrients.*
f) *the gut produces the chemical substances that break foods down.*
g) *the molecules are combined, heated, chewed, broken down, absorbed and used within the body's cells.*
h) *these concepts are symbiosis, secretion and motility.*
i) *to the movement of the gut.*

Exercise 2
Translate the expressions. Try to explain their meanings in English.

Profusion, relationship, mainstream culture, compare to, underpin, remarkably, versatile, profound effect, retained, striking similarities, adaptable, diverse, emphasis, rich foods, hearty dishes, enhance, condiments, sustain health, junk food, exposed to, ubiquitous, trigger, withdrawal, invariably, addictive, intentionally, compulsion, compulsively, banish, fads, failings, contradicting, seeming, enhancement, desire, diet-related illness, food corporations, maximise profit, shareholders, passionate, healthy and vibrant, complexity, diversity, sections, secreting organs, substantial, powerful, alter, significant, discreet, enteral, ingredients, chewed, broken down, absorbed, assimilation, linking, rickets, scurvy, beri beri, fixed with, interactions, distinctly, concepts, symbiosis, secretion, motility, distressed, independent, influenced, comprehensive view.

Exercise 3
Answer the following questions. Prepare short talks and/or dialogues on these topics.

1. What can you say about modern diets?
2. Which are the five key factors for dietary health?
3. Why is the traditional Chinese approach so inspiring?
4. What are the similarities of the traditional Chinese nutrition and the nutrition of the developed world?
5. What went wrong with modern diets? The rise of junk food.
6. Can you remember any diets we have been offered over the past half-century?
7. Describe the function of gastrointestinal system.
8. Talk about the transformation, absorption and assimilation of food.
9. Link single nutrients to major diseases (rickets, scurvy, beri beri)
10. What do you know about symbiosis, secretion and motility?

Vocabulary 1

Fill in the meanings in your mother language:

adaptable /əˈdæptəbəl/
addictive /əˈdɪktɪv/
approach /əˈprəʊtʃ/
arise /əˈraɪz/
astonishing /əˈstɒnɪʃɪŋ/
attempt /əˈtempt/
baffled /ˈbæfəld/
banish /bænɪʃ/
beri beri /beri/
bewildering /bɪˈwɪldərɪŋ/
break /breɪk/ **down** /daʊn/
cash /kæʃ/ **in st**
chestnut /ˈtʃesˌnʌt/
compare /kəmˈpeə/
complex /kɒmpleks/
complexity /kəmˈpleksɪtɪ/
comprehensive /ˌkɒmprɪˈhensɪv/
compulsion /kəmˈpʌlʃən/
concept /ˈkɒnsept/
condiment /ˈkɒndɪmənt/
conscious /kɒnʃəs/
contradict /ˌkɒntrəˈdɪkt/
corporation /kɔːpəˈreɪʃən/
countless /kaʊntlɪs/
damp /dæmp/
deficient /dɪˈfɪʃənt/
desire /dɪˈzaɪə/
digestible /dɪˈdʒɛstəbəl/
discreet /dɪˈskriːt/
distinctly /dɪˈstɪŋktlɪ/
diverse /ˈdaɪvɜːs/
diversity /daɪˈvɜːsɪtɪ/
dumpling /ˈdʌmplɪŋ/
emphasis /ˈemfəsɪs/
enhance /ɪnˈhɑːns/
enteral /ˈen.tə.rəl/

extensive /ɪk'stensɪv/
extraordinary /ɪk'strɔːdənrɪ/
fad /fæd/
failing /'feɪlɪŋ/
feed back /'fiːd.bæk/
genuine /'dʒenjʊɪn/
genuinely /'dʒenjʊɪnlɪ/
hearty /'hɑːtɪ/
infiltrate /'ɪnfɪlˌtreɪt/
intentionally /ɪn'tenʃənəli/
invariably /ɪn'veərɪəblɪ/
junk /dʒʌŋk/ **food** /fuːd/
lacking /'lækɪŋ/
machination /ˌmækɪ'neɪʃən/
mainstream /'meɪnˌstriːm/
manufacturer /ˌmænjʊ'fæktʃərə/
market /'mɑːkɪt/
miraculous /mɪ'rækjʊləs/
motility /ˌməʊ.'til.i.'tiː/
offal /'ɒfəl]/
originator /ə'rɪdʒ əˌneɪtə/
ostensibly /ɒ'stɛn sə bəli/
outset /'aʊtˌset/
passionate /pæʃənɪt/
pathway /'pɑːθˌweɪ]/
profit /'prɒfɪt/
profound /prə'faʊnd/
profusion /prə'fjuːʒən/
promote /prə'məʊt/
remarkably /rɪ'mɑːkəbəlɪ/
retailer /'riːteɪlə/
rich /rɪtʃ/
rickets /'rɪkɪts/
rise /raɪz/
science /'saɪəns/
scurvy /'skɜːvɪ/
secretion /sɪ'kriːʃən/
shareholder /'ʃeəˌhəʊldə/
spinal /'spaɪ.nəl/ **cord** /kɔːd/
stew /stjuː/
striking /'straɪkɪŋ/
support /sə'pɔːt/
sustain /sə'steɪn/
symbiosis /ˌsɪmbaɪ'əʊsɪs/
trigger /'trɪgə/
ubiquitous /juː'bɪkwɪtəs/
underpin /ˌʌndə'pɪn/
utterly /'ʌtəlɪ/
versatile /vɜːsəˌtaɪl/
vibrant /'vaɪbrənt/
virtually /'vɜːtʃʊəlɪ/
withdrawal /wɪð'drɔːəl/
work out /wɜːk/
wrapper /'ræpə/

Solution to Exercise 1a
1d, 2b, 3e, 4h, 5c, 6f, 7g, 8a

Solution to Exercise 1b
1a, 2c, 3b, 4g, 5d, 6h, 7e, 8f, 9i

Unit 2 - Symbiosis. Secretion.

As human beings, we are literally covered from top to toe, inside and out, with **bacteria and other micro-organisms**. Taking digestion as an example, it becomes clear that every human on the planet is his or her own little ecosystem.

Our bodies are made up of around ten trillion cells but we have about ten times as many micro-organisms, or microbes, as they are sometimes called, in our guts; as much as two kilograms. **These microbes can be bacteria, yeasts, fungi, or larger animals (protozoa).** They are known as the **gut flora** and may be **good for health (symbiotic)** or **bad (pathogenic)**.

In a healthy individual the vast majority of them are symbiotic (symbionts). **Symbionts** are **absolutely vital to healthy living**. Indeed, such is the role of these microbes in health that they have come to be known as the "forgotten organ". The crucial relationship that our bacteria have with health is one that is only just beginning to be appreciated scientifically.

Recent DNA sequencing research concluded that human digestion is dependent on a minimum of 1,000 species of bacteria, of which we probably have at least 200 in us at any of the time. What these bacteria look like and the potentially massive range of functions that they have within our bodies is beyond modern science.

Bacteria – our friends

Microbes clean our skin, help our babies to develop in the womb and line and protect our sinuses. And they form the bedrock of our digestion. **Symbiotic bacteria** are fundamental to health. **Antibiotics** that **upset the balance of gut flora** is linked to obesity as well as other major health problems such as **allergies, inflammatory bowel disease and asthma**.

The symbionts in our guts are constantly working on our behalf to enhance our health by:

- helping us **break down complex carbohydrates and sugars** (fibres and the like)
- stimulating and supporting **the immune system**
- **suppressing** the development of **harmful organisms**
- **producing useful nutrients** like **biotin and vitamin K** that we aren't normally able to produce for ourselves
- helping to **process fats**
- developing the **gut**

Bacteria – our enemies

We live in an age where there is a fashion for cleanliness. It is developments in **hygiene and sanitation** that have **protected us from** dreadful diseases such as **polio, cholera, and infectious bacteria such as Clostridium and Staphylococcus**, micro-organisms that have become infamous as hospital "super-bugs". These diseases used to kill people by the million; now they are much rarer in the Western world, largely because we have become cleaner.

This awareness of hygiene, combined with the awesome impact of antibiotics on infectious bacteria, has led to a philosophy of "anti-biosis" - humans constantly fighting pitched battles against other organisms – a philosophy that dominates medical thinking today.

Most **micro-organisms are essential for health,** a relationship known as **"probiosis".** It is inevitable that all these bacteria, including the good ones, are sourced from our environment and also from other humans in an important process called "seeding".

Seeding

Seeding **takes place from conception**. Some studies suggest that babies need bacteria for their **growth and survival in the womb.** Symbionts that are vital to health and development are working with us from the outset and they are **picked up from the uterus**. More bacteria are **picked up at birth** as the baby passes through its mother's **vagina** and into an area rich with digestive bacteria near her **bottom**. Further pro-biotic bacteria are then passed on through the **breast milk.**

The importance of this transmission of bacteria from mother to child and seeding of the baby's gut is revealed in statistics – babies born by caesarean section miss out on the vaginal bacteria and babies that aren't breast-fed miss out on bacteria from breast milk, leading to a higher incidence of disease in both groups.

After birth and weaning, little children then continue to pick up symbionts from the floor and from the soil; even from pets. It has been demonstrated that **soil bacteria** stimulate the release extra serotonin, a key neurotransmitter in the brain. Similarly, laboratory studies suggest that a range of major emotions, such as anxiety, are affected by the balance or our gut flora. Muck actually makes us all happier.

Seeding is a process that we should **continue throughout our lives.** One way to achieve this is to grow our own food. Fruit and vegetables produced on an allotment, or even in a window box, in good **organically managed soil, carry microbes that are beneficial to us** – our exposure to this good, uncontaminated local dirt is great.

We gain similar benefits from **regularly consuming** small amounts of **live fermented food** such as **sauerkraut, pickled and preserved vegetables, herring, yoghurt, buttermilk and beer**. Foods that are rich in bacteria are delicious and much cheaper than the sort of probiotic products that can be bought in the shops.

In short, if we:

- ate more **naturally preserved and fermented foods**
- ate, played and worked **more outside**
- gathered more **foods from hedgerows, and woodlands** with their rich accompaniment of **yeasts and bacteria**
- just used **normal soap** rather than toxic industrial "antibacterial" cleaners

we would be an altogether healthier and happier bunch.

Artificial sweeteners

Recent research has shown the commonly used artificial sweetener sucralose to have **significant destructive effect on gut symbionts**. The other major artificial sweetener aspartame is no better as once metabolised, it produces, among other chemicals, methanol, which is highly toxic to humans. Both products, which are used to sweeten "diet", "low-calorie", "sugar-free" and "weight loss" products, have been implicated in a wide range of debilitating diseases, including obesity.

Stevia, a naturally occurring low-calorie sweetener which has recently been declared "safe" for market, coincidentally at the same time as some major food companies came up with stevia-based products, has also had mixed reviews in terms of safety.

Exercise 1a
Match the column A with the column B. Try to learn the expressions and/or sentences by heart.

A

1. The microbes can be
2. The microbes are known as the gut flora
3. Antibiotics that upset the balance of gut flora is linked to
4. The symbionts in our guts
5. Developments in hygiene and sanitation have protected us from
6. Most micro-organisms are essential for health,
7. Babies born by caesarean section miss out on the vaginal bacteria
8. Fruit and vegetables produced in good organically managed soil,
9. We gain similar benefits from regularly consuming
10. Sucralose and aspartame which are used to sweeten "diet", "low-calorie", "sugar-free" and "weight loss" products,

B

a) a relationship known as "probiosis".
b) allergies, inflammatory bowel disease and asthma.
c) and babies that aren't breast-fed miss out on bacteria from breast milk, leading to a higher incidence of disease in both groups.
d) and may be good for health (symbiotic) or bad (pathogenic).
e) bacteria, yeasts, fungi, or larger animals (protozoa).
f) carry microbes that are beneficial to us.
g) have been implicated in a wide range of debilitating diseases, including obesity.
h) help us break down complex carbohydrates and sugars, support the immune system, suppress the development of harmful organisms, produce useful nutrients and help us to process fats.
i) live fermented food such as sauerkraut, pickled and preserved vegetables, herring, yoghurt, buttermilk and beer.
j) polio, cholera, and infectious bacteria such as Clostridium and Staphylococcus.

Secretion

Food provides both the **energy** for and the **substance** of, our bodies. In order to fulfil these functions, is has to be first **broken down**

into very small molecules in the gut, **then absorbed** through the membrane barrier that lines the stomach and intestines **into the blood stream**, and finally **taken to** where it is needed in **the body.**

To achieve the sort of molecule size that is easily absorbed into the blood stream, the typically **large nutritional molecules** of food have to be **broken down many times** over. This is initially a **mechanical process. Teeth** chomp through the food and break it into little pieces. The breaking down then continues as a series of **chemical processes** involving enzymes, emulsifiers and other chemicals.

Enzymes

Enzymes are **proteins** whose job is to make **chemical reactions** happen more **easily. Digestive enzymes** are very specific **for particular nutrient groups**, there are enzymes that break down particular nutrient groups; there are enzymes that break down **sugars and starches**, enzymes that break down **proteins**, and so on. They do this by seeking out particular types of chemical bonds and snipping them to produce smaller and smaller molecules.

Enzymes are not only very specific in terms of the molecules on which they act, but also **regarding the environment** in which they work. For example, **amylase**, an enzyme that is secreted by the **salivary gland,** works best in the slightly **alkaline** warm conditions that are found in the **mouth**. Similarly, **enzymes** that are secreted in the **stomach**, where it is very **acidic**, work best in this acidity, and at body temperature.

Other chemical groups that aid breakdown in the gut include:

- the **acid of the stomach** itself
- **emulsifiers** which help to break insoluble chemicals into tiny droplets that enzymes can then act upon **(bile is an example** of a key emulsifier);
- **alkalines** – secreted in the **bile**, they are important as they **neutralise** the acid from the stomach. This **protects the intestine** and enhances the environment for the action of other secretions.

This range of digestive secretions break down the main **nutritional macromolecules** that constitute the bulk of what we eat: carbohydrates, fat and protein. They are also instrumental in the **release, modification** and **absorption** of just about every other nutrient.

This has huge significance for the **character of our diets** because quite simply, a dish is not balanced unless it stimulates secretion. If the ingredients of a dish are not tailored for its digestion then the results can be distinctly unpleasant.

The **starting point** for secretion stimulation comes before a meal has even begun, in the **stimulation of appetite**. **Appetisers** come in different forms. In **Britain** it might be a small glass of aromatic and sweet **sherry**, **angostura bitters**, or aromatic and **bitter gin and tonic.** In **Germany herbal bitters** are traditionally drunk before a meal. In the **Mediterranean** salty **olives** or an intensely **herbal fish** or **garlic soup** are often eaten, and in **China** small **salty fish** or **spicy shellfish** or **chicken wings or feet** are popular. All of these dishes and drinks **stimulate secretion** in preparation for the larger meal to come.

In the meal itself the key to managing secretion is the general **balance of flavours in the dish. Spicy aromatics and bitterness** are particularly good at stimulating secretion in the gut. **Sourness** is also important as it has a key role in the stimulation of bile secretion for the digestion of fats.

Bitter herbs and spices such as **basil, juniper, fenugreek and rosemary** are used extensively in **southern European cuisine and Chinese and Japanese** cooking is characterised by the use of **bitter greens**. The cornerstones of the Chinese kitchen are aromatic **spring onion**, and **spicy ginger, garlic and chilli.** They are there first and foremost for their stimulation of secretion and promotion of digestive strength. But these bitter, aromatic and spicy foods have **another key function**: they have expansive and moving qualities, which means that **stimulate motility.**

Exercise 1b

Match the column A with the column B. Try to learn the expressions and/or sentences by heart.

A

1. Food has to be first broken down into very small molecules,
2. Enzymes are proteins
3. Amylase, an enzyme that is secreted by the salivary gland
4. Enzymes that are secreted in the stomach, where it is very acidic
5. Other chemical groups that aid breakdown in the gut include
6. Alkalines secreted in the bile
7. Digestive secretions break down the main nutritional macromolecules that constitute the bulk of what we eat:
8. A dish is not balanced
9. The starting point for secretion stimulation
10. In the meal itself the key to managing secretion
11. Bitter, aromatic and spicy foods

B

a) carbohydrates, fat and protein.

b) comes in the stimulation of appetite.

c) is the general balance of flavours in the dish.

d) *neutralise the acid from the stomach which protects the intestine.*
e) *stimulate motility.*
f) *the acid of the stomach, emulsifiers which help to break insoluble chemicals into tiny droplets and alkalines secreted in the bile.*
g) *then absorbed through the membrane barrier into the blood stream, and finally taken to where it is needed in the body.*
h) *unless it stimulates secretion.*
i) *whose job is to make chemical reactions happen more easily.*
j) *work best in this acidity, and at body temperature.*
k) *works best in the slightly alkaline warm conditions that are found in the mouth.*

Exercise 2
Translate the expressions. Try to explain their meanings in English.

Human beings, vast majority, symbionts, crucial, DNA sequencing research, concluded, fundamental, inflammatory bowel disease, suppressing, harmful organisms, process fats, essential, probiosis, inevitable, seeding, conception, growth and survival, womb, picked up, at birth, passed on, caesarean section, incidence, serotonin, neurotransmitter, anxiety, organically managed soil, fermented food, hedgerows, woodlands, accompaniment, artificial sweeteners, destructive effect, sweeten, debilitating diseases, coincidentally, molecule size, initially, chomp, emulsifiers, seeking out, salivary gland, insoluble chemicals, constitute, bulk, instrumental, tailored, distinctly, flavours, bitterness, sourness, promotion, expansive, motility.

Exercise 3
Answer the following questions. Prepare short talks and/or dialogues on these topics.

1. Why are symbionts vital to healthy living?
2. What is the function of the symbionts in our guts?
3. Why is hygiene important?
4. What is seeding?
5. Why should we eat foods that are rich in bacteria?
6. Characterise artificial sweeteners.
7. What happens with the food in your body?
8. What is the function of enzymes?
9. Secretion stimulation and stimulation of appetite.
10. Balance of flavours in the dish (spicy aromatics, bitterness, sourness)

Vocabulary 2

Fill in the meanings in your mother language:

accompaniment /əˈkʌmpənɪmənt/
acidic /əˈsɪd.ɪk/
acidity /əˈsɪdɪtɪ/
act /ækt/
alkaline /ˈæl.kəl.aɪn/

allotment /əˈlɒtmənt/
amylase /ˈæm.ɪ.leɪz/
angostura /ˌæŋgəˈstjʊərə/
anxiety /æŋˈzaɪ.ə.ti/
appetiser /ˈæpɪˌtaɪzə/
appreciate /əˈpriː.ʃi.eɪt/
aromatic /ˌærəˈmætɪk/
artificial /ˌɑː.tɪˈfɪʃ.əl/
sweetener /ˈswiːtənə/
aspartame /əˈspɑːˌteɪm/
awareness /əˈweənɪs/
awesome /ˈɔːsəm/
barrier /ˈbær.i.ər/
basil /ˈbæzəl/
bedrock /ˈbedˌrɒk/
behalf /bɪˈhɑːf/
beyond /bɪˈjɒnd/
bile /baɪl/
biotin /ˈbaɪətɪn/
bitter /ˈbɪtə/
bloodstream /ˈblʌd.striːm/
bond /bɒnd/
bottom /ˈbɒtəm/
bowel /ˈbaʊ.əl/
breast /brest/ **milk** /mɪlk/
bug /bʌg/
bulk /bʌlk/
bunch /bʌntʃ/
buttermilk /ˈbʌtəˌmɪlk/
caesarean section /sɪˌzeə.ri.ənˈsek.ʃən/
chomp /tʃɒmp/
Clostridium /kləˈstrɪ.dɪ.əm/
coincidentally /kəʊˌɪnsɪˈdentəlɪ/
conception /kənˈsep.ʃən/
conclude /kənˈkluːd/
crucial /ˈkruː.ʃəl/
cuisine /kwɪˈziːn/
debilitating /dɪˈbɪl.ɪ.teɪt.ɪŋ/
declare /dɪˈkleə/
delicious /dɪˈlɪʃəs/
destructive /dɪˈstrʌk.tɪv/
dominate /ˈdɒm.ɪ.neɪt/
dreadful /ˈdredfʊl/
droplet /ˈdrɒplɪt/
emotion /ɪˈməʊ.ʃən/
emulsifier /ɪˈmʌlsɪˌfaɪə/
enemy /ˈenəmɪ/
enzyme /ˈen.zaɪm/
expansive /ɪkˈspænsɪv/
fenugreek /ˈfɛnjʊˌgriːk/
flavour /ˈfleɪ.vər/
foremost /ˈfɔːˌməʊst/
fulfil /fʊlˈfɪl/
fundamental /ˌfʌn.dəˈmen.təl/
fungus /ˈfʌŋ.gəs/ pl **fungi**
ginger /ˈdʒɪndʒə/
green /griːn/
grow /groʊ/ **(grew, grown)**
hedgerow /ˈhedʒˌrəʊ/
herbal /ˈhɜː.bəl/
human /ˈhjuː.mən/ **being** /ˈbiː.ɪŋ/
impact /ˈɪm.pækt/
implicate /ˈɪm.plɪ.keɪt/
incidence /ˈɪnt .sɪ.dənts/
inevitable /ɪnˈevɪtəbəl/
infamous /ɪnfəməs/
inflammatory /ɪnˈflæm.ə.tər.i/
initially /ɪˈnɪʃ.əl.i/
insoluble /ɪnˈsɒl.jʊ.bl̩/
instrumental /ˌɪnstrəˈmentəl/
intestine /ɪnˈtes.tɪn/
juniper /ˈdʒuːnɪpə/
line /laɪn/
membrane /ˈmem.breɪn/
methanol /ˈmɛθəˌnɒl/
muck /mʌk/
neurotransmitter /ˌnjʊə.rəʊ.trænzˈmɪt.ər/
particular /pəˈtɪk.jʊ.lər/
pathogenic /ˌpæθ.əˈdʒen.ɪk/
pick /pɪk/ **up** /ʌp/
pickled /ˈpɪkəld/
pitched /pɪtʃt/ **battle** /ˈbætəl/
polio /ˈpəʊlɪəʊ/
preserved /prɪˈzɜːvd/
probiosis /proʊˈbaɪəʊsɪs/
protozoan /ˌprəʊ.təˈzəʊ.ən/ pl **protozoa**
range /reɪndʒ/
regarding /rɪˈgɑː.dɪŋ/
relationship /rɪˈleɪ.ʃən.ʃɪp/

release /rəˈliːs/
research /rɪˈsɜːtʃ/
reveal /rɪˈviːl/
review /rɪˈvjuː/
rosemary /ˈrəʊzmərɪ/
salivary /səˈlaɪ.vər.i/ **gland** /glænd/
sauerkraut /ˈsaʊəˌkraʊ/
seed /siːd/
seek /siːk/ **(sought, sought)**
sequence /ˈsiːkwəns/
serotonin /ˌse.rəˈtəʊ.nɪn/
sherry /ˈʃerɪ/
significance /sɪgˈnɪfɪkəns/
sinus /ˈsaɪ.nəs/ pl **sinuses**
snip /snɪp/
soil /sɔɪl/
sour /ˈsaʊə/
spicy /ˈspaɪsɪ/
Staphylococcus /ˌstæf.ɪl.əˈkɒk.əs/ pl **Staphylococci** /ˈkɒk.saɪ/
stevia /ˈstɛv i ə/
stomach /ˈstʌm.ək/
substance /ˈsʌb.stəns/
sucralose /ˈsu krəˌloʊs/
suppress /səˈpres/
sweeten /ˈswiːtən/
symbiotic /sɪmbɪˈɔtɪk/
tailored /ˈteɪləd/
tiny /ˈtaɪ.ni/
upset /ʌpˈset/
uterus /ˈjuː.tər.əs/ pl **uteri**
vital /ˈvaɪ.təl/
weaning /wiːnɪŋ/
wing /wɪŋ/
womb /wuːm/
woodland /ˈwʊdlənd/

Solution to Exercise 1a
1e, 2d, 3b, 4h, 5j, 6a, 7c, 8f, 9i, 10g

Solution to Exercise 1b
1g, 2i, 3k, 4j, 5f, 6d, 7a, 8h, 9b, 10c, 11e

Unit 3 - Motility. Emotion and digestion.

In any natural context **the essence of health is harmonious movement**. The same principle applies to our digestion. If our blood keeps circulating and the food moves smoothly through our guts, then we are healthy. If **blood and food stagnate, pain and disease** will occur.

The need to achieve this slow, constant movement of food through our bodies is revealed in the structure of our guts. The **digestive tract** is essentially **a long muscular tube,** divided into separate parts with **specific functions** which are reflected in their form.

Food is first **chewed and passed down the oesophagus** into the **stomach**, which is like **a muscular bag**. There, the food is **stored and broken down**, before slowly being **pushed into the small intestine** where it is further broken down, and **absorbed**. It then passes to the **colon and rectum**, where **water** is **reabsorbed** and further **digestive processes** take place. Finally, **waste** products are **expelled**.

So we eat food, it is broken down, transformed, absorbed, and finally excreted, a series of processes that rely on precisely controlled, smooth and **constant movement** from the top to the bottom of the gut. We need power for this movement, which is why the gut is so muscular.

Peristalsis

Gut muscles contract in sequential waves, **pushing the food** from one part of the digestive tract to the next, a precisely controlled process that is called peristalsis.

Peristalsis depends on the bewilderingly complex Enteric Nervous System (ENS). Like all complex systems, the ENS is easily disrupted and hence its function needs to be actively protected. **If this function is not protected** the result will be familiar in some form to most: **trapped wind, bloating, abdominal and gastric pain, poor absorption**. We can add the **constipation** and **diarrhoea** found in **Irritable Bowel Syndrome** (IBS) to the list of **poor motility symptoms.**

The **pain** from poor motility can be excruciating and crippling. The events in one part of the gut can also cause loss of motility in another. For example, it is not unusual to experience bloating and trapped wind, largely in the colon, having just eaten a meal. But this is a result of food that is still sitting in the stomach.

Most of us have experienced discomfort from poor motility; a significant proportion of the population experiences these symptoms frequently. Our digestive systems are under constant daily strain as the three major factors that impact on motility are very commonplace. And since **the functions of digestion** are so **intimately linked**, the **same factors** often also **impact on symbiosis and secretion**. These three factors are **emotion, climate and diet.**

Exercise 1a
Match the column A with the column B. Try to learn the expressions and/or sentences by heart.

A

1. If our blood keeps circulating and the food moves smoothly through our guts,
2. The digestive tract is essentially a long muscular tube,
3. Food is first chewed
4. In the stomach, the food is stored and broken down,
5. Food then passes to the colon and rectum,
6. Finally,
7. Gut muscles contract in sequential waves, pushing the food from one part of the digestive tract to the next,
8. Peristalsis depends on
9. If the Enteric Nervous System is not protected
10. The events in one part of the gut
11. Since the functions of digestion are so intimately linked,

B

a) *a precisely controlled process that is called peristalsis.*
b) *and passed down the oesophagus into the stomach.*

c) *before slowly being pushed into the small intestine.*
d) *can also cause loss of motility in another.*
e) *divided into separate parts with specific functions.*
f) *Enteric Nervous System.*
g) *the result will be trapped wind, bloating, abdominal and gastric pain, poor absorption, constipation and diarrhoea found in Irritable Bowel Syndrome.*
h) *the same factors often also impact on symbiosis and secretion.*
i) *then we are healthy.*
j) *waste products are expelled.*
k) *where water is reabsorbed and further digestive processes take place.*

Emotion and digestion

Many of **the nerves in the ENS** are hitched up to **gut muscles**; they are "motor" nerves, These are the nerves that **control peristalsis**. The digestive tract is made up of very nervous organs. The stomach is second only to the heart and the brain in the secretion of a special group of molecules called **neuropeptides**, molecules that are central to emotional reactions. The result of this is that strong emotions such as **stress and anxiety** are able to **inhibit motility.**

The kind of constant, **intense feelings** associated with stress and anxiety **activate the sympathetic nervous system**, our so called "fight, flight or freeze" nerves, which effectively shut down gut motility and secretion. **Blood leaves the gut** and surges to our arms, and legs, so that we can either defend our patch (fight), leg it (flight) or just plain panic (freeze). The result is not good for digestion

Mild examples of this sympathetic nervous reaction include pre-math butterflies and first-date appetite loss. But the constant nervous stimulation that we associate with stress can lead to extreme reactions like the **nervous vomiting and severe gut cramps**. While stress and anxiety inhibit motility and secretion, calm protects them.

Contrasting lifestyles

Many of us don't eat breakfast or lunch; or breakfast on the hoof, with working lunches and TV dinners increasingly the norm. This **constant stress, stimulation and distraction** erodes our digestive strength and motility, causing **stagnation, fatigue** and, in the long term, **potentially life-threatening disorders** such as cardiovascular disease. As part of our healthy diet we definitely need to create space for eating and digestion just like our ancestors did.

Climate and digestion

Scientifically speaking, it's rather tenuous to relate climate with healthy digestion. But, in fact, throughout history humans have linked their digestive health to their surroundings. And the effects of climate on digestion are palpable today. Ever lost your appetite in heat and humidity, or felt tired after lunch on a cold, damp, drizzly day? Or woken up feeling stodgy with a poor appetite on a damp morning?

The gut's highly muscular nature means that it requires a prodigious blood flow to work effectively, hence **digestion occupies up to 30% of our metabolism.** The **impact of the climate** on us **is intense,** yet our modern dietary culture and lifestyles are disconnected from it in direct contrast to our ancestors. To get back to a healthy diet, we need to re-establish our connection with climate. Cold salads and insipid clammy sandwiches should be made a thing of the past, and replaced with warm, nourishing, aromatic soups, stews and casseroles.

Food choices to match emotion and climate

We need to look at **the way in which specific foods affect the gut's workings**, which foods are good, and which foods do us harm. What we eat is what the digestive system exists to process and the nature of the food to be processed can either break down easily to help the gut with its work, or it can be stubborn and sit in our bellies, like a lump.

Easily broken-down food enhances motility and takes the strain off secretion. The gut muscles don't have to work too hard, peristalsis is smooth and blood circulation is uninhibited.

Overly rich, goopy, sticky or over-fibrous food, and substances that quickly upset the balance of the gut and its symbionts – like the classic **junk-food ingredients**: refined sugar, artificial sweeteners and white wheat flour – have the opposite effect. These sort of foods are either **too hard to break down**, or generate **irritating chemicals**, so that the gut has to work overtime to move them along. This causes a lot of **strain**. That's why many of us get a stomach ache after Christmas lunch. Our digestion is overwhelmed, the body normally shuts down and goes to sleep, and gut motility suffers.

Two groups of foods are particularly important, **fatty foods** and **raw fruit and vegetables**. Both of these food types are **hard-to-digest** but both are **essential ingredients** for a healthy diet, making processing for digestibility absolutely vital to avoid diet-relating illness.

Exercise 1b
Match the column A with the column B. Try to learn the expressions and/ or sentences by heart.

A

1. Many of the nerves in the ENS
2. Strong emotions such as stress and anxiety
3. Intense feelings
4. Blood leaves the gut and surges to our arms, and legs,
5. Constant nervous stimulation
6. Constant stress, stimulation and distraction erodes our digestive strength and motility,

7. Throughout history humans
8. The gut's highly muscular nature means
9. Easily broken-down food enhances motility
10. Overly rich, goopy, sticky or over-fibrous food, and substances that quickly upset the balance of the gut and its symbionts
11. Two groups of foods are particularly important,

B

a) activate the sympathetic nervous system.
b) and takes the strain off secretion.
c) are able to inhibit motility.
d) can lead to nervous vomiting and severe gut cramps.
e) causing stagnation, fatigue and, in the long term, potentially life-threatening disorders.
f) control peristalsis.
g) fatty foods and raw fruit and vegetables.
h) have linked their digestive health to their surroundings.
i) like the classic junk-food ingredients have the opposite effect.
j) so that we can either defend our patch (fight), leg it (flight) or just plain panic (freeze).
k) that it requires a prodigious blood flow to work effectively.

Exercise 2
Translate the expressions. Try to explain their meanings in English.

Motility principle, stagnate, constant movement, muscular tube, separate parts, small intestine, colon, rectum, expelled, constant, movement, peristalsis, disrupted, protected, bloating, constipation, diarrhoea, irritable bowel syndrome, discomfort, strain, intimately linked, impact on, hitched up, motor nerves, neuropeptides, inhibit motility, shut down, defend, butterflies, appetite loss, gut cramps, on the hoof, distraction, erodes, stagnation, fatigue, life-threatening disorders, surroundings, effects of climate, heat and humidity, felt tired, damp, drizzly, feeling stodgy, prodigious blood flow, impact of the climate, establish connection, nourishing, match, affect the gut's workings, do harm, nature of the food, be stubborn, overly rich, goopy, sticky, over-fibrous food, upset the balance, junk-food, generate, irritating chemicals, overwhelmed, essential ingredients, digestibility.

Exercise 3
Answer the following questions. Prepare short talks and/or dialogues on these topics.

1. What do you understand by the term motility?
2. What do you understand by the term peristalsis?
3. What is the relation between emotion and digestion?

4. Explain "fight, flight or freeze" reaction.
5. How can our lifestyles influence digestion?
6. What kinds of food are suitable for our digestion?

Vocabulary 3

Fill in the meanings in your mother language:

abdominal /æbˈdɒm.ɪ.nəl/
achieve /əˈtʃiːv/
ancestor /ˈænsestə/
belly /ˈbelɪ/
bloating /ˈbləʊ.tɪŋ/
butterfly /ˈbʌtəˌflaɪ/
calm /kɑːm/
clammy /ˈklæm.i/
colon /ˈkəʊ.lɒn/
commonplace /ˈkɒm.ən.pleɪs/
constant /ˈkɒn.stənt/
constipation /ˌkɒnt .stɪˈpeɪ.ʃən/
crippling /ˈkrɪplɪŋ/
defend /dɪˈfend/
diarrhoea /ˌdaɪ.əˈriː.ə/
digestibility /daɪˌdʒestəˈbɪlɪtɪ/
discomfort /dɪˈskʌm.fət/
disconnected /ˌdɪskəˈnektɪd/
disrupt /dɪsˈrʌpt/
distraction /dɪˈstræk.ʃən/
drizzly /ˈdrɪzlɪ/
erode /ɪˈrəʊd/
essence /ˈesəns/
essential /ɪˈsen.t ʃəl/
excruciating /ɪkˈskruː.ʃi.eɪ.tɪŋ/
expel /ɪkˈspel/
fatigue /fəˈtiːg/
feeling /ˈfiː.lɪŋ/
fight or flight /ˌfaɪt.ɔː.ˈflaɪt/
gastric /ˈgæs.trɪk/
generate /ˈdʒen.ər.eɪt/
goopy /ˈgu pi/
harmonious /hɑːˈməʊnɪəs/
hitch /hɪtʃ/
hoof /huːf/
humidity /hjuːˈmɪd.ɪ.ti/
increasingly /ɪnˈkriː.sɪŋ.li/
inhibit /ɪnˈhɪb.ɪt/
insipid /ɪnˈsɪpɪd/
intense /ɪnˈtens/
intimately /ˈɪntɪmɪtlɪ/
irritable /ˈɪr.ɪ.tə.bl̩/
irritating /ˈɪr.ɪ.teɪ.tɪŋ/
leg /leg/
lump /lʌmp/
motor /ˈməʊ.tər/
movement /ˈmuːv.mənt/
muscular /ˈmʌs.kjʊ.lər/
neuropeptide /ˌnjʊərəʊˈpɛptaɪd/
nourishing /ˈnʌrɪʃɪŋ/
oesophagus /ɪˈsɒf.ə.gəs/
opposite /ˈɒp.ə.zɪt/
overly /əʊvəlɪ/
overwhelm /ˌəʊ.vəˈwelm/
pain /peɪn/
palpable /ˈpælpəbəl/
panic /ˈpænɪk/
pass /pɑːs/
past /pɑːst/
patch /pætʃ/
peristalsis /ˌpɛrɪˈstælsɪs/
precisely /prɪˈsaɪslɪ/
processing /ˈprəʊsesɪŋ/
prodigious /prəˈdɪdʒəs/
raw /rɔː/
re-establish /ˌriː.ɪˈstæb.lɪʃ/
rectum /ˈrek.təm/ pl **recta**
relate /rɪˈleɪt/
sequential /sɪˈkwenʃəl/
shut /ʃʌt/ **down** /daʊn/
small /smɔːl/ **intestine** /ɪnˈtes.tɪn/
smoothly /ˈsmuːð.li/
stagnate /ˈstægˌneɪt/
stagnation /stægˈneɪʃən/
sticky /ˈstɪk.i/
stodgy /ˈstɒdʒɪ/
strain /streɪn/
stubborn /ˈstʌbən/

surge /sɜːdʒ/
sympathetic /ˌsɪm.pəˈθe.tɪk/
tenuous /ˈtenjʊəs/
throughout /θruːˈaʊt/
trapped /træpd/
tube /tjuːb/
uninhibited /ˌʌnɪnˈhɪbɪtɪd/
wave /weɪv/
wind /wɪnd/
working /ˈwɜːkɪŋ/

Solution to Exercise 1a
1i, 2e, 3b, 4c, 5k, 6j, 7a, 8f, 9g, 10d, 11h

Solution to Exercise 1b
1f, 2c, 3a, 4j, 5d, 6e, 7h, 8k, 9b, 10i, 11g

Unit 4 - Fatty foods. Raw foods and the importance of cooking 1.

A balanced nutritious diet should include **fatty foods,** particularly the increasingly appreciated **essential fatty acids (EFAs)** that are abundant in foods like the herring. EFAs **nourish the membranes of every cell** in our bodies, they constitute the **bulk of our nervous systems** and they underpin important **hormone** manufacture and secretion. But fats are rich foods and they **obstruct motility**; they are really hard to shunt along the gut. The answer to this problem has been to **combine fats with flavours** that help to **break down fat globules** and molecules, and also to include flavours that **stimulate motility** to move the fat along the gut.

Sour is the flavour that helps to break up fats. Sour flavours tend to be acidic, such as the acetic acid in vinegar. They will **raise the overall acidity** of a dish and thus the acidity of the stomach, which **stimulates the hormonal pathway**s that cause the **release of bile into the small intestine.** Bile has the effect of breaking up fat globules into **smaller droplets** which can then be more easily moved, broken down and absorbed. Sour should be combined with the motility-stimulating flavours that help to move the fat droplets along the gut: spicy aromatics and bitterness. These flavours must be combined with sourness in the digestion of fats, as sourness, though very good at helping to break down fats, is also astringent and so can have the effect of inhibiting motility.

Thus the **expanding movement achieved by aromatics and spice** and the **downward movement achieved by bitterness** work together to stimulate motility and balance out the inhibitory and contracting astringency of sourness. This is why **condiments that accompany fatty foods**, such as **chutneys and pickles** are **spicy and aromatic, sour and bitter**. These flavours are essential companions to fatty foods as they stimulate the processes that break up fat and move it along the gut. Compare this traditional approach to the way that we eat a modern-day high-street sausage roll or pie. Such products are normally eaten on their own, or sometimes with tomato ketchup that is so bland and sweet that is it more like jam.

Fatty foods + sourness + spicy aromatics = good motility

- **Sourness** often comes from **vinegar or lemon juice**
- **Aromatic spice and bitterness** might come from **juniper, allspice, turmeric, fenugreek, cumin, coriander, cayenne pepper and black peppercorns** (for example the mint sauce that is traditionally served with fatty lamb is a simple combination of sour vinegar and aromatic mint.)

Exercise 1a
Match the column A with the column B. Try to learn the expressions and/or sentences by heart.

A

1. Essential fatty acids nourish the membranes of every cell in our bodies,
2. Sour flavours will raise the overall acidity of a dish and thus the acidity of the stomach,
3. Bile has the effect of breaking up fat globules into smaller droplets
4. Sour should be combined with the motility-stimulating flavours
5. The expanding movement achieved by aromatics and spice

B

a) and the downward movement achieved by bitterness work together to stimulate motility.
b) that help to move the fat droplets along the gut: spicy aromatics and bitterness.
c) they constitute the bulk of our nervous systems and they underpin important hormone manufacture and secretion.
d) which can then be more easily moved, broken down and absorbed.
e) which stimulates the hormonal pathways that cause the release of bile into the small intestine.

Raw foods and the importance of cooking 1

Raw foods present **a different kind of digestive challenge** to fatty foods. Human beings are not designed to digest raw food. And this is reflected in the structure and function of our digestive systems. So today we find raw food **too tough;** it sits around in our guts, challenging the balance of our symbionts, **generating wind and obstructing motility**. And, in the case of fruit and vegetables, much of it pass through undigested. There are sound physiological reasons why humans find raw food hard to digest, which become obvious when we examine the digestive adaptations of other mammals. Wild cats, for example, eat almost exclusively raw meat and bones, and their digestive systems are fit for purpose

– extremely acidic in order to break down the fibrous connective tissue and kill the bugs that tend to fester in old meat. And, like raw meat with its resilient connective tissue, raw fruit and vegetables have **structures made up of molecules, cellulose and lignin**, which are so tough that we simply cannot digest them.

Plant eaters in the animal kingdom get around this problem by relying very heavily on fermentation. All mammalian herbivores have regions of their anatomy that are enlarged for the storage of huge numbers of symbiotic bacteria. These bacteria then have a chance to go to work on breaking down that tough, fibrous material, converting the plant matter into nutrients that the animals are then able to absorb and use. For cows, this fermentation vat is the stomach, giving them their characteristic barrel bellies. For rabbits and horses it's the caecum, the so-called hind gut, which contains a mixture of friendly fermenters. Rabbits even eat their own stools so that they get a chance to ferment their food twice. Closer to us on the evolutionary tree, primates have long intestines to house bacteria and to aid absorption: this is why they sport pot bellies. In addition, like herbivores that chew the cud, primates spend a long time chewing to break down the physical structures of the food. All of these **behavioural and anatomical adaptations** mean that different species tend to be very specialised in what they eat, as they are built to digest a relatively narrow range of foodstuffs.

Humans, by contrast, have a **hugely varied diet,** if we consider what is eaten in different parts of the globe. **Roots, seeds, fruits, vegetables, worms, grubs, insects, seafood, birds** and a wide range of **mammals** are all included. No animal on the planet matches humans in terms of the variety of foods that they consume. And, yet, if we ate large amounts of any of this food raw we would get a mighty stomach-ache or even food poisoning. To avoid this kind of digestive stress we have **a key biological adaptation** – we transform our food by **peeling, chopping, cooking and external fermentation**. The use of these processes means that effectively humans have always eaten their food **pre-digested**; we have to because we can't cope with tough, fibrous food.

Since **our stomachs aren't that acidic, our guts aren't that long and we don't have a specifically enlarged "fermentation vessel" part** like other mammal plant eaters, **we can't handle the food** the other mammals eat, **in its raw state**. However our energy-hungry brains, which require a quarter of all our energy, place and intense burden on our relatively weak digestions. Therefore, **cooking our food** has always underpinned our survival as human beings. Cooking means that we can eat food faster without having to chew as much, since the heat of cooking **breaks up larger molecules and structures in the**

food. We can also get more energy from it when it gets into our guts because we are relieved of the need to spend energy on breaking down remaining complex chemical structures. This is a great benefit as **digestion** already **consumes a third of our metabolic energy**.

Exercise 1b
Match the column A with the column B. Try to learn the expressions and/ or sentences by heart.

A

1. We find raw food too tough; it sits around in our guts,
2. Raw fruit and vegetables have structures made up of molecules, cellulose and lignin,
3. Humans have a hugely varied diet,
4. We have a key biological adaptation,
5. Cooking means that we can eat food faster without having to chew as much,

B

a) generating wind and obstructing motility.
b) roots, seeds, fruits, vegetables, worms, grubs, insects, seafood, birds and a wide range of mammals are all included.
c) since the heat of cooking breaks up larger molecules and structures in the food.
d) we transform our food by peeling, chopping, cooking and external fermentation.
e) which are so tough that we simply cannot digest them.

Exercise 2
Translate the expressions. Try to explain their meanings in English.

Essential fatty acids, abundant, nourish, hormone manufacture, obstruct motility, fat globules, sour flavours, overall acidity, release of bile, small intestine, moved, broken down, absorbed, spicy aromatics, bitterness, astringent, expanding movement, downward, condiments, traditional approach, bland, raw foods, human beings, too tough, pass through, digestive adaptations, mammals, fibrous, connective tissue, resilient, relying on, herbivores, converting, fermentation, caecum, species, narrow range, food poisoning, adaptation, transform, cope with, plant eaters, intense burden, complex chemical structures.

Exercise 3
Answer the following questions. Prepare short talks and/or dialogues on these topics.

1. Why are essential fatty acids appreciated?
2. Why is it suitable to combine fatty foods with flavours?
3. Why should sour be combined with spicy aromatics and bitterness?
4. Why do humans find raw food hard to digest?

5. Talk about behavioural and anatomical adaptations of mammalian herbivores (cows, rabbits, horses, primates).
6. Give examples of foods eaten in different parts of the globe (roots, seeds, fruits, vegetables, worms, grubs, insects, seafood, birds, mammals).
7. How to cope with tough, fibrous food (peeling, chopping, cooking and external fermentation) ?
8. Why is cooking so important?

Vocabulary 4

Fill in the meanings in your mother language:

abundant /ə'bʌn.dənt/
acetic /ə'si:tɪk/ **acid** /'æsɪd/
adaptation /ˌæd.əp'teɪ.ʃən/
allspice /ɔ:lˌspaɪs/
astringent /ə'strɪn.dʒənt/
barrel /'bær.əl/
bland /blænd/
burden /'bɜ:.dən/
caecum /'si:.kəm/
cayenne /keɪ'en/ **pepper** /pepə/
challenge /'tʃæl.ɪndʒ/
chop /tʃɒp/
chutney /tʃʌtnɪ/
companion /kəm'pænjən/
connective /kəˌnek.tɪv/
convert /kən'vɜ:t/
coriander /ˌkɒrɪ'ændə/
cud /kʌd/
cumin /'kʌmɪn/
distinctly /dɪ'stɪŋktlɪ/
evolutionary /ˌi:və'lu:ʃənərɪ/
fermentation /ˌfɜr.men'teɪ.ʃən/
fester /'festə/
fibrous /'faɪ.brəs/
globule/'glɒbju:l/
grub /grʌb/
herbivore /'hɜ:bɪˌvɔ:/
hind /haɪnd/ **gut** /gʌt/
lamb /læm/
lignin /'lɪgnɪn/
mammal /'mæm.əl/
mighty /'maɪtɪ/
obstruct /əb'strʌkt/
obvious /'ɒb.vi.əs/
pathway /'pɑ:θˌweɪ]/
peel /pi:l/
peppercorn /'pepəˌkɔ:n/
pie /paɪ/
pot belly /'pɒtˌbelɪ/
roll /rəʊl/
root /ru:t/
shunt /ʃʌnt/
sport /spɔ:t/
tough /tʌf/
turmeric /'tɜ:mərɪk/
vat /væt/
vinegar /'vɪn.ɪ.gər/
worm /wɜ:m/

Solution to Exercise 1a
1c, 2e, 3d, 4b, 5a

Solution to Exercise 1b
1a, 2e, 3b, 4d, 5c

Unit 5 - Raw foods and the importance of cooking 2. The flavour principle.

If we ate only raw food, our guts would consume even more energy digesting and we would have to chew for at least six hours a day. Appreciation of these **biological facts** is very important because, while

healthy motility and symbiotic balance underpins the **digestion** of all mammals alike, each species achieves these balances in a different way, through **different behaviours, different gut structures** and **different food choices**. To be healthy, we need to make uniquely human choices: that means cooking our food. **Cooked food** is **more digestible** and thus kinder to motility and absorption.

If the scientific and anthropological evidence clearly indicates that we should not be eating a diet mainly composed of raw food, why do so many restaurants menus, health retreats and books still advocate its consumption? **Raw foodism** is a classic example of a fad that is based on scientific language, but **not on sound scientific arguments**. To clarify, here are the key claims of the "raw food" diet and explanations as to why they are inaccurate:

1. **Claim: Raw food preserves vital enzymes, otherwise denatured by cooking**

Raw foodism suggests that humans need the help of enzymes in food to be able to digest it effectively. There is **no good scientific evidence** for this claim. Enzymes are proteins that are mostly denatured by our own stomach acid. The food-derived enzymes are in fact digested by the **special protease enzymes** secreted in our stomachs (which are not denatured by the stomach acid as they are specifically adapted to working in a very acidic environment). Rather than the enzymes helping us to digest, we digest the food enzymes themselves. Any "**vital enzymes**" which survive the stomach to get to the **small intestine**, and which aren't locked up in indigestible raw food material, probably would not work properly there either, as the small intestine is an **intensely alkaline** environment which would also distort and denature the plant enzymes.

It is also quite possible that as **our body temperature** (around 37ºC), is higher than the ambient temperature to which most plants that we eat are adapted, the plant enzyme function would be compromised. So any help that we might get from "vital enzymes" would be minuscule to the point of insignificance relative to the massive amount of digestive enzymes that we already produce for ourselves.

2. **Claim: Raw food is more nutritious as cooking destroys nutrients**

Cooking does destroy nutrients, but it also makes them more available than they would be from raw food, by **breaking down the tough or fibrous structures** of the food and allowing for **easier absorption**. So in real terms, cooked food is more nutritious than raw food. A specific example of a nutrient that is less easily absorbed from raw food because of its indigestibility is carotene from carrots. In addition, cooking helps to enhance the nutrient content of foods by **forming new essential nutrients**, such as lycopene from tomatoes.

3. Claim: Raw food benefits health through detoxication of the body

Although it sounds like it, "detoxification" is not a scientific term. It is used to explain away the fact that people feel awful on a raw-food diet because it is not healthy and sustaining. If worried about specific toxicity, why not eat food that is fresh, from non-toxic agriculture and cooked by boiling or steaming so that no toxins develop in the first place? Ironically, raw-food diets may actually be more toxic than cooked diets. **Cooking destroys toxins**: this is why we cook potatoes and beans. Also raw food upsets the symbiotic balance, which is why it makes us fart so much; and when the gut flora struggles it produces irritant chemicals that have a toxic effect.

The **raw food movement** started in the desert states of southern USA as a Caucasian adaptation to the searing and desiccating climate. Raw vegetables were felt to have a **hydrating and cooling effect** and were considered significant remedial foodstuff. But the same principle is not appropriate for cold and damp temperature climate at all. A high proportion of **raw-foodists** are suffering **low body mass and chronic fatigue.** Fifty percent of the women on the diet ceased to menstruate and men suffer low libidity; there is a very high level of **infertility** among both men and women. None of these are indicators of good health.

Exercise 1a
Match the column A with the column B. Try to learn the expressions and/or sentences by heart.

A

1. Cooked food is more digestible
2. Cooking does destroy nutrients,
3. Coking helps to enhance the nutrient content of foods
4. Cooking destroys toxins:
5. The raw food movement started in the desert states of southern USA
6. Raw vegetables were felt to have a hydrating and cooling effect
7. The same principle is not appropriate

B

a) and thus kinder to motility and absorption.
b) and were considered significant remedial foodstuff.
c) as a Caucasian adaptation to the searing and desiccating climate.
d) but it also makes them more available than they would be from raw food, by breaking down the tough or fibrous structures of the food and allowing for easier absorption.
e) by forming new essential nutrients, such as lycopene from tomatoes.

f) for cold and damp temperature climate at all.

g) this is why we cook potatoes and beans.

The flavour principle

The **basic flavours** are as follows:

- natural **sweetness** to **nourish symbionts**
- **sourness** to **cut through fats**
- **bitterness, spice and aromatics** to **stimulate secretion and motility**
- **salt** to **stimulate appetite**

In the days before the development of nutritional chemistry, flavour was the main tool for the analysis and classification of foods. **Individual foods** or **combinations** of foods were said to **strengthen**, **invigorate**, **cleanse**, **refresh**, **decongest**, **calm**, **move**, **heat**, **cool**, **cause sweating** and **nourish** the body, all according to their **flavour** or **blends** of flavours. This was the traditional language of diet. It would be impossible to summarise in a properly scientific way the interaction of all the chemicals in the foods that we ingest, or how they react with us once we have eaten them.

There are simply **too many chemicals and processes** to take into account, in any practical or accessible way. What we can do, however, is to continue to base our dietary system on flavour, as humans have done for millennia. All the **nutritional chemical classes** have their own **distinctive flavours** (**acids are sour, alkaloids are bitter, aromatic oils are aromatic, sugars are sweet, glutamates are savoury**) and flavours do reflect the chemical constituents of food, and hence their actions in terms of health, accurately.

There are slight variations in the classification of flavours in different countries and traditions, e.g. the **Chinese tradition** of five flavours:

- sweet
- salty/savoury
- sour
- bitter
- spicy/aromatic

Flavour – science and tradition

For a long time scientists have recognised **four flavour categories**: bitter, salty, sour and sweet. **Chinese** tradition **adds spicy/ aromatic** to this and **Ayurveda** (the traditional health practice of **India**) a further category – **astringent**.

Ancient Greek and Roman medical commentators, including **Hippocrates** and **Galen** (Galen was a Greek living in Rome), on whose work the institutional **Western European dietetic traditions** were largely based, recognised as many as **nine flavours** but their categories still displayed similar characteristic to those of the Chinese. Another flavour, **umami**, was officially recognised in 1908. This is the taste of glutamates and nucleotides, but, since umami is basically a flavour **enhancer that acts on salt** in particular, it tends not to occupy its own category in traditional systems.

However, to take account of the importance of savoury flavours such as umami in cooking, not just for salt, the salty category is referred to as **salty/savoury**. Interestingly, receptors on the tongue for another taste that is not included in traditional systems have just been discovered: **fat**. This emphasises the importance of this nutrient in human evolution and health. Like umami it would either act as a **flavour enhancer** in general or be classified as savoury (or sometimes sweet, especially when cooked)

Exercise 1b
Match the column A with the column B. Try to learn the expressions and/or sentences by heart.

A

1. The basic flavours are as follows:
2. In the days before the development of nutritional chemistry,
3. Individual foods or combinations of foods were said
4. All the nutritional chemical classes have their own distinctive flavours
5. For a long time scientists have recognised
6. Umami is basically a flavour enhancer
7. Receptors on the tongue for another taste

B

a) *(acids are sour, alkaloids are bitter, aromatic oils are aromatic, sugars are sweet, glutamates are savoury).*
b) *flavour was the main tool for the analysis and classification of food.*
c) *four flavour categories: bitter, salty, sour and sweet.*
d) *natural sweetness to nourish symbionts, sourness to cut through fats, bitterness, spice and aromatics to stimulate secretion and motility, salt to stimulate appetite.*
e) *that acts on salt in particular.*
f) *that is not included in traditional systems have just been discovered: fat.*
g) *to strengthen, invigorate, cleanse, refresh, decongest, calm, move, heat, cool, cause sweating and nourish the body.*

Exercise 2
Translate the expressions. Try to explain their meanings in English.

Consume, appreciation, underpins, mammals, behaviours, composed of, health retreats, advocate, clarify, inaccurate, denatured, specifically adapted, locked up, indigestible, alkaline, distort, ambient, compromised, insignificance, destroys nutrients, indigestibility, sounds like, feel awful, sustaining, boiling or steaming, upsets the balance, struggles, irritant chemicals, remedial foodstuff, infertility, indicators, sweetness, nourish, sourness, bitterness, strengthen, invigorate, cleanse, refresh, decongest, calm, move, sweating, blends, summarise, ingest, take into account, distinctive, constituents, accurately, savoury, spicy, recognised, astringent, displayed, flavour enhancer, take account of, receptors, emphasises, in general.

Exercise 3
Answer the following questions. Prepare short talks and/or dialogues on these topics.

1. What do we need to be healthy?
2. Why should we not be eating a diet mainly composed of raw food?
3. In real terms, is raw food more nutritious than cooked food?
4. May raw-food diets actually be more toxic than cooked diets?
5. What are the basic flavours?
6. Explain the terms: strengthen, invigorate, cleanse, refresh, decongest, calm, move, heat, cool, cause sweating and nourish the body.
7. What are the flavours of the nutritional chemical classes (acids, alkaloids, aromatic oils, sugars, glutamates)?

Vocabulary 5

Fill in the meanings in your mother language:

accurately /ˈæk.jʊ.rət.li/
advocate /ˈæd.vəˌkeɪt/
alkaloid /ˈæl.kə.lɔɪd/
ambient /ˈæm.bi.ənt/
awful /ˈɔːfʊl/
blend /blend/
carotene /ˈkærəˌtiːn/
Caucasian /kɔːˈkeɪ.ʒən/
cease /siːs/
claim /kleɪm/
clarify /ˈklær.ɪ.faɪ/
cleanse /klenz/
compromise /ˈkɒmprəˌmaɪz/
decongest /dɪ kənˈdʒest/
denature /diːˈneɪtʃə/
desert /ˈdezət/
desiccated /ˈdesɪˌkeɪtɪd/
destroy /dɪˈstrɔɪ/
distort /dɪˈstɔːt/
emphasise /ˈemfəˌsaɪz/
fart /fɑːt/
glutamate /ˈgluː.tə.meɪt/
inaccurate /ɪˈnæk.jʊ.rət/
indicator /ˈɪn.dɪ.keɪ.tər/
indigestible /ˌɪndɪˈdʒɛstəbəl/
infertility /ˌɪn.fəˈtɪl.ɪ.ti/
insignificance /ˌɪnsɪgˈnɪfɪkəns/
invigorate /ɪnˈvɪgəˌreɪt/
irritant /ˈɪr.ɪ.tənt/
libido /lɪˈbiːdəʊ/
locked /lɒkt/ **up** /ʌp/
lycopene /ˈlaɪkəˌpiːn/
minuscule /ˈmɪnəˌskjuːl/
move /muːv/
nourish /ˈnʌrɪʃ/
nucleotide /ˈnjuːklɪəˌtaɪd/
plant /plɑːnt/
protease /ˈprəʊ.tiː.eɪz/
recognise /ˈrɛk əgˌnaɪz/
refresh /rɪˈfreʃ/

relative /'rel.ə.tɪv/
remedial /rɪ'miːdɪəl/
retreat /rɪ'triːt/
savoury /'seɪvərɪ/
searing /'sɪərɪŋ/
strengthen /'streŋθən/
struggle /'strʌgəl/
sweating /swet.ɪŋ/
tool /tuːl/
umami /uː'mɑː.mi/
uniquely /juː'niːk.li/
upset /ʌp'set/

Solution to Exercise 1a
1a, 2d, 3e, 4g, 5c, 6b, 7f

Solution to Exercise 1b
1d, 2b, 3g, 4a, 5c, 6e, 7f

Unit 6 - Sweet. Salty/savoury.

We all have an instinctive love for this flavour, which exists for good reason. **Sweetness** reflects the **sugar content** of foods, which **provides the calories** to sustain us in our day-to-day lives.

This ongoing energetic sustenance means that in traditional terms sweetness is known as the strengthening **flavour** – the one that more than any other builds strength, and digestive strength in particular. As such, it is **ideal for staple foods** – those that form the foundation and **bulk of your healthy diet.** If you look at the table of staple foods, you will see that they are usually slightly sweet in nature. They might be referred to as sweet and "bland".

This **balance of sweetness with blandness** is particularly important for our **symbiotic bacteria** which we carry with us are like a special culture that **needs nurturing and maintaining**. Symbiotic bacteria require a certain amount of complex sugars, at a certain rate, to flourish. The benefit of good sweet-bland staples is that they provide that perfect amount and type of complex sugars that our symbiotic bacteria need. If they don't **get enough** of these foods, our **symbionts die off** and we become week.

The balance is delicate, however. If we eat **too much very sweet**-tasting refined sugar, then disease-causing (pathogenic) micro-organisms such as **candida yeasts** grow at a dangerous rate, edging out our symbiotic bacteria, weakening our digestion and **making us ill;** not to mention the havoc that such sugars also plays with our vital hormonal balances, particularly those of **insulin**, resulting in today's extraordinary levels of **obesity and diabetes.** Today virtually all **industrially processed food** is crammed with sugar, because food manufacturers know that **sweetness creates compulsion**.

Despite this, handled with care the sweet flavour can be used to enhance health. Sweetness is the flavour of staple products such as **oats, rye, barley**, older wheat varieties (such as **spelt**) and **potatoes**, and so underpins a healthy diet. And as it is the strengthening flavour it is particularly important for **recuperation** and **convalescence**. A chicken broth, made with barley and a few root vegetables, makes it the ideal tonic for the immune system as it battles infection, not to mention the boost it gives our symbionts which help us in the task. More than any other flavour, sweetness can sustain, recover and create health. But use it wisely, for it can also destroy health. It is up to us to manage this balance.

Sweet summary

- **Stimulates** and strengthens **digestion**
- Fuel for **metabolisms**
- Nourishes **symbiotic bacteria**

Food should only be slightly sweet; **refined sugar and artificial sweeteners** are very **destructive**

Exercise 1a
Match the column A with the column B. Try to learn the expressions and/ or sentences by heart.

A

1. Sweetness reflects the sugar content of foods,
2. The balance of sweetness with blandness
3. Symbiotic bacteria
4. If we eat too much very sweet-tasting refined sugar, then disease-causing micro-organisms such as candida yeasts
5. All industrially processed food is crammed with sugar,
6. Sweetness is the flavour of staple products such as oats, rye, barley, spelt and potatoes,
7. Sweetness can sustain,
8. Refined sugar and artificial sweeteners

B

a) *and so underpins a healthy diet.*
b) *are very destructive.*
c) *because food manufacturers know that sweetness creates compulsion.*
d) *grow at a dangerous rate, edging out our symbiotic bacteria, weakening our digestion and making us ill.*
e) *is particularly important for our symbiotic bacteria.*
f) *recover and create health.*
g) *require a certain amount of complex sugars, at a certain rate, to flourish.*
h) *which provides the calories to sustain us in our day-to-day lives.*

Salty/savoury

This flavour is dominated by one **chemical: salt**, an ingredient that rightly gets a bad press these days. There is **too much** of it in the Western diet, as it is added in prodigious quantities to just about **every food product** available because, just like the sweetness of refined sugar, **we crave it.** Unfortunately, high salt consumption is linked to raised levels of **heart disease, high blood pressure, dementia and strokes**, and this is why there are so many warnings against eating lots of salty foods.

There was a time when salt was a rare and treasured flavour enhancer **and medicinal substance. Certain foods, like seeds,** were – and still are – **processed with salt** in order to **stimulate the urinary system** and **strengthen digestion** and the **constitution**. For example black sesame seeds are widely used in Japanese and Chinese cooking as a traditional tonic to stimulate digestive function. Similarly, salt-fried aromatic seeds are used to stimulate digestive function in Ayurvedic medicine.

Generally speaking, **we should seek to limit it** to small but satisfying quantity; commercially produced bread, breakfast cereals, snacks and ready meals are all loaded with it and our palates have come to expect large amounts of salt in our food. Many foods for babies and children also have added salt.

However, if you get into the habit of eating **freshly prepared and cooked food,** you will find that you need to add **only a little salt** for taste. It will then act solely as a flavour enhancer and not as an addictive agent. It is also worth noting that some types of salt are better than others – a traditionally produced **sea salt** gives much more flavour and nutrition, and therefore smaller quantities are required than of the cheap mass produced stuff. Naturally salty/savoury foods fall into **three categories**, all of which tend to be rich in mineral salts and/or umami: foods from the sea, deeply savoury foods and flavour-enhancing sauces and condiments.

From the sea	Deeply savoury foods	Flavour-enhancers
Anchovies Mussels Oysters Seaweed	Celery stalk Duck Pigeon Pork	Brown sauce Mushroom ketchup Soy sauce Worcester sauce

Salty summary

- Can **nourish the constitution** in small quantities
- **Enhances other flavours**
- **Stimulates appetite**
- **Moves the bowel**

Use a small amount of really good quality salt and watch out for added salt in pre-prepared foods.

Exercise 1b
Match the column A with the column B. Try to learn the expressions and/or sentences by heart.

A

1. There is too much of salt in the Western diet, as it is added in prodigious quantities
2. High salt consumption is linked to raised levels
3. Seeds are – processed with salt
4. Commercially produced bread, breakfast cereals, snacks and ready meals are all loaded with salt

5. Naturally salty/savoury foods fall into three categories, all of which tend to be rich in mineral salts and/or umami:

B

a) and our palates have come to expect large amounts of salt in our food.
b) foods from the sea, deeply savoury foods and flavour-enhancing sauces and condiments.
c) in order to stimulate the urinary system and strengthen digestion and the constitution.
d) of heart disease, high blood pressure, dementia and strokes.
e) to just about every food product available because, just like the sweetness of refined sugar, we crave it.

Exercise 2
Translate the expressions. Try to explain their meanings in English.

Instinctive, content, provides, sustain, digestive strength, staple foods, blandness, nurturing, maintaining, flourish, delicate, sweet-tasting, candida yeasts, edging out, extraordinary levels, creates compulsion, underpins, recuperation and convalescence, destructive, prodigious quantities, crave, constitution, traditional tonic, salt-fried, get into the habit of, addictive agent, it is worth, condiments.

Exercise 3
Answer the following questions. Prepare short talks and/or dialogues on these topics.

1. What does sweetness reflect?
2. Why is the balance of sweetness with blandness particularly important for our symbiotic bacteria?
3. What do symbiotic bacteria require?
4. What happens when we eat too much very sweet-tasting refined sugar?
5. Why is sweetness considered particularly important for recuperation and convalescence?
6. Why are there so many warnings against eating lots of salty foods.
7. Why are certain foods (like seeds) processed with salt?
8. Why should we seek to limit salt to small but satisfying quantity?
9. Give examples of three categories of naturally salty/ savoury foods (foods from the sea, deeply savoury foods and flavour-enhancing sauces and condiments).

Vocabulary 6

Fill in the meanings in your mother language:

barley /ˈbɑːli/
boost /buːst/
broth /brɒθ/
candida /ˈkæn.dɪ.də/

celery /'selərɪ/ **stalk** /stɔ:k/
compulsion /kəm'pʌl.ʃən/
constitution /ˌkɒnstɪ'tju:ʃən/
convalescence /ˌkɒn.və'les.əns/
crammed /kræmd/
crave /kreɪv/
delicate /'delɪkət/
despite /dɪ'spaɪt/
die /daɪ/
die off /daɪ/
duck /dʌk/
edge /edʒ/ **out** /aʊt/
flourish /'flʌrɪʃ/
foundation /faʊn'deɪ.ʃən/
havoc /'hævək/
in particular /pə'tɪk.jʊ.lər/
mushroom /'mʌʃru:m/
ketchup /'ketʃəp/
mussel /'mʌsəl/
nurture /'nɜ:tʃər/
oats /əʊts/
ongoing /'ɒŋˌgəʊ.ɪŋ/
oyster /'ɔɪstə/
palate /'pælət/
particularly /pə'tɪk.jʊ.lə.li/
pigeon /'pɪdʒɪn/
recuperation /rɪˌkju:pər'eɪʃən/
rye /raɪ/
seaweed /'si:ˌwi:d/
sesame /'sesəmɪ/ **seed** /si:d/
soy /sɔɪ/ **sauce** /sɔ:s/
spelt /spelt/
staple /'steɪpl/
stroke /strəʊk/
stuff /stʌf/
sustenance /'sʌs.tɪ.nəns/
treasured /'treʒəd/
urinary /'jʊə.rɪ.nər.i/
warning /'wɔ:nɪŋ/
wheat /wi:t/

Solution to Exercise 1a
1h, 2e, 3g, 4d, 5c, 6a, 7f, 8b

Solution to Exercise 1b
1e, 2d, 3c, 4a, 5b

Unit 7 - Sour. Bitter.

In comparison with sweet and salty/savoury, there is relatively **little sour** in our diets. Sour is the **cooling and refreshing flavour**, an ideal antidote to our overheated constitutions and lifestyles. Hence, sourness in the diet is said to be **calming** and can be advantageously **used in times of stress**. Sometimes we talk about being "liverish", that is, **feeling obstructed** both digestively and emotionally. The dietary answer is to eat more **sour foods**, which **stimulate the liver and gall bladder**.

Some classic examples of **sour foods** are **crab apple, damson, hawthorn, sloe and rose tips**. Historically these were prepared as **sauces, jellies, purées or syrups** to **soothe and move the gut and liver**. Citrus fruits such as lemon and lime have a similar role. Further afield there are many such approaches to the sour flavour. An example of this is the sour of Chinese plum, ume in Japanese. This wonderful **fruit** is variously **juiced, pickled, preserved, smoked and made into wine.** The juice is light, sour and refreshing, especially when consumed in summer to counter the affect of heat in the body.

The **pickles and preserves** have a more intense sourness and this makes them particularly useful when consumed **after meals**, especially heavy fatty meals, to **disperse the fats and to aid digestion**. Similarly, in China, hawthorn is combined with cinnamon and other digestive herbs and made into sour sweets to be eaten after meals. These are widely available and particularly popular with children. **Rich, fatty food** provides the **calories** that we need to get through long winter days while also **enhancing satiety** so that we avoid the hunger cravings that so commonly affect those who struggle with their weight. In the age of the **calorie-controlled diet** the idea that **rich food actually helps us to reduce our body weight** might seem counter-intuitive; but study after study confirms this phenomenon. Rich food fills you up and if you eat it you will want to eat less overall.

We should always **accompany rich meals with sour ingredients**, condiments and dressings. Here are some **classic combinations** that follow the principle of combining the sour flavour with rich and fatty foods:

- **Cheese and pickle**
- **Coconut milk and lime**
- **Duck and orange**
- **Lamb and mint sauce** (made with vinegar)
- **Pie** and chutney – **chutney** fruits include **apple, apricot, grape, kiwi, mango and plum**
- **Olive oil and lemon** or balsamic vinegar
- **Pork and apple or cider**
- **Salmon and sorrel**

Sour summary

- Stimulates **bile release** to break down rich foods
- **Calms**
- Use **in winter** to **cut through the richer diet**
- Use **in summer to refresh** when hot

Exercise 1a
Match the column A with the column B. Try to learn the expressions and/ or sentences by heart.

A

1. Sourness in the diet is said to be calming
2. Some classic examples of sour foods
3. Historically sour foods were prepared as
4. The pickles and preserves are
5. Rich, fatty food provides the calories that we need to get through long winter days
6. We should always accompany rich meals
7. Here are some classic combinations:

B

a) and can be advantageously used in times of stress.
b) are crab apple, damson, hawthorn, sloe and rose tips.
c) cheese and pickle, coconut milk and lime, duck and orange, lamb and mint sauce, pie and chutney, olive oil and lemon, pork and apple, salmon and sorrel
d) particularly useful when consumed after meals,

especially heavy fatty meals, to disperse the fats and to aid digestion.

e) sauces, jellies, purées or syrups to soothe and move the gut and liver.

f) while also enhancing satiety so that we avoid the hunger cravings that so commonly affect those who struggle with their weight.

g) with sour ingredients, condiments and dressings.

Bitter

Bitterness is the most neglected of the five flavours. **Bitter greens** such as **dandelion, chicory, lettuce, kale and chard** are largely neglected by us today. Historically, the varieties of bitter vegetable that were grown in Europe, from **cucumber** to **cabbage**, were more **diverse** and much more bitter than they are today – the bitterness has been bred out of them in favour of sweetness. This change is to our detriment as **bitterness** is a **profoundly medicinal flavour**; a key ingredient in a wide range of phytochemicals with **antibacterial, antiviral, anti-inflammatory and diuretic properties**. Therefore, nearly every traditional **herbal remedy** tasted, and tastes, bitter.

The bitter flavour is much loved in many parts of the world. Bitterness is said to have a **calming effect**, especially when the weather is hot. Traditionally, this has encouraged a habit of consuming more bitter food in the height of summer. It is said to **enhance sleep, reduce irritability** and help to prevent the onset of "liverishness". In damper weather, bitters are said to compensate by **drying out** the body, as well as stimulating **movement of the bowel** to counter damp's stagnating effect. Bitterness can be found in many foods. **Leafy greens** tend to be bitter and grow all year round in one form or another. Similarly, seasonal greens, **courgette, cucumber, aubergine and broccoli** are all classified as **bitter vegetables.** The most significant bitter substance of all, however, is not a food but a drink – tea. **Tea**, an infusion of the leaves of the Camellia sinensis plant, is consumed in huge quantities by people worldwide. It is the worlds **greatest medicine** and its health properties are extensive.

Tea

With regards to digestion, tea is hugely significant and versatile. It regulates digestion as **its astringent tannic acid** protects against diarrhoea, while its **bitter components** (such as **alkaloids**) stimulate the bowel to **counter constipation.** Meanwhile, **antibacterial agents** maintain the balance of our **symbionts** and protect our **teeth from bacteriogenic erosion**. No wonder then that tea has been the traditional mealtime beverage in China for countless generations. It is drunk pure, in green or black forms.

There are ancient **tea-drinking cultures** that routinely drink **milky tea**, most notably the **Tibetans**, who add milk and butter to their infusions.

But there is a good reason for this. The Tibetan climate is so cold that they have to consume a rich diet day in day out to stay warm, and for religious reasons they eat little or no meat, hence the addition of butter in the tea. Furthermore, as the Tibetan plateau is so dry that digestion is relatively unobstructed, they can get away with consuming the rich drink without excessive digestive impact. Combining the rich dairy products with digestion-enhancing tea is a necessity for the Tibetans.

We should stop putting sugar in our tea. **Sugar rots our teeth** and **disturbs symbiotic balance** so its impact is obviously and directly opposed to the natural digestion-enhancing effects of tea. **Milk is similar**. Its proteins bind out the astringent and bitter tannins, and neuter other chemicals too, such as the catechins that protect our hearts.

Here is a list of **everyday bitter foods** to include in your diet:

Artichoke	Basil
Broccoli	Bay leaf
Buckwheat	Chervil
Celery	Chives
Chard	Coffee
Chicory	Dill
Dandelion	Fenugreek seed
Dark chocolate/cocoa	Juniper berry
Kale	Lemon zest
Lettuce	Marjoram
Millet	Mustard
Parsnip	Oregano
Rocket	Parsley
Rye	Rosemary
Watercress	Tea

Bitterness summary

- Moves the gut and **stimulates secretion and motility**
- Helps **push food down the bowel**
- **Counters** the pathogenic **effects of dampness**
- **Cools and calms**

Exercise 1b
Match the column A with the column B. Try to learn the expressions and/ or sentences by heart.

A

1. Bitterness is a profoundly medicinal flavour;
2. Bitterness is said to have a calming effect,
3. In damper weather, bitters are said to compensate by drying out the body, Seasonal greens, courgette, cucumber, aubergine and broccoli
4. Tea is the world's greatest medicine
5. Tea regulates digestion as its astringent tannic acid protects against diarrhoea,
6. Antibacterial agents maintain the balance of our symbionts
7. Sugar rots our teeth and disturbs symbiotic balance

B

a) a key ingredient in a wide range of phytochemicals

with antibacterial, antiviral, anti-inflammatory and diuretic properties.

b) *and its health properties are extensive.*

c) *and protect our teeth from bacteriologic erosion.*

d) *are all classified as bitter vegetables.*

e) *as well as stimulating movement of the bowel to counter damp's stagnating effect.*

f) *especially when the weather is hot.*

g) *so its impact is obviously and directly opposed to the natural digestion-enhancing effects of tea.*

h) *while its bitter components (such as alkaloids) stimulate the bowel to counter constipation.*

Exercise 2
Translate the expressions. Try to explain their meanings in English.

Comparison, cooling and refreshing, antidote, calming, advantageously, liver and gall bladder, approaches, pickled, preserved, smoked, counter the affect of, pickles and preserves, aid digestion, digestive herbs, available, to get through, enhancing satiety, hunger cravings, struggle with the weight, body weight, fills you up, sour ingredients, condiment, dressings, bile release, neglected, bitter greens, diverse, detriment, profoundly, medicinal, diuretic properties, herbal remedy, calming effect, habit, enhance sleep, reduce irritability, compensate, drying out, movement of the bowel, stagnating, infusion, health properties, with regards to, counter, constipation, bacteriogenic erosion, get away with, rots our teeth, disturbs impact, digestion-enhancing tannins, neuter, bay leaf, chervil, chives, dill, fenugreek seed, juniper berry, lemon zest, marjoram, parsley, rosemary, buck, wheat, chard, chicory, dandelion, kale, lettuce, millet, parsnip, rocket, rye, watercress, counters the effects, dampness.

Exercise 3
Answer the following questions. Prepare short talks and/or dialogues on these topics.

1. Why can sour be advantageously used in times of stress?
2. Which foods, stimulate the liver and gall bladder?
3. Give some classic examples of sour foods.
4. Why would you serve the pickles and preserves after meal?
5. Talk about classic combinations that follow the principle of combining the sour flavour with rich and fatty foods.
6. Talk about antibacterial, antiviral, anti-inflammatory and diuretic properties of bitterness.
7. Give examples of some bitter greens and bitter vegetables.
8. Tea and its health properties.

9. Why should we stop putting sugar and milk in our tea?
10. Which bitter foods should we include in our everyday diet?

Vocabulary 7

Fill in the meanings in your mother language:

advantageously /ˌæd.væn'teɪ.dʒəs.li/
afield /ə'fiːld/
anti /ænti/ **-inflamatory** / ɪn'flæmətəri/
antidote /æn.tɪ.dəʊt/
artichoke /'ɑːtɪtʃəʊk/
aubergine /'əʊbəʒiːn/
bacteriogenic /bæk'tɪəriədʒenɪk/
balsamic vinegar / bɔːlˌsæm.ɪk'vɪn.ɪ.gər/
bay /beɪ/ **leaf** /liːf/
berry /'berɪ/
bind /baɪnd/ **out** /aʊt/
breed /briːd/ **(bred, bred)**
broccoli /'brɒkəlɪ/
buckwheat /'bʌkˌwiːt/
cabbage /'kæb.ɪdʒ/
Camellia /kə'miː.li.ə/ **sinensis**
catechin /'kætəkɪn/
chard /tʃɑːd/
chervil /'tʃɜːvɪl/
chicory /'tʃikərɪ/
chives /tʃaɪvz/
coconut /'kəʊkənʌt/
counter /kaʊntə/
courgette /kɔː'ʒet/
crab /kræb/ **apple** /'æpl/
craving /'kreɪ.vɪŋ/
cucumber /kjuːˌkʌmbə/
damson /'dæm.zən/
dandelion /'dændɪˌlaɪən/
detriment /'detrɪmənt/
dill /dɪl/
disperse /dɪ'spɜːs/
diuretic /ˌdaɪ.jʊə 'ret.ɪk/
erosion /ɪ'rəʊ.ʒən/
get /get/ **away** /ə'weɪ/
hawthorn /'hɔː.θɔːn/
infusion /ɪn'fjuː.ʒən/
intuitive /ɪn'tjuːɪtɪv/
jelly /'dʒeli/
juniper /'dʒuːnɪpə/
kale /keɪl/
lamb /læm/
lemon /'lemən/ **zest** /zest/
lettuce /'letɪs/
lime /laɪm/
liverish /'lɪv.ər.ɪʃ/
marjoram /'mɑːdʒərəm/
millet /'mɪlɪt/
mustard /'mʌstəd/
neglect /nɪ'glekt/
neuter /'njuːtə/
oregano /ˌɒrɪ'gɑːnəʊ/
parsley /'pɑːslɪ/
parsnip /'pɑːsnɪp/
phenomenon /fə'nɒm.ɪ.nən/
pl **phenomena**
phytochemical /ˌfaɪtəʊ'kɛmɪkəl/
pickle /'pɪkl/
plum /plʌm/
purée /'pjʊəreɪ/
religious /rɪ'lɪdʒəs/
remedy /'rem.ə.di/
rocket /'rɒkɪt/
satiety /sə'taɪə.ti/
sloe /sləʊ/
soothe /suːð/
sorrel /'sɒr.əl/
syrup /'sɪrəp/
tannic /'tænɪk/ **acid** /'æsɪd/
tip /tɪp/
watercress /'wɔːtəˌkres/

Solution to Exercise 1a
1a, 2b, 3e, 4d, 5f, 6g, 7c

Solution to Exercise 1b
1a, 2f, 3e, 4b, 5h, 6c, 7g

Unit 8 - Spicy/aromatic. Using flavours to create a strong, health-giving diet 1

Spicy flavours and aromatic oils are vital. These are the **moving flavours** and many spicy and aromatic foods have a **warming quality,** and are therefore ideal for stimulating gut motility. When **digestion stagnates**, causing symptoms like **trapped wind** and **poor appetite**, dietary traditions throughout the world use spicy and aromatic food like **fennel seeds** as a matter of course to get moving again. Not all of the spicy and aromatic foods are warm, however; **coriander, marjoram and mint leaves** actually have **cooling and refreshing** properties.

Spicy and aromatic foods have another huge health benefit. The **stagnant, damp air**, especially when it is combined with **pollution** damages the health of the lungs. Spicy and aromatic foods are the principal dietary method of combating this effect. The oils in these foods help the **lungs** to move, to **expand and contrac**t freely, and to **shift phlegm**. This is why traditional **cough linctus** and **decongestants** are intensely aromatic. Aromatic and spicy foods have a range of intensities. The **chilli** and **pepper** that characterise strong **curries** and some Sichuanese dishes are the top end of the scale and are too strong for our purposes.

In the long term, regular consumption of large amounts of food this spicy damages health as it **irritates membranes** and causes **inflammation**. Instead, we need to include mild aromatic foods, herbs and spices as staples in our diet. Here are some common examples:

Vegetables	Spices	Leafy herbs
Celeriac	Cardamom	Basil
Fennel bulb	Cinnamon	Celery
Garlic	Coriander	Coriander
Leek	seed	leaf
Onion	Cumin	Mint
Radish	Fennel seed	Oregano
Watercress	Mustard seed	Rosemary
	Paprika	Thyme

Spicy/aromatic summary

- Stimulates **motility and circulation**
- **Counters obstructive effect** of damp and humidity
- **Warms** against the cold
- **Strengthens** the lungs

Mild aromatic herbs and spices stimulate and move the gut without irritating it.

Exercise 1a
Match the column A with the column B. Try to learn the expressions and/ or sentences by heart.

A

1. Many spicy and aromatic foods have a warming quality,
2. When digestion stagnates, causing symptoms like trapped wind and poor appetite,

3. Not all of the spicy and aromatic foods are warm, however;
4. The oils in spicy and aromatic foods
5. In the long term, regular consumption of large amounts of spicy food
6. Spicy/aromatic stimulates motility and circulation, counters obstructive effect of damp and humidity,
7. Mild aromatic herbs and spices

B

a) and are therefore ideal for stimulating gut motility.
b) coriander, marjoram and mint leaves actually have cooling and refreshing properties.
c) damages health as it irritates membranes and causes inflammation.
d) dietary traditions throughout the world use spicy and aromatic food like fennel seeds.
e) help the lungs to move, to expand and contract freely, and to shift phlegm.
f) stimulate and move the gut without irritating it.
g) warms against the cold, and strengthens the lungs.

Using flavours to create a strong, health-giving diet 1

Climate change means that the **annual cycle of seasonal weather** changes is less predictable than it used to be, which demands a special sort of adaptability and **intelligence**. Shielded by modern technology, we are increasingly loosing our ability to respond to what the weather throws at us, and we need to retrieve it.

Adapting diet for climate

Since **sweet and salty/savoury** are a more or less constant **part of every meal,** they tend to vary little. We should eat more **sweet, bland staples** in **winter** – such **as barley, chicken, potatoes, carrots and parsnips** – as our **calorific requirement rises**. It is the other three flavours – sour, bitter and spicy aromatics – that are the main tastes to consider in terms of variation and adaptability.

Bitterness and spicy aromatics constantly **stimulate motility** to counter the dietary inhibition of cold and damp. Meanwhile, **sour helps to cut through and break down the rich food** that we need in the relatively cold autumn, winter and spring. A healthy diet should be a **mix of at least four of the five flavours**, and as the weather gets more challenging, the flavours should get more intense.

A **good winter dish,** such as a **stew or casserole**, might easily include components that are strong in all five flavours; for example, parsnip, carrot, barley or potato (**sweet**); beef, stock, a fermented condiment such as Worcester sauce and seasoning (**salty/savoury**); juniper berry, rosemary, seasonal greens and parsley (**bitter**); black pepper, paprika and oregano (**spicy and aromatic**); and tomato, vinegar, wine, cider or a pickle accompaniment (**sour**). Most **traditional dishes** have a similar composition and include the three most important flavours: sour, bitter and aromatic. First, you need to know the flavour-based characteristics of a **wide range of ingredients**: meat, fish, vegetables, pulses, oils, spices, herbs, nuts and fruits. You also need to recognise the **overall properties** of the dishes that they constitute, from pancakes to chicken soup. Then you need to choose the right recipe for your circumstances, and **increase or diminish** the amount of **each flavour** according to your needs.

If it gets **colder**, you should eat **richer foods** like meat or fish, and plant fats such as hemp or olive oil. You should also increase the sour accompaniment (such as pickles) to **help digestion of the fats**. Consuming more aromatic spices will **warm the body** and **stimulate circulation**. In wet weather, we need to eat more aromatic spices and bitterness to stimulate motility in the gut. However, the spicy diet for cold weather needs to be **balanced** with cooling and refreshing flavours so that the gut does not get irritated. To achieve this, you need bitter and sour ingredients – spinach and yoghurt in curries, for example, or pickles, tomatoes, white wine or vinegar in chilli con carne. Similarly, you should eat lighter food such as stir-fries and salads that contain more sour and bitter ingredients to cool and refresh the body when the weather is very hot.

These are the **individual actions** of the three key flavours and how they act in combination:

Aromatic/spicy

- Warms and disperses cold and dampness
- Counters damp, humid weather and sluggish gut
- Aids digestion of fatty foods

Bitter

- Stimulates motility
- Counters damp, humid weather and sluggish gut
- Calms and cools in hot weather

Sour

- Breaks up fatty food
- Aids digestion of fatty foods
- Calms and cools in hot weather

Exercise 1b
Match the column A with the column B. Try to learn the expressions and/or sentences by heart.

A

1. We should eat more sweet, bland staples in winter
2. Bitterness and spicy aromatics constantly stimulate motility
3. Sour helps to cut through and break down the rich food

4. You need to know the flavour-based characteristics of a wide range of ingredients:
5. You also need to recognise the
6. The spicy diet for cold weather needs to be balanced

B

a) as our calorific requirement rises.
b) meat, fish, vegetables, pulses, oils, spices, herbs, nuts and fruits.
c) overall properties of the dishes that they constitute.
d) that we need in the relatively cold autumn, winter and spring.
e) to counter the dietary inhibition of cold and damp.
f) with cooling and refreshing flavours so that the gut does not get irritated.

Exercise 2
Translate the expressions. Try to explain their meanings in English.

Digestion, stagnates, trapped wind, cooling and refreshing, damp air, pollution, principal, combating, expand and contract, shift phlegm, decongestants, counters, celeriac, radish, cardamom, basil, inflammation, celery, rosemary, irritates, thyme, coriander, leaf, mint, cinnamon, coriander seed, cumin, watercress, fennel bulb, garlic, leek, strengthens, predictable, adaptability, respond, retrieve, variation, challenging, composition, recognise, overall properties, constitute, increase or diminish, accompaniment, dampness, sluggish.

Exercise 3
Answer the following questions. Prepare short talks and/or dialogues on these topics.

1. Why are spicy flavours and aromatic oils vital?
2. Why are cough linctus and decongestants intensely aromatic?
3. Why do we need to include mild aromatic foods in our diet?
4. Give examples of aromatic vegetables, spices and leafy herbs.
5. Which components should a good winter dish include?
6. Why do you need to know the flavour-based characteristics of a wide range of ingredients?
7. What are the individual actions of the three key flavours and how do they act in combination?

Vocabulary 8

Fill in the meanings in your mother language:

bulb /bʌlb/
cardamom /ˈkɑː.də.məm/
celeriac /səˈler.i.æk/
chilli /ˈtʃɪl i/ **con carne** /kɒn ˈkɑːnɪ/
cinnamon /ˈsɪnəmən/
combat /ˈkɒm.bæt/

cough /kɒf/
curry /ˈkʌrɪ/
cut /kʌt/ **through** /θruː/
decongestant /ˌdiː.kənˈdʒest.ənt/
diminish /dɪˈmɪn.ɪʃ/
fennel /ˈfenəl/
hemp /hɛmp/ **oil** /ɔɪl/
leaf /liːf/
leek /liːk/
linctus /ˈlɪŋk.təs/
mint /mɪnt/
overall /ˌəʊ.vəˈrɔːl/
pankake /ˈpænˌkeɪk/
phlegm /flem/
predictable /prɪˈdɪk.tə.blˌ/
pulse /pʌls/
radish /ˈrædɪʃ/
retrieve /rɪˈtriːv/
shield /ʃiːld/
shift /ʃift/
sluggish /ˈslʌg.ɪʃ/
spinach /ˈspɪn.ɪtʃ/
thyme /taɪm/

Solution to Exercise 1a
1a, 2d, 3b, 4e, 5c, 6g, 7f

Solution to Exercise 1b
1a, 2e, 3d, 4b, 5c, 6f

Unit 9 - Using flavours to create a strong, health-giving diet 2. How to put together a healthy meal 1.

The principles of food analysis can be applied not only to individual ingredients but also to whole dishes:

Climate type: Cold and damp

Food type: Rich and spicy, with a little sour and bitter to cut through the richness

Simple recipes	**Average recipes**	**More complex recipes**
Chestnut soup Spicy scrambled eggs	Kedgeree Sausage casserole	Boiled ham hocks with pease pudding Slow-roasted lamb and harissa

Climate type: Cold and dry
Food type: Rich and aromatic

Simple recipes	**Average recipes**	**More complex recipes**
Mushroom risotto Tuna, fennel and bean salad	Aromatic mussels with cider and bacon Lemon chicken	Casserole Chicken chasseur

Climate type: Hot and humid
Food type: Light, spicy and bitter

Simple recipes	**Average recipes**	**More complex recipes**
Spicy chicken broth with noodles Baked fish with herbs	Salmon and caper fish cakes Spicy stir fry	Chicken curry Dal

Climate type: Hot and dry
Food type: Light, sour and bitter

Simple recipes	**Average recipes**	**More complex recipes**
Aromatic chicken broth with noodles Nasturtium, chicken and pesto salad	Ceviche Basic stir fry	Falafel Grilled or barbecued sardines with salsa

Adapting diet for lifestyle and circumstance

Most of us have demanding and **stressful lifestyles**. Lack of sleep, illness, accidents and bereavement all have the same debilitating effect. **Adaptation** is relatively easy once you understand the principles. For example, when you are under great physical or emotional strain, there is a **need for a light, naturally sweet and digestible food** such as chicken soup with barley.

Here are some other examples:

Condition	Food type	Recipe examples
Convale scence	Light, gently aromatic food	Chicken broth with noodles
Tired/ worn out	Regular small amounts of richer food, more heavily spiced On a foundation of blander easily digested food	Boiled ham hocks with pease pudding Pancakes, potato salad, chestnut soup
Stressed/ anxious	Light and easy to digest food with a balance of all the flavours	Lemon chicken

Summary

- **Weather and environment** affect health and well-being. **Work out what sort of flavours and dishes you should be eating** at any particular time.
- **Dietary strategies** exist for conditions such as **fatigue, convalescence and emotional stress.** There are a number of websites for seasonal foods, food groups and recipes that can be adapted for your needs.
- **Complex situations** such as pregnancy require **detailed dietary rationales and input.** If you suffer from an illness, seek the help of an appropriately qualified health professional.

Exercise 1a
Match the column A with the column B. Try to learn the expressions and/ or sentences by heart.

A

1. The principles of food analysis
2. Rich and spicy food
3. In cold and dry climate
4. In hot and humid climate
5. In hot and dry climate
6. Lack of sleep, illness, accidents and bereavement
7. When you are under great physical or emotional strain,
8. Work out what sort of flavours and dishes
9. Dietary strategies exist for conditions
10. Complex situations such as pregnancy

B

a) all have the same debilitating effect.
b) can be applied not only to individual ingredients but also to whole dishes.
c) is suitable in cold and damp climate.
d) light, spicy and bitter food is suitable.
e) require detailed dietary rationales and input.

- *f) rich and aromatic food should be served.*
- *g) such as fatigue, convalescence and emotional stress.*
- *h) there is a need for a light, naturally sweet and digestible food such as chicken soup with barley.*
- *i) you need light, sour and bitter food.*
- *j) you should be eating at any particular time.*

How to put together a healthy meal 1

Recipes are **useful tools** as they represent the bigger picture in terms of **combinations of foods** and the **construction of dishes and meals**. They are also a great way to learn to cook, providing the kind of structure that is a perfect helping hand as we develop confidence in the kitchen. Recipes have a long history. Indeed, they are as old as written language itself. For a really good health-promoting diet, it is fine in principle to adapt the celebrity cookbooks. We should learn the **set of dietary principles** embodied in the understanding of flavour, and use these to build our own recipes, as well as to adapt ones that already exist.

Creating meals using the flavour principle

Using flavours to create a healthy meal is remarkably simple. Balance is the key, and to achieve balance we have to approach the flavours one by one. So **we start with a staple**, which is typically **sweet and bland**, but can be **savoury**. Then **add salty/savoury** flavour enhancers and **finish** with the appropriate **balance of bitter, sour, spice and aromatics** according to climate and lifestyle.

Start with a staple – sweet and bland

Staples are **the most fundamental** of foods, the foundations on which all dishes and diets are built, providing **starchy calories** that fuel us in our day-to-day activities. Because of **large-scale wheat consumption**, there is a **lack of variety** in the staples eaten in modern non-traditional diets.

Wheat

Wheat is a popular grain because modern varieties are **easily grown**, modern distribution has made it **relatively cheap** and, due to its high gluten content, it is a doddle to process industrially. **Gluten** is a **sticky, stretchy protein** that forms **when wheat is processed**. It helps food products pass through processing machines very easily, trapping air and facilitating efficient bread and pastry production. However, the very properties that make gluten so machine-friendly make it particularly **digestion-unfriendly**. Our enzymes and symbionts find it very **hard to break down**; so wheat, with its high gluten levels, is a staple that inhibits rather than promotes digestion.

People with **celiac disease** (gluten enteropathy) have a **total intolerance** to gluten and cannot eat any products containing wheat. And yet despite the basic digestive stubborness of wheat it is not uncommon for us to use wheat as the staple for all three of our daily meals; cereal or toast for breakfast, a sandwich for lunch and pasta, a pie or pizza for supper.

The effect of so **much wheat** in our diets is to slow us down – indeed, in traditional medicine it is used as a mild sedative and calmant – an effect that is not only undesirable, but has resulted in **epic levels of constipation.** This, combined with our modern inactive lifestyles, means that we aren't doing enough to stimulate healthy motility. Little exercise and a wheat-heavy diet make for an unhappy gut – a balance we need to compensate for when devising our diet. Fortunately, **other staples** are **much lighter** and therefore extremely good for digestion. They **should form the basis** of our diet. This greater digestibility can be due to a variety of reasons; they might have just **the right amount of fibre**, for example, and the **right sorts of proteins and starches** may be spot on for the **nourishment of our symbiotic bacteria.**

In most cases it is a mix of all three of these factors. With this principle of staples that **support, nourish and strengthen digestion** in mind, we can build a list of staples that are ideal for a healthy diet.

Grains	**Vegetables**	**Animal products**	**Beans** (well cooked)
Barley Buck wheat Corn Millet Oats Rice Rye	Carrot Leek Onion (well-cooked) Parsnip Pumpkin Sweet Potato/ Yam Turnip	Beef/ Lamb/ Chicken broth Chicken Cod/ Haddock Plaice Turkey	Aduki Bean sprouts Haricot Hyacinth Kidney Lentils Split peas

It is worth noting that **some meats, fish, beans and broths** are **included as staples**; they were and still are used to bulk out traditional diets. They are also **compatible with (healthy) modern weight-loss regimes**, thus indicating a strong correlation between traditional approaches and modern protocols that help to lose weight without damaging health. In dietary terms, the bogey foods, the foods that are most likely to make us fat, cause diabetes and damage hearts and blood vessels are refined sugar, refined wheat products and cheap industrially processed fat. If you follow the principle of using the **recommended staples** as a **foundation** for your own meal, without eating too much of bread, then you have taken a vital step towards **long-lasting health** and a consistent, **healthy weight.**

Exercise 1b
Match the column A with the column B. Try to learn the expressions and/or sentences by heart.

A

1. Recipes are useful tools
2. We should learn the set of dietary principles embodied in the understanding of flavour,
3. We start with a staple, then add salty/savoury flavour enhancers
4. Staples are the most fundamental of foods,
5. Because of large-scale wheat consumption,
6. Gluten is a sticky, stretchy protein
7. Our enzymes and symbionts find it very hard to break down;
8. People with celiac disease (gluten enteropathy)
9. The effect of so much wheat in our diets is to slow us down
10. Other staples are much lighter and
11. With this principle of staples that support, nourish and strengthen digestion in mind,
12. It is worth noting that some meats, fish, beans and broths
13. In dietary terms, the foods that are most likely to make us fat, cause diabetes and damage hearts and blood vessels
14. Follow the principle of using the recommended staples:

B

a) *an effect that has resulted in epic levels of constipation.*
b) *and finish with the appropriate balance of bitter, sour, spice and aromatics according to climate and lifestyle.*
c) *and use these to build our own recipes, as well as to adapt ones that already exist.*
d) *are included as staples.*
e) *are refined sugar, refined wheat products and cheap industrially processed fat.*
f) *as they represent the bigger picture in terms of combinations of foods and the construction of dishes and meals.*
g) *grains (barley, buckwheat, corn, millet, oats, rice, rye), vegetables (carrot, onion, parsnip, leek, pumpkin, sweet potato/Yam, turnip), animal products (beef/lamb/chicken broth, chicken, cod/haddock, plaice, turkey), beans (aduki, bean sprouts, haricot, hyacinth, kidney, lentils, split peas).*
h) *have a total intolerance to gluten and cannot eat any products containing wheat.*
i) *so wheat, with its high gluten levels, is a staple that inhibits rather than promotes digestion.*

j) that forms when wheat is processed.
k) the foundations on which all dishes and diets are built.
l) there is a lack of variety in the staples eaten in modern non-traditional diets.
m) they should form the basis of our diet.
n) we can build a list of staples that are ideal for a healthy diet.

Exercise 2
Translate the expressions. Try to explain their meanings in English.

Individual ingredients, whole dishes, scrambled eggs, sausage casserole, simple recipes, average, complex, spicy chicken broth with noodles, chicken curry, adapting diet, stressful lifestyles, physical or emotional strain, digestible food, debilitating effect, pancakes, potato salad, foundation, work out, dietary strategies, fatigue, convalescence, adapted, appropriately qualified, health professional, develop, confidence, health-promoting diet, dietary principles, adapt, achieve balance, according to climate and lifestyle, fundamental, foundations, lack of variety, gluten content, sticky, stretchy protein, processed, efficient, bread and pastry production, inhibits, promotes digestion, celiac disease, slow down, undesirable, compensate for, devising, nourishment, in mind, grains, barley, buckwheat, corn, millet, oats, rye, leek, parsnip, pumpkin, aduki, bean sprouts, haricot, hyacinth, kidney, lentils, turnip, lamb, cod/haddock, plaice, split peas, to bulk out, compatible, correlation, follow the principle.

Exercise 3
Answer the following questions. Prepare short talks and/or dialogues on these topics.

1. How can weather and environment affect health and well-being?
2. What are the principles of food analysis applied to whole dishes?
3. Talk about food types suitable for cold and damp and cold and dry climate.
4. Talk about food types suitable for hot and humid and hot and dry climate.
5. How to adapt diet for lifestyle and circumstance? Give some examples.
6. Work out what sort of flavours and dishes you should be eating at any particular time.
7. Why are recipes useful tools?
8. How to create meals using the flavour principle?
9. Advantages and disadvantages of wheat.
10. Talk about other staples, give examples of grains, vegetables, animal products and beans.

Vocabulary 9

Fill in the meanings in your mother language:

accompaniment /əˈkʌmpənɪmənt/
acidic /əˈsɪd.ɪk/
acidity /əˈsɪdɪtɪ/
act /ækt/
aduki /əˈduː.ki/
alkaline /ˈæl.kəl.aɪn/
allotment /əˈlɒtmənt/
amylase /ˈæm.ɪ.leɪz/
angostura /ˌæŋgəˈstjʊərə/
anxiety /æŋˈzaɪ.ə.ti/
appetiser /ˈæpɪˌtaɪzə/
appreciate /əˈpriː.ʃi.eɪt/
aromatic /ˌærəˈmætɪk/
artificial /ˌɑː.tɪˈfɪʃ.əl/
sweetener /ˈswiːtənə/
aspartame /əˈspɑːˌteɪm/
average /ˈæv.ər.ɪdʒ/
awareness /əˈweənɪs/
awesome /ˈɔːsəm/
barbecue /ˈbɑːbɪˌkjuː/
barrier /ˈbær.i.ər/
basil /ˈbæzəl/
bean /biːn/
bean /biːn/ **sprouts** /spraʊts/
bedrock /ˈbedˌrɒk/
beef /biːf/
behalf /bɪˈhɑːf/
bereavement /bɪˈriːv.mənt/
beyond /bɪˈjɒnd/
bile /baɪl/
biotin /ˈbaɪətɪn/
bitter /ˈbɪtə/
bloodstream /ˈblʌd.striːm/
bogey /ˈbəʊgɪ/
bond /bɒnd/
bottom /ˈbɒtəm/
bowel /ˈbaʊ.əl/
breast /brest/ **milk** /mɪlk/
bug /bʌg/
bulk /bʌlk/
bunch /bʌntʃ/
buttermilk /ˈbʌtəˌmɪlk/
caesarean section /sɪˌzeə.ri.ənˈsek.ʃən/
calmant /kɑːmənt/
caper /ˈkeɪpə/
carrot /ˈkærət/
casserole /ˈkæsəˌrəʊl/
celiac disease /ˈsiː.liː.æk.dɪˌziːz/
ceviche /səvɪːʃəɪ/
chicken /ˈtʃɪkɪn/
chomp /tʃɒmp/
Clostridium /kləˈstrɪ.dɪ.əm/
cod /kɒd/
coincidentally /kəʊˌɪnsɪˈdentəlɪ/
compatible /kəmˈpætəbəl/
conception /kənˈsep.ʃən/
conclude /kənˈkluːd/
confidence /ˈkɒnfɪdəns/
consistent /kənˈsɪstənt/
constipation /kɒnstɪˈpeɪʃən/
cookbook /ˈkʊkˌbʊk/
corn /kɔːn/
correlation /ˌkɒrɪˈleɪʃən/
crucial /ˈkruː.ʃəl/
cuisine /kwɪˈziːn/
dal /dɑːl/
debilitating /dɪˈbɪl.ɪ.teɪt.ɪŋ/
declare /dɪˈkleə/
delicious /dɪˈlɪʃəs/
destructive /dɪˈstrʌk.tɪv/
devise /dɪˈvaɪz/
doddle /ˈdɒdəl/
dominate /ˈdɒm.ɪ.neɪt/
dreadful /ˈdredfʊl/
droplet /ˈdrɒplɪt/
efficient /ɪˈfɪʃənt/
embody /ɪmˈbɒdɪ/
emotion /ɪˈməʊ.ʃən/
emulsifier /ɪˈmʌlsɪˌfaɪə/
enemy /ˈenəmɪ/
enteropathy /ˈentərɒpəθi/
enzyme /ˈen.zaɪm/
epic /epɪk/
expansive /ɪkˈspænsɪv/
facilitate /fəˈsɪlɪˌteɪt/

falafel /fəl'ɑːfəl/
fenugreek /'fɛnjʊˌgriːk/
flavour /'fleɪ.vər/
foremost /'fɔːˌməʊst/
fulfil /fʊl'fɪl/
fundamental /ˌfʌn.də'men.təl/
fungus /'fʌŋ.gəs/ pl **fungi**
ginger /'dʒɪndʒə/
green /griːn/
grow /groʊ/ **(grew, grown)**
haddock /'hædək/
ham /hæm/ **hock** /hɒk/
haricot /'hærɪkəʊ/
harissa /hə'rɪsə/
hedgerow /'hedʒˌrəʊ/
herbal /'hɜː.bəl/
human /'hjuː.mən/ **being** /'biː.ɪŋ/
hyacinth /'haɪ.ə.sɪnθ/
impact /'ɪm.pækt/
implicate /'ɪm.plɪ.keɪt/
incidence /'ɪnt.sɪ.dənts/
inevitable /ɪn'evɪtəbəl/
infamous /ɪnfəməs/
inflammatory /ɪn'flæm.ə.tər.i/
initially /ɪ'nɪʃ.əl.i/
input /'ɪnˌpʊt/
insoluble /ɪn'sɒl.jʊ.blˌ/
instrumental /ˌɪnstrə'mentəl/
intestine /ɪn'tes.tɪn/
kedgeree /ˌkɛdʒə'riː/
kidney /'kɪdnɪ/
lentil /'lentɪl/
line /laɪn/
membrane /'mem.breɪn/
methanol /'mɛθəˌnɒl/
millet /'mɪlɪt/ **grain** /greɪn/
muck /mʌk/
nasturtium /nə'stɜːʃəm/
neurotransmitter /ˌnjʊə.rəʊ.trænz'mɪt.ər/
noodle /'nuːdəl/
onion /'ʌnjən/
particular /pə'tɪk.jʊ.lər/
pathogenic /ˌpæθ.ə'dʒen.ɪk/
pease /piː/ **pudding** /'pʊdɪŋ/
pesto /'pes.təʊ/
pick /pɪk/ **up** /ʌp/
pickled /'pɪkəld/
pitched /pɪtʃt/ **battle** /'bætəl/
plaice /pleɪs/
polio /'pəʊlɪəʊ/
preserved /prɪ'zɜːvd/
probiosis /proʊ'baɪəʊsɪs/
protocol /'prəʊtəˌkɒl/
protozoan /ˌprəʊ.tə'zəʊ.ən/ pl **protozoa**
pumpkin /'pʌmpkɪn/
range /reɪndʒ/
rationale /ˌræʃə'nɑːl/
regarding /rɪ'gɑː.dɪŋ/
relationship /rɪ'leɪ.ʃən.ʃɪp/
release /rə'liːs/
research /rɪ'sɜːtʃ/
reveal /rɪ'viːl/
review /rɪ'vjuː/
rice /raɪs/
risotto /rɪ'zɒtəʊ/
rosemary /'rəʊzmərɪ/
salivary /sə'laɪ.vər.i/ **gland** /glænd/
salsa /'sælsə/
sauerkraut /'saʊəˌkraʊ/
sausage /'sɒsɪdʒ/
scrambled /'skræmbəld/ **eggs**
seed /siːd/
seek /siːk/ **(sought, sought)**
sequence /'siːkwəns/
serotonin /ˌse.rə'təʊ.nɪn/
sherry /'ʃerɪ/
significance /sɪg'nɪfɪkəns/
simple /'sɪmpəl/
sinus /'saɪ.nəs/ pl **sinuses**
snip /snɪp/
soil /sɔɪl/
sour /'saʊə/
spicy /'spaɪsɪ/
split /splɪt/ **peas** /piː/
spot /spɒt/ **on** /ɒn/
Staphylococcus /ˌstæf.ɪl.ə'kɒk.əs/ pl **Staphylococci** /'kɒk.saɪ/
stevia /'stɛv i ə/
stomach /'stʌm.ək/

stretchy /ˈstretʃɪ/
substance /ˈsʌb.stəns/
sucralose /ˈsu krəˌloʊs/
suppress /səˈpres/
sweeten /ˈswiːtən/
symbiotic /sɪmbɪˈɔtɪk/
tailored /ˈteɪləd/
tiny /ˈtaɪ.ni/
trap /træp/
tuna /ˈtjuːnə/
turkey /ˈtɜːkɪ/
turnip /ˈtɜːnɪp/
uterus /ˈjuː.tər.əs/ pl **uteri**
vital /ˈvaɪ.təl/
weaning /wiːnɪŋ/
wing /wɪŋ/
womb /wuːm/
woodland /ˈwʊdlənd/
worn /wɔːn/ **out** /aʊt/
yam /jæm/

Solution to Exercise 1a
1b, 2c, 3f, 4d, 5i, 6a, 7h, 8j, 9g, 10e

Solution to Exercise 1b
1f, 2c, 3b, 4k, 5l, 6j, 7i, 8h, 9a, 10m, 11n, 12d, 13e, 14g

Unit 10 - How to put together, and eat, a healthy meal 2. Time to cook.

Fresh read meat

Fresh read meat is definitely a nutritional friend. This nutritious food is and always has been a most **valued component of traditional diets**, and yet today it is consistently vilified as a dietary villain by medics, dietitians, politicians and faddists. We can be sure that there is currently **no good evidence linking** fresh **red meat to heart disease or cancer**. Indeed, there is really good evidence suggesting the opposite; fresh red meat is health-enhancing.

So what should we avoid meat-wise? First look out for the product of ropey agriculture. Animals raised predominantly on grain will have higher levels of omega 6 fats, which we know are linked to heart disease and cancer. Such animals also tend to be given antibiotics and other damaging drugs routinely. The evidence linking industrially processed meat to cancer is also strong. Such products are packed with preservatives and other pathogenic chemicals, so eat your meat fresh rather than relying on the cheapest supermarket snags.

Build on the staple – salty and savoury

Once you have **established the staple(s)** in your dish, it is time to **choose your salty/savoury component**. There is a wide range of options, apart from the addition of refined salt itself. The salty/savoury flavour component of a meal is important – it adds depth, **stimulates appetite and secretion**, and enhances the other flavours. Particularly fascinating in this respect is the "sixth flavour" umami.

Our greatest exposure to **umami** is through **industrially produced mono-sodium glutamate** (MSG, or E621 as it appears on the packet, which is added to most processed foods as a cheap, possibly addictive, flavour enhancer. Consumption of this chemical is not desirable as it **bumps up our sodium levels** and consequently our blood pressure; it may cause other disease and could be neurotoxic – there is a scientific debate raging on this front, so you will have to make your own mind up on this subject. Suffice is to say that, in healthy terms, industrially produced MSG is a dirty also-ran when we compare it with traditional, **health-enhancing, umami rich alternatives, such as seaweed and fermented foods**.

Seaweed

Seaweed is a fast emerging superfood and one of the main dietary reasons why the Japanese live so long. Be aware that if you have a thyroid condition exclude seaweed from your diet due to its iodine content.

Fermented foods

These are also often umami-rich and vital as part of a healthy diet. Fermented-foods are common to all of the world's truly sustaining traditional diets. A great way to include these foods in your diet is through sauces such as **anchovy sauce, Worcester sauce, mushroom ketchup and brown sauce** (traditionally produced – not the mass-produced stuff). It seems incredible that we have forgotten the importance of fermented sauces to nutrition in spite of their central place in traditional diets around the world. Consider the various Asian versions: **soy sauce, fish sauce, shrimp paste, miso, black bean sauce and oyster sauce,** among others. In many ways, choosing the savoury component of a meal is the most exciting bit. Use savoury products like anchovy sauce, mushroom ketchup, Worcester sauce, and fish sauce in your cooking and you will massively **enhance its flavour and nutritional content** – and you will have little or no need to add salt. Or how about using some good-quality bouillon or an organic stock cube instead?

Add sour, bitter, spicy and aromatic

The sweet and salty/savoury flavours lay the foundations of a meal. We now need to add the other three flavours – sour, bitter and spicy/aromatic. **Using the sour, bitter and spicy/aromatic flavours** is essentially diagnostic, and this is where you can truly become your own nutritionist. It's up to you to look at the season, the weather, what food is available, and to see how you feel within yourself, and eat accordingly; almost inevitably, regardless of what foods you choose, you will end up using **all three of these flavours in different proportions**, according to circumstance.

Exercise 1a

Match the column A with the column B. Try to learn the expressions and/or sentences by heart.

A

1. Fresh read meat
2. There is currently no good evidence
3. The evidence linking industrially processed meat

4. The salty/savoury flavour component
5. Our greatest exposure to umami
6. Traditional, health-enhancing, umami rich alternatives,
7. Fermented-foods are common to
8. Use savoury products like anchovy sauce, mushroom ketchup, Worcester sauce, and fish sauce in your cooking
9. The sweet and salty/savoury flavours
10. We now need to add the other three flavours

B

a) adds depth, stimulates appetite and secretion, and enhances the other flavours.
b) all of the world's truly sustaining traditional diets.
c) always has been a most valued component of traditional diets.
d) and you will massively enhance its flavour and nutritional content.
e) are seaweed and fermented foods.
f) is through industrially produced mono-sodium glutamate which is added to most processed foods as a cheap, possibly addictive, flavour enhancer.
g) lay the foundations of a meal.
h) linking fresh red meat to heart disease or cancer.
i) sour, bitter and spicy/aromatic.
j) to cancer is strong.

Time to cook

Like all of life's great skills, to be good at cooking we have to take the time to practise **recognition of food** and its value, and develop **connection, through smells, textures, colour and taste.** These values were recognised in traditional nutritional approaches. In centuries past, cooking had greater significance than just sticking a pan on a burner. Instead, it was revered as a series of complex, intriguing and delightful processes. So we really should see cooking not just as a way of heating our food, but as a form of preparation, or even the first stage of digestion.

Preparation
Chopping

Our healthy diet requires time to choose great ingredients, time to **cut them up carefully,** not just to make them look attractive but to **release flavours,** and time to prepare them in other ways.

Marinating

Marinating is an example of a key preparation method. **Marinades** tend to be **acidic**, setting up a **pre-digestion process** in which the acids start to **break down the complex molecules** of the food. This is a form of pre-digestion that is particularly helpful **for tough and**

rich foods; the marinating gives our digestion a valuable helping hand. It also introduces flavours to a dish early on, giving them a chance to **meld and mature.** The digestive effect of marinating can be so powerful that some dishes, such as the Mexican ceviche, require no heating at all, **the lime juice and spices** making the **fish tender enough to be eaten raw.** Pickled herring, that was once consumed in Britain and is still widely consumed in Scandinavian countries is based on the same principle.

Cooking is essential

Humans and hominids have been cooking, or "**thermally processing**" food for over a million years. We absolutely depend on heating up our food to be healthy, and so does every major traditional dietary culture in the world. Cooking foods **takes the complex molecules** that make up food structure and **breaks them down**. The cellulose packaging and fibrous scaffold of plant food is broken apart so that we can easily **access the nutrients within**, and soluble fibre, vital for motility, is generated. In **animal foods**, the structural proteins like **collagen** are **broken down** to **form soluble proteins** such as **gelatine**. Gelatine is a wonderfully nourishing nutrient that is specifically created by cooking.

In addition to making food digestible, cooking helps **flavours** in combinations of ingredients **to interact**, develop and mellow, Similarly, **nutrients from different foods** intermingle and **react**, enhancing each other's actions, an effect known as synergism. As a general rule, **the more tough and fibrous** a food is, **the more we need to cook it**. Foods such as **beans**, some **root vegetables** and **cheap cuts of meat** like shin of beef or oxtail, lend themselves to gentle, **slow cooking** in soups, stews and casseroles, and, once they have been cooked like this, they become extremely nutritius. The right cooking method turns cheap food into some of the most healthy food.

Of course, this kind of long cooking requires some planing. **Slow cookers**, **hay boxes** and the like are great in this respect, as are **warming ovens** that can be used to cook food over **several hours**. By contrast, when it comes to **lighter foods** like **grains, potatoes** and **whole fish**, and even lighter foods like **leafy greens** and chicken and **fish fillets**, we can ease the overall intensity of the cooking, from **baking to boiling to steaming to stir-frying**, to **maintain freshness** of nutrient content without compromising the taste of the food. So the method that we use to cook our food is important in terms of health and the availability of nutrients. There is a balance to be struck. **Some foods** actually become more **nutritious the longer that they are cooked**, most notably **bone stocks** and **tough cuts of meat**. **Dried beans** have to be cooked for a long time to be edible and other tough plant material such as **kale** is much more palatable if it has been cooked well.

Other foods are **more nutritious with less cooking**, for example, **vitamin C** which is thermally degradable - we have to cook plant foods to get to more of the nutrients from them, but if we cook them too much we will destroy a lot of the goodness. Therefore, a little bit of cooking can go a long way; just **five minutes of steaming or stir-frying makes a big difference. The cooking method** is also important, as nutrients may leach into the cooking water, or be destroyed at high temperatures. **Boiling** leaches more than **steaming** although this becomes incidental if **cooking water is used** in a sauce or retained for use in a bone stock. However, both these water-based methods are preferable to **baking** and **roasting**, which involve **temperatures higher** than the boiling point of water: an important difference, since when food is cooked **at a temperature above 100°C, cancer-causing chemicals are formed**.

Exercise 1b
Match the column A with the column B. Try to learn the expressions and/or sentences by heart.

A

1. We have to take the time to practise recognition of food and its value,
2. Cut the ingredients up carefully
3. Marinating introduces flavours to a dish
4. The lime juice and spices
5. Cooking foods
6. In animal foods, the structural proteins like collagen
7. Gelatine is a wonderfully nourishing nutrient
8. Nutrients from different foods intermingle and react,
9. Foods such as beans, some root vegetables and cheap cuts of meat like shin of beef or oxtail
10. When it comes to lighter foods like grains, potatoes and whole fish, leafy greens and chicken and fish fillets,
11. Some foods become more nutritious the longer that they are cooked,
12. Other foods are more nutritious with less cooking;
13. The cooking method is also important,
14. Water-based methods are preferable to baking and roasting,
15. When food is cooked at a temperature above 100°C,

B

a) *and develop connection, through smells, textures, colour and taste.*
b) *are broken down to form soluble proteins such as gelatine.*
c) *as nutrients may leach into the cooking water, or be destroyed at high temperatures.*

d) *cancer-causing chemicals are formed.*
e) *enhancing each other's actions, an effect known as synergism.*
f) *giving them a chance to meld and mature.*
g) *if we cook them too much we will destroy a lot of the goodness.*
h) *lend themselves to gentle, slow cooking in extremely nutritious soups, stews and casseroles.*
i) *make the fish tender enough to be eaten raw.*
j) *makes the complex molecules that make up food structure and breaks them down.*
k) *most notably bone stocks and tough cuts of meat.*
l) *takes the complex molecules that make up food structure and breaks them down.*
m) *that is specifically created by cooking.*
n) *to release flavours.*
o) *we can ease the overall intensity of the cooking, from baking to boiling, steaming, or stir-frying to maintain freshness of nutrient content.*
p) *which involve temperatures higher than the boiling point of water.*

Exercise 2
Translate the expressions. Try to explain their meanings in English.

Consistently, villain, faddists, currently, evidence, linking, ropey agriculture, predominantly, tend to, relying on, established, wide range of options, mono-sodium glutamate, processed foods, desirable, seaweed, fermented foods, be aware that, thyroid condition, iodine, content, sustaining, incredible, in spite of, organic stock cube, inevitably, regardless, proportions, recognition, connection, smells, textures, taste, approaches, significance, burner, revered, complex, chopping, release flavours, marinating, tough and rich foods, meld and mature, powerful, tender, scaffold, gelatine, interact, mellow, intermingle, synergism, tough and fibrous, slow cookers, baking, boiling, steaming, stir-frying, availability, bone stocks, palatable, thermally, degradable, nutrients, may leach, cooking water, roasting, cancer-causing chemicals.

Exercise 3
Answer the following questions. Prepare short talks and/or dialogues on these topics.

1. Compare the properties of fresh red meat and industrially processed meat.
2. Differences between foods containing industrially produced mono-sodium glutamate and umami rich alternatives, such as seaweed and fermented foods.
3. Talk about fermented foods as part of a healthy diet.
4. Using the sour, bitter and spicy/aromatic flavours.
5. Why is marinating a key preparation method?

6. Why is cooking essential?
7. How does cooking change plant and animal foods?
8. Differences between roasting, baking, boiling, steaming and stir-frying.
9. Foods that require slow cooking.
10. Foods that require less cooking.

Vocabulary 10

Fill in the meanings in your mother language:

also-ran /'ɔ:l.səʊ.ræn/
anchovy /'æntʃəvɪ/
bit /bɪt/
bouillon /'bu:jɒn/
bump /bʌmp/ **up** /ʌp/
burner /'bɜ:nə/
ceviche /səvɪ:ʃəɪ/
chop /tʃɒp/
degradable /dɪ'greɪ.də.bl̩/
delightful /dɪ'laɪtfəl/
fad /'fæd/
fillet /'fɪlɪt/
gelatine /'dʒeləti:n/
hay /heɪ/ **box** /bɒks/
incidental /ˌɪnsɪ'dentəl/
incredible /ɪn'kredəbəl/
inevitably /ɪn'evɪtəblɪ/
intermingle /ˌɪn.tə'mɪŋ.gl̩/
intriguing /ɪn'tri:gɪŋ/
introduce /ˌɪn.trə'dju:s/
iodine /'aɪəˌdi:n/
leach /li:tʃ/
leafy /'li:fi/ **greens** /gri:nz/
marinate /'mærɪˌneɪt/
mature /mə'tjʊər/
meld /meld/
mellow /'meləʊ/
mind /maɪnd/
miso /'mi:.səʊ/
monosodium glutamate / ˌmɒnəʊ'səʊdɪəm 'glu:təˌmeɪt/
oven /'ʌvən/
oxtail /'ɒks.teɪl/
oyster /'ɔɪstə/
palatable /'pælətəbl/
preservative /prɪ'zɜ:vətɪv/
recognition /ˌrek.əg'nɪʃ.ən/
retain /rɪ'teɪn/
revere /rɪ'vɪər/
ropey /'rəʊpɪ/
scaffold /'skæf.əʊld/
seaweed /'si:ˌwi:d/
shin /ʃɪn/
shrimp /ʃrɪmp/
slow /sləʊ/ **cooker** /'kʊkər/
snag /snæg/
soluble /'sɒljʊbəl/
strike /straɪk/ **(struck, struck)**
suffice /sə'faɪs/
synergism /'sɪnədʒɪzəm/
tender /'ten.dər/
thyroid /θaɪrɔɪd/
value /'væl.ju:/
vilify /'vɪlɪˌfaɪ]/
villain /'vɪlən/

Solution to Exercise 1a
1c, 2h, 3j, 4f, 5f, 6e, 7b, 8d, 9g, 10i

Solution to Exercise 1b
1a, 2n, 3f, 4i, 5l, 6b, 7m, 8e, 9h, 10o, 11k, 12g, 13c, 14p, 15d

Unit 11 - Seasonal cooking. Be-Your-Own-Nutritionist Food Tower.

How you cook your foods affects its qualities, and this means that different methods are more suited to different seasons:

- **Late autumn, winter, early spring** – rich food is needed for cold weather. Soups, stews and casseroles can be rich and easy to digest. Baking and roasting concentrate food to make it richer but harder to digest; they shouldn't be overused as high heat can form cancer-causing chemicals.
- **Late spring, early summer** – mix bakes, stews, and soups with lighter, moister steamed and boiled foods. The occasional well-dressed salad is fine.
- **Hot summer** – steamed and stir-fried food predominates, with some dressed salads. Use offal and bones for light soups, broths, stews, dips and patés.
- **Early autumn** – anything goes. The weather is changeable and there is a glut of vegetables and fruit. An Indian summer means more stir-fries, steamed veg and light grilling and braising. Early storms and rain mean soup, stews, casseroles and bakes.

Microwaving

Microwaves destroy a breathtaking proportion of the nutrients in food as the microwaves penetrate deep and blow them apart. Microwaving also produces **cancer-causing substances**, and, when cooking with plastic, so-called **oestrogenic or hormone-mimicking chemicals** which have been linked to a range of diseases and conditions including obesity, cancer, polycystic ovarian syndrome (PCOS) and endometriosis.

Time to eat

Eating well depends entirely on **good food** and the **promotion of parasympathetic nervous system function**. We should be steady and unflustered when we eat. So, stay calm, avoid rushing, enjoy yourself, seek good company and avoid intense distraction. Then you'll be able to relax and focus on the food itself and give the digestive process the respect that it deserves.

Time to digest

Once a **meal is prepared, cooked and eaten**, it is the job of our **digestive system** to extract the maximum benefit from the food. What our guts need is just a little time. The principle of **taking time to digest** is very much at odds with our modern lifestyles. We are left with three options in relation to our energy "budget" and the needs of our digestive systems: work on and muddle through (illness and chronic fatigue awaits); stop eating the sandwiches and eat more digestible food (preferable); or **eat great food then rest and digest** (perfect).

Cultures that routinely take naps after lunch are more healthy than typical Westerners. The most studied of these populations are around the

Mediterranean; the South of France, Italy, Greece, Malta etc. The people in these traditional cultures live longer, healthier, and happier lives due to their **habit of resting after lunch.** If we take a little time to allocate most of our energy to digestion after a meal, then we can concentrate harder, be more energetic, and live longer and healthier lives. We have to find **a sensible compromise**. Just sit back, close your eyes, cut out the surrounding stimuli – noise, lights, people – and digest. We also need to **make our food more digestible**. A working sandwich lunch is bad in this respect - preserved meats, salad and cheap mass-produced bread are extraordinarily hard to break down and absorb once we have eaten them.

They sit like a lump in our stomachs, sucking the vitality away from our brains. Instead, we should be **eating easy-to-digest staples**, with **good-quality proteins and fats, vegetables** and lots of **spicy, aromatic, bitter and sour flavours**; all adjusted according to the needs of the dish. Eating a well-balanced hot meal at lunchtime is not easy, when you are working in an office and reliant on local fast-food providers every day. It would be better to bring more food from home in wide-necked, insulated food flasks.

Exercise 1a
Match the column A with the column B. Try to learn the expressions and/or sentences by heart.

A

1. Different methods
2. In late autumn, winter and early spring
3. In late spring and early summer
4. In hot summer
5. Early autumn
6. Oestrogenic or hormone-mimicking chemicals
7. Eating well depends entirely
8. Once a meal is prepared, cooked and eaten.
9. The principle of taking time to digest
10. The people in traditional cultures live longer, healthier, and happier lives
11. We need to
12. We should be eating easy-to-digest staples, with good-quality proteins and fats, vegetables

B

a) and lots of spicy, aromatic, bitter and sour flavours; all adjusted according to the needs of the dish.
b) are more suited to different seasons.
c) due to their habit of resting after lunch.
d) have been linked to a range of diseases and conditions including obesity, cancer, polycystic ovarian syndrome and endometriosis.
e) is very much at odds with our modern lifestyles.

f) *it is the job of our digestive system to extract the maximum benefit from the food.*

g) *make our food more digestible.*

h) *means more stir-fries, steamed veg and light grilling and braising.*

i) *mix bakes, stews, and soups with lighter, moister steamed and boiled foods.*

j) *on good food and the promotion of parasympathetic nervous system function.*

k) *soups, stews and casseroles can be rich and easy to digest.*

l) *steamed and stir-fried food predominates, with some dressed salads.*

Be-Your-Own-Nutritionist Food Tower

Our understanding of flavour tells us what we should be eating, but not necessarily how much of each food. The best way is to **construct our own food tower**, broken down into different sections to represent the **balance of food groups** that we should be eating, and in what **proportions**.

Each level represents a food group, and the area that each food group takes up on the tower is roughly equal to the proportion of our diet that that particular food group should occupy. This means that there is great flexibility in terms of how we eat – the tower does not portray absolute dietary rules, just the **guidelines**. It is a movable feast that is designed to accommodate our changing nutritional needs and of course our climate.

Fresh fats (vegetable and animal)
Herbs, spices and medicinal foods
Seeds and nuts
Fruits
Meat, fish and eggs
Grains and beans
Fresh vegetables

How the tower differs from pyramids

The tower is a simple visual way of showing us what proportion of our diet should be taken up by different types of foods. If we compare it with other food pyramids we can see how much more nourishing age-old, traditional diets are. **Breakfast cereals**, for example, are **mass-produced** for industrial and commercial convenience and are therefore **nutritionally compromised.** While food corporation pyramids include factory food that we should definitely be avoiding, fad diets earnestly direct us away from these foods towards foods that are far too extreme and may lead to eating habits that will damage health.

Calorie-controlled diets tend to include far too much raw food and not enough nourishing fats. Diets that encourage broader consumption of richer foods for body-fat reduction, which can form part of a healthy weight-loss regime, often **fail to emphasize the importance of cooking** and combining these rich foods for digestibility. This can lead to basing the diet on **a limited range of foods**, which can be **harmful**; people end up eating too much steak and chicken breast rather than whole fish, offal, marrow, bone stocks and cheap cuts that lean, healthy, traditional populations have valued over millennia. As a result, many people on so called **low-carb diets** can risk **nutritional deficiencies**.

Exercise 1b
Match the column A with the column B. Try to learn the expressions and/ or sentences by heart.

A

1. Construct our own food tower, broken down into different sections
2. The tower does not portray absolute dietary rules,
3. Breakfast cereals are mass-produced
4. Calorie-controlled diets
5. Basing the diet on a limited range of foods
6. People end up eating too much steak and chicken breast
7. Many people on so called low-carb diets

B

a) can be harmful.
b) for industrial and commercial convenience and are therefore nutritionally compromised.
c) just the guidelines.
d) rather than whole fish, offal, marrow, bone stocks and cheap cuts.
e) risk nutritional deficiencies.
f) tend to include far too much raw food and not enough nourishing fats.
g) to represent the balance of food groups that we should be eating, and in what proportions.

Exercise 2
Translate the expressions. Try to explain their meanings in English.

Seasonal cooking, suited, rich food, soups, stews and casseroles, well-dressed salad, broths, stews, dips, patés, changeable, grilling and braising, penetrate deep, microwaving, linked to, polycystic ovarian syndrome, endometriosis, promotion of parasympathetic nervous system, distraction, extract benefit, odds with, options, take naps, habit of resting, concentrate harder, sensible compromise, local fast-food providers, food flasks, understanding, construct, proportions, equal to, dietary rules, guidelines, accommodate the needs, differs from, be taken up, compare with, nourishing, commercial, convenience, compromised, definitely, fad diets, encourage, fail, consumption, emphasize, digestibility, harmful, low-carb diets, nutritional deficiencies.

Exercise 3
Answer the following questions. Prepare short talks and/or dialogues on these topics.

1. What do you understand by the term seasonal cooking?
2. What are the dangers of microwaving?
3. What does eating well depend on?
4. Why would you recommend the habit of resting after lunch?
5. Why is eating a well-balanced hot meal at lunchtime important?
6. What is the best way to construct our own food tower?
7. How does the tower differ from pyramids?
8. What are the principles of a healthy weight-loss regime?

Vocabulary 11

Fill in the meanings in your mother language:

accommodate /ə'kɒm.ə.deɪt/
allocate /'æl.ə.keɪt/
apart /ə'pɑ:t/
await /ə'weɪt/
bake /beɪk/
base /beɪs/
be at odds /ɒdz/ **with** /wɪð/
blow /bləʊ/ **(blew, blown)**
braise /breɪz/
breathtaking /'breθˌteɪkɪŋ/
convenience /kən'vi:niəns/
deficiency /dɪ'fɪʃ.ənt .si/
deserve /dɪ'zɜ:v/
dip /dɪp/
direct /da ɪ'rekt/
earnest /'ɜ:nɪst/
endometriosis /ˌen.dəʊˌmi:.tri'əʊ.sɪs/
equal /'i:kwəl/
feast /fi:st/
flask /flɑ:sk/
flustered /'flʌstəd/
glut /glʌt/
guideline /'gaɪd.laɪn/
insulate /'ɪnsjəleɪt/
marrow /'mærəʊ/
medicinal /mə'dɪs.ɪ.nəl/
microwave /'maɪkrəʊˌweɪv/
mimick /'mɪmɪk/
muddle /'mʌdl/
occasional /ə'keɪ.ʒə.nəl/
occupy /'ɒkjʊˌpaɪ/
oestrogen /'i:.strə.dʒən/
ovarian /əʊ'veə.ri.ən/
paté /'pæteɪ/
penetrate /'pen.ɪ.treɪt/
polycystic /ˌpɒl.ɪ'sɪs.tɪk/
portray /pɔ:'treɪ/
reliant /rɪ'laɪənt/
roughly /'rʌf.lɪ/
rule /ru:l/
seasonal /'si:zənəl/
sensible /'sensɪbl/
suck /sʌk/
take /teɪk/ **a nap** /næp/
tower /taʊər/
well-dressed /ˌwel'drest/ (salad)

Solution to Exercise 1a
1b. 2k, 3i, 4l, 5h, 6d, 7j, 8f, 9e, 10c, 11g, 12a

Solution to Exercise 1b
1g, 2c, 3b, 4f, 5a, 6d, 7e

Unit 12 - Fresh fats. What we shouldn't be eating 1.

There is a distinctly proud place for fats and oils in this tower: from **animal fats**, such as **dripping, suet** and **butter**, to **plant fats**, like **olive oil** and **flax, walnut, rapeseed and sesame oils**. Fats are fundamental to health. These include not just the fats that are officially recognized as **health-enhancing**, such as **omega 3s and mono-unsaturates**, but also fats that have in recent decades been considered woefully unhealthy. In much of the **industrialized world**, our view of fat has become incredibly warped, in this bloated age of **obesity, excessive consumption** and cheap industrially manipulated **hydrocarbons**. But eaten in moderation, **good, fresh, natural fats** are very good food. They fill us up, suppressing our appetites so that we don't overeat and put on weight, and they provide **essential fatty acids** (EFAs), vital building blocks for our cells and nervous systems. For these reasons, long-living healthy folk all over the world depend on consuming appreciable amounts of fat for their well-being.

Saturated Fats

Contrary to the prevailing view, animal fat does not cause heart disease, while the omega 6 fats in margarine do. There is no evidence that eating less animal fat improves health or extends our lives; in fact, recent research links this important nutrient to well-being and happiness.

Butter

The best available evidence indicates that butter does not raise heart disease levels, while margarine – with its water content, colouring and industrially modified oils - seems insipid. Indeed, omega 6 fats such as those found in margarine, sunflower oil and a number of other plant fats have been linked to heart disease among other pathologies.

Herbs, spices and medicinal foods

These foods are extremely important and significantly under-represented in diets for health. They are so valuable because the vast majority of them have strong flavours and consequently **strong actions**. We should turn to these foods to achieve an effect in a dish, to create balance and compensate for prevailing clima, lifestyle, or emotion. **Medicinal foods** without strong flavours, such as **mushrooms, certain nuts, fruits and offal**, cross over with other food categories in the tower. They have a fundamental role in well-being, providing intense and sustaining nutrition for vibrant health and long life.

Seeds and nuts

Seeds and nuts (**walnuts, chestnuts, hazelnuts**) are valued as good snack foods and sources of valuable oils.

Fruit

We all know about **apples, pears, blackberries, strawberries and plums**. Most sets of food guidelines recommend more fruit but fruit fibre can be very hard to break down (like **bananas**, especially when they are not completely ripe), tropical fruits such as **pineapples and mangos** can be very sugary and create digestive imbalance, and the acidity of fruits such as apples, plums and **citrus** in the wrong context can easily **disturb the gut.** For this reason, many people with IBS struggle with raw fruit, much to their frustration, as it perceived in our culture as being particularly healthy. They are suffering from a common dietary error. In digestive terms, most **fruit should be eaten dried, or spiced and cooked**, especially when the weather is cold and damp.

Meat, fish and eggs

Seafoods, eggs, meat and offal are all wonderful foods that add vital richness to our diets in the face of busy lives and a cold, damp climate. For environmental sustainability, we need to rely more on plant foods, in particular plant fats and foods that are rich in protein. You can feel relaxed if animal foods make up 15-50% of your diet, although the less meat and fish that you eat then the more richness you have to make up from **plant sources** such as **oils, nuts, seeds and beans**.

Grains and beans

Beans are the protein-rich reason that we can get away with eating less meat. Because of their **protein content**, beans are much more substantial and filling than other plant foods. For example, **lentils** were routinely used to thicken or bulk our soups and stews, and fresh beans were regular fare. **Pulses** are also a major part of Japanese and Chinese diets (**bean sprouts, mung, hyacinth and aduki beans**) and the Mediterranean diet (**haricot, borlotti, black and broad beans, chickpeas**, etc.). Soaking dried beans well, then thoroughly rinsing them and boiling them with kelp can help to reduce generating tremendous wind. It is certainly essential to boil beans for a long time to deactivate poisonous lectins and enzyme inhibitors. **Grains** are also important staples, although not quite as exciting in medicinal terms as beans. If you intend to lose weigh you may need to modify your grain intake.

Fresh vegetables

This is an important part of the food tower. The bottom line it that we simply don't eat as enough fresh vegetables and yet they are foods that do so much to make us tick. These are definitely **worth including as a priority** in your diet. But otherwise we just need to get to know local veg when it is in season, grow it ourselves, head off to the greengrocer and, above all, eat the stuff.

Exercise 1a
Match the column A with the column B. Try to learn the expressions and/or sentences by heart.

A

1. Eaten in moderation,
2. Natural fats fill us up, suppressing our appetites
3. Contrary to the prevailing view, animal fat does not cause heart disease,
4. Omega 6 fats such as those found in margarine, sunflower oil and a number of other plant fats
5. Herbs, spices and medicinal foods are so valuable
6. Medicinal foods without strong flavours,
7. Seeds and nuts (walnuts, chestnuts, hazelnuts)
8. Fruit fibre can be very hard to break down
9. Tropical fruits such as pineapples and mangos can be very sugary and create digestive imbalance,
10. Seafoods, eggs, meat and offal are all wonderful foods
11. The less meat and fish that you eat
12. Because of their protein content,
13. Lentils are routinely used
14. Soaking dried beans well,
15. Grains are important staples,
16. Fresh vegetables are definitely

B

a) although not quite as exciting in medicinal terms as beans.
b) and the acidity of fruits such as apples, plums and citrus in the wrong context can easily disturb the gut.
c) are valued as good snack foods and sources of valuable oils.
d) beans are much more substantial and filling than other plant foods.
e) because the vast majority of them have strong flavours and consequently strong actions.
f) good, fresh, natural fats are very good food.
g) have been linked to heart disease among other pathologies.
h) like bananas, especially when they are not completely ripe.
i) so that we don't overeat and put on weight, and they provide essential fatty acids.
j) such as mushrooms, certain nuts, fruits and offal, cross over with other food categories in the tower.
k) that add vital richness to our diets in the face of busy lives and a cold, damp climate.
l) the more richness you have to make up from plant sources such as oils, nuts, seeds and beans.
m) then thoroughly rinsing them and boiling them with

kelp can help to reduce generating tremendous wind.

n) to thicken or bulk our soups and stews, and fresh beans are regular fare.

o) while the omega 6 fats in margarine do.

p) worth including as a priority in your diet.

What we shouldn't be eating 1

Salt, refined sugar and cheap fat are the mainstays of **industrial food**. They have been called **junk food**, and they really need to be avoided. Food industrialists pack their products with salt, sugar and fat for the simple reason that they know that these foods **create compulsion**. We find these simple, cheap ingredients incredibly hard to resits.

These manufacturers are playing on what was once a **human survival mechanism**. In the old hunter-gatherer and early agricultural days, human beings developed an obsession with two types of food that are rare, or difficult to find in nature: **calorie-dense foodstuffs like honey and fat**, and **mineral salts, sodium chloride** in particular, which, away from the sea at least, is also uncommon.To this end our behaviour was adapted to a dedicated hunt for sources of these foods, and salt licks (inland concentrations of salt), a trait that is **shared with other mammal species**. And consequently many animal species can be seen to congregate around salt licks, as well as to brave bee stings to steal honey from wild hives, and to seek out and relish seeds, fresh kills and other calorie-rich delights. Unfortunately for the human race, not only do we crave these foods but, because of their historical scarcity, they have a disproportionate effect on our metabolisms. Hence we are still geared up to **retain and nurture every calorie** of sugar or fructose that we can **as extra body fat,** rather than excrete it or burn it off.

This strategy was valuable in the past because our ancestors never knew when they would come across sugary foods again, but these days it means that **we gain and retain weight** as never before. We have to take care of our diet from the very beginning, because cravings for and addiction to salt, sugar and cheap modified fat are formed in early childhood, probably even in the womb. **Cook good fresh food**. Try **not to get addicted.** This principle is as relevant in our schools and workplaces as in our home kitchens. Cooking fresh food to avoid eating junk food is at the heart of this diet. Only then can we protect our digestion and our general physiology.

Hard-to-digest-foods

Hard-to-digest-foods include major food groups that can be viewed as **traditional**, such as **raw and cold food, preserved foods and very rich foods.** They may also be good quality, in that they are well produced but they are difficult to digest. These sorts of foods that can be part of a healthy diet should be eaten **in small quantities.**

Raw and cold foods

Human beings evolved **cooking.** We **process our food** before we eat it to make life **easier for our digestive systems**. Since we have always eaten warm food, **stomach enzymes** have evolved to work optimally at body temperature, **around 37 °C**. At this temperature the complex three dimensional shapes of the enzymes are just right to fit the chemical constituents of the food, like a key in a lock, and break them down. If we then go on to eat and drink **cold food and drinks**, the shapes of the **enzymes** distort – they no longer work since they can't **easily latch onto the molecules** that they are designed **to break down**. In this, very real chemical way, coldness inhibits digestion and it creates a de facto digestive paralysis. A paralysis that can be exaggerated and distinctly uncomfortable because **coldness** also **inhibits circulation**.

Exercise 1b
Match the column A with the column B. Try to learn the expressions and/or sentences by heart.

A

1. Salt, refined sugar and cheap fat have been called junk food,
2. Salt, sugar and fat
3. Human beings developed an obsession with two types of food that are rare, or difficult to find in nature:
4. We are still geared up
5. Cravings for and addiction to salt, sugar and cheap modified fat
6. Hard-to-digest-foods include major food groups
7. We process our food before we eat it
8. At body temperature, around 37 °C
9. If we eat and drink cold food and drinks, the shapes of the enzymes distort;
10. Coldness inhibits digestion and

B

a) and they really need to be avoided.
b) are formed in early childhood, probably even in the womb.
c) calorie-dense foodstuffs like honey and fat, and mineral salts, sodium chloride in particular.
d) coldness also inhibits circulation.
e) create compulsion.
f) that can be viewed as traditional, such as raw and cold food, preserved foods and very rich foods.
g) the complex three dimensional shapes of the enzymes are just right to fit the chemical constituents of the food.
h) they no longer work since they can't easily latch onto the molecules that they are designed to break down.

i) to make life easier for our digestive systems.

j) to retain and nurture every calorie of sugar or fructose that we can as extra body fat, rather than excrete it or burn it off.

Exercise 2

Translate the expressions. Try to explain their meanings in English.

Dripping, suet, flax, walnut, rapeseed, fundamental, health-enhancing, excessive consumption, in moderation, suppressing, overeat, depend on, prevailing view, extends, recent research, industrially modified oils, sunflower oil, vast majority, consequently, compensate for, sustaining nutrition, walnuts, chestnuts, hazelnuts blackberries, strawberries, plums, pineapples, mangos, perceived, suffering from, rely on, get away with, substantial, filling, poisonous, intend, greengrocer, create compulsion, hard to resits, human survival mechanism, obsession with, behaviour, dedicated, hunt for, consequently, congregate, seek out, relish, crave, scarcity, disproportionate, retain nurture, gain and retain weight, cravings, addiction, general physiology, preserved foods, rich foods, process our food, three dimensional shapes of the enzymes, chemical constituents, distort, latch, designed, inhibits digestion, exaggerated, distinctly.

Exercise 3

Answer the following questions. Prepare short talks and/or dialogues on these topics.

1. Why are fats fundamental to health?
2. Give examples of animal fats and plant fats.
3. The importance of good, fresh, natural fats.
4. Compare butter and margarine.
5. Why are herbs, spices and medicinal foods so valuable?
6. Give examples of medicinal foods, seeds and nuts. Why are they important?
7. The importance of fruit and vegetables.
8. Why should we eat meat, fish and eggs?
9. Give examples of grains and beans. Why are they important?
10. What do you understand by the term junk food?
11. Describe a human survival mechanism.
12. What causes that we gain and retain weight?
13. When are cravings for and addiction to salt, sugar and cheap modified fat formed?
14. What happens when we eat raw and cold foods?

Vocabulary 12

Fill in the meanings in your mother language:

appreciable /əˈpriːʃəbl/
blackberry /ˈblækbəri/
borlotti bean /bɔːˈlɒt.iˌbiːn/
brave /breɪv/
calorie /ˈkæləri/ **-dense** /dens/
chickpea /ˈʧɪkˌpiː/
congregate /ˈkɒŋgrɪgeɪt/
constituent /kənˈstɪt.ju.ənt/
contrary /ˈkɒn.trə.ri/
cross /krɒs/ **over** /ˈəʊvər/
deactivate /ˌdiˈæk.tɪ.veɪt/
delight /dɪˈlaɪt/
disproportionate /ˌdɪsprəˈpɔːʃənət/
disturb /dɪˈstɜːb/
dripping /ˈdrɪpɪŋ/
evolve /ɪˈvɒlv/
exaggerate /ɪgˈzæʤəˌreɪt/
extend /ɪkˈstend/
fare /feər/
folk /fəʊk/
greengrocer /ˈgriːnˌgrəʊsər/
head /hed/ **off** /ɒf/
hive /haɪv/
hunt /hʌnt/
hunter-gatherer /ˌhʌn.təˈgæð.ər.ər/
in moderation /ˌmɒd.ərˈeɪ.ʃən/
inhibitor /ɪnˈhɪb.ɪ.tər/
junk /dʒʌŋk/
latch /læʧ/
lectin /ˈlɛktɪn/
mainstay /ˈmeɪnsteɪ/
margarine /ˌmɑːdʒəˈriːn/
mung bean /ˈmʌŋˌbiːn/
obsession /əbˈseʃən/
paralysis /pəˈræl.ə.sɪs/ pl **paralyses**
perceive /pəˈsiːv/
pineapple /ˈpaɪnæpl/
prevailing /prɪˈveɪ.lɪŋ/
rapeseed /ˈreɪpˌsiːd/
relish /ˈrelɪʃ/
resit /ˌriːˈsɪt/
richness /ˈrɪtʃˌnɪs/
ripe /raɪp/
salt /sɔːlt/ **lick** /lɪk/
scarcity /ˈskeəsəti/
soaking /ˈsəʊkɪŋ/
sprout /spraʊt/
sting /stɪŋ/
sue /suː/
sunflower /ˈsʌnflaʊər/
sustainability /səˈsteɪ.nəˈbɪl.ɪ.ti/
tick /tɪk/
trait /treɪt/
tremendous /trɪˈmendəs/
warped /wɔːpt/
woeful /ˈwəʊfəl/

Solution to Exercise 1a
1f, 2i, 3o, 4g, 5e, 6j, 7c, 8h, 9b, 10k, 11l, 12d, 13n, 14m, 15a, 16p

Solution to Exercise 1b
1a, 2e, 3c, 4j, 5b, 6f, 7i, 8g, 9h, 10d

Unit 13 - What we shouldn't be eating 2

Combinations to counter cold food and drink

Savoury food

Chilli, paprika, cayenne pepper, garlic, horseradish, mustard seed (commonly seen in traditional recipes that are served cold, such as gazpacho, ceviche, cold beef sandwiches).

Sweet food

Allspice, cinnamon, clove, dried ginger, fresh ginger, mace, nutmeg These all **work well with sweet flavours**, making them particularly compatible with iced offenders like **sorbet, ice cream** and cold winter and summer **cocktails.** A good chef for foodie will undoubtedly be able to add to this list.

Combinations to counter raw food

Bananas, for example, are fibrous and starchy and severely **obstruct motility,** particularly in children. Sautéed with **nutmeg** and a tiny pinch of **dried ginger**, they are a delicious and much more digestible child-friendly food. For **salads**, it is essential to add a **spicy dressing** to stimulate motility and secretion, hence the convention of adding **black pepper** and/or **mustard** to dressings.

Preserved foods

Similarly important is the chemical resilience of food; some foods are very **resistant** to their large molecules being broken down in the gut, which means that **motility and adsorption are inhibited**. Others have artificial or natural **preservatives** and **inhibit the actions of bacteria and fungi** in general. These preservatives therefore inhibit our own **gut symbionts**, whose digestive action is such an essential component of human gut function.

An informative way to test a food's chemical resilience is to mush it up and place on a shelf, then set **how easily the microbes around it settle and grow,** breaking down the nutrients to sustain that growth.

Those microbes and our gut symbionts use a similar suite of enzymes, and other chemicals and secretions, to break down food so the length of time it takes a **food to go rotten** is an appropriate **indicator of how digestible** it might be to us. We now know that **artificial preservatives** are linked to a number of very **serious and fatal diseases**, due at least in part to their **effects on digestive symbionts**. As far as our healthy diet is concerned, it is absolutely clear that we shouldn't be keen on artificially preserved foods.

This principle should also be applied to a different group of foods, foods that have been produced in such a way that they are naturally preserved. The **preservation process** such as **smoking**, protects these foods against the effects of bacteria and moulds and, at the same time, renders them harder for us to break down. The main foods are **cheese, cured and smoked meats, and pastry.**

Cheese

It is controversial to say that cheese might be harmful to health. Cheese tastes good; it is a concentrated food, packed with fat, protein, salt and sugars, exactly what our bodies have evolved to crave. There is no denying that cheese is **difficult to digest**. It is a food that is high-fat and therefore rich, but sour accompaniments alone, such as pickle, cannot compensate for this, because it has other stubborn constituents that the digestive system struggles with.

Casein, a **milk protein**, and **lactose**, a **milk sugar**, both of which are prevalent in cheese, are very hard to break down in the human gut, particularly in the case of adults, many of whom lack the **specific**

enzyme, lactase, that **breaks down the milk sugar.** It is this very indigestibility that has made cheese so useful to us in the past. By turning fresh milk into cheese, we create a **store of fat and protein that could last for years**; bacteria and moulds struggle to digest it too. Eating cheese might have broad implications for our health. It can **obstruct motility**, causing **bloating and fatigue**, potentially further-reaching **inflammatory conditions** and severe diseases such as **bladder cancer**. One of the reasons for the popularity of cheese is its **calcium content**, which is relatively high. Calcium consumption is important for the development and maintenance **of strong bones** but it **seems to be a myth** that dairy consumption alone **protects us against osteoporosis.**

There are **many foods other than dairy products** that have **high levels of calcium** and the other nutrients necessary for strong bones, and these foods are much easier for our bodies to break down and assimilate than cheese. The calcium content attributed to specific foods varies greatly in different sources, and depends on how foods are grown, processed or tested.

Food	**Approx. calcium level** (mg/100g portion
Kelp	1, 200
Hard cheese, Sesame seeds	680
Sardines, Tofu	510
Almonds, Amaranth, Figs (dried), Parsley	210-250
Kale (cooked)	180
Black beans, Chickpeas, Pistachio nuts, Quinoa, Sunflower seeds, Watercress	140-170
Milk, Yoghurt	120
Broccoli, Cottage cheese, Eggs, Salmon	40-80

Exercise 1a

Match the column A with the column B. Try to learn the expressions and/or sentences by heart.

A

1. Chilli, paprika, cayenne pepper, garlic, horseradish or mustard seed
2. Allspice, cinnamon, clove, dried ginger, fresh ginger, mace, and nutmeg
3. Bananas, sautéed with nutmeg and a tiny pinch of dried ginger,
4. For salads, it is essential to add
5. Preserved foods are very resistant
6. Artificial or natural preservatives
7. An informative way to test a food's chemical resilience
8. The length of time it takes a food to go rotten
9. Artificial preservatives are linked to a number of very serious and fatal diseases,
10. The preservation process such as smoking, protects these foods

against the effects of bacteria and moulds

11. Casein, a milk protein, and lactose, a milk sugar, both of which are prevalent in cheese,
12. By turning fresh milk into cheese,
13. Eating cheese
14. One of the reasons for the popularity of cheese
15. There are many foods other than dairy products that have high levels of calcium

B

a) *a spicy dressing to stimulate motility and secretion.*

b) *and, at the same time, renders them harder for us to break down.*

c) *are seen in traditional recipes that are served cold, such as gazpacho, ceviche, or cold beef sandwiches.*

d) *are a delicious and digestible child-friendly food.*

e) *are very hard to break down in the human gut, particularly in the case of adults, many of whom lack the specific enzyme, lactase, that breaks down the milk sugar.*

f) *can obstruct motility, causing bloating and fatigue, potentially inflammatory conditions and severe diseases.*

g) *due to their effects on digestive symbionts.*

h) *inhibit the actions of bacteria and fungi in general.*

i) *is an appropriate indicator of how digestible it might be to us.*

j) *is its calcium content, which is relatively high.*

k) *is to mush it up and place on a shelf, then set how easily the microbes around it settle and grow.*

l) *we create a store of fat and protein that could last for years.*

m) *which are much easier for our bodies to break down and assimilate than cheese.*

n) *which means that motility and adsorption are inhibited.*

o) *work well with sweet flavours, making them particularly compatible with sorbet, ice cream and cold cocktails.*

Preserved meats and smoked foods

Like cheese, these products were developed in pre-refrigeration times as a way of **prolonging** their **shelf life**, and, like cheese, they are hard for us to digest. They are the opposite of healthy. Studies have repeatedly **linked** the consumption of **preserved and smoked foods** to a range of **cancers** and official agencies recently **warned parents** not to give their children **ham, salami or bacon** sandwiches in their lunch boxes. It is sensible to limit such ingredients in our diets.

The key is to **use them in small quantities** to add richness and depth of flavour and always to **combine them with** other ingredients such as **lemon juice, cider, vinegar** and the like so that their richness can **disperse** in the dish and so that the **acids and antioxidants**, can start to break them down before we come to eat them. Above all, where it comes to foods like ham and bacon, **quality matters**. A preservative-free naturally produced product made from very high-quality meat is a much healthier option than a sort of ham-like, died-pink, preservative-packed alternative.

Pastry

Pastry, a combination of **fat and wheat flour**, is hard to digest by design. It is another food that fails the chemical resilience test; left out, it just sits there for weeks. In the old days, this property was very useful indeed, because pastry was used as food packaging. So why do we eat so much pastry now? Because it's full of fat and is delicious. But this, combined with the **high gluten content** of the flour, makes it particularly **tough on digestion**.

We should eat relatively **little pastry** as part of a **healthy** diet. It is so heavy that it bogs us down in our cold climate. When we do eat pastry, as a special treat, of course, it should always combined with digestion-enhancing accompaniments. Pastry can be healthy as long as it remains a relatively small part of overall diet. And only if it is made in a traditional way, with **suet or butter and spelt.** It remains, however, a rich food, so the strategies for enhancing digestibility are important.

Combinations for hard-to-digest foods

Cheese

To counter its stubborn fat cheese needs a **sour condiment**. To counter its stubborn protein it needs **spice**. This is why a good spicy pickle is traditionally combined with cheese. Ideally, make your own and use lots of **vinegar** and sour ingredients like **green tomatoes**, combined with mild aromatic spices like **cinnamon** and **cloves**, with something with a bit of **punch** like a **chilli**.

Pastry

A similar **pickle** enhances the digestibility of pastry, composed as it is of stubborn fat (shortening, industrially modified fat, butter, suet or other fat) and stubborn protein (gluten). Another strategy is to accompany pies and pastries with a **spiced fruit jelly** or **purée**.

Preserved and smoked meats and fish

The crucial flavours for these foods are **sour**, made more palatable by **spice**. When preparing **smoked mackerel**, for example, **marinade it in lemon** juice first, even in only for a few minutes. The acids in the juice react with the protein and fat of the fish, effectively predigesting it. Then add plenty of **black pepper** to stimulate gut motility. The same principle is classically applied to smoked **salmon**. For **bacon** or

ham, **mustard** is a typical spicy condiment, combined with the sour of **gherkin, sauerkraut** or other **pickled vegetables**. Also, try the **tomato ketchup**. It is an ideal accompaniment to these hard-to-digest foods.

Exercise 1b
Match the column A with the column B. Try to learn the expressions and/or sentences by heart.

A

1. Studies have repeatedly linked
2. Official agencies recently warned parents
3. The key is to use preserved and smoked foods in small quantities
4. Pastry, a combination of fat and wheat flour,
5. The high gluten content of the flour,
6. Pastry can be healthy
7. To counter its stubborn fat
8. To counter its stubborn protein
9. A similar pickle enhances the digestibility of pastry,
10. The crucial flavours for preserved and smoked meats and fish
11. When preparing smoked mackerel,
12. The acids in the juice react with
13. For bacon or ham,

B

a) and always to combine them with lemon juice, cider, vinegar and the like so that their richness can disperse in the dish.
b) are sour, made more palatable by spice.
c) as it is composed of stubborn fat (shortening, industrially modified fat, butter, suet or other fat) and stubborn protein (gluten).
d) as long as it remains a relatively small part of overall diet.
e) cheese needs a sour condiment.
f) is hard to digest.
g) it needs spice.
h) makes pastry particularly tough on digestion.
i) marinade it in lemon juice first.
j) mustard is a typical spicy condiment, combined with the sour of gherkin, sauerkraut or other pickled vegetables.
k) not to give their children ham, salami or bacon sandwiches in their lunch boxes.
l) the consumption of preserved and smoked foods to a range of cancers.
m) the protein and fat of the fish, effectively predigesting it.

Exercise 2
Translate the expressions. Try to explain their meanings in English.

Counter, horseradish, gazpacho, ceviche, allspice, cinnamon, clove, ginger, mace, nutmeg, compatible with, offender, chef, sautéed, nutmeg, pinch, spicy dressing, convention, preseved foods, chemical resilience, resistant, inhibited, artificial or natural preservatives, bacteria and fungi, mush up, microbes settle and grow, artificial preservatives, serious and fatal diseases, preservation process, smoking, moulds, denying, sour accompaniments, pickles, compensate for, stubborn constituents, prevalent, indigestibility, implications, bloating, fatigue, quinoa, inflammatory conditions, bladder cancer, calcium content, dairy consumption, assimilate, attributed, kelp, cottage cheese, watercress, chickpeas, parsley, figs, almonds, amaranth, kale, shelf life, opposite, sensible to limit, vinegar, disperse, pastry, resilience test, special treat, digestion-enhancing, accompaniments, overall diet, stubborn fat, punch, shortening, suet, fruit jelly, purée, crucial, gherkin, sauerkraut, pickled vegetables, accompaniment.

Exercise 3
Answer the following questions. Prepare short talks and/or dialogues on these topics.

1. List savoury and sweet ingredients suitable for cold foods and drinks.
2. Which combinations can counter raw food?
3. What are advantages and disadvantages of preserved foods?
4. What do you think about eating cheese?
5. Why shouldn't children eat preserved meats and smoked foods?
6. Why are the strategies for enhancing digestibility of pastry important?
7. Talk about combinations for hard-to-digest foods (cheese, pastry, preserved and smoked meats and fish).

Vocabulary 13

Fill in the meanings in your mother language:

attribute /ˈæt.rɪ.bjuːt/
bladder /ˈblæd.ər/
bog /bɒg/ **down** /daʊn/
chef /ʃef/
clove /kləʊv/
condition /kənˈdɪʃən/
convention /kənˈvenʃən/
cottage /ˈkɒt.ɪdʒ/ **cheese** /tʃiːz/
deny /dɪˈnaɪ/
dressing /ˈdres.ɪŋ/
dried /draɪd/
foodie /ˈfuːdi/
gazpacho /gæsˈpætʃ.əʊ/
gherkin /ˈgɜː.kɪn/
horseradish /ˈhɔːsˌræd.ɪʃ/
implication /ˌɪm.plɪˈkeɪ.ʃən/
kelp /kelp/
mace /meɪs/
matter /ˈmæt.ər/
mush /mʌʃ/
myth /mɪθ/

nutmeg /ˈnʌtmeg/
offender /əˈfen.dər/
option /ˈɒp.ʃən/
pastry /ˈpeɪstrɪ/
pinch /pɪntʃ/
prevalent /ˈprev.əl.ənt/
punch /pʌntʃ/
quinoa /kɪnˈwɑː/
resilience /rɪˈzɪl.i.əns/
salmon /ˈsæm.ən/
sauté /ˈsəʊteɪ/
settle /ˈset.l̩/
shortening /ˈʃɔːtənɪŋ/
sorbet /ˈsɔː.beɪ/
spelt /spelt/
suet /ˈsuː.ɪt/
suite /swiːt/
treat /triːt/
undoubtedly /ʌnˈdaʊtɪdli/

Solution to Exercise 1a
1c, 2o, 3d, 4a, 5n, 6h, 7k, 8i, 9g, 10b, 11e, 12l, 13f, 14j, 15m

Solution to Exercise 1b
1l, 2k, 3a, 4f, 5h, 6d, 7e, 8g, 9c, 10b, 11i, 12m, 13j

Unit 14 - How and where to get the best food. Well produced/organic food. Specialist retailers.

Now that you have got a good idea of what you want to cook, and how to cook it, it is vital to know **where and how to get the food**. There are three principles, all of which are key to our building a healthy relationship with food:

- seasonal
- local
- well produced

Eating seasonally

In the days before the development of refrigeration and the advent of air freight, food had to be seasonal. There was no alternative. Inevitably, this dictated the pattern of food shopping and eating: what was available, what had grown well from year to year and what suited purses and household needs.

Today, nearly every **food is available year round** and cookbooks rarely have significant seasonal content. Therefore we tend to decide what to eat from a recipe, then go out and buy the ingredients, without looking out of the window or referencing a calendar. This modern habit of ours has an inherent **lack of sensitivity** that detaches us from our **health, climate and environment**. It means that we are effectively eating to other countries' seasons and food varieties. We ought to be considering it now, as there are compelling health arguments involved.

In **late autumn and winter, starch root vegetables, nuts and seeds**, intense **bitter greens** (like kale and Brussels sprouts) and **fatty meat and fish,** together with preserved foods such as **pickled, salted and fermented fish,** are most available. Which is just what we need, when the climate is persistently cold and damp, warranting **rich, sustaining food** and **strong bitter, spicy and sour** flavours to help us **digest it.**

In **late spring, summer and early autumn, lighter greens**, **fresh beans** and **soft fruit** can be eaten in abundance straight out of the field, combined with the right mix of **refreshing sour** flavours and **cooling aromatic herbs**, or **warming aromatic herbs and spices**, according to the prevailing weather. So, despite the current unnatural abundance of unseasonal imported food, we would do well to eschew it by choice. In the age of the internet, ignorance can no longer be an excuse; there are many good **websites** with accurate information of seasonal food availability and **local providers.** If we follow this seasonal route, over time our dietary culture will regain its sophistication, particularly in relation to climate and health. It remains to us to create, rediscover and adopt equivalent strategies.

Locally grown food

The key thing about local, seasonal food is that it is more likely to be fresh, and **fresh means nutritious**, since, with a few notable exceptions, as soon as food is picked, captured or slaughtered it starts to degrade nutritionally. The actions of **sunlight, temperature and chemical processes** like the **oxidising atmosphere break up** certain vital nutrients such as **vitamin C and omega 3 oils** so that they lose their nutritional benefit. There is no doubt that **the fresher food is, the more likely it is to retain high levels of the delicate nutrients** that give our food that health-enhancing "X-factor". Sustained on food that has not lost too much of its natural nutritional goodness, the body becomes much more resilient; **immunity is strong,** the constitution is protected and we are far better able to deal with our day-to-day challenges.

There is an **exception** to the seasonal, local food rule, and that's for vegetables and fruit that are grown in heated and lit **greenhouses** hydroponically. This system extends the growing season of foods considerably, meaning that a wide variety of vegetables such as **tomatoes and cucumbers** can be produced in countries where previously they might have had to be imported. There is **a lack of r**eally good, unbiased **research comparing the nutritional value** of hydroponic foods with foods grown in a natural way. Microbes, worms, fungi and other small organisms in soil produce chemicals and interact with plants in ways which have not yet been explored, so we do not know they might be of benefit. These **vital soil organisms** are deliberately **kept out of hydroponic systems**, meaning that the range of chemical nutrients that hydroponic plants are exposed to is very low indeed. This can only be reflected in the food itself, resulting in a lowered nutritional diversity.

Exercise 1a
Match the column A with the column B. Try to learn the expressions and/or sentences by heart.

A

1. There are three principles, all of which are key to

2. Today, nearly every food is available year round
3. This modern habit of ours
4. In late autumn and winter,
5. We need rich, sustaining food
6. In late spring, summer and early autumn, lighter greens, fresh beans and soft fruit can be eaten
7. If we follow this seasonal route,
8. As soon as food is picked, captured or slaughtered
9. The actions of sunlight, temperature and chemical processes like the oxidising atmosphere
10. Sustained on food that has not lost too much of its natural nutritional goodness,
11. There is an exception and that's for
12. The range of chemical nutrients that hydroponic plants

flavours and cooling or warming aromatic herbs and spices, according to the prevailing weather.

f) detaches us from our health, climate and environment.

g) starch root vegetables, nuts and seeds, intense bitter greens, fatty meat and fish and preserved foods are most available.

h) it starts to degrade nutritionally.

i) our building a healthy relationship with food: seasonal, local, well produced.

j) our dietary culture will regain its sophistication, particularly in relation to climate and health.

k) the body becomes much more resilient.

l) vegetables and fruit that are grown in heated and lit greenhouses hydroponically.

B

a) and cookbooks rarely have significant seasonal content.

b) and strong bitter, spicy and sour flavours to help us digest it.

c) are exposed to is very low, resulting in a lowered nutritional diversity.

d) break up certain vital nutrients such as vitamin C and omega 3 oils.

e) combined with the right mix of refreshing sour

Well produced/organic food. Specialist retailers.

In nutritional terms, the more food that we can eat that is produced organically or according to an **organic/chemical-free style**, the better. The rule of good purchase is to buy the best quality that you can afford. In an ideal world, home grown food is the best around. It is **harvested and immediately eaten**. It is only in modern times, since the advent of petrochemical-boosted agriculture, that the passion for home-grown food has diminished. Food used to be much more expensive and people once made a huge effort to make savings where they could by recycling scraps through keeping pigs and chickens, and growing vegetables and fruit. It was often a matter of survival. But it created habits that lingered into the next generations.

How to get food from abroad

Not all food, however, can be home-grown or local. Many foods that form part of a balanced, intelligently combined and nutritious diet don't grow well in this country. We have no option other than to source them from elsewhere. It is not just **spices** that we have obsessively sourced from foreign climes. Other important foreign foodstuffs include **grains**, like **rice and millet**, **seeds** such as **quinoa, sesame and sunflower**, and **nuts** like **macadamia and cashew**.

Many **medicinal foods** come from abroad. Today, despite transient obsessions with a limited number of "super foods", genuine medicinal foods have declined in our consciousness to become far to small part of our own culture, yet they are undoubtedly **crucial elements** of a balanced and healthy diet.

How to become an expert

In the last few decades, we have seen the **consumption of ready meals** and industrially produced food sky-rocket, to the point where many of us are almost completely disconnected from what we eat. This massive shift in the dietary habits of our society has **large implications for health**.

Emulsifiers, trans-fats, flavourings, modified corn starch and the like that tend to be so abundant in factory-produced foods are unequivocally **toxic to us.** As are the vast quantities of salt and sugar used in these products. It is easy to see how **damaging products** like **ready-made pizza, oven chips and pre-fabricated curries** are for us; they are loaded with chemical additives, modified fat, sugar and salt.

Fromage frais

Let's take an important mass-produced "health food" as an example: fromage frais. Nothing is more minutely scrutinised than the foods that our children eat. Yet this particular "health food" is often marketed specifically for children and it frequently slips through the net.

There is a significant range of fromage frais **on the market** today. They are **promoted** as being **high in calcium** with **added vitamins**, **good for growth** and **good for bones**. Yet **we should be suspicious** of mass-produced flavoured versions such as strawberry fromage frais. Fromage frais has only one major ingredient in its production – cow's **milk**; we should buy it as such. If we want to turn it into strawberry fromage frais **at home,** it's easy. We **add strawberries**. A fruit that, if it is not in season, can easily be taken out of the freezer. And if we want to sweeten it up a bit, how about some lovely local honey? You can also add a few aromatic spices such as **nutmeg,**

mace, or dried ginger to help cut through the richness of the diary.

The **mass-produced stuff** routinely contains added **sugar, water, fructose** (that is extra sugar), **colour** (unspecified), concentrated **juices and extracts**, **gum stabilizers, modified starches, flavourings** (also unspecified), and **acidity regulators.** This is only one of the items that demonstrate how virtually any industrial food product has a deeply toxic nature, often in direct **contrast to the health claims made on the packaging**. Further examination of the ingredients reveals why:

- **Sugar and refined fructose** – ingredients linked to diabetes, obesity, heart attacks and stroke
- **Modified maize starch** – a cheap thickener of little nutritional value
- **Colour, stabilizers, flavourings** – typically nutritionally useless
- **Processed concentrated juices and extracts**, many of which remain unspecified on the packaging.

The natural version is also very convenient, because fromage frais is a fermented product and keeps well in the fridge, similarly, honey sits on the shelf and most fruit can be stored in the freezer. All in all, then, we can see that **natural fromage frais** is not only far **healthier**, but also more **cost-effective** that the mass-produced flavoured versions.

This means that, at the most, **additive-laden factory food** should be a **rare treat,** because it can never be as healthy as fresh, locally sourced, seasonal, well-produced and home-processed food. If we get into the habit of **choosing our own ingredients and cooking them at home,** not only will our food be fresher and more nutritious, but we will also avoid a bevy of hidden and not-so-hidden industrial additives that do so much damage on our health. This means that each of us, in our own way, needs to become a **food expert.** You should rebuild your connection with what you eat, and understand how it is impacted by climate, lifestyle and environment.

Exercise 1b
Match the column A with the column B. Try to learn the expressions and/ or sentences by heart.

A

1. The more food that we can eat that
2. The rule of good purchase is
3. Food used to be much more expensive
4. Keeping pigs and chickens, and growing vegetables and fruit
5. Many foods that form part of a balanced, intelligently combined and nutritious diet
6. Spices, grains, like rice and millet, seeds such as quinoa, sezame and

sunflower, and nuts like macadamia and cashew
7. Genuine medicinal foods
8. Emulsifiers, trans-fats, flavourings, modified corn starch and the like
9. Ready-made pizza, oven chips and pre-fabricated curries
10. There is a significant range of fromage frais on the market promoted as being
11. The mass-produced stuff routinely contains
12. Sugar and refined fructose are ingredients
13. Modified maize starch
14. Colour, stabilizers and flavourings
15. Choosing our own ingredients and cooking them at home, not only will our food be fresher and more nutritious,

B

a) *added sugar, water, fructose, colour, concentrated juices and extracts, gum stabilizers, modified starches, flavourings and acidity regulators.*
b) *and people once made a huge effort to make savings where they could.*
c) *are loaded with chemical additives, modified fat, sugar and salt.*
d) *are typically nutritionally useless.*
e) *are undoubtedly crucial elements of a balanced and healthy diet.*
f) *but we will also avoid additives that do so much damage on our health.*
g) *don't grow well in this country.*
h) *form an important part of a nutritious diet.*
i) *high in calcium with added vitamins, good for growth and good for bones.*
j) *is a cheap thickener of little nutritional value.*
k) *is produced organically the better.*
l) *linked to diabetes, obesity, heart attacks and stroke.*
m) *that tend to be so abundant in factory-produced foods are unequivocally toxic to us.*
n) *to buy the best quality that you can afford.*
o) *was often a matter of survival.*

Specialist retailers

We should not ignore a very important source of products and information – the specialist retailer. These are the real experts. Many of us are already lucky enough to know that an **experienced butcher, fishmonger or stall holder** will be able to share valuable **advice on the provenance** of his goods. Also, he can supply a greater variety of produce such as cheap cuts, bones and offal, which spoils easily – and teach us how to cook it. These cheap foods are some of the most nutritious around, and yet they are often entirely absent in supermarkets.

Bones

Bone stocks are the bedrock of virtually every **traditional cuisine** in the world, and yet bones and carcasses can be readily obtained only from a good butcher. By choosing to shop at our local butcher and buying these sorts of ingredients we can get cheap, exceptional food.

Supermarkets

It is clever to buy foods like **rice, barley, flour, beans, noodles, pasta, honey, maple syrup and tea** in bulk from a local **wholesaler**, cutting costs and reducing the need to go out and buy them all the time.

The internet

For specialist items like **mushrooms, gou qi zi (wolf-berry fruit),** certain **teas and spices**, the internet if often the place to turn to, as long as you can establish the reputation of the supplier and end up with a high quality and good-value product. Through making these small but vital **choices about when and where we shop**, we can transcend the modern barriers that we are all too often placed between us and our food. Barriers that exist, for example, in the form of cellophane and packaging. And barriers to real understanding of our food, which are erected in other ways, too, such as shipping it from wherever it is cheapest, regardless of seasonality and quality of production.

To-be-your-own-nutritionist **shopping list**

Staples	They are chosen for their digestibility and ability to provide sustenance. If you are focused on diet for weight/ fat loss then you will need to adapt and expand these lists of foods creatively to include a wider range of fat- and protein-rich alternatives.
Fats and oils	These fall into two categories: **Fats for cooking** – clarified butter/ghee, dripping or tallow, lard, goose or duck fat, coconut oil **Fats for eating** – butter, dripping, hemp oil, rapeseed oil, sesame oil, walnut oil, cobnut oil, olive oil
Fermented foods	There are a lot of options here: soy sauce, Thai fish sauce, black bean sauce, anchovy sauce, Worcester sauce, mushroom ketchup, vinegars (cider, red and white wine, rice wine), yoghurt, chorizo (fermented sausage), hard cheese and miso, pickles, sauerkraut, real ale, local organic cider.
Veg, fruit and mushrooms	These should be seasonal when eaten fresh. When sourced from the wild, market gardens, farmers' markets, home-grown or gifted from allotments they inevitably will be. Some, but not all greengrocers use local producers.
Bread	This needs to be a high-quality artisanal loaf. Alternatively, you may be into home baking.
Meat, fish and eggs	It is best to focus on cheap cuts and offal, including kidney, liver and tongue, pork belly, beef shin and good-quality sausages. Bones for stocks come from good butchers. Fish – aim for variety,

	cook with whole fish (gutted of course), use the bones for stocks. Eggs – organic eggs are the most nutritious. Quail eggs are a revered constitutional tonic.
Beans	The best beans are fresh or dried. As far as tinned beans are concerned, some researches suggest that the plastic linings of the tins release chemicals such as BPA which may cause cancer, and other illnesses.
Snacks/ Appetisers	**Snacks** – clients often wonder about snacks, especially for children. It is important not to snack too much or digestion never gets a rest and becomes weak, with consequent illness. Here are some ideas: **Nuts and seeds** (like walnuts, chestnuts, pumpkin and sesame seeds), good **bread and butter**/dripping, **dried fruit, soup, pancakes, dried meat** or **fermented sausage**, **relish, potted meat, pâté, corn on the cob**. Raw fruit should be limited, local and eaten only in season; raw fruit in the depths of winter is likely to weaken digestion.
	Chinese snacks are hugely varied and typically highly digestible, although modern versions often contain too much sugar. Examples include steamed buns, lychees, dumplings, noodles, persimmon cakes, smashed-bean buns. **Sushi** is a brilliant snack if out and about, especially in summer (the cold, raw food element is mitigated by the hot wasabi and the spice of the preserved ginger) **Appetisers** – you can choose from a wide range of foods, from olives and walnuts to spicy pickles and salted fish.
Condiments	These add vital digestibility value to food, especially rich dishes. Here are some **examples:** brown sauce, home made tomato ketchup, spiced damson purée, curry chutney, real ale chutney, apple and tomato chutney, wholegrain mustard, pesto and spiced beetroot pickle. It is best to make mint and horseradish sauces from fresh ingredients as they go off easily.
Tea and other infusions	Green tea is much kinder to digestion than black, but overall tea is a very healthy drink. Other infusions of herbs and spices are valuable for digestion, too.

Summary

- Eat mostly **cooked food**
- **Serve** food and drink **warm or hot**
- Eat protein and fat from a wide variety of sources. Eat a richer diet as the weather **gets colder -more hearty food**!
- Ensure, as far as possible, that you eat **fresh and well-produced food**
- **Balance the flavours** for climate and circumstance, focusing on bitter, sour and spicy/aromatic
- Eat **fermented foods** daily
- Severely restrict or, even better, **cut out refined sugar** (including fructose), **artificial sweeteners** and **refined wheat flour**
- **Cut out** industrially processed foods like **margarine** and **ready meals**

- **Restrict cheese**, pasteurised cow's **milk** and **preserved foods**, especially those with chemical preservatives.

Exercise 1c
Match the column A with the column B. Try to learn the expressions and/ or sentences by heart.

A

1. An experienced butcher, fishmonger or stall holder
2. Cheap cuts, bones and offal, which spoil easily
3. The internet if often the place to turn to,
4. Staples are chosen for their digestibility
5. Fats for cooking are e.g.
6. Fats for eating are e.g.
7. There are a lot of options of fermented foods:
8. It is best to focus on
9. It is important not to snack too much
10. Chinese snacks
11. Here are some ideas of a good snack:
12. Brown sauce, home made tomato ketchup, spiced damson purée, curry chutney, real ale chutney, apple and tomato chutney, wholegrain mustard, pesto and spiced beetroot pickle
13. Green tea is much kinder to digestion
14. Restrict or, even better, cut out
15. Restrict cheese, pasteurised cow's milk and preserved foods,

B

a) add vital digestibility value to food, especially rich dishes.
b) and ability to provide sustenance.
c) are some of the most nutritious around, and yet they are absent in supermarkets.
d) as long as you can establish the reputation of the supplier and end up with a high quality and good-value product.
e) butter, dripping, hemp oil, rapeseed oil, sesame oil, walnut oil, cob nut oil, olive oil
f) cheap cuts and offal, including kidney, liver and tongue, pork belly, beef shin and good-quality sausages.
g) clarified butter/ghee, dripping or tallow, lard, goose or duck fat, coconut oil.
h) especially those with chemical preservatives.
i) include steamed buns, lychees, dumplings, noodles, persimmon cakes, or smashed-bean buns.
j) nuts and seeds (like walnuts, chestnuts, pumpkin and sesame seeds), good bread and butter/dripping, dried

fruit, soup, pancakes, dried meat or fermented sausage, relish, potted meat, pâté, corn on the cob.

k) *or digestion never gets a rest and becomes weak, with consequent illness.*

l) *refined sugar (including fructose), artificial sweeteners and refined wheat flour.*

m) *soy sauce, Thai fish sauce, black bean sauce, anchovy sauce, Worcester sauce, mushroom ketchup, vinegars (cider, red and white wine, rice wine), yoghurt, chorizo, hard cheese and miso, pickles, sauerkraut, real ale, local organic cider.*

n) *than black, but overall tea is a very healthy drink.*

o) *will be able to share valuable advice on the provenance of his goods.*

Exercise 2

Translate the expressions. Try to explain their meanings in English.

Rule of, purchase, afford, home grown food, harvested, diminished, effort, make savings, survival, option, sourced from, transient, obsessions, genuine consciousness, crucial elements, disconnected, shift, dietary habit, simplifications, abundant, unequivocally, scrutinised, marketed, promoted, suspicious, reveals, modified maize starch, convenient, cost-effective, rare treat, get into the habit of, impacted by, specialist retailer, butcher, fishmonger, stall holder, provenance, spoil, bone stocks, traditional cuisine, obtained, barley, noodles, pasta, maple syrup, wholesaler, turn to, establish reputation, supplier, transcend, packaging, shipping, provide sustenance, focused on, adapt, expand, ghee, dripping, tallow, lard, coconut oil, hemp oil, rapeseed oil, cob nut oil, anchovy sauce, chorizo, miso, ale, cider, allotments, inevitably, greengrocers, artisanal, tinned, quail, revered, constitutional, gutted, pork belly, beef shin, appetisers, wasabi, mitigated, persimmon, smashed, dumplings, steamed, buns, lychees, weaken, digestion, potted meat, pâté, corn on the cob, pancakes, pumpkin, infusions, go off, beetroot, pesto, wholegrain, mustard, damson purée, curry chutney, hearty food, restrict, cut out, condiments.

Exercise 3

Answer the following questions. Prepare short talks and/or dialogues on these topics.

1. What do we mean by organically produced food?
2. Which medicinal foods come from abroad?
3. Give examples of foods loaded with chemical additives, modified fat, sugar and salt.
4. Why is it better to prepare the foods that our children eat at home?
5. What does mass-produced stuff routinely contain?

6. Where to shop (specialist retailers, supermarkets, the internet)?
7. How to create a good shopping list?
8. Talk about the principles of healthy eating.

Vocabulary 14

Fill in the meanings in your mother language:

abundance /əˈbʌndəns/
advent /ˈædvent/
ale /eɪl/
appetiser /ˈæpɪˌtaɪzə/
argument /ˈɑːg.jʊ.mənt/
artisanal /ɑː.ˈtɪ.zə.nəl/
beef /biːf/ **shin** /ʃɪn/
beetroot /ˈbiːtruːt/
bevy /ˈbev.i/
boost /buːst/
brilliant /ˈbrɪl.i.ənt/
bun /bʌn/
butcher /ˈbʊtʃər/
cake /keɪk/
capture /ˈkæp.tʃər/
carcass /ˈkɑːkəs/
cellophane /ˈseləfeɪn/
chorizo /tʃɔːˈriːzəʊ/
chutney /ˈtʃʌtni/
clarify /ˈklærɪfaɪ/
cobnut /ˈkɒb.nʌt/
compelling /kəmˈpelɪŋ/
consciousness /ˈkɒn.ʃəs.nəs/
constitutional /ˌkɒnstɪˈtjuːʃənəl/
corn /kɔːn/ **on the cob** /kɒb/
damson /ˈdæm.zən/ **purée** /ˈpjʊəreɪ/
decline /dɪˈklaɪn/
degrade /dɪˈgreɪd/
deliberately /dɪˈlɪb.ər.ət.li/
detach /dɪˈtætʃ/
diversity /daɪˈvɜː.sɪ.ti/
dripping /drɪpɪŋ/
duck /dʌk/
erect /ɪˈrekt/
eschew /ɪsˈtʃuː/
exception /ɪkˈsep.ʃən/
explore /ɪkˈsplɔːr/
ferment /fəˈment/
fishmonger /ˈfɪʃˌmʌŋ.gər/
freight /freɪt/
fromage frais /ˈfrɒmɑːʒ ˈfreɪ/
genuine /ˈdʒenjuɪn/
ghee /giː/
goose /guːs/
gou qi zi /ˈgəʊdʒɪ/
gutted /ˈgʌtɪd/
harvest /ˈhɑːvɪst/
hemp /hɛmp/ **oil** /ɔɪl/
holder /ˈhəʊldər/
hot /hɒt/
implication /ˌɪm.plɪˈkeɪ.ʃən/
inevitably /ɪˈnev.ɪ.tə.bli/
inherent /ɪnˈher.ənt/
laden /ˈleɪdən/
lard /lɑːd/
linger /ˈlɪŋgər/
loaf /ləʊf/
lychee /ˈlaɪ.tʃiː/
maple /ˈmeɪpl/ **syrup** /ˈsɪrəp/
minute /maɪˈnjuːt/
mitigate /ˈmɪtɪgeɪt/
notable /ˈnəʊ.tə.bl̩/
obsession /əbˈseʃ.ən/
organic /ɔːˈgæn.ɪk/
passion /ˈpæʃən/
persimmon /pəˈsɪm.ən/
persistent /pəˈsɪstənt/
pickle /ˈpɪkl/
pork /pɔːk/ **belly** /ˈbeli/
potted /ˈpɒtɪd/ **meat** /miːt/
provenance /ˈprɒv.ən.əns/
quail /kweɪl/
quinoa /kɪnˈwɑː/
real /ˈrɪəl/
reference /ˈref.ər.ənt s/
relish /ˈrelɪʃ/
rever /rɪˈvɪər/

rocket /'rɒkɪt/
scrap /skræp/
scrutinise /'skruː.tɪ.naɪz/
seasonal /'siːzənəl/
sensitivity /ˌsent.sɪ'tɪv.ɪ.ti/
sky /skaɪ/
slaughter /'slɔːtər/
slip /slɪp/
smash /smæʃ/
sophistication /səˌfɪstɪ'keɪʃən/
stall /stɔːl/
steam /stiːm/
survival /sə'vaɪ.vəl/
sushi /'suːʃi/
suspicious /sə'spɪʃ.əs/
tallow /'tæl.əʊ/
Thai /taɪ/ **fish** /fɪʃ/ **sauce** /sɔːs/
the wild /waɪld/
thickener /'θɪk.ən.ər/
tomel /toʊməl/
tongue /tʌŋ/
tonic /'tɒnɪk/
transcend /træn'send/
unbiased /ʌn'baɪəst/
vast /vɑːst/
warrant /'wɒr.ənt/
wasabi /wə'sɑː.bi/
wholesaler /'həʊlˌseɪlər/
wolf /wʊlf/ **-berry** /'beri/ **fruit** /fruːt/

Solution to Exercise 1a
1i, 2a, 3f, 4g, 5b, 6e, 7j,
8h, 9d, 10k, 11l, 12c

Solution to Exercise 1b
1k, 2n, 3b, 4o, 5g, 6h, 7e, 8m,
9c, 10i, 11a, 12l, 13j, 14d, 15f

Solution to Exercise 1c
1o, 2c, 3d, 4b, 5g, 6e, 7m, 8f,
9k, 10i, 11j, 12a, 13n, 14l, 15h

Unit 15 - How to loose weight

Insulin

It is this hormone -more than any other- that instructs fat cells to take in the building blocks of fat from the blood stream, to lay on the fat, and then to retain it. This **laying-on** and **retention of fat** is what **results in obesity**. The pathological **effects of insulin** are widely accepted in scientific circles.

The key to weigh loss is to **reduce consumption of foods** that strongly **stimulate the release of insulin**. The food group that does this more than any other is **carbohydrate**, the group that **contains sugars and starches. If we don't eat enough** calories, especially in the form of **protein and fat,** then our **metabolisms slow down.** We **become tired,** listless and less active and we **burn fewer calories**. We also want to eat more because we're **permanently hungry** as our diet is not satisfying and doesn't fill us up properly.

What this means is that, in the real world **people cannot maintain calorie-restricted diets**; the endless gnawing hunger that accompanies them grinds them down and in the end most people will become **locked into a cycle of yo-yo dieting,** unsustainable exercise regimes and obesity. Because of the **action of insulin**, **carbohydrate** rather than dietary fat is the main food group that is **converted into body fat**, since it is dietary carbohydrate that **stimulates the release of insulin**. This released insulin caused by the consumption of carbohydrates like **sugar** is mainstream physiological science.

Carbohydrates

The worst carbohydrates of all are the **refined sugar and white wheat flour.** Once you start eating these foods, it is very hard to stop. But to lose the weight and reduce body fat, **you must stop.**

The solution

The first step in any weight-loss/fat-reduction plan is to:

- **cut out refined sugar and white flour** completely. That means **no white bread, sweets, sugary drinks or puddings.** And just about **no processed food** – this includes even apparently healthier items like baked beans. If you look at the labels on these foods you will see that nearly all of them contain sugar.

For those with stubborn **predispositions to weight gain** another step may be needed, which is to:

- radically reduce or **eliminate** from your diet all **refined grains, starches and sugars,** effectively cutting out the broader carbohydrate groups **that raise blood insulin levels when ingested**. (This means that you will no longer be eating a small number of staple foods that form part of typically healthy traditional diets, such as **white rice**).
- cut out all processed foods to **avoid additives** such as **maize starch and fructose.**

Taking these steps, the vast majority of people will loose weight.

A word on fructose

Fructose, found in large amounts **in fruit and processed foods,** is a sugar that does not raise blood insulin the way that other sugars do. But it is just as big a cause of obesity, since **once consumed, most fructose is metabolised into fat**. Much of this fat is deposited in the liver. Fructose also **turns off the body's appetite control system, resulting in overconsumption of food** in general. Because fructose levels are high in fruit, you **should cut out fruit juice** altogether if you are trying to lose weight. Overall, fruit juice, especially from concentrate, tends not to be a healthy drink as it provides a relatively large volume of very **acidic liquid**, combined with **high sugar** levels. **Fructose** is also **added to** many processed foods, such as children's **yoghurts**, and is a major component of **corn syrup**, a food manufacturers' favourite.

Exercise 1a
Match the column A with the column B. Try to learn the expressions and/or sentences by heart.

A

1. Insulin is a hormone that instructs
2. This laying-on and retention of fat
3. The key to weigh loss is to
4. The food group that does this
5. If we don't eat enough calories, especially in the form of protein and fat,
6. We're permanently hungry
7. Because of the action of insulin, carbohydrate rather than dietary fat
8. It is dietary carbohydrate
9. The first step in any weight-loss/fat-reduction plan is to:
10. For those with predispositions to weight gain another step may be needed,
11. Cut out all processed foods
12. Fructose, found in large amounts in fruit and processed foods,
13. Fructose also turns off the body's appetite control system,
14. Because fructose levels are high in fruit,
15. Fruit juice, especially from concentrate,

B

a) *as our diet is not satisfying and doesn't fill us up properly.*
b) *cut out refined sugar and white flour completely.*
c) *fat cells to take in the building blocks of fat from the blood stream, to lay on the fat, and then to retain it.*
d) *is carbohydrate, the group that contains sugars and starches.*
e) *is just as big a cause of obesity, since once consumed, most fructose is metabolised into fat.*
f) *is the main food group that is converted into body fat.*
g) *is what results in obesity.*
h) *provides a relatively large volume of very acidic liquid, combined with high sugar levels.*
i) *reduce consumption of foods that strongly stimulate the release of insulin.*
j) *resulting in overconsumption of food in general.*
k) *that stimulates the release of insulin.*
l) *then our metabolisms slow down.*
m) *to avoid additives such as maize starch and fructose.*
n) *to eliminate from your diet all refined grains, starches and sugars that raise blood insulin levels when ingested.*
o) *you should cut out fruit juice altogether if you are trying to lose weight.*

How to loose weight 2

There is a much smaller group of people who will still struggle to lose weight even on this stricter regime. In this case, **most carbohydrate** has to be **cut out of the diet,** including starchy vegetables like **potatoes, whole grains and beans**. This means that many of recommended staples need to be cut out too, such as **oats, barley, rye, spelt, carrots, parsnips and pumpkins. Fruit** should also be **restricted**. This is a specific strategy applied in cases where fat is particularly difficult to shed, normally as a result of **genetic and hormonal predisposition**, rather than an approach to general healthy living. Once you have lost fat and have **regained a healthy body shape** and weight you can experiment with **reintroducing healthy starchy staples**. It is important to appreciate, though, that if you have a strong tendency to retain fat, you will never be able to eat dietary carbohydrate in the quantities that others seem to manage.

Beyond this, you may be part of the very small group of people whose hormonal predisposition or addictive tendencies causes a stubborn **propensity to gain and retain body fat.** You will be in a position where, no matter how hard you try, even by following a severely carbohydrate-restricted diet you will struggle to regain a healthy body shape. At this point, if you haven't already sought it, you need **professional help** and ongoing support from a nutritionist who already appreciates the true causes of and solutions to fat gain and loss.

There are a number of strategies such as the use of certain supplements that may help, but they require experienced supervision and guidance to be employed safely. A **low-carb diet** is inevitably a richer diet as its **protein and fat content** is **higher** than usual, which presents issues of digestibility that will now be familiar. The typical **consequence** of a **fat- and protein-rich diet** is that **motility is affected**, which may be why, especially in the early stages, low-carb dieters experience **nausea and stomach-aches** or feel a bit rotten. The answer is to prepare their meals for digestibility. We know from good traditional principles that **fat** needs to be **accompanied by sour and aromatic flavours, vegetables** need to be **cooked** and, while **fatty and protein-rich foods** are well suited to our damp climate, we need to add a bit of **spice and bitterness** to assist motility.

Artificial sweeteners in a low-carb diet

These **chemicals** have a highly **destructive influence** on the gut flora and disrupt **hormonal homoeostasis**; they are not recommended. Some have been linked to obesity, with people who drink **artificially sweetened lemonade** consuming **more calories** than those who drink conventional soda.

Summary

- **Carbohydrate restriction** is the key, so that **food is predominantly** from **protein and fat** sources with non-starchy vegetables.

- Remember to use good traditional principles to **enhance digestibility of the richer food.**
- Take it **step by step**. If one step doesn't work, move onto the next one and see how far you have to go to lose weight:

Step 1:

Cut out refined sugar, fructose, refined wheat and processed foods.

Step 2:

Cut out all refined grains (like white rice), fruit juice and alcoholic drinks.

Step 3:

Cut out most carbohydrates, including potatoes, whole grains and beans.

Step 4:

Restrict fruit and starchy vegetables normally considered healthy, like carrots.

Step 5:

Seek professional help. You have a strong hormonal or genetic predisposition to weight gain that needs a more detailed diet plan and ongoing assessment.

Exercise 1b

Match the column A with the column B. Try to learn the expressions and/or sentences by heart.

A

1. There is a much smaller group of people
2. In this case, most carbohydrate has to be cut out of the diet,
3. Recommended staples need to be cut out too,
4. Once you have lost fat and have regained a healthy body shape and weight
5. You may be part of the very small group of people
6. A low-carb diet is a richer diet as its
7. The typical consequence of a fat- and protein-rich diet
8. Fat needs to be accompanied
9. Artificial sweeteners
10. Carbohydrate restriction is the key,
11. Cut out
12. Cut out
13. Cut out
14. Restrict fruit and starchy vegetables

B

a) *all refined grains (like white rice), fruit juice and alcoholic drinks.*
b) *by sour and aromatic flavours.*
c) *have a highly destructive influence on the gut flora and disrupt hormonal homoeostasis.*
d) *including starchy vegetables like potatoes, whole grains and beans.*
e) *is that motility is affected.*

f) *like carrots.*

g) *most carbohydrates, including potatoes, whole grains and beans.*

h) *protein and fat content is higher than usual.*

i) *refined sugar, fructose, refined wheat and processed foods.*

j) *so that food is predominantly from protein and fat sources with non-starchy vegetables.*

k) *such as oats, barley, rye, spelt, carrots, parsnips, pumpkins and fruit should also be restricted.*

l) *who will still struggle to lose weight even on strict regime.*

m) *whose hormonal predisposition or addictive tendencies causes a stubborn propensity to gain and retain body fat.*

n) *you can experiment with reintroducing healthy starchy staples.*

Exercise 2

Translate the expressions. Try to explain their meanings in English.

Take in, lay on, retain the fat, accepted, reduce consumption, stimulate the release, contains sugars and starches, slow down, permanently, satisfying, fill up, properly, maintain diets, unsustainable, exercise regimes, converted, completely, apparently, contain, eliminate, maize starch, fructose, cause of obesity, deposited, turns off, appetite control system, resulting in overconsumption, large volume, acidic liquid, favourite, struggle to lose weight, starchy vegetables, whole grains and beans, oats, barley, rye, spelt, carrots, parsnips, pumpkins, predisposition, approach, regain body shape, appreciate, addictive tendencies, propensity, ongoing support, solutions, supervision and guidance, motility is affected, feel rotten, artificial sweeteners, destructive influence, conventional, predominantly, enhance, whole grains.

Exercise 3

Answer the following questions. Prepare short talks and/or dialogues on these topics.

1. Describe the function of insulin in our body.
2. What causes yo-yo dieting?
3. Steps in weight-loss/ fat-reduction plans.
4. Explain the danger of high levels of fructose.
5. In which case must potatoes, whole grains and beans be cut out of the diet?
6. Describe a low-carb diet.
7. Talk about the step by step strategy to lose weight.

Vocabulary 15

Fill in the meanings in your mother language:

apparently /əˈpær.ənt.li/
employ /ɪmˈplɔɪ/
fill /fɪl/ **up** /ʌp/
gnawing /ˈnɔː.ɪŋ/ **pain** /peɪn/

grind /graɪnd/
guidance /ˈgaɪ.dəns/
lay /leɪ/ **on** /ɒn/
listless /ˈlɪst.ləs/
lock /lɒk/ **into** /ˈɪntə/
predisposition /ˌpriːdɪspəˈzɪʃən/
propensity /prəʊˈpensəti/
result /rɪˈzʌlt/
satisfying /ˈsætɪsfaɪɪŋ/
shed /ʃed/
suit /suːt/

Solution to Exercise 1a
1c, 2g, 3i, 4d, 5l, 6a, 7f, 8k, 9b, 10n, 11m, 12e, 13k, 14o, 15h

Solution to Exercise 1b
1l, 2d, 3k, 4n, 5m, 6h, 7e, 8b, 9c, 10j, 11i, 12a, 13g, 14f

Unit 16 - Herbs, spices and medicinal foods. Spices

Each foodstuff is listed along with its **flavours**, its **actions** on digestion and its **relationship** with areas other than digestion, such as the lungs and nervous system.

Herbs

When they are picked **fresh**, they have the maximum level of light aromatic oils and therefore maximum effect. The annual or deciduous herbs can be used fresh or the leaves can be **preserved** in **oil, frozen** or **dried** to be used in cooking all year round.

Basil	**Pungent, bitter and slightly sweet**, stimulates **motility**, **secretion** and **flora**. Also said to **strengthen the lungs.**
Bay leaf	**Pungent and bitter**, stimulates **motility** and **secretion**
Bitter orange peel	As in **marmalade**, bitter slightly sweet and aromatic, stimulate **appetite**, secretion and **gut flora**. Used in stocks, soups and sweets.
Caper (berry or bud-pickled)	**Mildly pungent**. Traditionally used in the Mediterranean for healthy **joints**, the pungency cuts through obstructiveness of damp. Classically combined **with rich meats, sauces and cured fish.**
Camomile	**Slightly bitter and sweet**, **soothes** digestion.
Chervil	**Bitter and slightly sweet**, used to **balance strong spices.**
Chives	**Pungent** and slightly **bitter**, stimulates **motility** and **secretion**.
Coriander leaf	**Bitter and aromatic**, stimulates **motility** and **secretion**. **Refreshing** and balances strong spices.
Dandelion leaf	**Bitter**, counters hot weather and very spicy food. A noted **diuretic**, it can help with fluid retention. **All parts** of the dandelion plant have a culinary use. The flowers can be eaten and the root taken as an infusion.
Dill leaf	**Aromatic and slightly bitter**, stimulates **appetite**
Lavender flower	**Aromatic and slightly sweet**. The French cook with lavender. Famously **calming**, it soothes the gut to clear wind and gently strengthen digestion.
Liquorice	**Very sweet and slightly bitter**, strengthens **digestion** overall.
Lovage	**Bitter and aromatic**, stimulates **motility** and **secretion**, good in **stews.**
Marjoram	**Bitter and aromatic, astringent** (can settle an over active bowel) and **calming** for digestion overall.
Mint	**Aromatic**. Like coriander leaf, this is one of the **refreshing** aromatic herbs, so it is good in summer, or in combination with very **spicy foods or lamb**.

Nasturtium (leaves, flowers and seeds)	**Bitter, pungent and sweet**. The flowers and leaves are broadly equivalent, with bitter and pungent flavours stimulating **motility** – particularly good for rich foods, eaten on a hot day i.e. **barbecues**. Nasturtium seeds can be pickled and are **equivalent to capers.**
Oregano	**Slightly aromatic and bitter,** stimulates **motility**. Classically combined with **cheese or pork sausage**.
Parsley leaves and seeds	**Slightly aromatic and bitter**, stimulates **secretion** and **motility** and is a mild **diuretic**.
Peppermint	**Aromatic and slightly sweet**. Cools excess spice and soothes the gut. **Relieves nausea**. Also said to **strengthen the lungs.**
Rose and rosewater	**Sweet, aromatic and slightly bitter**. **Calms and soothes the gut,** stimulating motility, especially where there is emotional stress involved or we are feeling liverish.
Rosemary	**Bitter and aromatic,** stimulates **motility** – renowned for treatment of **trapped wind**. Said to calm the effects of **emotional stress** on the gut.
Saffron	**Sweet, bitter and aromatic**, regulates **digestion** overall.
Sage	**Bitter and aromatic**, warms and moves the gut to counter rich foods. It is said to **soothe the gut and promote healing.**
Savory	**Aromatic, bitter and slightly sweet**, stimulates **motility** and **secretion** and it is said to strengthen **the lungs**. Winter savory is traditionally combined with Jerusalem artychokes to mitigate their flatulence-inducing properties.
Sorrel	**Sour**, a mild **diuretic**, **counters hot weather** and very spicy food.
Sweet Cicely	The **leaves and seeds** have an aniseedy flavour that mellows sour flavours, so a good **summer herb**. The aromatic components also combine well with rich ingredients like **eggs**.
Tarragon	**Bitter and slightly aromatic**, stimulates **motility and secretion.**
Thyme	**Bitter and aromatic**, stimulates **motility** to counter sluggish digestion, especially in combination with fatty foods. Traditionally said to **dry out mucous lungs**.

Exercise 1a
Match the column A with the column B. Try to learn the expressions and/or sentences by heart.

A

1. Basil stimulates motility, secretion and flora
2. Bay leaf
3. Bitter orange peel, used in stocks, soups and sweets,
4. Caper (berry or bud-pickled), used in the Mediterranean for healthy joints,
5. Camomile, slightly bitter and sweet,
6. Chervil, bitter and slightly sweet,
7. Chives pungent and slightly bitter,
8. Coriander leaf, bitter and aromatic,
9. Dandelion leaf, bitter, a noted diuretic,
10. Dill leaf, aromatic and slightly bitter,
11. Lavender flower, aromatic and slightly sweet,

12. Liquorice, very sweet and slightly bitter,
13. Lovage, bitter and aromatic, good in stews,
14. Marjoram, bitter and aromatic is
15. Mint is one of the refreshing aromatic herbs,
16. Nasturtium (leaves, flowers and seeds), bitter, pungent and sweet,
17. Oregano, slightly aromatic and bitter,
18. Parsley leaves and seeds, slightly aromatic and bitter,
19. Peppermint, aromatic and slightly sweet,
20. Rose and rosewater, sweet, aromatic and slightly bitter,
21. Rosemary, bitter and aromatic,
22. Sage, bitter and aromatic,
23. Savory, aromatic, bitter and slightly sweet,
24. Sorrel, sour, a mild diuretic,
25. Sweet Cicely mellows sour flavours;
26. Thyme, bitter and aromatic,

B

a) and is said to strengthen the lungs.
b) astringent and calming for digestion overall.
c) calms and soothes the gut.
d) cools excess spice and soothes the gut.
e) counters hot weather and very spicy food.
f) counters hot weather and very spicy food.
g) good in summer, or in combination with very spicy foods or lamb.
h) is combined with rich meats, sauces and cured fish.
i) is said to soothe the gut and promote healing.
j) is used to balance strong spices.
k) said to dry out mucous lungs, stimulates motility especially in combination with fatty foods.
l) soothes digestion.
m) soothes the gut to clear wind and gently strengthen digestion.
n) stimulate motility, particularly good for rich foods, eaten on a hot day i.e. barbecues.
o) stimulates appetite, secretion and gut flora.
p) stimulates appetite.
q) stimulates motility and secretion.
r) stimulates motility and secretion and it is said to strengthen the lungs.
s) stimulates motility and secretion.
t) stimulates motility and secretion.
u) stimulates motility and secretion.
v) stimulates motility, classically is combined with cheese or pork sausage.
w) stimulates motility, renowned for treatment of trapped wind.

x) *stimulates secretion and motility and is a mild diuretic.*

y) *strengthens digestion overall.*

z) *the aromatic components also combine well with rich ingredients like eggs.*

Spices

Allspice (pimento, Jamaica pepper)	Aromatic. A **gentle digestive stimulant** said to **ease flatulence and stomach ache.**
Aniseed	Aromatic and sweet, warms **and stimulates motility and gut flora. Soothes** the gut to **release flatulence**.
Caraway seed	Aromatic and sweet, warms **and stimulates** motility and gut flora. It **stimulates appetite** and is said to **treat diarrhoea and trapped wind.**
Cardamom	Aromatic. Stimulates **appetite and motility**. Traditionally used to **counteract nausea**, muddy **headaches** and **gut pain.**
Cayenne pepper (red pepper)	Very spicy. A form of **chilli pepper** that is often ground into a powder. Often added to sauces and condiment recipes and **balanced with sour cooling flavours**.
Chilli pepper	Very spicy, stimulates **motility** but **needs balancing** with other **refreshing and cooling** herbs and foods.
Cinnamon bark	Strongly aromatic and spicy too, stimulates appetite. A traditional **cold and diarrhoea remedy** as it is slightly **astringent**.
Cinnamon twig	**Aromatic and bitter**, regulates **digestion overall** and stimulates the **lungs**.
Clove	**Pungent**, warms the digestion to specifically counter the stagnation of damp and coldness. Stimulates **appetite** and regulates intestinal **motility** to **relieve nausea and trapped wind.**
Coriander seed	**Aromatic**. Regulates **motility** to **relieve trapped wind** and **diarrhoea**, especially in children.
Cumin	**Aromatic and sweet**, warms digestion and stimulates **motility and symbionts.**
Dill seeds	**Aromatic**. Traditionally this is the herb of choice for **colic in children** as it gently regulates motility.
Fennel seed	**Aromatic and sweet**, stimulates **motility** and **warms digestion**. Promotes **appetite** and **relieves spasm**, as in **trapped wind**. Considered a very important mild spice for regulating motility in **babies and children**.
Fenugreek seed	Very **bitter, aromatic,** warms digestion. Used to **alleviate lower-abdominal pain.**
Galangal root	**Spicy**, more or less **equivalent to fresh ginger.**
Garlic	**Spicy and aromatic**, strongly stimulates **motility** and is said to **strengthen the lungs**. Proven to **promote symbiotic bacteria** while killing pathogenic bacteria.
Ginger (fresh root)	**Spicy** and **slightly sweet**, regulates **stomach motility** and **secretion**, hence its role in soothing nausea.
Ginger (dried)	**Strongly spicy**. **Warms** and stimulates motility.
Horseradish	**Strongly spicy**. Strongly stimulates **motility**, hence its **combination with rich meats** such as beef.
Juniper berry	Slightly **aromatic and bitter**, stimulates motility **to aid digestion of rich food**. A great way to introduce tasty bitterness to a dish. Try adding it to **stews and casseroles**.

Mace	**Aromatic** and **slightly sweet**, warms and stimulates **motility**. Regulates **symbionts** to keep out the bad guys.
Mustard seeds	Spicy and aromatic, **warms digestion** and stimulates **motility**.
Nutmeg	**Aromatic**, warms and stimulates **motility**. Regulates **symbionts** just like mace.
Paprika	**Bitter**, **aromatic** and **slightly sweet**, stimulates **secretion** and **motility**.
Pepper, black and white	Very **spicy**, **counters stagnation** caused by cold and damp.
Star anise	**Sweet and aromatic**, promotes **motility** and **gut symbionts**. A mild spice to combine with **puddings and rich meat** like pork and beef.
Turmeric	**Bitter and pungent**, stimulates **motility** and **secretion**. Used for **reducing pain from trapped wind and bloating**
Vanilla	Sweet, a gentle flavouring that **strengthens symbionts** and stimulates **secretion**.

Exercise 1b
Match the column A with the column B. Try to learn the expressions and/ or sentences by heart.

A

1. Allspice is a gentle digestive stimulant
2. Aniseed
3. Caraway seed
4. Cardamom
5. Cayenne pepper (red pepper)
6. Chilli pepper
7. Cinnamon bark
8. Cinnamon twig
9. Clove
10. Coriander seed
11. Cumin
12. Dill seeds
13. Fennel seed
14. Fenugreek seed
15. Garlic promotes symbiotic bacteria,
16. Ginger
17. Horseradish
18. Juniper berry
19. Mace
20. Mustard seeds
21. Nutmeg
22. Paprika
23. Pepper, black and white
24. Star anise
25. Turmeric
26. Vanilla

B

a) chilli pepper that is often ground into a powder.
b) counters stagnation caused by cold and damp.
c) is a mild spice to combine with puddings and rich meat like pork and beef.
d) is a traditional cold and diarrhoea remedy.
e) is considered a very important mild spice for regulating motility in babies and children.
f) is the herb of choice for colic in children as it gently regulates motility.
g) is used for reducing pain from trapped wind and bloating, stimulates motility and secretion.

h) *is used to alleviate lower-abdominal pain.*
i) *is used to counteract nausea, muddy headaches and gut pain.*
j) *regulates digestion overall and stimulates the lungs.*
k) *regulates motility to relieve trapped wind and diarrhoea, especially in children.*
l) *regulates stomach motility and secretion, hence its role in soothing nausea.*
m) *regulates symbionts just like mace.*
n) *said to ease flatulence and stomach ache.*
o) *stimulates appetite and is said to treat diarrhoea and trapped wind.*
p) *stimulates appetite and regulates intestinal motility to relieve nausea and trapped wind.*
q) *stimulates motility but needs balancing with other refreshing and cooling herbs and foods.*
r) *stimulates motility to aid digestion of rich food.*
s) *stimulates secretion and motility.*
t) *strengthens symbionts and stimulates secretion.*
u) *strongly stimulates motility and is said to strengthen the lungs.*
v) *strongly stimulates motility, hence its combination with rich meats.*
w) *warms and stimulates motility and gut flora.*
x) *warm digestion and stimulate motility.*
y) *warms and stimulates motility and regulates symbionts.*
z) *warms digestion and stimulates motility and symbionts.*

Exercise 2

Translate the expressions. Try to explain their meanings in English.

Herbs, relationship, deciduous, basil, pungent, bay leaf, orange peel, marmalade, gut flora, stocks, caper, camomile, sooth, chervil, chives, coriander, refreshing, dandelion, counters, fluid retention, root, infusion, dill, lavender, liquorice, lovage, marjoram, astringent, mint, rosemary, trapped wind, feeling liverish, rose, peppermint, nasturtium, savory, mitigate, flatulence, sage, counter, saffron, thyme, mucous lungs, tarragon, sweet Cicely, mellows, sorrel, allspice, pimento, flatulence, aniseed, caraway seed, cardamom, counteract nausea, ground into a powder, cinnamon bark, remedy, astringent, cinnamon twig, clove, coriander seed, cumin, dill seeds, colic, fennel seed, relieves spasm, fenugreek seed, alleviate, galangal root, ginger, horseradish, juniper berry, mace, mustard seeds, nutmeg, paprika, pepper, star anise, turmeric, vanilla.

Exercise 3
Prepare short talks and/or dialogues on these topics.

1. Characterise basil, bay leaf, bitter orange peel.
2. Characterise caper, camomile, chervil, chives, coriander leaf.
3. Characterise dandelion leaf, dill leaf.
4. Characterise lavender flower, liquorice, lovage.
5. Characterise marjoram, mint, nasturtium, oregano.
6. Characterise parsley, peppermint, rose and rosewater, rosemary.
7. Characterise saffron, sage, savory, sorrel, sweet Cicely, tarragon, thyme.
8. Characterise allspice, aniseed, caraway seed, cardamom, cayenne pepper.
9. Characterise chilli pepper, cinnamon bark, cinnamon twig, clove, coriander seed.
10. Characterise cumin, dill seeds, fennel seed, fenugreek seed, garlic, ginger.
11. Characterise horseradish, juniper berry, mace, mustard seeds.
12. Characterise nutmeg, paprika, black and white pepper, star anise, turmeric, vanilla.

Vocabulary 16

Fill in the meanings in your mother language:

alleviate /ə'liː.vi.eɪt/
anise /'ænɪs/
aniseed /'æn.ɪ.siːd/
bark /bɑːk/
bud /bʌd/
calming /kɑːm.ɪŋ/
camomile /'kæm.ə.maɪl/
caraway /'kærəˌweɪ/
colic /'kɒlɪk/
culinary /'kʌlɪnərɪ/
deciduous /dɪ'sɪd.ju.əs/
flatulence /'flæt.jʊ.lənts/
galangal /gə'læŋgəl/
gentle /'dʒen.tlˌ/
ground /graʊnd/
Jamaica /dʒə'meɪkə/ **pepper** /'pepər/
lavender /'lævəndər/
liquorice /'lɪk.ər.ɪs/
lovage /'lʌv.ɪdʒ/
marmalade /'mɑːməleɪd/
mucous /'mjuː.kəs/
muddy /'mʌdi/
paprika /pæ'priːkə/
peppermint /'pepəmɪnt/
pimento /pɪ'mentəʊ/
proven /'pruː.vən/
pungent /'pʌndʒənt/
refreshing /rɪ'freʃɪŋ/
rose /rəʊz/
rosewater /rəʊz'wɔːtər/
saffron /'sæfrən/
sage /seɪdʒ/
sooth /suːð/
spice /spaɪs/
star /stɑːr/
sweet /swiːt/ **Cicely** /'sɪsəlɪ/
tarragon /'tærəgən/
twig /twɪg/
vanilla /və'nɪlə/
winter /'wɪn.tər/ **savory** /'seɪvəri/

Solution to Exercise 1a

1a, 2q, 3o, 4h, 5l, 6j, 7s, 8t, 9e, 10p, 11m, 12i, 13u, 14b, 15g, 16n, 17v, 18x, 19d, 20c, 21w, 22i, 23r, 24f, 25z, 26k,

Solution to Exercise 1b

1n, 2w, 3o, 4i, 5a, 6q, 7d, 8j, 9p, 10k, 11z, 12f, 13e, 14h, 15v, 16l, 17u, 18r, 19y, 20x, 21m, 22s, 23b, 24c, 25g, 26t

Unit 17 - Medicinal vegetables. Medicinal beans.

Super-fresh vegetables provide vital nutrition for the metabolism and substance of our bodies.

Celery stalk	Slightly **salty and bitter**, **balances very hot dry weather**. Also ideal to **balance the warming and drying nature** of strongly **aromatic spices**.
Chard	**Bitter and sweet**, traditionally said to **soothe the lungs** and cool excessive spice.
Chicory/ Endive	**Bitter and sweet**, a wonderful **summer vegetable for hot dry weather.**
Cress	Aromatic, **an ideal summer food that also balances strong spices.**
Fennel bulb	Sweet and aromatic, **soothes digestion and stimulates motility.**
Leek	**Aromatic and sweet**, stimulates **motility** and **counters the stagnating effect** of cold damp climate.
Nettle	**Sweet and bitter**. This should be viewed as a **fresh vegetable, especially in spring** when the tips are tender. Rich in **nutrients**, it is viewed as a **blood tonic**, while the **bitterness** means that traditionally it is used as a mild **diuretic** to **regulate the urinary system.**
Onion	**Aromatic and sweet**, stimulates **motility** and is said to **strengthen the lungs.**
Radish	Strongly **aromatic, stimulates the stomach** and is said to **strengthen the lungs.**
Rocket	**Aromatic and bitter**, stimulates **appetite** and **motility**, **a great green leaf for year-round consumption.**
Seaweed	**Salty savoury** and **mineral** rich, seaweed is considered one of the key foods responsible for the **health and longevity of the Japanese.** Be careful if you have a thyroid problem as they are high in iodine.
Spring onion	Aromatic, **stimulates** the **stomach** and the lungs, one of the great Eastern culinary vegetables.
Watercress	**Aromatic** and slightly **bitter**, very nutritious, stimulates motility and secretion.

Medicinal grains

Baked, sprouted, fermented and boiled, they deserve much higher status on our plates than the ever-present wheat.

Barley	This **sweet grain** is particularly **good for stomach health.** It is **cooling, calming and moistening** and stimulates motility while nourishing symbionts. Also consumed as **barley water. Barley couscous** is available.
Buckwheat	**Calms the stomach** and stimulates **motility**. Sweet in flavour, it **nourishes symbionts.**
Millet	**Sweet and bitter**, stimulates **motility and nourishes symbionts.**
Oats	**Sweet, nourishes symbionts.** It **strengthens** the **nervous system,** so it is calming in regular small quantities.

Rice	Sweet, a **most digestible grain.** It is likely that **white rice** is **healthier** than wholegrain as it contains much lower **levels of** compounds like **phytic acid that affect iron absorption**. **Rice has starches that break down** at just the right rate to **nourish digestion** and be healthily absorbed – no wonder it underpins the diet of the most healthy people on earth.
Rye	**Bitter, encourages motility** and, as a mild **diuretic**, the excretion of excess body fluids.
Spelt	An **ancient form of wheat**. It contains **much lower levels of gluten** than modern varieties and a better nutritional profile. This makes it much **more digestible** than the modern stuff. People who tend to suffer bloating and significant gut pain after eating normal wheat bread often find that they can **tolerate spelt bread. Spelt pasta** is also available.
Wheat bran	**Sweet, mellow** and **strengthening for digestion.**

Exercise 1a
Match the column A with the column B. Try to learn the expressions and/or sentences by heart.

A

1. Medicinal vegetables
2. Celery stalk, salty and bitter, balances very hot dry weather
3. Chard, bitter and sweet, is traditionally said
4. Chicory/Endive, bitter and sweet, is
5. Cress, aromatic, is an ideal summer food
6. Fennel bulb, sweet and aromatic,
7. Leek, aromatic and sweet,
8. Nettle, sweet and bitter, a fresh vegetable, especially in spring
9. Onion, aromatic and sweet,
10. Radish, strongly aromatic,
11. Rocket, aromatic and bitter,
12. Seaweed, salty savoury and mineral rich, is
13. Spring onion, aromatic, one of the great Eastern culinary vegetables,
14. Watercress, aromatic and slightly bitter, very nutritious,
15. Medicinal grains, baked, sprouted, fermented and boiled,
16. Barley, sweet grain, is cooling, calming and moistening
17. Buckwheat, sweet in flavour,
18. Millet, sweet and bitter,
19. Oats, sweet, nourishes symbionts,
20. Rice, sweet, a most digestible grain,
21. Rye, bitter, encourages motility and,
22. Spelt, an ancient form of wheat,
23. Wheat bran, sweet, mellow,

B

a) a wonderful summer vegetable for hot dry weather.

b) and is ideal to balance the warming and drying nature of strongly aromatic spices.

c) *and stimulates motility while nourishing symbionts.*
d) *and strengthens the nervous system.*
e) *as a mild diuretic, the excretion of excess body fluids.*
f) *calms the stomach, stimulates motility, and nourishes symbionts.*
g) *considered one of the key foods responsible for the health and longevity of the Japanese.*
h) *contains much lower levels of gluten than modern varieties.*
i) *has starches that break down at just the right rate to nourish digestion and be healthily absorbed.*
j) *is strengthening for digestion.*
k) *is viewed as a blood tonic, and is used to regulate the urinary system.*
l) *provide vital nutrition for the metabolism and substance of our bodies.*
m) *soothes digestion and stimulates motility.*
n) *stimulates appetite and motility, a great green leaf for year-round consumption.*
o) *stimulates motility and counters the stagnating effect of cold damp climate.*
p) *stimulates motility and is said to strengthen the lungs.*
q) *stimulates motility and nourishes symbionts.*
r) *stimulates motility and secretion.*
s) *stimulates the stomach and is said to strengthen the lungs.*
t) *stimulates the stomach and the lungs.*
u) *that also balances strong spices.*
v) *they deserve much higher status on our plates than the ever-present wheat.*
w) *to soothe the lungs and cool excessive spice.*

Medicinal beans

Beans are splendid food. Many of them have particular **medicinal properties** that make them especially useful in **strengthening and maintaining our health,** and countering the effects of our climate.

Aduki bean	Both sweet and sour, strengthens **digestion and soothes the stomach so it protects against the effects of excess spice.**
Black bean	Sweet and mild, strengthens **digestion and the constitution.**
Broad bean	Sweet and mild, **stimulates motility and nourishes gut flora.**
Cocoa	Bitter and sweet, **stimulates motility and secretion.**
Green bean	Sweet and mild, strengthens **digestion.**
Soy bean, black (fermented)	Sweet and mild, strengthens **digestion and the constitution.**
White bean	Sweet and mild, strengthens **digestion.**

Medicinal fruit

Fruits often have **strong flavour** and therefore **strong effects** on digestion and the rest of our health. Excessive consumption of **raw fruit depletes digestive strength**. The best way to deal with fruit is **to cook it, or combine it** intelligently to enhance the digestibility of other foods.

Crab apple (and other sour apple varieties)	Sour and sweet. **Stimulates secretion, particularly to help in digestion of rich meats such as pork or goose.**
Elderberry	Bitter and sweet, **soothes and regulates the intestine.**
Goji berries (wolfberry/ gou qi zi)	Sweet and rich, **a constitutional tonic. Add to soups, stews, stocks and casseroles** and combine with light aromatic spices.
Hawthorn berry	Sour and sweet. **Is used in China to relieve indigestion, particularly from eating too much meat and greasy food.**
Lemon zest	Bitter and aromatic, **balances the effect of very spicy food and stimulates secretion.**
Lychee	Sweet and sour, strengthens **symbionts.**
Pear	Sweet and cooling. **Steamed with cloves it is said to clear the phlegm from the lungs.**
Persimmon	Bitter and astringent, regulates the stomach. **Renowned for its use as a relief for belching and hiccough.**
Rosehip	Sour and slightly sweet. **Stimulates the gall bladder** to **cut through fat and gently stimulates motility.**

Medicinal Mushrooms

Many types of mushroom are used in traditional cooking including the **chestnut, button, field and boletus varieties.** Others, such as **shiitake, maitake, and oyster mushrooms** are renowned as dietary medicines. Mushrooms have a strengthening **effect** on the body, both for digestion and the general constitution. Indeed their medicinal benefits are unique, probably because they are primary decomposers, **extracting and creating nutrients** that cannot be found in other type of organism.

Boletus edulious (porcini/ ceps)	Sweet, **regulates the immune system and nourishes symbionts.**
Button/ chestnut	Sweet, **stimulates the appetite and nourishes digestion.**
Oyster	Sweet, **a strong immune tonic.**
Portobello	Sweet and savoury, **a strong blood tonic**.
Shiitake	Sweet, **an important blood and constitutional tonic**. One of the most popular mushrooms in the world and revered by the Chinese and Japanese.

Medicinal meat, fish and eggs

When sourcing meat, fish and eggs, quality is very important. If animals have been well looked after, allowed to roam and given access to a varied diet, the meat will have fewer toxic contaminants and a much healthier range of nutrients. This is a crucial dietary principle: **healthy animals mean healthy humans.**

Carp	Sweet and nourishing. A **strong tonic for blood and digestion**.
Chicken	Sweet, nourishes symbionts. It is **nourishing and easy to digest.**
Eggs	**Chicken** and **duck** eggs are **sweet, rich and strengthening. Quail** eggs are a revered constitutional tonic.
Herring	Sweet and rich. Although **an oily fish**, it is **light enough to be easily digested** and a digestive tonic. Also **traditionally said to benefit the lungs**.
Mackerel	Sweet and rich. **An important tonic for digestion and blood.**
Mussels	Salty. **A constitutional tonic, said to be good for fertility and longevity.**

Offal	Includes **brains, heart, sweetbreads, liver, kidneys and pluck** (lungs and intestines of sheep). Traditionally speaking, the organs are said to nourish the corresponding organ in the human body; chicken liver strengthens the human liver, for example.
Oysters	Salty and sweet. **Nourish vitality, blood, and the constitution**. Said to be **good for fertility and longevity.**
Quail	Sweet, **nourishes symbionts**.
Rabbit (wild)	Sweet, **nourishes symbionts.**
Sardines	Sweet and rich. An **important tonic for digestion and blood**.

Exercise 1b
Match the column A with the column B. Try to learn the expressions and/or sentences by heart.

A

1. Medicinal beans (Aduki bean, black bean, broad bean, green bean, soybean, white bean)
2. Fruits often have strong flavour
3. Crab apple (and other sour apple varieties)
4. Elderberry
5. Goji berries a constitutional tonic; can be
6. Hawthorn berry
7. Lemon zest
8. Lychee, sweet and sour,
9. Pear steamed with cloves
10. Persimmon, bitter and astringent,
11. Rosehip, sour and slightly sweet,
12. Boletus edulious, and button/chestnut
13. Oyster, sweet,
14. Portobello, sweet and savoury,
15. Shiitake is one of the most popular mushrooms in the world
16. Medicinal meat, fish and eggs:
17. Carp, sweet and nourishing
18. Chicken is
19. Chicken and duck eggs
20. Herring, although an oily fish,
21. Mackerel, sweet and rich,
22. Mussels, salty, a constitutional tonic,
23. Offal (includes brains, heart, sweetbreads, liver, kidneys and pluck)
24. Oysters, salty and sweet, nourish vitality, blood, and the constitution
25. Quail, and wild rabbit, sweet,
26. Sardines, sweet and rich

B

a) added to soups, stews, stocks and casseroles and combine with light aromatic spices.
b) and are said to be good for fertility and longevity.
c) and revered by the Chinese and Japanese.
d) and therefore strong effects on digestion and the rest of our health.
e) are an important tonic for digestion and blood.

f) *are said to nourish the corresponding organ in the human body.*

g) *are sweet, rich and strengthening; quail eggs are a revered constitutional tonic.*

h) *balances the effect of very spicy food and stimulates secretion.*

i) *have particular medicinal properties that make them especially useful in strengthening and maintaining our health.*

j) *healthy animals mean healthy humans.*

k) *is a strong blood tonic.*

l) *is a strong immune tonic.*

m) *is a strong tonic for blood and digestion.*

n) *is an important tonic for digestion and blood.*

o) *is light enough to be easily digested.*

p) *is said to be good for fertility and longevity.*

q) *is said to clear the phlegm from the lungs.*

r) *is used in China to relieve indigestion, particularly from eating too much meat and greasy food.*

s) *nourish symbionts.*

t) *nourishing and easy to digest.*

u) *regulate the immune system and nourish symbionts.*

v) *renowned for its use as a relief for belching and hiccough.*

w) *soothes and regulates the intestine.*

x) *stimulates secretion, particularly to help in digestion of rich meats such as pork or goose.*

y) *stimulates the gall bladder to cut through fat and gently stimulates motility.*

z) *strengthens symbionts.*

Exercise 2

Translate the expressions. Try to explain their meanings in English.

Celery stalk, chard, chicory, endive, cress, soothe, fennel bulb, leek, nettle, blood tonic, urinary system, onion, radish, rocket, seaweed, year-round consumption, longevity, thyroid problem, spring onion, watercress, moistening, barley couscous, buckwheat, millet, nourishes, oats, rice, wholegrain, right rate, underpins, rye, spelt, ancient, stuff, tend to, suffer bloating, tolerate, wheat bran, mellow, aduki bean, excessive, depletes, crab apple, goose, elderberry, intestine, constitutional tonic, goji berries, hawthorn berry, greasy, lemon zest, lychee, pear, cloves, phlegm, persimmon, renowned for, relief belching, hiccough, rosehip, gall bladder, cut through fat, gently, chestnut, button, field and boletus, shiitake, maitake, oyster mushrooms, decomposers, extracting and creating nutrients, boletus edulious, portobello, shiitake, blood tonic, roam, access, crucial dietary principle, carp, quail, herring, benefit, mussels, fertility, longevity, offal, brains, heart, sweetbreads, liver, kidneys, plucks, quail, rabbit.

Exercise 3
Answer the following questions. Prepare short talks and/or dialogues on these topics.

1. Characterise celery stalk, chard, chicory, cress.
2. Characterise fennel bulb, leek, nettle, onion, radish.
3. Characterise rocket, seaweed, spring onion, watercress.
4. Characterise barley, buckwheat, millet, oats.
5. Characterise rice, rye, spelt, wheat bran.
6. Characterise crab apple, elderberry, goji berries, hawthorn berry.
7. Characterise lemon zest, lychee, pear, persimmon, rose hip.
8. Characterise boletus edulious, oyster, portobello, shiitake.
9. Characterise carp, chicken, eggs, herring, mackerel, mussels.
10. Characterise offal, oysters, quail, wild rabbit, sardines.

Vocabulary 17

Fill in the meanings in your mother language:

belch /beltʃ/
boletus /bəʊˈliːtəs/
edulious /ˌedʒʊˈli.əs/
broad /brɔːd/ **bean** /biːn/
button /ˈbʌtən/ **mushroom** /ˈmʌʃ.ruːm/
carp /kɑːp/
cep /sep/
couscous /ˈkuːskuːs/
cress /kres/
decomposer /ˌdiː.kəmˈpəʊz.ər/
deplete /dɪˈpliːt/
edulious /ˌedʒʊˈli.əs/
elderberry /ˈel.dəˌber.i/
endive /ˈendaɪv/
fennel /ˈfenəl/ **bulb** /bʌlb/
goji, gou qi /ˈgəʊdʒɪ/
greasy /ˈgriːsi/
herring /ˈherɪŋ/
hiccough, also **hiccup** /ˈhɪkʌp/
longevity /lɒnˈdʒev.ə.ti/
mackerel /ˈmæk.rəl/
maitake /meɪˈtɑː.ki/
mild /maɪld/
nettle /ˈnetl/
pear /peə/
phytic /ˈfaɪ tɪk/ **acid** /ˈæsɪd/
pluck /plʌk/
porcino /pɔːˈtʃiːnəʊ/ pl. **porcini**
portobello /ˈpɔːtəbɛləʊ/
rabbit /ˈræbɪt/
roam /rəʊm/
rosehip /rəʊzhɪp/
shiitake /ʃɪˈtɑː.ki/
soybean /ˈsɔɪˌbiːn/
splendid /ˈsplendɪd/
spring /sprɪŋ/ **onion** /ˈʌn.jən/
sprouted /spraʊtəd/
sweet bread /ˈswiːt.bred/
wheat /wiːt/ **bran** /bræn/
wild /waɪld/

Solution to Exercise 1a
1l, 2b, 3w, 4a, 5u, 6m, 7o, 8k, 9p, 10s, 11n, 12g, 13t, 14r, 15v, 16c, 17f, 18q, 19d, 20i, 21e, 22h, 23j

Solution to Exercise 1b
1i, 2d, 3x, 4w, 5a, 6r, 7h, 8z, 9q, 10v, 11y, 12u, 13l, 14k, 15c, 16j, 17m, 18t, 19g, 20o, 21n, 22p, 23f, 24b, 25s, 26e

Unit 18 - Medicinal nuts and seeds

These provide a number of particularly important nutrients, most notably their **essential oils**.

Almond	Sweet and slightly bitter, it is said to strengthen **the lungs.**
Chestnut	Sweet, a **digestive and constitutional tonic**.
Flax seeds	Rich and oily. A vegetable source of **omega 3 oils**, it improves motility in the large intestine to **relieve constipation.**
Hazelnut	Sweet and rich, can **strengthen gut symbionts**.
Hempseeds	Sweet, they **moisten, soothe and nourish the gut.** Hemp oil is a wonderful locally produced tonic.
Sezame, black	Sweet and rich, **a constitutional tonic.**
Walnut	Sweet, bitter and rich, a **constitutional tonic** and ideal winter food.

Medicinal oils and fats

Fats can come from plant and animal sources. **Plant oils**, fresh, cold-pressed and produced without chemicals, are precious foods. Organic production is particularly important for plant oils because many **pesticides are fat-soluble.** Not all of these oils are suitable for **frying**, because **high temperatures** can alter their chemical structure and reduce their health benefits. But **boiling is fine**, so they can be used in **soups, stews and casseroles,** as well as **dressings, mayonnaise and dips. Animal fats** are just as valuable. They contain a wide range of **essential nutrients** including **omega 3 essential fatty acids** and vitamins. Similarly, in **eggs, butter** and clarified butter or **ghee**, animal fats provide vital nutrients for vegetarians. Animal fats are also very **important for cooking** as they are partly saturated and therefore stable at high temperatures. **Plants fats,** by contrast, tend to **distort** when they get hot, forming cancer- and heart-disease-causing **trans fats** and other pathogenic chemicals.

Butter	Sweet and rich, **a strong tonic for the blood, membranes and nervous system**.
Clarified butter/ Ghee	This is effectively cooked butter. The cooking process **removes the milk solids and water**, making it more stable at high temperatures and less likely to burn – it is **ideal for frying.** Sweet and rich, **it nourishes nerves and membranes** and is relatively easy to digest.
Coconut oil	Sweet and rich. This is a saturated plant fat but one that we should love rather than fear. **A tonic for the blood and nervous system**. The molecules are small and easy to digest. It is also great to cook with, as its molecules are stable at high temperatures.
Beef dripping/ suet	Delicious and rich.
Flax oil	Sweet and moistening, an omega 3-rich oil that **soothes the gut**. Traditionally used in the **treatment of constipation.**
Goose fat/ Duck fat	Sweet and moistening. These two fats deserve a mention because they are **lighter than most other animal fats** because they contain high levels of mono-unsaturated fats, just like olive oil, making them easier to digest.

Hemp oil	Sweet and rich, this is one of the most digestible oils. Now widely available, it has a fabulous **balance of essential fatty acids** and is a revered traditional ingredient. This oil is not stable at high temperatures and so it is not a good frying oil.
Olive oil (fresh extra virgin)	Sweet and moistening, **nourishes all of the body's membranes**. The fresher this oil is, the easier it is to digest as it contains some wonderful **light aromatic components**.
Rape seed oil	Sweet and rich, this oil is packed with **omega 3 fats** and is a great dietary option. Go for the good stuff, though, fresh, **cold-pressed and well-produced** as there are all sorts of problems with "Canola" which is produced with high chemical inputs.
Sezame oil	Sweet and moistening, this oil is an all-round good performer. In particular, it **enhances the fluidity and flexibility of membranes**, resulting in **skin nourishment** and **cardiovascular benefits**. Sezame can be used for cooking as it tends to form less nasties at higher temperatures than other polyunsaturated oils.

Medicinal condiments

There are a number of simple products and foods **stimulating appetite** and **enhancing digestion**. Each dietary tradition has its own particular foodstuffs.

Cider vinegar	Sour and slightly pungent, **refreshes and stimulates appetite.**
Miso	Salty/savoury and slightly sour, strengthens **digestion** in small amounts.
Soy sauce	Sweet and salty/savoury, **stimulates appetite** and regulates the stomach to **reduce nausea**.
Yeast (natural, not fast acting)	Sour, sweet and bitter, **stimulates secretion, motility and gut symbionts.** Consume in small amounts to avoid candida.

Others that are worthy of mention are **Thai fish sauce**, **mushroom ketchup**, **Worcester sauce**, **anchovy paste or sauce** and **black bean sauce**; they are all salty/savoury and contain **fermented ingredients**. Therefore, they are highly nutritious and stimulate the appetite.

Exercise 1
Match the column A with the column B. Try to learn the expressions and/or sentences by heart.

A

1. Almond, sweet and slightly bitter,
2. Chestnut
3. Flax seeds
4. Hazelnut
5. Hempseeds
6. Sezame, sweet and rich,
7. Walnut,
8. High temperatures can alter chemical structure
9. Plant oils can be used in soups, stews and casseroles,
10. Animal fats are also very important for cooking
11. Plants fats tend to distort when they get hot,
12. Butter
13. Ghee is ideal for frying,
14. Coconut oil, a tonic for the blood and nervous system
15. Flax oil soothes the gut;
16. Goose and duck fats,

17. Hemp oil
18. Olive oil (fresh extra virgin)
19. Rape seed oil, sweet and rich,
20. Sezame oil enhances the fluidity and flexibility of membranes,
21. Medicinal condiments are products and foods
22. Cider vinegar, sour and slightly pungent,
23. Miso, salty/savoury and slightly sour,
24. Soy sauce, sweet and salty/savoury,
25. Yeast (natural, not fast acting), sour, sweet and bitter,
26. Thai fish sauce, mushroom ketchup, Worcester sauce, anchovy paste or sauce and black bean sauce

B

a) *are highly nutritious and stimulate the appetite.*
b) *are lighter than most other animal fats because they contain high levels of mono-unsaturated fats.*
c) *as they are partly saturated and therefore stable at high temperatures.*
d) *as well as dressings, mayonnaise and dips.*
e) *can strengthen gut symbionts.*
f) *forming cancer- and heart-disease-causing trans fats.*
g) *has a fabulous balance of essential fatty acids and is a revered traditional ingredient.*
h) *improve motility in the large intestine to relieve constipation.*
i) *is a constitutional tonic.*
j) *is a digestive and constitutional tonic.*
k) *is a strong tonic for the blood, membranes and nervous system.*
l) *is also great to cook with, as its molecules are stable at high temperatures.*
m) *is packed with omega 3 fats and is a great dietary option.*
n) *is said to strengthen the lungs.*
o) *moisten, soothe and nourish the gut.*
p) *nourishes all of the body's membranes.*
q) *nourishes nerves and membranes and is relatively easy to digest.*
r) *of plant oils, and reduce their health benefits.*
s) *refreshes and stimulates appetite.*
t) *resulting in skin nourishment and cardiovascular benefits.*
u) *stimulates appetite and regulates the stomach to reduce nausea.*
v) *stimulates secretion, motility and gut symbionts.*
w) *stimulating appetite and enhancing digestion.*
x) *straightens digestion in small amounts.*
y) *sweet, bitter and rich, is a constitutional tonic.*
z) *traditionally is used in the treatment of constipation.*

Exercise 2
Translate the expressions. Try to explain their meanings in English.

Notably, almond, chestnut, flax seeds, relieve constipation, hazelnut, hempseeds, moisten, constitutional, walnut, precious, alter, boiling, dressings, dips, partly saturated, stable, distort, clarified, solids, coconut oil, beef dripping, suet, flax oil, goose, duck, deserve a mention, hemp oil, revered, olive oil, rape seed oil, dietary option, canola, inputs, nasties, fluidity, flexibility, foodstuffs, cider vinegar, miso, Soy sauce, yeast, fast acting, be worthy of.

Exercise 3
Answer the following questions. Prepare short talks and/or dialogues on these topics.

1. Characterise almond, chestnut, flax seeds, hazelnut, hempseeds, sezame, walnut.
2. Characterise butter, ghee, coconut oil, flax oil, hemp oil, olive oil, rape seed oil, sezame oil.
3. Characterise cider vinegar, miso, soy sauce, yeast.

Vocabulary 18

Fill in the meanings in your mother language:

all-round /ˈɔlˈraʊnd/
almond /ˈɑːmənd/
candida /ˈkændɪdə/
canola /kəˈnəʊlə/
cold /kəʊld/ **-pressed** /ˈprest/
fabulous /fæbjʊləs/
fear /fɪə/
flax /flæks/
flexibility /ˌflek.sɪˈbɪl.ə.ti/
fluidity /fluːˈɪdɪtɪ/
foodstuff /ˈfuːdˌstʌf/
hazelnut /ˈheɪzəlˌnʌt/
mention /ˈmen.ʃən/
moisten /ˈmɔɪ.sən/
nasties /ˈnɑːstɪs/
partly /ˈpɑːt.lɪ/
performer /pəˈfɔːmə/
range /reɪndʒ/
rape /reɪp/
relieve /rɪˈliːv/
solid /ˈsɒlɪd/
source /sɔːs/
stable /ˈsteɪ.blˌ/
valuable /ˈvæl.jʊ.blˌ/
vegetarian /ˌvedʒɪˈteərɪən/
virgin /ˈvɜːdʒɪn/
walnut /ˈwɔːlˌnʌt/

Solution to Exercise 1
1n, 2j, 3h, 4e, 5o, 6i, 7y, 8r, 9d, 10c, 11f, 12k, 13q, 14l, 15z, 16b, 17g, 18p, 19m, 20t, 21w, 22s, 23x, 24u, 25v, 26a

Chapter IV

Good cooking made easy. Recipes.

Unit 1 - Planning the menu. First courses.

If you are planning a company dinner, then it is important to **plan the menu** so that it is **well balanced**

in texture, colour and flavour. When you are thinking about the dishes you should also bear in mind **the time you can set aside** to prepare them. Once you have decided what to cook, try to work out **a rough time-scale** for the cooking, taking into account any **dishes which can be frozen, chilled or marinated well in advance**. Decide which dishes really do need attention just before they are served and be prepared for this.

Cutting down on preparation time

Organization is the key to success when it comes to cooking. Disaster can result from an **overcrowded work surface** leaving little or no space for **transferring hot pots** from the stove, no room to **roll out the pastry**, or worse, meaning that the bowl or dish near the edge is knocked on to the floor scattering the contents everywhere. So, try to **keep the kitchen tidy** – keep the dish washing to a minimum or stack it in the **dishwasher** as you work, put all the scraps and unwanted peelings or wrappers in the disposal or **garbage can** and keep the food preparation as neat as possible.

There are a few practical hints which can often help with the most basic preparation. **Chopping onions**, for example can be quicker in the onion is cut in half, laid flat on the board, then cut into slices in one direction. Holding the slices firmly together cut across them to give small pieces. If the onion should be finely chopped, then make the slices thin; for chunky pieces make the slices thicker. A quick way of chopping **parsley** is to put the washed and trimmed herb into a coffee mug, then snip at it with a pair of scissors – the pieces will not be evenly tiny, but usually good enough for a quick garnish or to flavour casseroles, soups and sauces. Kitchen **scissors** can be invaluable for **trimming the edges off pastry**, for cutting out pastry leaves for decoration, and for **trimming excess fat** from meat. They are also ideal for **snipping chives and scallions**, for **cutting** fish fillets and bacon **into strips** and for lots of similar tasks.

Food **mixers and blenders** are very commonplace pieces of equipment. Remember to use the mixer for preparing **creamed mixtures** of all types, for **beating egg whites**, for **whipping cream**, for **making batters and mayonnaise**. You can also turn to the food mixer if you are creaming savoury butters, **rubbing the fat** into flour to make pastry or similar mixtures and preparing a range of **frostings**. If you have a large food mixer then it will probably cope with **bread dough, fruit cakes** and even **mashed potatoes**. The blender is invaluable when it comes to making **sauces, soups and purées**. This piece of equipment can also be used for **making bread crumbs**, for **crushing ice cubes**, and for **chopping or mincing** dry ingredients like **nuts and herbs**. For **pâtés, dips** and other similar creamy mixtures, turn to the blender, you will find life much easier than if you spend hours battling with a **grinder, sieve or food masher**. The **food processor** is a compact piece of equipment which will carry out most of the tasks, like **chopping onions, slicing vegetables and grating cheese.** For making cakes and pastry, even bread dough, and food puréeing, blending and grinding, there is no better utensil in the kitchen. Many of the new models are designed to be easy to **assemble** and simple to clean.

Microwave ovens offer a speedy solution to many cooking processes. For example rice and vegetables can be cooked quite successfully in the microwave along with fish dishes and some chicken dishes. **Pressure cookers** have been around for years but they still play an important part when it comes to **cooking the tougher cuts of meat** quickly and successfully. For **steaming vegetables**, making steamed puddings and for a broad range of other recipes you can use the pressure cooker with confidence. **Slow cookers** work on a completely different principle – these employ a very **low temperature** to cook food slowly over a period of many hours. Successful for **meat casseroles** and **dried legume dishes**, these cookers are very helpful.

Exercise 1a
Match the column A with the column B. Try to learn the expressions and/or sentences by heart.

A

1. Once you have decided what to cook, try to work out a rough time-scale for the cooking,
2. Organization is the key to success
3. An overcrowded work surface leaves little or no space
4. Keep the kitchen tidy –
5. Kitchen scissors can be invaluable for trimming the edges off pastry, for trimming excess fat from meat,
6. Remember to use the mixer for preparing creamed mixtures of all types,
7. If you have a large food mixer then it will probably cope with
8. The blender can also be used for
9. The food processor is a compact piece of equipment
10. There is no better utensil in the kitchen
11. Rice and vegetables can be cooked quite successfully in the microwave
12. Pressure cookers play an important part
13. Slow cookers employ a very low temperature

B

a) along with fish dishes and some chicken dishes.
b) bread dough, fruit cakes and even mashed potatoes.
c) for beating egg whites, for whipping cream,

and for making batters and mayonnaise.

d) *for making cakes and pastry, even bread dough, and food puréeing, blending and grinding.*

e) *for snipping chives and scallions, or for cutting fish fillets and bacon into strips.*

f) *for transferring hot pots from the stove, and no room to roll out the pastry.*

g) *making bread crumbs, for crushing ice cubes, and for chopping or mincing dry ingredients like nuts and herbs.*

h) *put all the scraps and unwanted peelings or wrappers in the disposal or garbage can.*

i) *taking into account any dishes which can be frozen, chilled or marinated well in advance.*

j) *to cook food slowly over a period of many hours.*

k) *when it comes to cooking the tougher cuts of meat, for steaming vegetables or making steamed puddings.*

l) *when it comes to cooking.*

m) *which will carry out most of the tasks, like chopping onions, slicing vegetables and grating cheese.*

First courses

The food should be chosen to complement the main dish, offering a contrast in texture and flavour. The portions should be **small and attractively presented**. If the main course is a cold dish, then a hot appetizer may be welcome. In warmer weather, or if the main dish is a heart-warming hotpot, for example, it may be preferable to offer a light, **cool savoury cocktail** or a splendid platter of **mixed hors d'oeuvre.** Offer some **hot crisp toast, warm crusty bread** or nutty **whole wheat rolls** with the appetizer. Remember to prepare the garnishes, butter dish and bread basket in advance.

Pâtés, terrines and pies

There are lots of pâtés and terrines which **require time** more than culinary skill when it comes to their preparation. You can find many recipes for **fish, meat**, variety meats, **poultry, game and vegetables** in traditional pies, rich pâtés and light vegetable-based terrines. Some are **encased in pastry**. A food processor or blender are invaluable when you are preparing the ingredients, otherwise, a good **sharp knife** and large **chopping board** are quite adequate. Once al the ingredients are prepared and mixed, most terrines and pâtés need fairly lengthy cooking. Depending on the texture, the pâté may need **weighting down and chilling** for several hours before it is served. The recipes are incredibly **versatile** – they can be served for **the first course**, for **the main course** or as a **light lunch or supper dish**. For **picnics, buffet meals** or as a filling **snack**, pâtés, terrines and pies are all excellent foods to offer.

The accompaniments you serve depend upon the occasion: for a light snack some **crisp crackers, celery** and **tomatoes** would complement a simple pâté. **Hot toast or rolls** with pâté make a substantial appetizer, or hot crusty bread, pâté and salad go to make a tasty lunch. Pies and terrines can be served with salads, bread and **baked potatoes** to make **substantial meals**.

Fish and seafood

Seafood is particularly versatile - it can be used to make hot or cold dishes **for all occasions**, from inexpensive meals to the most elaborate dinner party dishes. There is often a tendency to shy away from cooking fish because of the **preparation** involved – **cleaning, filleting and skinning**. Alternatively the common varieties of fish are available frozen in the most convenient forms.

Broiled, baked, poached or fried, fish and shellfish can be turned into any number of light or satisfying meals. To poach fish, white **wine or cider** can be used in some recipes or a **court bouillon or fish stock** can be used in others. You can prepare your own stock: **boil** fish **trimmings – heads, tails, skin and bones** – in plenty of water with a roughly chopped **onion, parsley springs, bay leaf** and a few **peppercorns** for about 30-40 minutes. **Strain and reduce** as necessary. For anyone who is diet conscious, whether simply **counting the calories** or trying to reduce the fat content of daily meals, then **fish is an excellent standby.** Poached very simply with the minimum of fish stock or broiled with just a little lemon juice, white fish is a low-calorie food. For extra flavour fresh herbs and vegetables can also be used. Special occasions offer an opportunity to prepare some **shellfish** specialities using **crab, lobster, shrimp or scallops**. The simplest way is to serve these seafood poached and dressed, with mayonnaise and lemon.

Poultry and game

Nowadays, **chicken and turkey** are available in the form of pieces, **boneless breasts, breast fillets** or in the shape of boneless **rolls of meat**. These poultry require little preparation before cooking. **Game** on the other hand is both seasonal and more expensive. Recipes most often include **guinea hen, pheasant, squab (small pigeon), duck, goose and hare and partridge.**

Meat dishes

Times and techniques for **roasting** meat are fairly personal; some people favour **rare meat** while others will eat only **well-cooked roasts**. Whether you opt for a quick roasting method or a slower method depends on individual preference but also on **the quality** of the meat.

Calculating the cooking time by weight is a good starting point when you are roasting meat. Check the roast as it cooks, using a **meat skewer** to pierce it or a meat **thermometer**. If you are roasting meat in a hot oven, have a piece of **cooking foil** at hand to cover the roast should it become too brown.

In addition to roasts, meat dishes also include **casseroles and hotpots, steaks and croquettes.**

Exercise 1b
Match the column A with the column B. Try to learn the expressions and/or sentences by heart.

A

1. The food for first courses should be chosen
2. The portions should be small
3. Offer some hot crisp toast, warm crusty bread
4. You can find many recipes
5. A food processor or blender are invaluable
6. Depending on the texture, the pâté
7. Pâtés, terrines and pies can be served
8. The accompaniments you serve depend upon the occasion:
9. Hot toast or rolls with pâté make a substantial appetizer,
10. Pâtés, terrines and pies
11. Preparation of fish and seafood involves
12. Broiled, baked, poached or fried, fish and shellfish
13. To poach fish, white wine or cider can be used in some recipes
14. Boil fish trimmings – heads, tails, skin and bones with
15. Poached with the minimum of fish stock
16. Special occasions offer an opportunity to prepare some shellfish specialities
17. Chicken and turkey are available
18. Game recipes most often include
19. Some people favour rare meat
20. Check the roast as it cooks,
21. Have a piece of cooking foil at hand

B

a) *a roughly chopped onion, parsley springs, bay leaf and a few peppercorns; then strain and reduce as necessary.*
b) *and attractively presented.*
c) *can be turned into any number of light or satisfying meals.*
d) *cleaning, filleting and skinning.*
e) *for a light snack some crisp crackers, celery and tomatoes.*
f) *for fish, meat, poultry, game and vegetables in traditional pies, rich pâtés and light vegetable-based terrines.*
g) *for the first course, for the main course or as a light lunch or supper dish, for picnics, buffet meals or as a filling snack.*
h) *guinea hen, pheasant, squab (small pigeon), duck, goose and hare and partridge.*

i) *hot crusty bread, pâté and salad will make a tasty lunch.*

j) *in the form of pieces, boneless breasts, breast fillets or rolls of meat.*

k) *may need weighting down and chilling for several hours before it is served.*

l) *or a court bouillon or fish stock can be used in others.*

m) *or broiled with just a little lemon juice, white fish is a low-calorie food.*

n) *or nutty whole wheat rolls with the appetizer.*

o) *otherwise, a good sharp knife and large chopping board are quite adequate.*

p) *served with salads, bread and baked potatoes make substantial meals.*

q) *to complement the main dish, offering a contrast in texture and flavour.*

r) *to cover the roast should it become too brown.*

s) *using crab, lobster, shrimp or scallops.*

t) *while others will eat only well-cooked roasts,*

u) *using a meat skewer to pierce it or a meat thermometer.*

Exercise 2

Translate the expressions. Try to explain their meanings in English.

Texture, flavour, bear in mind, set aside, chilled, in advance, overcrowded work surface, roll out the pastry, knocked on, scattering, dish washing, scraps, peelings, wrappers, garbage can, chopping onions, garnish, trimming, snipping chives and scallions, strips, mixers and blenders, beating egg whites, whipping cream, rubbing the fat, make pastry, frostings, bread dough, mashed potatoes, purées, bread crumbs, crushing ice cubes, chopping or mincing, grinder, sieve, food processor, carry out, slicing vegetable, grating cheese, blending and grinding, assemble, microwave ovens, pressure cookers, steaming vegetables, first courses, complement, the main dish, texture and flavour, appetizer, cool savoury cocktail, hors d'oeuvre, crisp toast, crusty bread, whole wheat rolls, bread basket, poultry, game, pies, encased in pastry, a food processor or blender, chopping board, weighting down and chilling, the first course, the main course, buffet meals, crisp crackers, baked potatoes, substantial meals, all occasions, cleaning, filleting and skinning, broiled, baked, poached or fried, court bouillon, fish stock, parsley springs, bay leaf, peppercorns, strain and reduce, an excellent standby, broiled, crab, lobster, shrimp or scallops, turkey, breast fillets, boneless rolls of meat, guinea hen, pheasant, pigeon, duck, goose, hare, partridge, favour, rare meat, meat skewer, to pierce, hot oven, croquettes.

Exercise 3
Answer the following questions. Prepare short talks and/or dialogues on these topics.

1. Why is planning of the menu important?
2. How can you cut down on preparation time?
3. What is the use of scissors, food mixers, blenders?
4. What is the use of microwave ovens, pressure cookers, slow cookers?
5. First courses (e.g. pâtés, terrines and pies).
6. Preparation of fish and seafood.
7. Preparation of poultry and game.
8. Times and techniques for roasting meat.

Vocabulary 1

Fill in the meanings in your mother language:

accompaniment /ə'kʌm pə nɪ mənt/
alternatively /ɔ:l'tɜ:nətɪvlɪ/
appetizer /'æpɪˌtaɪzə/
assemble /ə'sem.bəl/
at hand /hænd/
attention /ə'ten.ʃən/
basket /'bɑ:skɪt/
batter /'bætə/
battle /bætəl/
bay /beɪ/ **leaf** /li:f/
beat /bi:t/
blend /blend/
blender /'blendə/
board /bɔ:d/
bowl /bəʊl/
breast /brest/
broil /brɔɪl/
buffet /bʊfeɪ/
can /kən/
carry out /'kær iˌaʊt/
casserole /'kæsəˌrəʊl/
celery /'selərɪ/
chill /tʃɪl/
chives /tʃaɪvz/
chop /tʃɒp/
chunky /tʃʌŋkɪ /
cider /'saɪdə/
cocktail /'kɒkˌteɪl/
commonplace /'kɒmənˌpleɪs/
complement /'kɒmplɪˌment/
confidence /'kɒnfɪdəns/
conscious /'kɒnʃəs/
content /'kɒntent/
convenient /kən'vi:nɪənt/
course /kɔ:s/
court /kɔrt/ **bouillon** /'bu:jɒn/
crab /kræb/
cracker /'krækə/
cream /kri:m/
crisp /krɪsp/
croquette /kroʊ'kɛt/
crumb /krʌm/
crush /krʌʃ/
crusty /'krʌstɪ/
cube /kju:b/
culinary /'kʌlɪnərɪ/
cut /kʌt/ **down** /daʊn/
cut /kʌt/
dip /dɪp/
disaster /dɪ'zɑ:stə/
dish /dɪʃ/
dishwasher /'dɪʃˌwɒʃə/
disposal /dɪ'spəʊzəl/
dough /dəʊ/
dress /dres/
duck /dʌk/
elaborate /ɪ'læb ər ɪt/
employ /ɪm'plɔɪ/
encase /ɪn'keɪs/
evenly /'i:vənlɪ/
excellent /eksələnt/

favour /ˈfeɪvə/
fillet /ˈfɪlɪt/
filling /ˈfɪlɪŋ/
finely /ˈfaɪnlɪ/
firmly /ˈfɜːmlɪ/
flat /flæt/
flavour /ˈfleɪvə/
food /fuːd/ **processor** /ˈprəʊsesə/
frosting /ˈfrɒstɪŋ/
game /geɪm/
garbage /ˈgɑːbɪdʒ/
garnish /ˈgɑːnɪʃ/
goose /guːs/
grate /greɪt/
grind /graɪnd/
grinder /ˈgraɪndə/
guinea /ˈgɪni/ **hen** /hɛn/
hare /heə/
heart-warming /ˈhartˌwɔr mɪŋ/
herb /ɜːrb/
hint /hɪnt/
hors d'oeuvre /ɔr ˈdɜrvr/
incredibly /ɪnˈkredəbəlɪ/
inexpensive /ˌɪnɪkˈspensɪv/
ingredient /ɪnˈgriːdɪənt/
invaluable /ɪnˈvæljʊəbəl/
knock /nɒk/
leave /liːv/
legume /lɪˈgjuːm/
lengthy /ˈleŋθɪ/
lobster /ˈlɒbstə/
marinate /ˈmærɪˌneɪt/
mash /mæʃ/
mashed /ˈmæʃt/
mayonnaise /ˌmeɪəˈneɪz/
microwave /ˈmaɪkrəʊˌweɪv/
mince /mɪns/
mixture /ˈmɪkstʃə/
mug /mʌg/
neat /niːt/
nutty /ˈnʌtɪ/
occasion /əˈkeɪʒən/
opt /ɒpt/
oven /ˈʌvən/
overcrowded /ˌəʊvəˈkraʊdɪd/
parsley /ˈpɑːslɪ/
particularly /pəˈtɪkjʊləlɪ/
partridge /pɑːtrɪdʒ/
pastry /ˈpeɪstrɪ/
pâté /pate/
peelings /ˈpiːlɪŋz/
peppercorn /ˈpepəˌkɔːn/
pheasant /ˈfezənt/
pie /paɪ/
pierce /pɪəs/
pigeon /ˈpɪdʒɪn/
platter /plætə/
poach /pəʊtʃ/
pot /pɒt/
poultry /ˈpəʊltrɪ/
preferable /ˈprefrəbəl/
preference /ˈprefrəns/
pressure /ˈpreʃə/ **cooker** /ˈkʊkə/
purée /ˈpuːrɪ/
range /reɪndʒ/
rare /reə/
recipe /ˈresɪpɪ/
roasting /ˈrəʊstɪŋ/
roll /rəʊl/ **out** /aʊt/
roll /rəʊl/
rough /rʌf/
rub /rʌb/
satisfying /ˈsætɪsfaɪɪŋ/
savoury /ˈseɪvərɪ/
scallion /ˈskæljən/
scallop /ˈskɒl əp/
scatter /ˈskætə/
scissors /ˈsɪzəz/
scrap /skræp/
seafood /ˈsiːˌfuːd/
seasonal /ˈsiːzənəl/
set aside /əˈsaɪd/
shellfish /ˈʃelˌfɪʃ/
shrimp /ʃrɪmp/
shy /ʃaɪ/ **away from**
sieve /sɪv/
skewer /ˈskjʊə/
skin /skɪn/
slice /slaɪs/
slow cooker /ˈkʊkə/

snip /snɪp/
speedy /ˈspiːdɪ/
splendid /ˈsplendɪd/
spring /sprɪŋ/
squab /skwɒb/
stack /stæk/
standby /ˈstænbaɪ/
steak /steɪk/
steam /stiːm/
stock /stɒk/
stove /stəʊv/
strain /streɪn/
strip /strɪp/
substantial /səbˈstænʃəl/
surface /ˈsɜːfɪs/
tail /teɪl/
take into account /əˈkaʊnt/
tendency /ˈtendənsɪ/
terrine /təˈrin/
texture /ˈtekstʃə/
thermometer /θəˈmɒmɪtə/
tidy /ˈtaɪdɪ/
time-scale /ˈtaɪmˌskeɪl/
tough /tʌf/
transfer /ˈtræns fər/
trim /trɪm/
trimming /ˈtrɪmɪŋ/
turkey /ˈtɜːkɪ/
utensil /juːˈtensəl/
versatile /ˈvɜːsəˌtaɪl/
weight /weɪ/ **down**
whip /wɪp/
white /waɪt/
whole wheat /ˈhəʊlˈwiːt/
wrapper /ˈræpə/

Solution to Exercise 1a
1i, 2l, 3f, 4h, 5e, 6c, 7b, 8g, 9m, 10d, 11a, 12k, 13j

Solution to Exercise 1b
1q, 2b, 3n, 4f, 5o, 6k, 7g, 8e, 9i, 10p, 11d, 12c, 13l, 14a, 15m, 16s, 17j, 18h, 19t, 20u, 21r

Unit 2 - Lunch and supper dishes. Desserts.

Vegetables and eggs are both economical and easy to prepare so these ingredients often form the backbone of many light meals. Traditional favourites have been a simple **cheese omelette, poached eggs** or a quick dish of **scrambled eggs with toast.** Remember to try and keep the diet balance in your lunches and suppers as well as in the main meal, so make a simple **green salad** if you have time. Alternatively, prepare a few sticks of scrubbed **celery**, sticks of **carrot** and an **apple** to add a little freshness to the snack.

Have some crusty **whole wheat bread**, crisp savoury **bran crackers** or a **slice of whole wheat toast** as an accompaniment. Fresh **fruit juice or sparkling spring water** will quench the thirst without increasing the calorie content. Don't be afraid of using **canned cooked rice, canned tomatoes** or **mushrooms, tuna fish** or prepared bottled or frozen **mussels** for example. A jar of mayonnaise is another good standby; **frozen chopped or leaf spinach** and some **rolls, brioches or croissants** are all useful ingredients to keep in the freezer.

Vegetable dishes

The role of vegetables is not merely that of adding colour, texture and a filling ingredient to the main dish. The fact that freezers are now a commonplace appliances means that a **wide range of vegetables** are available **all the year round – cauliflowers, zucchini, green and lima beans, carrots, peas and corn** are just a few types of vegetables for which we no longer rely on seasonal availability. However, it is good to make the most of fresh items in the market. Look out for seasonal produce – **baby carrots, young leeks, new beans and fresh peas** – buy those which are unblemished, bright and fresh. Often it is not necessary to **peel** good quality new vegetables, so just **scrub or scrape** early carrots, potatoes and zucchini and they will retain their goodness and flavour to the full.

Vegetables can be a supper dish, a vegetarian main dish or tasty appetizer and they go well with **a roast, broiled steaks, chops or burgers**. With fish, poultry, pies and quiches you may like to serve some mushrooms, zucchini, cauliflower or spinach.

Salads

There are one or two guidelines to follow when **preparing a salad.** Firstly, if there are lots of crisp vegetables included, then make sure that they are at their best – fresh, **crisp lettuce**, crisp **green celery** and **bright scallions**. Avoid any ingredients which are limp or damaged. If the salad consists of cooked ingredients as well as fresh ones, then make sure that these too are in tip-top condition.

Cooked meats should be perfectly cooked and **lightly seasoned** before cooking to bring out their flavour to the full. **Eggs and fish** should be cooked until they are just ready, **not overcooked** or they will be dry and unappetizing. Prepare the fresh ingredients as near to serving the salad as possible: tear lettuce leaves into pieces with your fingers, slice or chop other ingredients evenly and cut meats, fish or eggs into similar-sized pieces. If the salad includes **rice, pasta or potatoes**, then it may be advantageous to prepare them in advance and allow the mixed ingredients to stand for a while so that the flavours combine and **mingle with the dressing.**

Salad dressings will bring out the flavour of the main ingredients, at the same time moistening and enhancing them with seasoning or herbs. If the salad is meant to be a **crisp green one**, then prepare **the dressing in advance** but toss it with the ingredients at the very last second. If, on the other hand, the salad includes **rice, pasta or potatoes**, then it may be best to **pour the dressing over the hot**, freshly cooked ingredients and leave them to **marinate until cold**, so that the flavours are thoroughly mingled, or enhanced by the dressing. A note about **dressings** – whether made from a simple **mixture of oil and vinegar,** seasoned and flavoured with just a little **mustard**, or **concocted** from cream, eggs and lemon juice, the dressing should always be tasted before it is poured over the salad. **Bottled mayonnaise** is a good standby, but other creamy dressings can be prepared from **sour cream**, heavy cream or plain yoghurt.

Mustard, garlic, herbs and spices can all be used to flavour salads.

Exercise 1a
Match the column A with the column B. Try to learn the expressions and/ or sentences by heart.

A

1. Traditional favourites have been
2. Alternatively, prepare a few sticks of scrubbed celery,
3. Have some crusty whole wheat bread, crisp savoury bran crackers or a slice of whole wheat toast
4. Fresh fruit juice or sparkling spring water
5. Don't be afraid of using
6. Frozen chopped or leaf spinach and some rolls, brioches or croissants
7. A wide range of vegetables are available all the year round –
8. Look out for baby carrots, young leeks, new beans and fresh peas
9. Vegetables go well with
10. With fish, poultry, pies and quiches you may
11. Tear lettuce leaves into pieces with your fingers, slice or chop other ingredients evenly
12. If the salad is meant to be a crisp green one,
13. If, on the other hand, the salad includes rice, pasta or potatoes,
14. Dressings can be made from a simple mixture of oil and vinegar, seasoned and flavoured with just a little mustard,
15. Creamy dressings can be prepared from sour cream, heavy cream or plain yoghurt;

B

a) *a roast, broiled steaks, chops or burgers.*
b) *a simple cheese omelette, poached eggs or a quick dish of scrambled eggs with toast.*
c) *and cut meats, fish or eggs into similar-sized pieces.*
d) *are all useful ingredients to keep in the freezer.*
e) *as an accompaniment.*
f) *canned cooked rice, canned tomatoes or mushrooms, tuna fish or prepared bottled or frozen mussels.*
g) *cauliflowers, zucchini, green and lima beans, carrots, peas and corn.*
h) *mustard, garlic, herbs and spices can all be used to flavour salads.*
i) *or concocted from cream, eggs and lemon juice.*
j) *pour the dressing over the hot ingredients and leave them to marinate until cold.*
k) *serve some mushrooms, zucchini, cauliflower or spinach.*

l) *sticks of carrot and an apple to add a little freshness to the snack.*
m) *then prepare the dressing in advance but toss it with the ingredients at the very last second.*
n) *which are unblemished, bright and fresh.*
o) *will quench the thirst without increasing the calorie content.*

Rice and pasta

Rice and pasta are among the most versatile of ingredients to keep in store. These filling ingredients can be served **hot or cold,** as **accompaniments** or as part of the **main dish**. Combined **with herbs, spices, cheese, oil and nuts**, they are quickly turned into a wide variety of supper dishes and snacks. There are several different types of rice available in the markets. Ordinary **white long-grain rice** is the most popular. Bring the water to **a boil**, add the rice, **stir** once and **cover** the pan very tightly. Leave to **simmer** gently for about 12 to 15 minutes or until the grains are tender and all water has been absorbed. **Fluff** the rice before serving it. **Converted rice**, which is **partially cooked**, takes about 3 to 5 more cooking than ordinary rice. There are lots of other types of white rice available: pre-seasoned **rice**, where the grains are enclosed in a perforated **boilable bag**, ready to be lowered into boiling water for the stated time; **canned**, partially cooked rice is also available, ready to be **heated** before **serving**.

Basmati or bashmati and patna rices are flavourful varieties of long-grain white rice, much used in Indian dishes. They are prized for their dry, fluffy texture and grains that remain separate when cooked. **Brown** rice retains **the outer bran and germ** that are removed to make white rice. Brown rice has more flavour and a nuttier texture than white rice and it requires longer cooking in more water. **Wild rice**, which is really a cereal grain, is also available.

There are lots of different shapes of dried pasta available. **Dried pasta** requires cooking - about 12 to 15 minutes – in plenty of boiling salted water. A little oil can be added to the cooking water to prevent the pasta from **sticking together** and from **boiling over** during cooking. The drained pasta can be tossed with herbs and oil, butter or Parmesan cheese and served very simply. Alternatively, if it is to be served **cold**, it should be **rinsed** under cold water immediately it is **drained**, then left to drain thoroughly. **Baked stuffed pasta** dishes are also particularly delicious and very popular for preparing in advance, then chilling or freezing until they are finally baked and served.

Dressings and sauces

There are a few basic techniques to master, and then you will find sauce-making a simple task. Many hot sauces rely on the preparation of a **roux**: a mixture of **fat and flour**, cooked for a few minutes to make a thin paste, then combine with liquid which is poured into the pan as the sauce is stirred continuously. Other method of thickening sauces include the addition of **egg yolks**. There is a danger of the **sauce curdling** if it is cooked over too high a heat or for too long. **Mayonnaise**-type sauces are thickened by adding **oil to beaten yolks** – this is refereed to as a liaison. For success, the ingredients should all be at **the same temperature** before use. The eggs should be thoroughly beaten with the seasonings, then the **oil added very slowly at first**, in a steady stream later as the mixture thickens. Finally, lemon juice is added to both stabilize and flavour the mixture. For **fruit sauces, purées** and those dressings which require chopped ingredients, then there is no real substitute for the blender or food processor. For more conventional methods, a good **heavy-based saucepan, wooden spoon** and **whisk** are necessary.

Exercise 1b
Match the column A with the column B. Try to learn the expressions and/or sentences by heart.

A

1. Combined with herbs, spices, cheese, oil and nuts,
2. Bring the water to a boil, add the rice, stir once and cover the pan very tightly;
3. Pre-seasoned rice, where the grains are enclosed in a perforated boilable bag,
4. Basmati and patna rices
5. Brown rice retains the outer bran and germ
6. Dried pasta requires cooking
7. A little oil can be added to the cooking water
8. Many hot sauces rely on the preparation of a roux: a mixture of fat and flour,
9. Mayonnaise-type sauces
10. The eggs should be thoroughly beaten with the seasonings,

B

a) *are prized for their dry, fluffy texture and grains that remain separate when cooked.*
b) *are thickened by adding oil to beaten yolks.*
c) *cooked for a few minutes and combined with liquid as the sauce is stirred continuously.*
d) *in plenty of boiling salted water.*
e) *ready to be lowered into boiling water for the stated time.*
f) *rice and pasta are quickly turned into a wide variety of supper dishes and snacks.*
g) *that are removed to make white rice.*
h) *then leave to simmer gently and fluff the rice before serving it.*

i) *then the oil added very slowly at first, in a steady stream later as the mixture thickens.*

j) *to prevent the pasta from sticking together and from boiling over during cooking.*

Desserts

People have different ideas about the sweet dishes – some save a space for the sweet dishes, others prefer **light fruit salad** as a substitute to the richer alternatives. If you plan to serve a **cheese course**, then decide whether this is to be offered before the dessert, between the main dish and the sweet, or at the end of the meal, just before the coffee. It is always a good idea to offer some **crisps, light cookies** with the dessert if it is a creamy one. You might like to serve a **pitcher of cream** with the dessert too. Plain **yoghurt** can be combined with fresh **fruits, nuts** and a little **sugar** or **honey**. Fresh fruit salads can be served unsweetened given that the combination of fruits is one which already has sweeter ingredients – like **figs, mangos** and **peaches** – with the tart ones.

Iced desserts

Ice creams, **sherbets**, and other frozen desserts are often the simplest to prepare. They can be made in advance (and need to be) ready for taking to the table at the last minute. The recipes suggest using an electric **ice cream maker**, but the ices can be prepared just as successfully by hand. The important thing to remember is that if you want to make a very smooth ice cream, it will need to be **whisked several times** during freezing to break down the ice crystals which are formed. Take the mixture out of the freezer when it is half frozen and whisk it thoroughly. If you have a food processor, then it is ideal for this. Put the mixture back into the freezer, and repeat the whisking process at least once more. Before serving, put the ice cream into the refrigerator for about 30 minutes, so that it will be **soft enough to scoop**. If the dessert is a moulded one, dip the container briefly in hot water, dry it and unmould **the dessert**. The ices can be served in fruits, in the form of **soufflés**. Some chopped toasted nuts, crushed macaroons or **crushed caramel** can also be **sprinkled over** the ice cream.

Exercise 1c

Match the column A with the column B. Try to learn the expressions and/or sentences by heart.

A

1. Decide whether a cheese course is to be offered
2. It is always a good idea to offer some
3. Plain yoghurt can be combined with
4. If you want to make a very smooth ice cream, it will need to be
5. Before serving, put the ice cream into the refrigerator for about 30 minutes

6. Some chopped toasted nuts, crushed macaroons or crushed caramel

B

a) *before the dessert, between the main dish and the sweet, or at the end of the meal, just before the coffee.*
b) *can also be sprinkled over the ice cream.*
c) *crisps, light cookies with the dessert if it is a creamy one.*
d) *fresh fruits, nuts and a little sugar or honey.*
e) *so that it will be soft enough to scoop.*
f) *whisked several times during freezing to break down the ice crystals which are formed.*

Exercise 2
Translate the expressions. Try to explain their meanings in English.

Favourites, poached eggs, scrambled eggs, sticks of scrubbed celery, freshness, crusty, crisp, bran crackers, slice of whole wheat toast, sparkling spring water, quench the thirst, canned tomatoes, tuna fish, chopped or leaf spinach, rolls, brioches or croissants, appliances, cauliflowers, zucchini, corn, leeks, unblemished, peel, scrub or scrape, a roast, broiled steaks, chops or burgers, quiches, lettuce, scallions, limp, seasoned, tear into pieces, advantageous, mingle with, moistening, toss, pour, mustard, filling, accompaniments, long-grain rice, bring to a boil, stir, cover, simmer, pre-seasoned, boilable bag, be heated, flavourful, prized for, fluffy texture, remain separate, outer bran and germ, sticking together, boiling over, rinsed, drained, stuffed pasta, roux, curdling, beaten yolks, steady stream, saucepan, wooden spoon, whisk, substitute, cookies, a pitcher of cream, figs, mangos, peaches, tart, by hand, smooth, be whisked, to scoop, moulded, chopped toasted nuts, crushed, sprinkled over.

Exercise 3
Answer the following questions. Prepare short talks and/or dialogues on these topics.

1. Give examples of light meals.
2. Suggest some vegetable dishes.
3. How to prepare salads and dressings.
4. Describe different types of rice available in the markets.
5. How to prepare rice and pasta correctly?
6. Basic techniques to master preparation of dressings and sauces.
7. Give examples of desserts and iced desserts.

Vocabulary 2

Fill in the meanings in your mother language:

add /æd/
advantageous /ˌædvənˈteɪdʒəs/
appliance /əˈplaɪəns/
availability /əˌveɪləˈbɪlɪtɪ/

backbone /ˈbækˌbəʊn/
bashmati /bɑsˈmɑ ti/
bean /biːn/
boil /bɔɪl/
bottled /ˈbɒtəld/
bran /bræn/
brioche /ˈbriːəʊʃ/
burger /ˈbɜːgə/
canned /kænd/
carrot /ˈkærət/
cauliflower /ˈkɒlɪˌflaʊə/
cereal /ˈsɪərɪəl/
concoct /kənˈkɒkt/
conventional /kənˈvenʃənəl/
convert /kənˈvɜːt/
cookie /ˈkʊkɪ/
corn /kɔːn/
croissant /ˈkrwʌsɒŋ/
curdle /ˈkɜːdəl/
damaged /ˈdæmɪdʒd/
delicious /dɪˈlɪʃəs/
dessert /dɪˈzɜːt/
dressing /ˈdresɪŋ/
dried /draɪd/
early /ˈɜːlɪ/
enclose /ɪnˈkləʊz/
enhance /ɪnˈhɑːns
fig /fɪg/
fluff /flʌf/
fluffy /ˈflʌfɪ/
freezer /ˈfriːzə/
freshness /freʃnɪs/
gently /ˈdʒentlɪ/
germ /dʒɜːm/
goodness /ˈgʊdnɪs/
grain /greɪn/
guideline /ˈgaɪdˌlaɪn/
heated /hiːtɪd/
heavy /ˈhevɪ/ **cream** /kriːm/
item /ˈaɪtəm/
jar /dʒɑː/
leaf /liːf/
leek /liːk/
lettuce /ˈletɪs/
liaison /lɪˈeɪzɒn/
lima /ˈlaɪmə/ **bean** /biːn/
limp /lɪmp/
macaroon /ˌmækəˈruːn/
mango /ˈmæŋgəʊ/
master /ˈmɑːstə/
merely /ˈmɪəlɪ/
mingle /ˈmɪŋgəl/
moisten /ˈmɔɪsən/
mould /məʊld/
mushroom /ˈmʌʃruːm/
mussel /ˈmʌsəl/
mustard /ˈmʌstəd/
omelette /ˈɒmlɪt/
ordinary /ˈɔːdənrɪ/
pan /pæn/
pasta /ˈpæstə/
paste /peɪst/
Patna /ˈpætnə/
pea /piː/
peach /piːtʃ/
peel /piːl/
pitcher /pɪtʃə/
plain /pleɪn/ **yogurt** /ˈjəʊgət/
poached /pəʊtʃd/ **eggs**
pour /pɔː/
preseasoned /ˌpriːˈsiːzənd/
prize /praɪz/
quench /kwentʃ/
quiche /kiʃ/
rely /rɪˈlaɪ/
retain /rɪˈteɪn/
rinse /rɪns/
roux /ruː/
saucepan /ˈsɔːspən/
scoop /skuːp/
scrambled /ˈskræmbəld/ **eggs**
scrape /skreɪp/
scrub /skrʌb/
seasoned /ˈsiːzənd/
seasoning /ˈsiːzənɪŋ/
shape /ʃeɪp/
sherbet /ˈʃɜːbət/
simmer /ˈsɪmə/
snack /snæk/
soufflé /ˈsuːfleɪ/

sour /ˈsaʊə/ **cream** /kriːm/
sparkling /ˈspɑːklɪŋ/
spice /spaɪs/
spinach /ˈspɪn ɪtʃ/
stabilize /ˈsteɪbɪˌlaɪz/
stand /stænd/
state /steɪt/
steady /ˈstedɪ/
stick /stɪk/ of **celery** /ˈselərɪ/
stick /stɪk/ **together** /təˈgeðə/
stir /stɜː/
store /stɔː/
stream /striːm/
stuffed /stʌft/
substitute /ˈsʌbstɪˌtjuːt/
supper /ˈsʌpə/
tart /tɑːt/
taste /teɪst/
tear /tɪə/
tender /ˈtendə/
thicken /ˈθɪkən/
thin /θɪn/
thoroughly /ˈθʌrəlɪ/
tightly /ˈtaɪtlɪ/
tip-top /ˌtɪpˈtɒp/
toss /tɒs/
tuna /ˈtjuːnə/
unappetizing /ˌʌnəˈpɪˌtaɪzɪŋ/
unblemished /ʌnˈblemɪʃt/
vinegar /ˈvɪnɪgə/
whisk /wɪsk/
wild /waɪld/
wooden /ˈwʊdən/ **spoon** /spuːn/
yolk /jəʊk/
zucchini /tsuːˈkiːnɪ/

Solution to Exercise 1a
1b, 2l, 3e, 4o, 5f, 6d, 7g, 8n, 9a, 10k, 11c, 12m, 13j, 14i, 15h

Solution to Exercise 1b
1f, 2h, 3e, 4a, 5g, 6d, 7j, 8c, 9b, 10i

Solution to Exercise 1c
1a, 2c, 3d, 4f, 5e, 6b

Unit 3 - Recipes 1

1
Chestnut soup
Serves about 6
Ingredients

- 50 g butter
- 3 shallots, finely chopped
- 2 celery stalks, finely chopped
- 1-2 cooking apples, peeled and roughly chopped
- 2 tins chestnut purée
- 1 litre vegetable stock
- 1 tsp sugar
- ½ tsp mace
- 45 ml medium dry sherry
- salt and pepper

Method

Melt the butter and fry the shallots for 5 minutes. Add the celery and apple. Cover the pan and sweat the vegetables over a gentle steam for 10 minutes. Add the chestnuts and pour in the stock, mace, sugar, salt and pepper. Bring to a gentle boil, then cover pan, and cook for 30 minutes. Liquidise. Gently rewarm and add the sherry just before the serving. This recipe doubles as a winter delight and a particularly nourishing dish for vegetarians. And it is well balanced, with representatives of all the flavours, bitter (celery), salt, sweet (chestnut and sugar), sour (apples) and aromatic/ spicy (cherry, mace, black pepper). The nourishing quality of the dish comes from the chestnuts, which are a famous sweet digestive and constitutional tonic. The addition of a small amount of sugar enhances the tonic sweetness of the chestnuts.

Variations

Steam fresh chestnuts, peel them, then whizz them up with a bit of stock to make the purée. You can also adapt the recipe in particularly perishing weather by adding more aromatic spices to counter penetrating cold and damp. Cinnamon, nutmeg and a little dried ginger are perfectly suitable.

2
Spicy scrambled eggs
Serves 2
Ingredients

- 4 organic eggs, beaten
- 4 spring onions or 1 red onion, finely chopped
- 2 cloves garlic, finely chopped or minced
- 1 green chilli, finely chopped - optional
- ½ tsp garam masala
- ½ tsp mustard seeds
- ¼ tsp turmeric
- 4 medium tomatoes, chopped
- small handful coriander

Method

Fry the onions, garlic and chilli (if using) for about 5 minutes until the onions are soft and translucent. Add the spices and cook for a further 3 minutes. Add the chopped tomatoes and continue to cook until they start to break up. Pour in the eggs and continue to stir until they are cooked to your liking, adding the coriander about a minute before serving.

Scrambled eggs are convenient and nutritious. But they are particularly rich, which is why they've had a bad press over the years, blamed for cholesterol trouble and high levels of allergy and intolerance. The picture would be different if we combined them intelligently with a good mix of aromatic vegetables, herbs and spices to stimulate digestion. Which is precisely what this recipe does, with garam masala, mustard seeds, turmeric and chilli to cut through the richness and stimulate secretion. Garlic and onion boost motility to get the gut moving. Because of the intensity of the spices, we use the sourness of the tomato and the freshness of the coriander to cool and mellow the dish.

Variations

In this recipe, the scrambled eggs have been taken down the spicy route to compensate for their richness. But not everyone gets on with strong spices, in which case you might prefer herby eggs. If you have them in your garden, pick a handful of fresh aromatic herbs, chop them up and combine them with some black pepper. Particularly good herbs to combine with eggs are sweet Cicely, tarragon and thyme.

3
Kedgeree
Serves 2-4
Ingredients

- 2 eggs
- 6 spring onions, finely chopped
- 2 bay leaves

- 115 g butter
- 1 clove garlic finely chopped
- 680 g un-dyed smoked haddock (it's worth a couple of minutes to pin bone it)
- 170 g basmati rice
- 2 heaped tsp curry powder (or 1 tsp each of ground coriander, cumin and turmeric)
- juice of 1 lemon
- 2 handfuls chopped coriander
- a small finger of grated ginger

Method

Hard-boil the eggs for 8 to 10 minutes, remove and plunge in cold water to stop the cooking process. Put the haddock in a frying pan with the 2 bay leaves, cover with water and simmer for around 5 minutes. Cook the basmati rice in water for 10 minutes, and drain. Now melt the butter in a pan on a low heat. Slowly cook the spring onions and garlic until translucent. Add the curry powder or spices and cook for a further 3 minutes. Add the rice to the pan and stir through with the lemon juice, gently warming it through. Fold the fish and coriander in until it is all nicely warm and ready to serve. This is a seriously tasty dish. But eggs, butter and smoked haddock take some digesting. Smoking any type of food is a way of preserving it. It partially cooks it and changes its chemical structure to make it harder to digest, not only for bacteria and moulds, but for us too. This means that although the smoky flavour is delightful, we need lots of sour and aromatic ingredients to help the fish to break down once we've eaten it. The same principle applies to the butter and the eggs. Sourness is provided by the lemon, while aromatic flavours come from ginger, garlic, spring onion, coriander, cumin and turmeric. Turmeric also provides bitterness to strongly stimulate motility, and coriander leaf plays an increasingly familiar role here as it balances out the heating action of the spices.

Variations

The sour and bitter flavours of this dish can be enhanced by adding lemon zest. Parsley will add bitterness and boost the refreshing action of the coriander leaf. More bitterness is great if you are prone to a sluggish bowel. If you like a bit more spice, paprika and mustard seeds are mild to combine well with the other spices. And you could try cooking the rice with saffron. Freely diced carrot and peas can be added to bring sweetness the dish, a particularly child-friendly ruse!

4
Sausage casserole
Serves 4
Ingredients

- 8 medium-sized good-quality sausages (two per person), pork, beef and lamb sausages are all suitable.
- 1 medium-sized onion chopped

- 4 shallots, roughly chopped
- 2 crushed garlic cloves
- 2 medium-sized potatoes peeled and diced into cubes
- 2 red peppers, sliced
- 400 g tin chopped tomatoes
- ½ pint chicken stock
- 400 g tin lentils
- 1 tbs of cider vinegar
- 1 sprig chopped rosemary
- knob of butter

Method

Melt the butter in a large heavy bottomed casserole dish on a medium heat on top of the stove. Pierce the sausages then brown all over. Remove from the dish, then put the onions, shallots and garlic in. Cook slowly for about 5 minutes or until they start to become tender. Add the cubed potatoes and fry for a further 5 minutes, taking care not to burn the onions and garlic. Add the chicken stock gradually, stir well and add the sausages. Add half the rosemary and all of the other ingredients. The liquid should cover the sausages, and reduce down during cooking as much as half. Continue to cook on the stove for a few minutes, gradually increasing the heat until the pot is simmering. Taste the sauce, if it's too acidic, add a pinch or two of brown sugar. Cook uncovered for about an hour in the oven at 180°C. Remove from the oven, garnish with the remaining rosemary and serve with fresh broad beans and rice or polenta. This is the ideal winter dish. It is not only thrifty, combining cheap meat and pulses, it is also nourishing and filling. This sort of rich aromatic food is perfectly suited to cold and damp weather, underpinned as it is by pungent, expansive onions, garlic and rosemary, with the sourness of vinegar to cut through the fat and richness.

Variations

You could add more spice or more aromatic herbs, particularly if you're not cooking for children. This would be particularly beneficial if using pork sausages, as they are so obstructive to motility. Good herbs to add are a classic bouquet garnish of bay, thyme and sage. Good spices are paprika, star anise and mustard seeds.

5

Boiled ham hocks with pease pudding

Serves 4-6

Ingredients for the ham hocks

- 4 fresh ham hocks
- 2 onions, roughly chopped
- 2 carrots, roughly chopped
- 2 sticks celery, roughly chopped
- 4 or 5 black peppercorns, whole
- 3 cloves
- 2 bay leaves

For the peas pudding

- 350 g yellow slit peas, soaked overnight
- 1 onion, fined diced
- 1 garlic clove, finely chopped

- a small tied bunch of thyme, rosemary, bay and sage, butter and seasoning

Method

Line a bowl with a square of muslin cloth. Rinse the soaked peas and mix them with the garlic, onion and herbs. Place them in the lined bowl and tightly twist and tie the cloth to make a parcel. Reserve the butter and seasoning. Put the muslin parcel, ham hocks and all the other ingredients in a deep saucepan. Cover with cold water, bring to the boil and simmer for around 2 to 3 hours until the meat is wonderfully tender and falling of the bone. Scrape the pease pudding from the cloth, remove the herbs and mash with the reserved butter and seasoning.

Additions

Add whole baby carrots, small leeks and a fennel bulb half an hour before the end of cooking. Serve these as an accompaniment. Use the strained stock as a gravy. Serve the dish with English mustard.

The combination of rich, salty or preserved meat with pulses is popular throughout the world. Think mutton and lentils, cassoulet, or bacon and peas. This is the original poor man's hearty meal and uses the principle of combining rich, flavoursome meat with pulses to marry flavour, fat and richness with the bulk and protein of the beans.

Boiling enhances the digestibility of the hock as it disperses its richness into the broth, in contrast to baking or roasting which concentrates the fats in the meat, exaggerating the work that the bile salts, digestive enzymes and symbionts have to do to break it down. It thus employs precisely the same elegant nutritional principles as any bone stock; the balanced combination of celery, carrot and onion together with other aromatic spices (cloves and peppercorns) and herbs (garlic, thyme, rosemary, bay and sage).

Using a range of herbs broaders the health-enhancing effect of the dish; bay, sage, and thyme are all bitter so stimulate bowel movement in response to preserved meat, while rosemary specifically counters the symptom of trapped wind – a particular problem when consuming large amounts of beans.

Variations

Suffice it to say that these are plenty of recipes along these lines out there in traditional cuisines around the world. They might be with mutton, pork, duck or beef and a range of pulses from lentils to haricot beans. All of them provide nutritious, delicious and cheap food. From this diet's perspective, there are a few issues that are important. The first is to take time to cook the dish in the first place, as the preparation of the beans and the bone stock is time-intensive. The second is to use plenty of really fresh herbs to refresh the balance out the effects of the spices, broaden the flavour profile and raise the automatic oil content of the dish. And finally, the spices are important to cut through the fatty intensity of the meat.

6
Slow-roasted lamb and harissa
Ingredients

- lamb shoulder
- 2 tbsp harissa sauce (this is a rough guide – spiciness varies between different products)
- 1 tbsp soy sauce
- 1 tsp mustard
- 1 tbsp balsamic vinegar
- 1 tbsp honey
- vegetables for steaming to serve

Method

Mix a paste of harissa, soy sauce, mustard, balsamic vinegar and a dollop of honey. Smear this all over the lamb shoulder and leave to marinade for an hour. Place in a roasting dish on the middle shelf of the oven at around 140°C. Cook for 4 to 5 hours. Serve it with plenty of steamed vegetables like broccoli, asparagus, kale or chard. The leftovers make fantastic salad ingredients. This dish is a classic winter warmer. Harissa is a spicy North African sauce based on piri piri: chilli peppers, tomatoes and paprika. Other ingredients vary depending on the brand and region of origin. It is traditionally used as an appetiser and plays a crucial role in this recipe as lamb is among the richest of meats. The other spicy ingredient, mustard, enhances this effect. The sour flavour of the harissa and the vinegar also enhances digestibility by cutting through the lamb fat, while sweet honey nourishes friendly bacteria.

Variations

Overall, this is a very hot and rich dish and needs balancing if you struggle with very spicy food. This balance is best achieved with refreshing aromatic herbs like mint, chervil or coriander. You could also mix yoghurt with cucumber, a strategy that is only recommended with very spicy dishes as it does significantly slow motility. The lamb also combines well with bitter greens like rocket, dandelion or chicory.

Vocabulary 3

Fill in the meanings in your mother language:

anise /'ænɪs/
asparagus /ə'spærəgəs/
bacon /'beɪkən/
baking /'beɪkɪŋ/
balsamic /bɔl'sæm ɪk/
vinegar /'vɪnɪgə/
be to sb's liking /'laɪkɪŋ/
beef /bi:f/
bile /baɪl/
blame /bleɪm/
boiling /'bɔɪlɪŋ/
bottom /'bɒtəm/
bouquet /bu:'keɪ/
brand /brænd/
break /breɪk/ **up** /ʌp/
broad /brɔ:d/ **bean** /bi:n/
broaden /'brɔ:dən/
broccoli /'brɒkəlɪ/

broth /brɒθ/
brown /braʊn/
bulb /bʌlb/
bulk /bʌlk/
bunch /bʌntʃ/
cassoulet /ˌkæsəˈleɪ/
chard /tʃɑːd/
chervil /ˈtʃɜːvɪl/
chestnut /ˈtʃesˌnʌt/
chicory /ˈtʃikərɪ/
chilli /ˈtʃɪlɪ/
chilli /ˈtʃɪlɪ/ **pepper** /pepə/
cider /ˈsaɪdə/ **vinegar** /ˈvɪnɪgə/
cinnamon /ˈsɪnəmən/
cloth /klɒθ/
clove /kləʊv/
coriander /ˌkɒrɪˈændə/
cover /kʌvə/
cucumber /kjuːˌkʌmbə/
cumin /ˈkʌmɪn/
curry /ˈkʌrɪ/
cut /kʌt/ **through** /θruː/
dandelion /ˈdændɪˌlaɪən/
dice /daɪs/
dollop /ˈdɒləp/
double /ˈdʌbəl/
drain /dreɪn/
exaggerate /ɪgˈzædʒəˌreɪt/
fall /fɔːl/
fennel /ˈfenəl/
fold /fəʊld/ **in** /ɪn/
fry /fraɪ/
garam masala /ˌgɑː.rəm.məˈsɑː.lə/
ginger /ˈdʒɪndʒə/
gradually /ˈgrædjuəlɪ/
grate /greɪt/
gravy /ˈgreɪvɪ/
haddock /ˈhædək/
ham /hæm/ **hock** /hɒk/
handful /ˈhændfʊl/
haricot /ˈhærɪkəʊ/ **bean** /biːn/
harissa /həˈrɪsə/
heaped /hiːpt/
increase /ɪnˈkriːs/
kale /keɪl/
kedgeree /ˌkɛdʒəˈriː/
knob /nɒb/
lamb /læm/
leftover /ˈleftˌəʊvə/
lemon /ˈlemən/ **zest** /zest/
lentil /ˈlentɪl/
line /laɪn/
liquidise /ˈlɪkwɪˌdaɪz/
mace /meɪs/
marry /ˈmærɪ/
medium /ˈmiːdɪəm/
medium /miːdɪəm/ **-sized** /saɪzd/
melt /melt/
minced /ˈmɪnst/
mint /mɪnt/
muslin /ˈmʌzlɪn/
mutton /ˈmʌtən/
nourishing /ˈnʌrɪʃɪŋ/
nutmeg /ˈnʌtmeg/
optional /ˈɒpʃənəl/
origin /ɒrɪdʒɪn/
paprika /pæˈpriːkə/
parcel /ˈpɑːsəl/
perish /ˈperɪʃ/
pin /pɪn/ **bone** /bəʊn/
pint /paɪnt/
piri piri /ˌpiːriˈpiːri/
plunge /plʌndʒ/
polenta /pəʊˈlɛntə/
pork /pɔːk/
powder /ˈpaʊdə/
precisely /prɪˈsaɪslɪ/
prone /prəʊn/
pudding /ˈpʊdɪŋ/
pulse /pʌls/
pungent /pʌndʒənt/
red pepper /ˈpepə/
reduce /rɪˈdjuːs/
reserve /rɪˈzɜːv/
richness /ˈrɪtʃˌnɪs/
rocket /ˈrɒkɪt/
rosemary /ˈrəʊzmərɪ/
roughly /ˈrʌflɪ/
ruse /ruːz/
saffron /ˈsæfrən/

sage /seɪdʒ/
saucepan /ˈsɔːspən/
sausage /ˈsɒsɪdʒ/
seed /siːd/
serving /ˈsɜːvɪŋ/
shallot /ʃəˈlɒt/
sliced /slaɪst/
smear /smɪə/
smoked /sməʊkt/
soaked /səʊkt/
spicy /ˈspaɪsɪ/
split /splɪt/
sprig /sprɪg/
square /skweə/
stalk /stɔːk/
star /stɑː/
suffice /səˈfaɪs/
sweat /swet/
sweet /swiːt/ **Cicely** /ˈsɪsəlɪ/
tarragon /ˈtærəgən/
tbsp, table spoonful /ˈspuːnˌfʊl/
thrifty /ˈθrɪftɪ/
thyme /taɪm/
tie /taɪ/
tin /tɪn/
translucent /trænzˈluːsənt/
trouble /ˈtrʌbəl/
tsp, tea spoonful /ˈspuːnˌfʊl/
turmeric /ˈtɜːmərɪk/
twist /twɪst/
un-dyed /ˈdaɪd/
underpin /ˌʌndəˈpɪn/
whizz /wɪz/
whole /həʊl/

Unit 4 - Recipes 2

1
Mushroom risotto
Serves 4
Ingredients

- 1 tbsp dried porcini mushrooms
- olive oil
- 1 onion, chopped
- 2 garlic cloves, finely chopped
- 225 g chestnut mushrooms, sliced
- 350 g arborio rice or pearled spelt
- 150 ml dry white wine
- 1.2 litres hot best vegetable stock
- handful chopped fresh parsley
- 25 g butter
- salt and freshly ground black pepper
- freshly grated parmesan, to serve

Method

Soak the mushrooms in a little hot water for 10 minutes. In a heavy-based pan fry the onion and garlic in a little olive oil for around 2 minutes. Add the chestnut mushrooms and cook for a further 2 minutes. Stir in the rice and make sure it is well coated with the cooking oil. Pour in the wine, simmer and stir until it has all been absorbed. Begin to add the stock, a ladleful at a time, maintaining a simmer and adding a fresh ladle of stock as the last one is absorbed. Continue adding the stock in this way until it has all been absorbed and the rice is tender or to your liking. Roughly chop the soaked mushrooms, add those, the soaking water, parsley and butter to the risotto and stir through. Put a lid on the dish and allow it to sit for just a few minutes before serving with the grated parmesan. Any dish that uses mushrooms as this one does is medicinal, such is their nutritional value. In this case the mushrooms form the basis for a light dish suited to cold, dry winter weather, suffused as it is with the aromatics of the onion, garlic, parsley and pepper that warm and stimulate circulation in the gut. Balancing this expansiveness is the astringency of the wine, while the bitterness of the parsley adds depth of flavour and stimulates secretion.

Variations

It is possible to get arborio rice and pearled spelt in a good health-food store. Spelt is richer than rice and will require more spice for balance. This can be provided with some extra black pepper or paprika. Spice can be used to compensate for extra dampness in the climate too. If you are eating this dish in summer, add some bitter greens such as dandelion, chicory, rocket or nasturtium. The bitterness helps to cool the warmth of the aromatics.

2
Tuna, fennel and bean salad
Serves 4
Ingredients

- 1 small head fennel, fronds removed
- 1 medium red onion, quartered
- 2 cloves garlic
- 2 x 400 g cannellini beans, drained and rinsed
- extra-virgin olive oil
- juice of half a lemon
- handful fresh flatleaf parsley leaves, chopped
- 2 x 200 g cans tuna steak in spring water or olive oil, drained
- 60 g black olives (pitted, if preferred)

Method

Trim and quarter the fennel and reserve the fronds. Put in a roasting dish with the quartered onion and a couple of garlic cloves. Give them a generous drizzle of olive oil and bake in the oven at around 180°C for 20 minutes. Slice the baked onion and fennel finely and place in a bowl with the beans and parsley. Whisk two tablespoons of olive oil with the lemon juice; stir it in the salad. Leave to stand for a few minutes. Meanwhile, drain the tins of tuna and gently stir the fish and the olives into the salad. Serve with the reserved fennel fronds to garnish. This is the ideal working lunch for cold, dry winter's days. Digestion is assisted by the fact that the salad is largely cooked. In addition, mild aromatics from the fennel, onion, garlic and parsley, stimulate gut motility and secretion; and olive oil and tuna add richness, balanced by a little lemon juice, to make the dish sustaining through the cold winter afternoon.

Variations

If you're at home or can get to a frying pan, it is just as good, and perhaps more convenient, to fry off the garlic, fennel and onion with olive oil for 10 minutes, rather that baking it. You can also add whatever fresh herbs you might have to hand, such as rosemary, marjoram, basil, coriander or tarragon. These add wonderful aromatic depth to the dish. You can also add a little extra spice such as some deseeded chilli or cumin seeds.

3

Aromatic mussels with cider and bacon

Serves 2

Ingredients

- 1 kg mussels, scrubbed and debearded
- 1 tbsp olive oil
- knob of unsalted butter
- 100 g streaky bacon, roughly chopped
- 1 bunch spring onions sliced
- 2 sprigs thyme, leaves removed
- 1 bay leaf
- 250 ml medium-sweet cider
- 1 tsp wholegrain mustard
- 2-3 tbsp crème fraîche
- seasoning
- 2 handfuls chopped flat-leaf parsley
- a pinch of chilli flakes

Method

Discard any mussels that don't close when tapped on a hard surface. In a large heavy bottomed saucepan, heat the olive oil and butter until the butter begins to foam. Add the bacon and cook for 4 minutes, then stir in the spring onions. Add the thyme and the bay leaf and continue to cook for 2 minutes. Turn the heat right up and add the mussels, giving the pan a good shake and turning the mussels over in the cooking juices. Pour in the cider and stir in the mustard. Put a lid on the pan and allow it to steam for 3 minutes giving the pan a good shake every minute. Remove the lid and discard any mussels that haven't opened. Stir in the crème fraîche and warm through for a further 30 seconds. Stir in the parsley and chilli flakes, season and serve. Mussels are a constitutional tonic food, full of minerals and nutrients, and therefore great to eat, but they are very rich. Similarly, the other rich ingredients – butter, bacon, crème fraîche – are variously fatty and sweet and therefore delicious, but they all tend to cause sluggish motility in the gut, just like the mussels. It is therefore very important to combine these rich ingredients with aromatic, moving and dispersing herbs and spices to stimulate secretion and get the gut moving. Spring onion, parsley, thyme, bay, mustard and a little bit of chilli do just such a job, warming and stimulating the intestines. As a counterbalance to this strong stimulus, cider is sour and astringent, calming the excesses of the spice and creating balance in the dish.

Variations

You may prefer to use white wine instead of cider as it is not quite as astringent. Even less astringent are rice wine and sherry which also go well with mussels. Using coconut cream instead of crème fraîche and coriander leaf instead of parsley takes the dish in a South-East Asian direction.

4
Lemon chicken
Serves 4-6
Ingredients

- 1 large chicken, jointed into 8-10 pieces
- olive oil
- 1 head garlic, halved horizontally
- thyme sprigs
- splash of sherry vinegar
- 2 tbsp dark soy sauce
- 3 tbsp honey
- 1 lemon, finely sliced (ideally with a mandolin)
- a handful flat-leaf parsley, finely chopped
- seasoning

Method

Season the chicken with salt and pepper and heat the olive oil in a large frying pan. Brown the chicken pieces in batches with the garlic and thyme for 2 to 3 minutes on each side. Return all the chicken to the pan, add the sherry vinegar and bubble until reduced by half. Drizzle over the soy sauce and honey and shake the pan to mix. Pour in a good splash of hot water and add the lemon slices. Let the liquid reduce down until syrupy, around 10 minutes. Check to make sure the chicken is cooked through. Sprinkle with the parsley. The ingredients provide a classic balanced combination of all of the flavours – sweet (chicken and honey), sour (lemon and vinegar), salty/savoury (soy sauce), bitter (lemon zest and pith and parsley) and aromatic/pungent (garlic, thyme, parsley and seasoning). Served with rice and some steamed greens, lemon chicken is incredible easy to digest.

Variations

This simple recipe can be whipped up in no time, but if you're really pressed, don't bother jointing the chicken. Just brown the chicken skin all over in a wok, bung in the other ingredients, pop on the lid and leave it to cook. If you have more time, get a chicken with giblets and boil up a small stock on the side with a couple of bay leaves. This stock, added to the sauce and reduced, adds lots of nutrition and depth of flavour. Indeed, with a little of stock, the recipe can be converted into a one-pot meal, with root vegetables and fresh herbs placed around the chicken in a big pan or wok. You could also add a bit more spice. Smoked paprika is particularly good, creating a lovely mellow depth of flavour.

5
Cassoulet
Serves 8+ and keeps well in the fridge
Ingredients

- 5 tbsp olive oil
- 5 belly pork ribs
- 100 g bacon pieces
- 3 cloves, crushed
- 2 onions, finely chopped
- 3 garlic cloves, finely chopped

- 1 carrot, diced
- 2 celery sticks, finely chopped
- 1 leek, finely sliced
- 1 litre chicken stock
- 1 tin plum tomatoes, finely chopped
- 1 tbsp of lemon juice
- 3 tins white haricot beans, drained (or 600 g beans, cooked from dry)
- 4 confit duck legs
- 4 bay leaves and a handful each of chopped thyme and sage
- salt and black pepper
- a handful of chopped flat-leaf parsley

Method

Heat the olive oil in a pan and add the belly pork ribs. Fry the pork until it is browned all over, then remove it from the pan. Now add the bacon, cloves, onions, garlic, carrot, celery and leek to the pan and fry until the onion is translucent. Return the pork to the pan with these ingredients and add the lemon juice, stock, tomatoes, bay, thyme, sage, and duck, bring to the boil and simmer for 1 ½ hours with the lid off so that the sauce thickens over time. Add the beans and simmer it for a further 30 minutes. Add salt, pepper and flat-leaf parsley to taste. It can then be served hot, although due to its high fat content the cassoulet is often allowed to cool and, once a layer of fat has risen to the top and solidified, it is skimmed off to reduce the fatty, cloying nature of the dish. It is then reheated to serve. Cassoulet derives its name from the French world "cassolé" which is the name of the earthenware ovenproof dish in which this type of food is normally cooked. It is a classic and appears in many guises, featuring other rich meats such a pork, mutton, goose, sausages and pancetta. But they all exist within a framework that combines fatty meats with beans, creating a nutritious, sustaining but not over-rich concoction. "Pleasant food", if you like, although such is the cultural depth of cassoulet that it can be found on all menus regardless of class. This recipe is typical, with a good chicken bone stock and pork ribs thrown in to add extra nutrition. Its flavour profile is predominantly aromatic rather than spicy, the onion, garlic, bay, thyme and sage are just about enough to stimulate gut motility in the face of this hearty fare. The aromatics are helped in this task by sourness (lemon, tomato) and bitterness (celery, sage). Otherwise this is first and foremost a naturally sweet dish with beans, onions, carrot, leek and meat cooking down over time to produce a deep enriching flavour that suits our energy-hungry winter metabolism.

Variations

The internet, long-standing chefs and classic French cook-books all have multiple versions of cassoulet. Sweet aromatic veg, lovely rich meat and bones, a good stock, fresh aromatic herbs and lots of beans. For damper winter days it is worth experimenting with more intense flavours, especially spice. Particularly good are allspice, aniseed, caraway, clove, fennel, juniper, mustard seed, paprika and star anise, although these need to be matched with the choice of meat. The same effect can be achieved by adding a spicy sausage such as chorizo or merguez. Of course, it is also great to use different types of bean, particularly other pale, soft and sweet varieties such as butter beans.

6
Chicken chasseur
Serves 4
Ingredients

- 1 tsb olive oil
- 25 g butter
- 4 chicken legs
- 1 onion, chopped
- 2 garlic cloves, finely chopped
- 200 g chestnut mushrooms
- 2 thyme sprigs
- 225 ml red wine
- 2 tbsp tomato purée
- 500 ml best chicken stock

Method

In a large heavy-bottomed casserole pan, heat the olive oil and half the butter. When the butter is bubbling, fry the chicken on both sides until browned. Remove the chicken, add the rest of the butter to the pan and begin to soften the onion. When the onion is translucent and soft, add the garlic and then the mushrooms and the thyme. Continue to cook for a further 3 to 4 minutes before adding the wine and the tomato purée. Once this has begun to reduce after around 5 minutes then add the chicken back to the pan before adding the stock. Put a lid on the pan and cook gently over a low heat for around an hour. Remove the chicken legs and keep warm. Reduce the sauce over a high heat for a few minutes before serving. It is rich (chicken, chicken stock, butter, olive oil and wine) and nourishing (chestnut mushrooms), but not strongly spiced, relying instead on aromatic flavours from onion, garlic and thyme to stimulate motility and secretion.

Variations

A simple version of this recipe involves fish fillets and the other ingredients sealed in a foil parcel and thrown on top of a barbecue. This is ideal for those who find barbecued food rich and cloying – definitely a healthy alternative! Otherwise, the dish can be made more complex by precooking wine or stock with butter, a small diced onion, a teaspoon of black peppercorns and a heaped teaspoon of juniper berries for 15 minutes. The resulting sauce is then poured hot over the fresh whole fish in a hot pan, which is cooked in the oven for 5 to 10 minutes. The advantage of this more complex method is that it gives the bitter aromatics and spice of the juniper and black pepper time to infuse the sauce. This creates more depth and potency of flavour for enhanced digestion and satisfaction.

Vocabulary 4

Fill in the meanings in your mother language:

arborio /ɑrˈbɔr iˌoʊ/ **rice** /raɪs/
astringent /əˈstrɪndʒənt/
barbecue /ˈbɑːbɪˌkjuː/
basil /ˈbæz əl/
batch /bætʃ/
belly /belɪ/
bubble /ˈbʌbəl/
bung /bʌŋ/
butter /ˈbʌtə/ **bean** /biːn/
cannellini /ˌkænɪˈlɪːnɪ/ **bean** /biːn/
caraway /ˈkærəˌweɪ/
cassolé /ˌkæsəˈle/
chef /ʃef/
chicken /ˈtʃɪkɪn/ **chasseur** /ʃæˈsɜː/
chorizo /tʃɔːˈriːzəʊ/
cloying /ˈklɔɪɪŋ/
coconut /ˈkəʊkəˌnʌt/
concoction /kənˈkɒkʃən/
confit /kɔ̃fi/
cook-book /kʊkˌbʊk/
crème fraîche /ˈkrɛm ˈfrɛʃ/
debeard /di bɪəd/
deseed /disiːd/
discard /dɪsˈkɑːd/
drizzle /ˈdrɪzəl/
earthenware /ˈɜːθənˌweə/
excess /ekses/
expansive /ɪkˈspænsɪv/
fare /feə/
flat /flæt/ **leaf** /liːf/
foam /fəʊm/
foil /fɔɪl/
foremost /ˈfɔːˌməʊst/
frond /frɒnd/
frying /fraɪɪŋ/ **pan** /pæn/
generous /dʒenrəs/
giblets /ˈdʒɪblɪts/
ground /graʊnd/
guise /gaɪz/
heavy /hevɪ/ **-based** /beɪst/
infuse /ɪnˈfjuːz/
joint /dʒɔɪnt/
juniper /ˈdʒuːnɪpə/
ladle /ˈleɪdəl/
ladleful /ˈleɪd l fʊl/
mandolin /ˌmændəˈlɪn/
marjoram /ˈmɑːdʒərəm/
matched /mætʃt/
merguez /mɜrˈdʒəːz/
mix /mɪks/
nasturtium /nəˈstɜːʃəm/
ovenproof /ˈʌvənˌpruː/
pancetta /pænˈtʃɛtə/
parmesan /ˈpɑːmɪˌzæn/
pearled /pɜːld/ **spelt** /spɛlt/
pinch /pɪntʃ/
pith /pɪθ/
pitted /ˈpɪtɪd/
plum /plʌm/ **tomatoe** /təˈmɑːtəʊ/
pop /pɒp/
porcino /pɔːˈtʃiːnəʊ/ pl. **porcini**
potency /ˈpəʊtənsɪ/
quarter /ˈkwɔːtə/
remove /rɪˈmuːv/
rib /rɪb/
satisfaction /ˌsætɪsˈfæk.ʃən/
seal /siːl/
season /ˈsiːzən/
shake /ʃeɪk/
skim /skɪm/
solidified /səˈlɪdɪˌfaɪd/
splash /splæʃ/
spring /sprɪŋ/ **water** /ˈwɔːtə/
sprinkle /ˈsprɪŋkəl/
streaky /ˈstriːkɪ/
suffuse /səˈfjuːz/
syrupy /ˈsɪrəpɪ/
tap /tæp/
throw /θrəʊ/
tuna /ˈtjuːnə/
turn /tɜːn/ **up** /ʌp/
wholegrain /ˈhəʊlˈgreɪn/
wok /wɒk/

Unit 5 - Recipes 3

1
Baked fish with herbs
Serves 2-4
Ingredients

- a whole fish, head on, scaled and gutted (mackerel, bream, mullet, bass, gurnard or pollock)
- a knob of butter and 2 tbsp olive oil
- l large fennel bulb, sliced
- ½ white onion, diced
- 2 cm fresh root ginger, finely sliced
- a generous handful of chopped fresh coriander
- 1 large mug chilli deseeded and finely chopped
- ½ cup dry white wine
- 3 slices lemon
- generous pinch of salt
- ½ tbs black pepper

Method

Sauté the fennel, onion, ginger and chilli in the olive oil and butter for 5 minutes, just to soften them a bit. Put all the ingredients in a foil-covered dish and place in an oven at 170℃ for 10 to 20 minutes until the fish is moist and just cooked; cooking time will depend on the size and type of the fish. Serve with rice, soy sauce and lightly sautéed fresh veg. This is a quick, convenient and common way to cook fish and produces a marvellously light, refreshing result. The refreshing coolness of the dish comes from the sourness of the wine and lemon and the cool aromatics of the fresh coriander, while the lemon pith provides a little bitter undertone which also stimulates motility and refreshes the palate in hot weather. As a rule, sour constricting astringency from the lemon and wine needs to be balanced with expansive spice to stimulate motility and give warm satisfaction, a task achieved by ginger, chilli and black pepper in this case. Onion and fennel round out the flavours in the recipe by providing sweet aromatics to stimulate appetite and nourish digestion. This can be a cheap recipe to put together, using less popular whole fish varieties. The use of whole fish instead of fillets adds a little richness and depth of flavour to this dish as the nutrients from the head and bones infuse the sauce.

2
Salmon and caper fish cakes
Serves 1
Ingredients

- tin of wild salmon or grilled salmon steak
- 1 tsp capers, rinsed and drained
- 120 g mashed potato
- bag of watercress
- 3 big pinches cayenne pepper
- 3 tbsp olive oil
- semolina
- mayonnaise

Method

If using tinned salmon drain it well in a sieve, pressing it down with the back of a spoon. Then place it in a bowl with the capers and potato. Chop three quarters of the watercress and add a large tablespoon to the bowl. Add some salt and the cayenne pepper and mix everything well together. Sprinkle some semolina onto a plate, then divide the salmon mix into six. Shape them into rounds using your hands, coating each one fully with semolina. Heat the oil in a wok or large frying pan and when it is very hot, add the fishcakes and cook them briefly – about 2 minutes on each side. Serve with remaining watercress and mayonnaise.

The lightness of this dish makes it ideal for hot and humid weather, as it is not particularly rich and fatty while the spice of the pepper, combined with the pungent bitterness of watercress strongly stimulates appetite and motility.

Variations

In drier hot weather, refreshing aromatic herbs such as mint, coriander and marjoram can be added to the mix. If it is more humid and damp, try using a little sweet chilli sauce as a condiment. In colder weather, more richness is required which can be provided by adding extra mayonnaise.

3
Basic stir-fry
Serves 4
Ingredients

- 300 g fresh beef, filleted chicken or tofu
- 2 cm fresh ginger root
- 1 clove garlic
- 1 chilli, deseeded
- 6 spring onions
- soy sauce
- 5 tbsp sunflower oil
- 2 handfuls mushrooms
- 2 handfuls seasonal veg
- 2 handfuls seasonal greens
- 2 tsp toasted sesame oil
- a handful chopped fresh basil

Method

Heat half the sunflower oil in a wok. Add the meat or tofu and sear it. If using chicken make sure it is clearly cooked through but still tender. Remove the meat or tofu from the wok, add mushroom and spices to the wok. Heat and stir for 3 minutes. Add the meat and cook for a further 30 seconds. Remove from the heat and stir in the basil and the toasted sesame oil. Add soy sauce at the end to taste. The stir-fry works on the basis that even a little bit of cooking 'opens up' our food, breaking it down enough to give our digestive systems a helping hand. It also allows flavours to mellow, mingle and mature.

In this recipe there are some of the stalwarts of the Chinese kitchen cupboard: chilli, garlic, ginger, spring onion and soy sauce. Garlic, chilli and ginger help it through strongly stimulating gut circulation, motility and secretion so that the lightly cooked vegetables can be easily broken down and absorbed. The spring onion adds a strong aromatic to the same effect while the soy sauce adds savoury depth to stimulate appetite. Adding a little bit of toasted sesame oil at the end of cooking is a good trick with stir fries, especially when cooking with tofu. It adds richness, especially in the cold months.

Variations

Stir-fry has exceptional variety as a dish, just about any vegetable, mushroom and meat can be used. The key thing is the principles that underlie the dish: light cooking to enhance digestion and develop flavours, and the right herbs and spices to assist digestion.

4
Chicken curry
Serves 4
Ingredients

- 4 chicken thighs, preferably free-range or organic
- 3 tbsp coconut oil or ghee
- 1 tsp yellow or brown mustard seeds
- 1 large onion, sliced
- 3 garlic cloves, finely sliced
- 1 x 400 ml canned coconut milk

For the marinade:

- 1 tsp paprika
- ½ tsp ground turmeric or 2 cm piece of turmeric root
- 1 ½ tbsp ground coriander
- 1 tsp ground cumin
- 1 tsp cayenne pepper
- 1 tbsp lemon juice
- ½ tsp raw sea salt
- 75 ml water

Method

Mix all the marinade ingredients together and add the chicken pieces. They are best left to marinate for at least an hour but preferably overnight. Heat the oil or ghee in a deep frying pan and add the mustard seeds. When they start to pop and jump about in the pan, add the onion and garlic. Cook until they're soft and translucent, then add the chicken and any extra paste from the marinade. Fry over a gentle heat for about 8 minutes, turning the chicken occasionally. Then add the coconut milk. Increase the heat slightly and bring to a simmer. Cook for a further 10-12 minutes until the sauce has thickened slightly and serve with rice or flat bread.

5
Dal
Serves 3
Ingredients

- cooking fat – coconut oil (if vegan)
- ghee/clarified butter (if vegetarian)
- 1 medium yellow onion, quartered
- 25 g grated coconut/ coconut cream
- 3 cloves garlic, sliced
- 2 chillies, deseeded and finely diced
- 1 tbsp fresh ginger root, minced
- 2 tsp garam masala
- 1 tsp cinnamon
- ½ tsp turmeric

- ¼ tsp ground coriander
- 240 ml light chicken or vegetable stock or water
- 400 g tomatoes, diced
- 230 g pumpkin, peeled and diced
- 360 g cooked black-eyed peas
- 70 g spinach, chopped
- some finely shredded mint

Method

Combine onion, coconut, garlic, chillies, ginger, garam masala, cumin, cinnamon, salt, turmeric, coriander and 3 tbsp (45ml) stock in a blender. Purée mixture to a paste, scraping down the sides of the blender as necessary. Heat the cooking fat in a large saucepan, and then add the spice paste and cook, stirring often, for 10 minutes. Add remaining stock, tomatoes and pumpkin. Cook over medium heat, stirring often, until pumpkin is just tender: about 20 minutes. Mix in black-eyed peas and spinach. Continue to cook, stirring often, for 5 more minutes. Remove from heat. Taste and adjust seasonings; stir in the mint just before serving. This is a spice-heavy dish that often forms part of a vegetarian menu. Interestingly, since it is a vegetarian stalwart, from this diet's perspective its value lies not so much in its spices as in its cooking fat and protein content. This is because vegetarian diets often lack necessary richness, the sort of richness supplied by coconut oil or ghee and beans. Ghee and coconut oil are both high in short-chain saturated fats, the sort that are easy to digest and strongly nourish blood, membranes and the nervous system. Because they are saturated, they are perfect for frying spices, maintaining their chemical structure even at high temperature. Meanwhile, beans are a great source of vegetarian protein. On their own, the combination of the saturated fat and the beans would present something of a digestive challenge.

But not with the plethora of herbs and spices that accompany them in this dish. The standard Asian pungent and spicy ingredients onion, garlic, ginger and chilli cut through the fat and stimulate secretion and motility. Garam masala, also used in this recipe, literally translates as 'hot mixture of spices' since most of the spices involved tend to be mellow in flavour: cloves, cinnamon, nutmeg, cardamom, cumin and coriander seeds. The ingredients of garam masala vary according to the region of origin and the taste of the chef. So have a look at the packet when you buy the pre-prepared stuff in case you have a flavour preference or don't like very spicy food as some brands will include chilli.

Variations

If you don't like very spicy food, leave out the chilli and cut down on garlic. Or you can make your own garam masala with just a few mild spices like cumin, coriander, cardamom and star anise. Other dal recipes include different pulses such as green, black or yellow lentils and split peas. All of these mush down nicely and are delicious.

6

Nasturtium, chicken and pesto salad

Ingredients

- Leftover chicken or sautéed chicken breast
- pesto
- nasturtium flowers
- lemon juice
- black pepper
- watercress

Method

Cover the chicken with generous amounts of pesto, then squeeze on a little lemon juice and black pepper. Top with a few nasturtium flowers and sprigs of watercress. Serve with macaroni or gnocchi while it is still hot. This is light summer food at its simplest. Like all of this diet's salads, its major components, chicken and macaroni or gnocchi are cooked, so that even in the hottest and driest weather much of the work is done for our digestive systems by the cooking process. Accompanying these ingredients is a little extra sweetness from the olive oil of the pesto. Basil (in the pesto), black pepper and the watercress provide spicy aromatics, lemon juice, a refreshing sourness to counter the heat of the weather, and nasturtium flowers, a zingy bitterness, again ideally suited to compensating for hot weather.

Variations

The best way to add variety to this dish is by making your own pesto. Olive oil can be substituted with rapeseed or hemp oil and basil replaced with parsley or coriander. Nasturtium leaves can be used as well as the flowers and other bitter salad greens used instead of, or alongside, the watercress.

7

Ceviche

Serves about 3

Ingredients

- 500 g fresh sea bass fillet, cut into 1 cm pieces
- 60 ml freshly squeezed lemon juice
- ½ a small red onion, finely diced
- 1 fresh tomato chopped and seeded
- 1 mild chilli, seeded and finely chopped
- 1 tsp salt
- ¼ tsp freshly ground black pepper
- 1 small pinch cayenne pepper
- ¼ handful chopped dill

Method

Place the fish, onion, tomato, chilli, black pepper, cayenne pepper and dill in a ceramic, glass or porcelain dish. Pour the lemon and lime juice over them and mix it all up well. Leave in the fridge for about 3 hours, gently mixing every hour. Do not leave for more than 3 hours or the fish will lose too much of its firmness.

8
Falafel
Serves 1-2
Ingredients

- 1 400 g tin chickpeas, drained and rinsed, or 200 g dried chick peas, soaked overnight
- 1 small onion, finely chopped
- 2 cloves garlic, finely chopped
- 1 small bunch parsley, stalks removed, leaves finely chopped
- 1 small bunch coriander, stalks removed, leaves finely chopped
- 1 tsp ground cumin
- ¼ tsp chilli flakes (optional)
- 2-3 tbsp plain flour
- lemon juice

Method

Combine the chickpeas, onion and garlic in a food processor. Add the herbs, cumin, chilli and a small pinch of sea salt, and pulse to a coarse paste. Add the flour a little at a time until the mixture comes together roughly in a ball. Put it into a bowl, cover and refrigerate for a couple of hours. Pre-heat the oven to 200℃. Roll the falafel mix into golf-ball-sized rounds. Line a baking tray with lightly oiled baking parchment, line up the balls so they don't touch and bake for around 20 minutes. Squeeze on fresh lemon juice before eating. Serve with a cooked grain and lightly cooked vegetables or some bitter leaves and a spicy pickle. Tahini (sesame paste) thinned with water and lemon juice is also a delicious accompaniment.

Falafel is an ancient dish illustrating a key principle of traditional cuisine. A bland, fibrous stable (chickpeas) is overlaid by intense and balanced flavours to make it appetising and easy to digest. In this case, sweet (chickpeas, onion), aromatic/spicy (onion, garlic, cumin and chilli), bitter (parsley, coriander), sour (lemon juice) and salt make up the flavour combination. The dish probably originated in Egypt and spread through Arabic and Mediterranean countries, all characterised by their hot and dry climates. In these countries it is often served in a flat bread such as pitta with a green salad. Falafel is prepared and served in a wide variety of ways throughout the world. Classic spices that can be used are ground cumin and coriander seed, cayenne pepper and paprika.

9
Grilled or barbecued sardines with salsa
Serves 4
Ingredients

- 8 sardines
- 3 tbsp olive oil
- 2 sprigs thyme leaves picked
- 2 cloves of garlic, finely chopped
- sea salt and ground pepper

Method

Combine the olive oil, garlic, thyme and seasoning. Rub the mixture all over the sardines, inside and out. If barbecuing them, place them in a fish basket and grill them over hot coals for a couple of minutes on each side until they are crisp and bubbling. Or place them under a hot grill for 3 to 4 minutes each side until the skin begins to darken. Serve with the tomato salsa.

The salsa
Ingredients

- 250 g fresh tomatoes, finely chopped
- 1 small onion, finely chopped
- 3 mild chillies, finely chopped
- small handful of coriander, finely chopped
- salt to taste
- lime juice to taste
- 1 tbsp water

Method

Mix all the ingredients together in a bowl. Best left for at least a couple of hours to infuse. The main principle that this recipe demonstrates is the use of an aromatic rub and a spicy sour salsa to help digest the rich oily meat of the fish. These stimulate gut motility and bile secretion, helping to avoid tiring sluggishness.

Vocabulary 5

Fill in the meanings in your mother language:

alongside /ə'lɒŋˌsaɪd/
appetising /'æpɪˌtaɪzɪŋ/
baking /'beɪkɪŋ/ **tray** /treɪ/
bass /beɪs/
black-eyed been /ˌblæ k.aɪd'biːn/
bream /briːm/
butter /'bʌtər/
caper /'keɪpə/
ceviche /səvɪːʃəɪ/
chickpea /'tʃɪkˌpiː/
coarse /kɔːs/
coating /'kəʊtɪŋ/
cut /kʌt/ **down** /daʊn/
dal /dɑːl/
darken /'dɑːkən/
dill /dɪl/
falafel /fəl'ɑːfəl/
firmness /fɜːmnəs/
flat flæt/ **bread** /bred/
free /friː/ **-range** /reɪndʒ/
ghee /giː/
gnocchi /'njɒk.i/
gurnard /'gɜːnəd/
gutted /'gʌtɪd/
head on /ˌhed'ɒn/
hemp /hɛmp/ **oil** /ɔɪl/
jump /dʒʌmp/ **about** /ə'baʊt/
lemon /'lemən/
lime /laɪm/
literally /'lɪtərəli/
macaroni /ˌmækər'əʊni/
mackerel /'mæk.rəl/
mature /mə'tjʊər/
mellow /'meləʊ/
moist /mɔɪst/
mullet /'mʌl.ɪt/
mush /mʌʃ/
organic /ɔː'gæn.ɪk/
overlaid /ˌoʊ vər'leɪd/
palate /'pælət/

parchment /ˈpɑːtʃmənt/
pesto /ˈpes.təʊ/
pick /pɪk/
plain /pleɪn/ **flour** /ˈflaʊə/
plate /pleɪt/
plethora /ˈpleθərə/
pollock /ˈpɒlək/
pumpkin /ˈpʌmpkɪn/
rapeseed /ˈreɪpˌsiːd/
raw /rɔː/
round /raʊnd/
salmon /ˈsæm.ən/
salsa /ˈsælsə/
sauté /ˈsəʊteɪ/
scale /skeɪl/
sea /siː/ **bass** /beɪs/
sea /siː/ **salt** /sɔːlt/
sear /sɪər/
semolina /ˌsem.əlˈiː.nə/
sesame /ˈsesəmɪ/ **oil** /ɔɪl/
short /ʃɔːt/ **-chain** /tʃeɪn/ **saturated** /ˈsætʃəreɪtɪd/ **fats** /fæts/
shred /ʃred/
sluggish /ˈslʌgɪʃ/
soften /ˈsɒfən/
spoon /spuːn/
squeeze /skwiːz/
stable /ˈsteɪbəl/
stalwart /ˈstɔːlwət/
stir-fry /ˈstɜː.fraɪ/
sunflower /ˈsʌnflaʊər/ **oil** /ɔɪl/
tahini /təˈhiːnɪ/
thigh /θaɪ/
tiring /ˈtaɪərɪŋ/
toast /təʊst/
undertone /ˈʌndətəʊn/
watercress /ˈwɔːtəˌkres/
zing /zɪŋ/

THEORETICAL PART

Chapter I

Human body in health and disease

Unit 1 - Cardiovascular system

The heart is made up of many **interconnected branching fibres** or cells that form the **walls** of the **two atria and two ventricles**. Some of these cells are specialized to **conduct electrical impulses**. Others have **contraction** as their main role. All of these cells are **nourished** through a profuse **network of blood vessels**.

Anatomy and physiology of the heart

Anatomy

The **coronary arteries** are the sole suppliers of arterial blood of the heart, delivering **200-250 mL of blood** to the **myocardium** each minute **during rest**.

The left main coronary artery supplies the **left ventricle, interventricular septum, and part of the right ventricle. The right** coronary artery supplies the **right atrium and ventricle, part of the left ventricle, and the conduction system**.

In addition, many **connections (anastomoses)** exist between **arterioles** to provide **backup (collateral)** circulation. These anastomoses play a key role in providing **alternative routes** of blood flow in the event of **blockage** in one or more of the coronary vessels. Coronary **capillaries** allow for the **exchange of nutrients and metabolic wastes** and they merge to form coronary veins; these veins deliver most of the blood to the **coronary sinus**. The coronary sinus empties directly into the right atrium and is the major vein draining the myocardium.

Physiology

The heart can be thought of as **two pumps** in one. **One** is a **low-pressure** pump (right atrium and right ventricle) and supplies blood to the **lungs**. The **second** is a **high-pressure** pump (left atrium and left ventricle) and supplies **blood to the body**. The **right atrium** receives venous blood **from the systemic circulation** and from the **coronary veins**; most of this de-oxygenated blood in the right atrium then passes to the **right ventricle.**

Contraction of the right ventricle pushes blood against the **tricuspid valve** and through the **pulmonic valve**; this allows the blood to **enter the lungs** via the **pulmonary arteries**. From the pulmonary arteries, the de-oxygenated blood enters the **capillaries in the lungs** where **gas exchange** takes place.

From the lungs the blood travels through four **pulmonary veins** back to the **left atrium**. The **mitral (bicuspid)** valve opens, and blood flows to the **left ventricle**. As the left ventricle contracts, blood is pushed against the bicuspid valve and against the **aortic valve**, which allows blood to enter the aorta. From the **aorta**, blood is distributed first **to the heart itself** and then throughout the **systemic arterial circulation.**

Cardiac cycle

The pumping action of the heart is a product of **rhythmic, alternate contraction (systole)** and **relaxation (diastole)** of the atria and ventricles. These **heartbeats** occur about **70 times per minute** in resting adults and these rhythmic contractions of the heart chambers are responsible for **blood movement**.

Stroke volume

The stroke volume is the amount of **blood ejected** from the heart with each **ventricular contraction** and depends on three factors: **pre-load** (the volume of **blood returning** to the heart), **after-load** (the **resistance** against which the heart muscle must pump) and **myocardial contractility.**

Myocardial contractility

The unique function of the **myocardial muscle** fibres and the influence of the **autonomic nervous system** play a major role in the function of the heart. **Ischaemia** or various drugs can **decrease** myocardial **contractility**; ischaemia can decrease the total number of working myocardial cells. (This occurs in myocardial infarction.) Hypoxia or the administration of beta-blockers can decrease the ability of the separate myocardial cells to contract.

Cardiac output

Cardiac output is the **amount of blood pumped** by the ventricles **per minute**. Cardiac output can increase by increasing the heart rate, stroke volume, or both.

Nervous system control of the heart

The **autonomic** nervous system also controls the behaviour of the heart, greatly influencing the **heart rate, conductivity, and contractility.** The autonomic nervous system **innervates** the atria and ventricles. The **parasympathetic** nervous system mainly is concerned with

vegetative functions. In contrast, the **sympathetic** nervous system helps prepare the body to **respond to stress**. These sympathetic and parasympathetic control systems work in a **check-and-balance** manner and stimulate the heart to increase or decrease cardiac output according to the **metabolic demands** of the body.

Parasympathetic control

Parasympathetic control of the heart is through the **vagus nerve**; control by these fibres has a continuous restraining **influence on the heart**, primarily by **decreasing the heart rate** and, to a lesser extent, **contractility**. Strong parasympathetic stimulation can decrease the heart rate to 20 or 30 beats per minute, yet such stimulation generally has little effect on stroke volume.

Sympathetic control

Sympathetic nerve fibres originate in the **thoracic region of the spinal cord** and form groups of **nerve fibres called ganglia.** Their post-ganglionic fibres **release** the chemical **noradrenaline**, which stimulates an **increase** in the heart rate. Noradrenaline also stimulates an increase in the force of **muscle contraction**; sympathetic stimulation of the heart causes **coronary arteries** to **dilate** and causes **constriction** of **peripheral vessels**. These two effects, dilation and constriction help to **increase blood and oxygen supply** to the heart.

Hormonal regulation of the heart

Impulses from the sympathetic nerves are sent to the **adrenal medulla**. In response, the adrenal medulla secretes the **hormones adrenaline** and **noradrenaline** into the **circulating blood** in response to increased **physical activity**, emotional **excitement or stress**. Adrenaline causes **blood vessels to constrict** in the **skin, kidneys, gastrointestinal tract,** and other organs (viscera) and causes **dilation** of **skeletal and coronary blood vessels.**

Role of electrolytes

Myocardial cells are bathed in an **electrolyte solution**. The major electrolytes that affect cardiac function are **calcium, potassium, and sodium. Magnesium** plays an important role as well.

Exercise 1

Match the column A with the column B. Try to learn the expressions and/or sentences by heart.

A

1. The heart is made up of many interconnected branching fibres or cells
2. Some of these cells are specialized to conduct electrical impulses,
3. All of these cells are nourished
4. Many connections (anastomoses) exist between arterioles to provide collateral circulation;

5. The right atrium receives venous blood from the systemic circulation and from the coronary veins;
6. Contraction of the right ventricle pushes blood against the tricuspid valve and through the pulmonic valve;
7. From the pulmonary arteries,
8. From the lungs the blood travels through four pulmonary veins back to the left atrium;
9. From the aorta, blood is distributed first to the heart itself
10. The pumping action of the heart is a product of
11. The stroke volume is the amount of blood
12. The unique function of the myocardial muscle fibres
13. Hypoxia or the administration of beta-blockers
14. Cardiac output is the amount of blood
15. The autonomic nervous system also controls the behaviour of the heart,
16. The autonomic nervous system
17. The parasympathetic nervous system mainly is concerned with vegetative functions;
18. Parasympathetic control of the heart is through the vagus nerve;
19. Sympathetic nerve fibres originate in the thoracic region of the spinal cord
20. Their postganglionic fibres release
21. Impulses from the sympathetic nerves are sent to the adrenal medulla; the adrenal medulla
22. Myocardial cells are bathed in an electrolyte solution;

B

a) *and form groups of nerve fibres called ganglia.*
b) *and the influence of the autonomic nervous system play a major role in the function of the heart.*
c) *and then throughout the systemic arterial circulation.*
d) *can decrease the ability of the separate myocardial cells to contract.*
e) *control by these fibres has a continuous restraining influence on the heart.*
f) *ejected from the heart with each ventricular contraction*
g) *greatly influencing the heart rate, conductivity, and contractility.*
h) *in contrast, the sympathetic nervous system helps prepare the body to respond to stress.*
i) *innervates the atria and ventricles.*
j) *most of this de-oxygenated blood in the right atrium then passes to the right ventricle.*
k) *others have contraction as their main role.*

l) *pumped by the ventricles per minute.*

m) *rhythmic, alternate contraction (systole) and relaxation (diastole) of the atria and ventricles.*

n) *secretes the hormones adrenaline and noradrenaline into the circulating blood in response to increased physical activity, emotional excitement or stress.*

o) *that form the walls of the two atria and two ventricles.*

p) *the chemical noradrenaline, which stimulates an increase in the heart rate.*

q) *the de-oxygenated blood enters the capillaries in the lungs where gas exchange takes place.*

r) *the major electrolytes that affect cardiac function are calcium, potassium, sodium and magnesium.*

s) *the mitral (bicuspid) valve opens, and blood flows to the left ventricle.*

t) *they play a key role in providing alternative routes of blood flow in the event of blockage in one or more of the coronary vessels.*

u) *this allows the blood to enter the lungs via the pulmonary arteries.*

v) *through a profuse network of blood vessels.*

Exercise 2

Translate the expressions. Try to explain their meanings in English.

Interconnected, branching, fibres, atria, ventricles, contraction, nourished, coronary arteries, delivering, interventricular, septum, conduction, connections, backup, merge, empties, coronary veins, de-oxygenated, resting adults, heart chambers, stroke volume, ejected, resistance, contractility, ischaemia, hypoxia, beta-blockers, separate, cardiac output, per minute, autonomic, heart rate, conductivity, contractility, innervates, parasympathetic, vegetative functions, sympathetic, demands, vagus nerve, continuous, restraining, influence, decreasing, extent, thoracic region, spinal cord, nerve fibres, ganglia, dilate, peripheral vessels, adrenal medulla, emotional excitement, kidneys, gastrointestinal tract, viscera, dilation, electrolyte solution, calcium, potassium, sodium, magnesium.

Exercise 3

Answer the following questions. Prepare short talks and/or dialogues on these topics.

1. Describe the anatomy of the heart.
2. Describe the physiology of the heart.
3. Explain the terms cardiac cycle, stroke volume, myocardial contractility and cardiac output.

4. How does the nervous system control the heart?
5. What do you know about hormonal regulation of the heart?

Vocabulary 1

Fill in the meanings in your mother language:

ability /ə'bɪl.ɪ.ti/
addition /ə'dɪʃ.ən/
adrenal /ə'dri:.nəl/
adrenaline /ə'dren.əl.ɪn/
affect /ə'fekt/
afterload /ˌɑ:f.tər.'ləʊd/
allow /ə'laʊ/
alternate /'ɔ:ltəˌneɪt/
alternative /ɒl'tɜ:.nə.tɪv/
amount /ə'maʊnt/
anastomosis /əˌnæs.tə'məʊ.sɪs/
aortic /eɪ'ɔ:.tə/
aortic /eɪ'ɔ:.tɪk/ **valve** /vælv/
arterial /ɑ:'tɪə.ri.əl/
artery /'ɑ:tərɪ/
atrium /'eɪ.tri.əm/ pl **atria**
autonomic /'ɔ.t̬ə'nɑm.ɪk/
backup /'bæk.ʌp/
balance /'bæl.əns/
beta /'bi:.tə/ **-blocker** /blɒk.ə/ **agents** /'eɪ.dʒənts/
bicuspid valve /baɪ'kʌs.pɪdˌvælv/
blockage /'blɒk.ɪdʒ/
blood /blʌd/ **vessel** /'ves.əl/
calcium /'kæl.si.əm/
capillary /kə'pɪl.ər.i/
cardiac /'kɑ:.di.æk/ **output** /'aʊt.pʊt/
cause /kɔ:z/
chamber /'tʃeɪm.bə/
check /tʃek/
collateral /kə'læt.ər.əl/
conduct /kən'dʌkt/
conduction /kən'dʌk.ʃən/
conductivity /ˌkɒn.dʌk'tɪv.ɪ.ti/
connection /kə'nek.ʃən/
constrict /kən'strɪkt/
continuous /kən'tɪn.ju.əs/
contractility /ˌkən.træk'tɪ.lə.ti/
contraction /kən'trækʃən/
coronary /'kɒr.ən.ər.i/
decrease /dɪ'kri:s/
deliver /dɪ'lɪv.ər/
demand /dɪ'mɑ:nd/
deoxygenated /dɪ'ɒk.sɪ.dʒə.neɪ.təd/
diastole /daɪ'æs.tə.li/
dilate /daɪ'leɪt/
drain /dreɪn/
eject /ɪ'dʒekt/
electrolyte /ɪ'lek.trə.laɪt/
empty /'emp.ti/
exchange /ɪks'tʃeɪndʒ/
excitement /ɪk'saɪt.mənt/
extent /ɪk'stent/
flow /fləʊ/
force /fɔ:s/
ganglion /'gæŋ.gli.ən/ pl **ganglia**
gastrointestinal /ˌgæs.trəʊˌɪn.tes'taɪ.nəl/
generally /'dʒen.ə r.əl.i/
heart /hɑ:t/ **rate** /reɪt/
heartbeat /'hɑ:t.bi:t/
hypoxia /haɪ'pɒk.sɪə/
increase /ɪn'kri:s/
influence /'ɪn.flʊ.əns/
innervate /'ɪn.ə.veɪt/
interconnect /ˌɪn.tə.kə'nekt/
interventricular /ˌɪn.tə'ven'trɪk.jə.lər/
ischaemia /ɪ'ski:.mi.ə/
kidney /'kɪd.ni/
magnesium /mæg'ni:.zi.əm/
manner /'mæn.ər/
medulla /meˌdʌl.ə/
merge /mɜ:dʒ/
minute /maɪ'nju:t/
mitral valve /'maɪ.trəlˌvælv/
movement /'mu:v.mənt/
myocardial /ˌmaɪ.əʊ'kɑ:.di.əl/
infarction /ɪn'fɑ:k.ʃən/
myocardial /maɪ.əˌkɑ:.di.əl/
myocardium /ˌmaɪ.ə'kɑ:.di.əm/

network /'net.wɜːk/
noradrenaline /ˌnɔːr.ə'dren.ə.lɪn/
nourished /nʌr.ɪʃt/
originate /ə'rɪdʒ.ɪ.neɪt/
parasympathetic /'pær.
əˌsɪm.pə'θet.ɪk/
pass /pɑːs/
peripheral /pə'rɪf.ər.əl/
postganglionic /pəʊstˌgæŋ.glɪ'ɒːnɪk/
potassium /pə'tæs.i.əm/
preload /ˌpriː'ləʊd/
prepare /prɪ'peə/
pressure /'preʃ.ə/
pulmonary /'pʊl.mə.nə.ri/
pulmonic /pʌl'mɒn.ɪk/
pump /pʌmp/
push /pʊʃ/
region /'riː.dʒən/
regulation /ˌreg.jʊ'leɪ.ʃən/
relaxation /ˌriː.læk'seɪ.ʃən/
release /rə'liːs/
resistance /rɪ'zɪs.tənts/
respond /rɪ'spɒnd/
resting /'rest.ɪŋ/
restrain /rɪ'streɪn/
route /ruːt/
separate /'sep.ər.ət/
septum /'sep.təm/
sinus /'saɪ.nəs/ pl **sinuses**
skeletal /'skel.ɪ.təl/
sodium /'səʊ.di.əm/
solution /sə'luː.ʃən/
spinal /'spaɪ.nəl/ **cord** /kɔːd/
stimulate /'stɪm.jʊ.leɪt/
stimulation /ˌstɪm.jʊ'leɪ.ʃən/
stroke /strəʊk/ **volume** /'vɒl.juːm/
supplier /sə'plaɪ.ər/
supply /sə'plaɪ/
systemic /sɪ'stem.ɪk/
systole /'sɪs.tə.li/
thoracic /θəˌræs.ɪk/
tricuspid valve /traɪ'kʌs.pɪdˌvælv/
unique /juː'niːk/
vagus /'veɪ.gəs/ pl **vagi**
valve /vælv/
vegetative /'vedʒ.ɪ.tə.tɪv/
vein /veɪn/
ventricle /'ven.trɪ.kl̩/
vessel /'ves.əl/
viscera /'vɪs.ər.ə/
volume /'vɒl.juːm/
waste /weɪst/

Solution to Exercise 1
1o, 2k, 3v, 4t, 5j, 6u, 7q, 8s, 9c, 10m, 11f, 12b, 13d, 14l, 15g, 16i, 17h, 18e, 19a, 20p, 21n, 22r

Unit 2 - Nervous system

Anatomy and physiology of the nervous system

The nervous system is divided into **two parts**. These two parts are the **central nervous system (CNS)** and the **peripheral nervous system (PNS)**. The ability of the human body to maintain a **state of balance (homeostasis)** is chiefly the result of the nervous system's **ability to coordinate and regulate** the body's activities. The CNS consists of the **brain and spinal cord.**

Cells of the nervous system

The **cells** of the nervous system include **neurons** and **connective tissue cells known as neuroglia. Each neuron** has three main parts: (1) the **cell body**; (2) one or more **branching projections, called dendrites**; and (3) a **single, elongated projection**, known as an **axon. Dendrites transmit impulses to** the cell bodies whilst **axons transmit impulses away from** the cell bodies.

Bundles of parallel axons with their associated **sheaths** are white and are called **white matter. In the PNS,** bundles of axons and their sheaths are called **nerves**. Collections of nerve cells are greyer in colour and are called **grey matter.** The **outer surface** of the **cerebrum and the cerebellum** consists of **grey matter,** which forms the cerebral cortex and the cerebellar **cortex**.

Types of neurons

Neurons are classified as **sensory neurons**, **motor** neurons or inter-neurons. Sensory neurons **transmit** impulses **to** the **spinal cord and brain from** all parts of **the body**. **Motor neurons** transmit impulses in the opposite direction, **away from the brain and spinal cord. Inter-neurons** (called **central** or **connecting** neurons) conduct impulses **from sensory neurons to motor neurons**; **sensory** neurons also are called **afferent** neurons and **motor** neurons are called **efferent** neurons.

Impulse transmission

The **transmission of nerve impulses** in the nervous system is **similar to the conduction of electrical impulses through the heart**.

Synapse

The membrane-to-membrane contact that **separates** the **axon endings** of one **neuron** from the **dendrites** of **another neuron** is known as a **synapse**. Several substances have been identified as **neurotransmitters**. Well known neurotransmitters include **acetylcholine, noradrenaline, adrenaline and dopamine**.

Reflexes

One type of route **travelled by nerve impulses** is a reflex or **reflex arc**. A **reflex** is the **basic unit** of the nervous system that is capable of **receiving a stimulus** and **generating a response**.

Individual reflexes vary in complexity; some function to **remove the body from painful stimuli**, some **prevent the body from suddenly falling** or moving as a result of external forces, and others are responsible for **maintaining a relatively constant blood pressure**, body **fluid pH**, blood **carbon dioxide level** and **water intake**. All reflexes are **homoeostatic**; that is, they function to **maintain healthy survival.**

Blood supply

The arterial **blood supply to the brain** comes from the **vertebral arteries** and the **internal carotid arteries**. The **veins that drain blood from the head** form the **venous sinuses** (these are **spaces in the dura mater** surrounding the brain); eventually they **drain into the internal jugular veins**.

Ventricles

Each **cerebral hemisphere** contains a **large space** (known as a **lateral ventricle**) that is **filled with cerebrospinal fluid (CSF)**.

Divisions of the brain

The major divisions of the adult brain are the **brain-stem (medulla, pons, mid-brain and the site of the reticular formation), cerebellum, diencephalon (hypothalamus and thalamus)** and **cerebrum**.

Exercise 1
Match the column A with the column B. Try to learn the expressions and/or sentences by heart.

A

1. The nervous system is divided into
2. The CNS consists of
3. The cells of the nervous system
4. Each neuron has three main parts:
5. Dendrites transmit impulses to the cell bodies
6. Bundles of parallel axons with their associated sheaths
7. Collections of nerve cells are called grey matter; the outer surface of the cerebrum and the cerebellum
8. Neurons are classified as
9. Sensory neurons transmit impulse
10. Motor neurons transmit impulses
11. Sensory neurons also are called afferent neurons
12. The membrane-to-membrane contact that separates the axon endings of one neuron
13. Well known neurotransmitters include
14. A reflex is the basic unit of the nervous system
15. Some reflexes function to remove the body from painful stimuli, some prevent the body from suddenly falling
16. The arterial blood supply to the brain
17. The veins that drain blood from the head form the venous sinuses (these are spaces in the dura mater surrounding the brain)
18. Each cerebral hemisphere contains a large space (known as a lateral ventricle)
19. The major divisions of the adult brain are the brain-stem (medulla, pons, mid-brain and the site of the reticular formation),

B

a) *(1) the cell body; (2) one or more branching projections, called dendrites; and (3) a single, elongated projection, known as an axon.*

b) *acetylcholine, noradrenaline, adrenaline and dopamine.*

c) *and motor neurons are called efferent neurons.*

d) *and still others are responsible for maintaining a relatively constant blood pressure, body fluid pH, blood carbon dioxide level and water intake.*

e) *are white and are called white matter.*

f) *cerebellum, diencephalon (hypothalamus and thalamus) and cerebrum.*

g) *comes from the vertebral arteries and the internal carotid arteries.*

h) *consists of grey matter, which forms the cerebral cortex and the cerebellar cortex.*

i) *eventually they drain into the internal jugular veins.*

j) *from the dendrites of another neuron is known as a synapse.*

k) *in the opposite direction, away from the brain and spinal cord.*

l) *include neurons and connective tissue cells known as neuroglia.*

m) *sensory neurons, motor neurons or inter-neurons.*

n) *that is capable of receiving a stimulus and generating a response.*

o) *that is filled with cerebrospinal fluid (CSF).*

p) *the brain and spinal cord.*

q) *the central nervous system (CNS) and the peripheral nervous system (PNS).*

r) *to the spinal cord and brain from all parts of the body.*

s) *whilst axons transmit impulses away from the cell bodies.*

Exercise 2

Translate the expressions. Try to explain their meanings in English.

Chiefly, ability to coordinate, regulate, brain and spinal cord, connective tissue, neuroglia, cell body, projections, dendrites, elongated projection, axon, transmit, bundles, parallel sheaths, collections, outer surface, cortex, sensory, motor, opposite direction, afferent, efferent neurons, separates axon endings, synapse, neurotransmitters, route, capable, generating a response, complexity, painful stimuli, carbon dioxide level, water intake, maintain healthy survival, vertebral arteries, carotid arteries, dura mater, jugular veins, hemisphere, cerebrospinal fluid, brain-stem (medulla, pons, mid-brain and the site of the reticular formation), cerebellum, diencephalon (hypothalamus and thalamus) and cerebrum.

Exercise 3

Answer the following questions. Prepare short talks and/or dialogues on these topics.

1. Describe the anatomy of the nervous system (CNS) and (PNS).
2. Characterize the cells of the nervous system and types of neurons.
3. Explain the terms impulse, transmission, synapse and reflexes.
4. Talk about blood supply to the brain and divisions of the brain.

Vocabulary 2

Fill in the meanings in your mother language:

acetylcholine /ˌæs.ɪ.taɪlˈkəʊliːn/
afferent /ˈæf.ər.ənt/
axon /ˈæk.sɑn/
blood /blʌd/ **pressure** /ˈpreʃ.ər/
brain /breɪn/
brainstem /ˈbreɪn.stem/
branch /brɑːntʃ/
bundle /ˈbʌn.dl/
capable /ˈkeɪ.pə.bl̩/
carbon /ˈkɑː.bən/ **dioxide** /
daɪˈɒk.saɪd/
carotid /kəˌrɒt.ɪd/
cell /sel/ **body** /ˈbɒd.i/
central /ˈsen.trəl/
cerebellar /ˌser.ɪˈbel.ər/
cerebellum /ˌser.əˈbel.əm/
cerebral /ˈser.ɪ.brəl/
cerebrospinal /ˌser.əbrəˈspaɪ.nəl/
cerebrum /sɪˈriː.brəm/
chiefly /ˈtʃiː.fli/
collection /kəˈlekʃən/
complexity /kəmˈplek.sɪ.ti/
connect /kəˈnekt/
connective tissue /kəˌnek.tɪvˈtɪʃ.uː/
consist /kənˈsɪst/
constant /ˈkɒn.stənt/
coordinate /kəʊˈɔː.dɪ.neɪt/
cortex /ˈkɔː.teks/ pl
cortices /ˈkɔː.tɪ..siːz/
dendrite /ˈden.draɪt/
diencephalon /ˌdaɪ.enˈsef.əˌlɒn/
direction /da ɪˈrek.ʃən/
division /dɪˈvɪʒ.ən/
dopamine /ˈdəʊ.pə.mɪːn/
dura mater /ˌdjʊə.rəˈmeɪ.tər/
efferent /ˈef.ər.ənt/ **neuron** /ˈnjʊə.rɒn/
elongated /ˈiː.lɒŋ.geɪ.tɪd/
ending /ˈen.dɪŋ/
eventually /ɪˈven.tju.əl.i/
external /ɪkˈstɜː.nəl/
fall /ˈfɔːl/
fluid /ˈfluː.ɪd/
generate /ˈdʒen.ər.eɪt/
hemisphere /ˈhem.ɪ.sfɪər/
homeostasis /ˌhəʊ.mi.əʊˈsteɪ.sɪs/
homeostatic /ˌhəʊ.mi.əʊˈstæt.ɪk/
hypothalamus /ˌhaɪ.pəʊˈθæl.ə.məs/
identify /aɪˈden.tɪ.faɪ/
impulse /ˈɪm.pʌls/
individual /ˌɪn.dɪˈvɪd.ju.əl/
intake /ˈɪn.teɪk/
internal /ɪnˈtɜː.nəl/
interneuron /ˌɪntəˈnjʊər.ɒn/
jugular /ˈdʒʌg.jʊ.lə/
lateral /ˈlæt.rəl/
maintain /meɪnˈteɪn/
matter /ˈmæt.ər/
membrane /ˈmem.breɪn/
midbrain /mɪd.breɪn/
motor /ˈməʊ.tər/
moving /ˈmuːvɪŋ/
nervous /ˈnɜː.vəs/ **system** /sɪstəm/
neuron /ˈnjʊə.rɒn/
neurotransmitter /ˌnjʊə.
rəʊ.trænzˈmɪt.ər/
opposite /ˈɒp.ə.zɪt/
outer /ˈaʊ.tər/
painful /ˈpeɪn.fəl/
parallel /ˈpær.ə.lel/
part /pɑːt/
pons /pɒnz/
prevent /prɪˈvent/
projection /prəˈdʒek.ʃən/
reflex /ˈriː.fleks/ **arc** /ɑːk/
regulate /ˈregjʊˌleɪt/
responsible /rɪˈspɒnt.sɪ.bl̩/
result /rɪˈzʌlt/
reticular /rɪˈtɪk.jʊ.lər/
formation /fɔːˈmeɪ.ʃən/
sensory /ˈsen.sər.i/
sheath /ʃiːθ/
space /speɪs/
state /steɪt/
stimulus /ˈstɪm.jʊ.ləs/ pl **stimuli**
substance /ˈsʌb.stəns/

suddenly /ˈsʌd.ən.li/
surface /ˈsɜː.fɪs/
survival /səˈvaɪ.vəl/
synapse /ˈsaɪ.næps/
thalamus /ˈθæl.ə.məs/
tissue /ˈtɪʃ.uː/
transmission /trænzˈmɪʃ.ən/
transmit /trænzˈmɪt/
vary /ˈveə.ri/
vertebral /ˈvɜː.tɪ.brə/
white /waɪt/ **matter** /ˈmæt.ər/

Solution to Exercise 1
1q, 2p, 3l, 4a, 5s, 6e, 7h, 8m, 9r, 10k, 11c, 12j, 13b, 14n, 15d, 16g, 17i, 18o, 19f

Unit 3 - Endocrine system

Anatomy and physiology of the endocrine system

The endocrine system is composed of **ductless glands** and **tissues that produce and secrete hormones**. The **major** endocrine glands are **the pituitary, thyroid, and parathyroid glands; the adrenal cortex and medulla; the pancreatic islets; and the ovaries and testes. Other** specialized groups of cells are found in the **kidneys** and the mucosa of the **gastrointestinal tract.**

Endocrine gland functions

Endocrine glands secrete hormones **directly into the bloodstream** and serve to **regulate** various **metabolic functions**. The products of endocrine glands travel **via the blood (or tissue fluids**) so are able to **exert their effects** on the entire body. This **integrated** chemical and coordination **system** enables **reproduction, growth** and **development**, and the regulation of **energy**. Target organs and body tissues have **hormone receptors** and are able to respond to a certain hormone.

Hormone receptors

Most hormones can be categorized as **proteins, polypeptides, derivatives of amino acids, or lipids**. Each hormone may affect a **specific organ or tissue, or** it may have a **general effect** on the entire body. **Steroid hormones** are manufactured by **endocrine cells** from cholesterol, and include **cortisol, aldosterone, oestrogen, progesterone and testosterone. Nonsteroid** hormones are synthesized chiefly **from amino acids** and include **insulin and parathyroid hormone**, amongst others.

Hormones affect only cells with **appropriate receptors** and act to initiate specific cell functions or activities. Cells with fewer receptor sites bind with less hormone. Abnormalities can result in **endocrine disorders.**

Regulation of hormone secretion

All hormones operate with **feedback systems** that help to maintain an **optimal internal environment**. These feedback systems are either positive or negative. An example of **positive feedback** can be found in **childbirth**. The hormone **oxytocin** stimulates and enhances **labour contractions**. The contractions intensify and increase until the baby is outside the birth canal. When the stimulus to the pressure receptors ends, oxytocin production stops. Labour contractions also stop. **Negative feedback** is the mechanism most commonly used to **maintain homoeostasis** and works by reversing a change in a controlled condition such as blood glucose levels. On the other hand, **hormone production** is stimulated **when serum levels of the hormone fall.** For example, the **hypothalamus receptors** monitor blood levels of thyroid hormones. Low blood levels of thyroid-stimulating hormone (TSH) cause the release of TSH-releasing hormone from the hypothalamus. This, in turn, causes the release of **TSH** from the **anterior pituitary**. TSH **travels to the thyroid**, where it promotes the production of thyroid hormones. These, in turn, regulate the **metabolic rate and body temperature.**

Specific disorders of the endocrine system

Disorders of the endocrine system **arise from** the effects of an **imbalance** in the production of one or more hormones. The clinical effects are determined by the **degree of dysfunction**. They are also determined by the individual's **age and gender.**

Disorders of the pancreas: diabetes mellitus

Diabetes mellitus is a **systemic disease of the endocrine system** that usually results from a **dysfunction of the pancreas**. It is a complex disorder of **fat, carbohydrate, and protein metabolism**. Diabetes mellitus is **potentially lethal** and can put the patient at risk for several kinds of true **medical emergencies.**

Anatomy and physiology of the pancreas

The pancreas is important in the absorption and use of carbohydrates, fat, and protein, and is the **chief regulator of glucose levels** in the blood. The healthy pancreas has **exocrine and endocrine** functions. Exocrine glands secrete substances **through a duct** onto the inner surface of an organ or the outer surface of the body; **endocrine glands** are those that **secrete chemicals** directly (not through a duct) **into the bloodstream**. The exocrine portion consists of **acini (glands that produce pancreatic juice)** and **a duct system** that carries the pancreatic juice **to the small intestine**. The **endocrine portion** consists of pancreatic islets (**islets of Langerhans**) that **produce hormones.**

Insulin

Primary functions of insulin

- To increase **glucose transport** into cells
- To increase glucose **metabolism** by cells
- To increase **liver glycogen** levels
- To **decrease blood glucose concentration** toward normal levels

Glucagon

Glucagon has two major effects. One effect is to **increase blood glucose** levels, which it does by **stimulating the liver to release glucose stores. The other effect** is to **stimulate gluconeogenesis** (glucose formation) through the **breakdown of fats and fatty acids.**

Growth hormone

Growth hormone (GH) is produced and secreted by the **anterior pituitary** gland. GH secretion is **triggered** by many physiological stimuli such as **exercise, stress, sleep, and hypoglycaemia.**

Regulation of glucose metabolism

Under normal conditions, the body maintains the **serum glucose level** in the blood **at 3.9-6.1 mmol/L.**

Dietary intake

The **three** main **organic components** of food are **carbohydrates, fats and proteins** (food also contains minerals and vitamins). Carbohydrates are found in all **sugary, starchy foods**. They are the **first food substances** to enter the **bloodstream** after a meal is ingested. If not "burned" for immediate energy, **glucose is stored** in the **liver and muscles as glycogen** or **converted into fat by adipose tissue.**

Exercise 1

Match the column A with the column B. Try to learn the expressions and/or sentences by heart.

A

1. The endocrine system is composed of
2. The major endocrine glands are
3. Endocrine glands secrete hormones
4. This integrated chemical and coordination system
5. Most hormones can be categorized as
6. Each hormone may affect a specific organ or tissue,
7. Steroid hormones are manufactured by endocrine cells from cholesterol,
8. Non-steroid hormones are synthesized chiefly from amino acids and
9. Cells with fewer receptor sites bind with less hormone;
10. All hormones operate with feedback systems
11. An example of positive feedback can be found in childbirth;
12. Negative feedback is
13. Hormone production is stimulated
14. Disorders of the endocrine system
15. Diabetes mellitus is a systemic disease of the endocrine system
16. It is a complex disorder of
17. The pancreas is important in the absorption and use of carbohydrates, fat, and protein,
18. The healthy pancreas
19. Endocrine glands are those

20. The exocrine portion consists of acini (glands that produce pancreatic juice)
21. The endocrine portion consists of
22. Primary functions of insulin are:
23. One effect of glucagon is to increase blood glucose levels, which it does by stimulating the liver to release glucose stores;
24. Growth hormone (GH) is produced and secreted by the anterior pituitary gland;
25. The three main organic components of food are
26. Glucose is stored in the liver and muscles as glycogen,

B

a) *abnormalities can result in endocrine disorders.*
b) *and a duct system that carries the pancreatic juice to the small intestine.*
c) *and include cortisol, aldosterone, oestrogen, progesterone and testosterone.*
d) *and is the chief regulator of glucose levels in the blood.*
e) *arise from the effects of an imbalance in the production of one or more hormones.*
f) *carbohydrates, fats and proteins (food also contains minerals and vitamins).*
g) *directly into the bloodstream and serve to regulate various metabolic functions.*
h) *ductless glands and tissues that produce and secrete hormones.*
i) *enables reproduction, growth and development, and the regulation of energy.*
j) *fat, carbohydrate, and protein metabolism.*
k) *has exocrine and endocrine functions.*
l) *include insulin and parathyroid hormone.*
m) *its secretion is triggered by many physiological stimuli such as exercise, stress, sleep, and hypoglycaemia.*
n) *or converted into fat by adipose tissue.*
o) *or it may have a general effect on the entire body.*
p) *pancreatic islets (islets of Langerhans) that produce hormones.*
q) *proteins, polypeptides, derivatives of amino acids, or lipids.*
r) *that help to maintain an optimal internal environment.*
s) *that secrete chemicals directly (not through a duct) into the bloodstream.*
t) *that usually results from a dysfunction of the pancreas.*
u) *the hormone oxytocin stimulates and enhances labour contractions.*
v) *the other effect is to stimulate gluconeogenesis (glucose formation) through the breakdown of fats and fatty acids.*

w) *the pituitary, thyroid, and parathyroid glands; the adrenal cortex and medulla; the pancreatic islets; and the ovaries and testes.*

x) *to increase glucose transport into cells, to increase glucose metabolism by cells, to increase liver glycogen levels and to decrease blood glucose concentration toward normal levels.*

y) *used to maintain homoeostasis.*

z) *when serum levels of the hormone fall.*

Exercise 2
Translate the expressions. Try to explain their meanings in English.

Ductless glands, tissues, secrete, pituitary, thyroid, parathyroid glands, adrenal cortex and medulla, pancreatic islets, ovaries and testes, bloodstream, via, tissue fluids, exert their effects, integrated, target organs, proteins, polypeptides, derivatives of amino acids, or lipids, general effect, entire body, cortisol, aldosterone, oestrogen, progesterone, testosterone, appropriate receptors, initiate, bind with, endocrine disorders, feedback, internal environment, oxytocin stimulates, enhances labour contractions, reversing a change in serum levels, blood levels, in turn, anterior pituitary, metabolic rate, arise from, imbalance, determined, degree of dysfunction, age and gender, systemic disease, dysfunction, fat, carbohydrate, and protein metabolism, potentially lethal, medical emergencies, absorption and use, exocrine and endocrine function, outer surface, acini, duct system, small intestine, increase blood glucose, release glucose stores, stimulate gluconeogenesis, breakdown of fats and fatty acids, triggered by serum glucose level, dietary intake, carbohydrates, fats and proteins, sugary, starchy foods, ingested, glucose is stored, converted into adipose tissue.

Exercise 3
Answer the following questions. Prepare short talks and/or dialogues on these topics.

1. Describe the anatomy and physiology of the endocrine system.
2. Talk about hormone receptors and regulation of hormone secretion.
3. Talk about diabetes as a specific disorder of the endocrine system.
4. Anatomy and physiology of the pancreas.
5. Functions of insulin; effects of glucagon; regulation of glucose metabolism.
6. Main organic components of food.

Vocabulary 3

Fill in the meanings in your mother language:

abnormality /ˌæb.nɔːˈmæl.ə.ti/
absorption /əbˈzɔːp.ʃən/
acinus /ˈæs.ɪ.nəs/ pl **acini** /ˈæs.ɪ.naɪ/

act /ækt/
activity /æk'tɪv.ɪ.ti/
adipose /'æd.ɪ.pəʊz/
aldosterone /'ɔːl.dəs.tər.əʊn/
amino acid /əˌmiː.nəʊ'æs.ɪd/
anterior /æn'tɪərɪə/
appropriate /ə'prəʊ.pri.ət/
arise /ə'raɪz/
bind /baɪnd/
birth /'bɜːθ/ **canal** /kə'næl/
bloodstream /'blʌd.striːm/
breakdown /'breɪk.daʊn/
carbohydrate /ˌkɑː.bəʊ 'haɪ.dreɪt/
categorize /'kæt.ə.gər.aɪz/
chemical /'kem.ɪ.kəl/
chief /tʃif/
childbirth /'tʃaɪld.bɜːθ/
cholesterol /kə'les.tər.ɒl/
complex /kɒm.pleks/
component /kəm'pəʊ.nənt/
composed /kəm'pəʊzd/ **of** /əv/
condition /kən'dɪʃən/
convert /kən'vɜːt/
cortisol /'kɔː.tɪ.sɒl/
degree /dɪ'griː/
derivative /dɪ'rɪv.ə.tɪv/
determine /dɪ'tɜː.mɪn/
development /dɪ'vel.əp.mənt/
diabetes /ˌdaɪə'biː.tiːz/
mellitus /mə'laɪ.təs/
disorder /dɪ'sɔː.dər/
ductless gland /ˌdʌkt.ləs'glænd/
dysfunction /dɪs'fʌŋk.ʃən/
effect /ɪ'fekt/
emergency /ɪ'mɜː.dʒənt .si/
enable /ɪ'neɪ.bl̩/
endocrine /'en.də.krɪn/
enhance /ɪn'hɑːns/
entire /ɪn'taɪə/
environment /ɪn'vaɪə .rən .mənt/
exercise /'ek.sə.saɪz/
exert /ɪg'zɜːt/
exocrine /'ek.səʊ.kraɪn/
fat /fæt/
fatty /'fæt.i/ **acids** /'æs.ɪds/
feedback /'fiːd.bæk/
gender /'dʒen.dər/
gland /glænd/
glucagon /gluːkə.gən/
glucose /'gluː.kəʊs/
glycogen /'glaɪ.kəʊ.dʒən/
growth /grəʊθ/
hormone /'hɔː.məʊn/
hypoglycaemia /ˌhaɪ.pəʊ .glaɪ'siː.mi.ə/
imbalance /ˌɪm'bæl.ənt s/
immediate /ɪ'miː.di.ət/
in /ɪn/ **turn** /tɜːn/
ingest /ɪn'dʒest/
initiate /ɪ'nɪʃ.i.eɪt/
inner /'ɪn.ər/
integrated /'ɪn.tɪ.greɪ.t̬ ɪd/
intensify /ɪn'tensɪˌfaɪ/
islets /'aɪ.ləts/ **of Langerhans** /'læŋəˌhæns/
juice /dʒuːs/
labour /'leɪ.bər/
lethal /'liː.θəl/
level /'lev.əl/
lipid /'lɪp.ɪd/
major /'meɪ.dʒər/
manufacture /ˌmæn.jʊ'fæk.tʃər/
metabolism /mə'tæb.əl.ɪ.zəm/
nonsteroid /ˌnɒn.stɛ'rɔɪd/
oestrogen /'iː.strə.dʒən/
ovary /'əʊ.vər.i/
oxytocin /ˌɒk.sɪ'təʊ.sɪn/
pancreas /'pæŋ.kri.əs/
pancreatic /ˌpæŋ.krɪ'æ.tɪk/ **islets** /'aɪ.ləts/
pancreatic /pæŋ.kri'æt.ik/
parathyroid gland /ˌpær.ə'θaɪ.rɔɪdˌglænd/
pituitary gland /pɪ'tjuː.ɪ.tər.iˌglænd/
polypeptide /ˌpɒl.ɪ'pep.taɪd/
portion /'pɔː.ʃən/
potentially /pə'ten.ʃəl.i/
progesterone /prəʊ'dʒes.tər.əʊn/
promote /prə'məʊt/
protein /'prəʊ.tiːn/
receptor /rɪ'sep.tər/

reproduction /ˌriː.prəˈdʌk.ʃən/
reverse /rɪˈvɜːs/
secrete /sɪˈkriːt/
serum /ˈsɪə.rəm/ pl **sera**
serve /sɜːv/
small /smɔːl/ **intestine** /ɪnˈtes.tɪn/
starchy /ˈstɑː.tʃi/
store /stɔːr/
synthesize /ˈsɪnθɪˌsaɪz/
target /ˈtɑː.gɪt/
temperature /ˈtem.prə.tʃər/
testis /ˈtes.tɪs/ pl **testes** /ˈtes.tiːz/
testosterone /ˌtesˈtɒs.tər.əʊn/
thyroid /ˈθaɪə.rɔɪd/
transport /ˈtræn.spɔːt/
trigger /ˈtrɪg.ər/
via /ˈvaɪə/

Solution to Exercise 1
1h, 2w, 3g, 4i, 5q, 6o, 7c, 8l, 9a, 10r, 11u, 12y, 13z, 14e, 15t, 16j, 17d, 18k, 19s, 20b, 21p, 22x, 23v, 24m, 25f, 26n

Unit 4 - Diabetes mellitus 1

Process of digestion

Before food compounds can be **used** by body cells, they must be **digested** and **absorbed** into the **bloodstream**. Digestion begins **in the mouth** and is accomplished by **physical** forces (**chewing**) and **chemical (enzymatic)** forces. This begins the process that reduces the food to **soluble molecules and particles** small enough to be absorbed. After food is **swallowed** it enters the **stomach**. There, various **nutrients** are absorbed into the **circulatory system**. These nutrients include **glucose, salts, water**, and some other substances (**alcohol** and certain other **drugs**). The remaining material (**chyme**) is **shunted** from the stomach into the **intestine** for further digestion.

The **duodenum** signals the release of **hormones** that mobilize the **pancreas** to contribute its molecule-splitting **enzymes** and the **gallbladder** to release **bile salts.** These enzymes and salts **neutralize acids** and help **emulsify fats. Carbohydrates** are absorbed as **simple sugars**, **fats** are absorbed as **fatty acids** and **glycerol**, and **proteins** are absorbed as **amino acids. These nutrients** are then carried from the intestine to the **liver** by way of the **portal vein**. **Water** and **remaining salts** are absorbed **from food residues** reaching the **colon**.

When **blood glucose** level begins to **fall**, the **liver releases glucose back** into the circulating blood. Thus, the liver removes glucose from the blood when it is excess after dietary intake and returns it to the blood when it is **needed between meals.** If the muscles are not exercised after a meal, much of the **glucose** transported into the muscle cells by insulin is **stored as muscle glycogen**. The stored glycogen must be used by the muscle **for energy**.

The brain is quite different from other body tissues with regard to glucose uptake. The cells of the brain do not have adequate storage capacity. The **brain** normally uses **only glucose for energy**. Thus it is **essential** that **serum glucose** be **maintained** at a level that provides adequate energy to these tissues.

When the serum glucose level **falls too low**, signs and symptoms of **hypoglycaemia** can develop quickly. These include progressive **irritability, altered mental states, fainting, convulsions**, and even **coma**.

The four mechanisms for achieving adequate blood glucose **regulation** are as follows:

- The **liver** functions as a blood glucose buffer system, it **removes glucose** from the blood **when it is in excess** (and stores it as glycogen), and **returns** glucose to the blood when the **glucose concentration and insulin secretion decline.**
- **Insulin and glucagon** function as a **feedback control system**. They work to maintain normal serum glucose concentrations. When serum **glucose levels rise, insulin is secreted to lower them** towards normal. On the other hand, when **serum glucose levels fall, glucagon is secreted to raise** the serum glucose level towards normal.
- **Low serum glucose** levels stimulate the **sympathetic nervous system** to **secrete adrenaline.** Adrenaline, and, to a lesser degree, noradrenaline have a glucagon-like effect that promotes liver glycogenolysis.
- **GH and cortisol** play a role in less immediate regulation of serum glucose levels. They are **secreted in response to more prolonged hypoglycaemic episodes**. (For example this might be a late overnight fast). They tend to increase the rate of glucose production. They tend to decrease the rate of glucose use.

Type 1 diabetes mellitus

Type 1 diabetes is characterized by **inadequate production of insulin by the pancreas**. It may occur any time after birth but it usually occurs in **teenagers** and young adults. **Heredity** is a factor in type 1 diabetes. Type 1 diabetes requires lifelong treatment with **insulin injections**, exercise, and diet regulation. The symptoms include **polyuria, polydipsia, dizziness, blurred vision, and rapid, unexplained weight loss**.

Type 2 diabetes mellitus

Type 2 diabetes is usually characterized by a **decrease in the production of insulin** by the **pancreatic beta cells** and **diminished tissue sensitivity to insulin**. The disease most often occurs in adults over 40 years of age and in those who are overweight; **obesity** predisposes a person to this form of diabetes. Most patients with type 2 diabetes require **oral hypoglycaemic medications, exercise**, and **dietary regulation** to control their illness. A small number of patients require insulin injection. **Fatigue, changes in appetite, and tingling, numbness, and pain in the extremities** are also indicators.

Exercise 1
Match the column A with the column B. Try to learn the expressions and/or sentences by heart.

A

1. Before food compounds can be used by body cells,
2. Digestion begins in the mouth
3. This begins the process that reduces the food
4. After food is swallowed
5. The chyme is shunted from the stomach
6. The duodenum signals the release of hormones
7. Carbohydrates are absorbed as simple sugars, fats are absorbed as fatty acids and glycerol,
8. These nutrients are then carried from the intestine to the liver by way of the portal vein;
9. The brain is quite different from other body tissues with regard to glucose uptake,
10. Signs and symptoms of hypoglycaemia
11. The liver removes glucose from the blood when it is in excess (and stores it as glycogen),
12. Insulin and glucagon work to
13. When serum glucose levels rise,
14. When serum glucose levels fall,
15. Low serum glucose levels stimulate
16. GH and cortisol are secreted
17. Type 1 diabetes is characterized
18. Type 1 diabetes requires lifelong treatment
19. The symptoms include
20. Type 2 diabetes is usually characterized
21. Most patients with type 2 diabetes require
22. Fatigue, changes in appetite, and tingling,

B

a) *and is accomplished by physical forces (chewing) and chemical (enzymatic) forces.*
b) *and proteins are absorbed as amino acids.*
c) *and returns glucose to the blood when the glucose concentration and insulin secretion decline.*
d) *because the cells of the brain do not have adequate storage capacity.*
e) *by a decrease in the production of insulin by the pancreatic beta cells and diminished tissue sensitivity to insulin.*
f) *by inadequate production of insulin by the pancreas.*
g) *glucagon is secreted to raise the serum glucose level towards normal.*

h) *in response to more prolonged hypoglycaemic episodes.*

i) *include progressive irritability, altered mental states, fainting, convulsions, and coma.*

j) *insulin is secreted to lower them towards normal.*

k) *into the intestine for further digestion.*

l) *it enters the stomach.*

m) *maintain normal serum glucose concentrations.*

n) *numbness, and pain in the extremities are also indicators.*

o) *oral hypoglycaemic medications, exercise, and dietary regulation to control their illness.*

p) *polyuria, polydipsia, dizziness, blurred vision, and rapid, unexplained weight loss.*

q) *that mobilize the pancreas to contribute its molecule-splitting enzymes and the gallbladder to release bile salts; these enzymes and salts neutralize acids and help emulsify fats.*

r) *the sympathetic nervous system to secrete adrenaline.*

s) *they must be digested and absorbed into the bloodstream.*

t) *to soluble molecules and particles small enough to be absorbed.*

u) *water and remaining salts are absorbed from food residues reaching the colon.*

v) *with insulin injections, exercise, and diet regulation.*

Exercise 2

Translate the expressions. Try to explain their meanings in English.

Compounds, chewing, enzymatic, soluble, particles, swallowed, chyme, shunted, intestine, duodenum, release, contribute, gallbladder, bile salts, emulsify fats, portal vein, residues, colon, dietary intake, exercised, stored, muscle glycogen, uptake, storage capacity, progressive irritability, altered mental states, fainting, convulsions, coma, in excess, decline, rise, lower towards normal, promotes, in response to, overnight fast, the rate of, decrease, inadequate, heredity, lifelong treatment, polyuria, polydipsia, dizziness, blurred vision, weight loss, diminished sensitivity, overweight, predisposes, fatigue, tingling, numbness, pain in the extremities, indicators.

Exercise 3

Answer the following questions. Prepare short talks and/or dialogues on these topics.

1. How would you describe the process of digestion?
2. What are the mechanisms for achieving adequate blood glucose regulation?
3. What are the signs and symptoms of type 1 diabetes mellitus?
4. What are the signs and symptoms of type 2 diabetes mellitus?

Vocabulary 4

Fill in the meanings in your mother language:

absorbed /əbˈzɔːbd/
accomplished /əˈkʌm.plɪʃt/
achieve /əˈtʃiːv/
adequate /ˈæd.ə.kwət/
altered /ˈɒl.tərd/
beta /ˈbiː.tə/ **cells** /selz/
bile /baɪl/
blurred /blɜːd/
buffer /ˈbʌf.ər/
capacity /kəˈpæs.ə.ti/
chew /tʃuː/
chyme /kaɪm/
circulate /ˈsɜː.kjʊ.leɪt/
colon /ˈkəʊ.lɒn/
coma /ˈkəʊ.mə/
compound /ˈkɒm.paʊnd/
contribute /kənˈtrɪb.juːt/
convulsion /kənˈvʌl.ʃən/
decline /dɪˈklaɪn/
digest /daɪˈdʒest/
digestion /daɪˈdʒes.tʃən/
diminish /dɪˈmɪn.ɪʃ/
dizziness /ˈdɪz.ɪ.nəs/
duodenum /ˌdjuː.əˈdiː.nəm/
enzymatic /ˌen.zaɪˈmə.tɪk/
episode /ˈep.ɪ.səʊd/
essential /ɪˈsen.tʃəl/
excess /ekˈses/
extremity /ɪkˈstrem.ɪ.ti/
faint /feɪnt/
fast /fɑːst/
fatigue /fəˈtiːg/
gallbladder /ˈgɔːlˈblæd.ər/
glycerol /ˈglɪs.ə.rɒl/
glycogenolysis /ˌglaɪ.kə.dʒɪˈnɒ.lɪ.sɪs/
heredity /həˈred.ə.ti/
hypoglycaemic /ˌhaɪ.pəʊ.glaɪˈsiː.mik/
inadequate /ɪˈnæd.ɪ.kwət/
indicator /ˈɪn.dɪ.keɪ.tər/
insulin /ˈɪn.sjʊ.lɪn/
intestine /ɪnˈtes.tɪn/
irritability /ˌɪr.ɪ.təˈbɪl.ɪ.ti/
lifelong /ˈlaɪf.lɒŋ/
lower /ˈləʊ.ə/
mental /ˈmen.təl/
neutralize /ˈnjuː.trə.laɪz/
noradrenaline /ˌnɔːr.əˈdrɛn.ə.lɪn/
numbness /ˈnʌm.nəs/
overnight /ˌəʊ.vəˈnaɪt/
overweight /ˌəʊ.vəˈweɪt/
particle /ˈpɑː.tɪ.kl̩/
polydipsia /ˌpɒl.ɪˈdɪp.sɪ.ə/
polyuria /ˌpɒl.ɪˈjʊə.rɪ.ə/
portal /ˈpɔː.təl/ **vein** /veɪn/
predispose /ˌpriː.dɪˈspəʊz/
progressive /prəˈgres.ɪv/
prolonged /prəˈlɒŋd/
regard /rɪˈgɑːd/
remain /rɪˈmeɪn/
require /rɪˈkwaɪər/
residue /ˈrez.ɪ.djuː/
response /rɪˈspɒns/
secretion /sɪˈkriː.ʃən/
sensitivity /ˌsent.sɪˈtɪv.ɪ.ti/
shunt /ʃʌnt/
soluble /ˈsɒljʊbəl/
splitting /ˈsplɪt.ɪŋ/
storage /ˈstɔː.rɪdʒ/
swallow /ˈswɒl.əʊ/
sympathetic /ˌsɪm.pəˈθe.tɪk/
tend to /tend/
tingling /ˈtɪŋ.gl.ɪŋ/
treatment /ˈtriːt.mənt/
unexplained /ˌʌnɪkˈspleɪnd/
uptake /ˈʌp.teɪk/
use /juːz/
vision /ˈvɪʒ.ən/

Solution to Exercise 1

1s, 2a, 3t, 4l, 5k, 6q, 7b, 8u, 9d, 10i, 11c, 12m, 13j, 14g, 15r, 16h, 17f, 18v, 19p, 20e, 21o, 22n

Unit 5 - Diabetes mellitus 2

Effects of diabetes mellitus

Most effects of diabetes mellitus can be attributed to one of the following three effects of decreased insulin levels:

- **Decreased use of glucose** by the body cells, with a resultant increase in the serum glucose level
- Markedly increased mobilization of fats from the fat storage areas, causing **abnormal fat metabolism**, which may result in the short term in **ketoacidosis** and in the long term in severe **atherosclerosis**
- **Depletion of protein** in body tissues and muscle wasting

Loss of glucose in the urine

When the amount of **glucose** entering the kidneys **rises above the kidneys' ability to reabsorb it**, a significant portion of the glucose "spills" into the urine. The effect is dehydration.

Acidosis in diabetes

The **shift from carbohydrate to fat metabolism** results in the formation of **strongly acidic ketone bodies** (called ketoacids). Continuous production of ketoacids leads to a metabolic acidosis. This **acidosis**, along with the usually **severe dehydration** can lead to **death**. Treatment of this condition can be lifesaving. Diabetes mellitus is a systemic disease with many **long-term complications**, including the following:

- **blindness**
- **kidney** disease
- **peripheral neuropathy**, which results in nerve damage to the **hands and feet** and an increased incidence of foot infections
- **autonomic neuropathy**, which damages the **nerves controlling voluntary and involuntary** functions and may affect sexual function, bladder and bowel control, and blood pressure
- **heart disease** and **stroke**
- high blood glucose and blood fat levels contribute to **atherosclerosis**
- people with diabetes have a risk of developing **cardiovascular disease** and are likely to have a stroke
- **peripheral vascular disease** (also secondary to atherosclerosis), which results in the need for amputations

Management

The treatment of diabetes mellitus consists of drug therapy (insulin or oral hypoglycaemic agents), diet regulation, and exercise.

Insulin

Genetically engineered human insulin is available in rapid-, intermediate-, and long-acting preparations. Insulin is **administered by injection**; it is a **protein** that **would be digested** if it were consumed orally. Another way for the patient to self-administer insulin is with an insulin **infusion pump**. The patient must regularly monitor the glucose level to ensure adequate medication control.

Diabetic emergencies

Three life-threatening conditions may result from diabetes mellitus: hypoglycaemia (insulin shock), hyperglycaemia (diabetic ketoacidosis) and hyperosmolar hyperglycaemic non-ketotic coma (HHNK).

Hypoglycaemia

Hypoglycaemia is a syndrome related to blood glucose levels **bellow about 4 mmol/L**. The condition may also occur in patients who are not diabetic and is usually the result of excessive response to glucose absorption, physical **exertion, alcohol** or **drug** effects, **pregnancy** and **lactation**, or **decreased dietary intake**. In diabetics, hypoglycaemic reactions are usually caused by the following:

- too **much insulin** (or oral hypoglycaemic medication)
- decreased dietary intake (a **delayed or missed meal**)
- unusual or **vigorous physical activity**
- administration of certain **antibiotics**

Less common causes and **predisposing factors** include the following:

- chronic **alcoholism** (alcohol depletes liver glycogen stores)
- **adrenal gland dysfunction**
- **liver disease** (i.e. hepatic insufficiency or failure)
- **malnutrition**
- **pancreatic tumour**
- **cancer**
- **hypothermia**
- **sepsis**
- administration of **beta-blockers**
- administration of **salicylates in ill infants** or children
- intentional **overdose** with **insulin, oral hypoglycaemic agents** or **salicylates**

Signs and symptoms

The signs and symptoms usually **appear quickly** (often within minutes). In the early stages, the patient may complain of extreme hunger. He or she may demonstrate one or more of the following signs and symptoms:

- **nervousness**, trembling
- **irritability**
- psychotic (**combative**) **behaviour**
- **weakness** and poor coordination
- **confusion**
- **appearance of intoxication**
- **weak, rapid pulse**
- **cold, clammy skin**

- **drowsiness**
- **seizures**
- **coma** (in severe cases)

Hypoglycaemia should be suspected in any diabetic patient with behavioural changes, confusion, abnormal neurological signs, or unconsciousness. This condition is a **true emergency** that requires **immediate administration of glucose** to prevent permanent brain damage or death.

Diabetic ketoacidosis

Diabetic ketoacidosis (DKA) results from an absence of or resistance to insulin. **Common causes of diabetic ketoacidosis:**

- **Inadequate insulin** dose
- **Failure to take** insulin
- **Infection**
- Increased stress (**trauma, surgery**)
- **Increased dietary intake**
- **Decreased metabolic rate**
- Other, less common predisposing factors, including significant **emotional stress, alcohol** consumption (often associated with hypoglycaemia), and **pregnancy**

Signs and symptoms

The signs and symptoms are usually related to diuresis and acidosis. They are normally slow in onset (over 12-48 h) and include the following:

- **diuresis**
- **warm, dry skin**
- **dry mucous membranes**
- **tachycardia, thready pulse**
- **postural hypotension**
- **weight loss**
- **polyuria**
- **polydipsia**
- **acidosis**
- **abdominal pain** (usually generalized)
- **anorexia, nausea, vomiting**
- **acetone breath** odour (fruity odour)
- **Kussmaul respirations** in an attempt to reduce carbon dioxide levels
- **decreased level of consciousness**

DKA patients are seldom deeply comatose. Patients who are unresponsive should be assessed for another cause, such as head injury, stroke or drug overdose.

HHNK coma

HHNK (**hyperosmolar hyperglycaemic non-ketotic coma)** is a **life threatening** emergency that most often occurs in older patients with **type 2 diabetes** or in patients with undiagnosed diabetes.

HHNK tends to develop slowly. Often **over several days**, and it has a **high mortality rate**. Early signs and symptoms include **polyuria and polydipsia**. Associated signs and symptoms may include **orthostatic hypotension, dry mucous membranes, and tachycardia**. CNS dysfunction may result in **lethargy,**

confusion and coma. Precipitating factors include the following:

- **advanced age**
- pre-existing **cardiac or renal disease**
- **inadequate insulin** secretion or action (type 2 diabetes)
- increased insulin requirements (**stress, infection, trauma, burns, myocardial infarction**)
- **medication** use
- **supplemental parenteral and enteral feedings**

Exercise 1
Match the column A with the column B. Try to learn the expressions and/ or sentences by heart.

A

1. Most effects of diabetes mellitus can be attributed to
2. Markedly increased mobilization of fats from the fat storage areas causes abnormal fat metabolism,
3. When the amount of glucose entering the kidneys rises above the kidneys' ability to reabsorb it,
4. The shift from carbohydrate to fat metabolism
5. Continuous production of ketoacids leads to a metabolic acidosis;
6. Long-term complications of diabetes mellitus include the following:
7. Insulin is administered by injection;
8. Three life-threatening conditions may result from diabetes mellitus:
9. Hypoglycaemia is a syndrome related to
10. The condition in patients who are not diabetic is usually the result of
11. In diabetics, hypoglycaemic reactions are usually caused by:
12. Less common causes of hypoglycaemia and predisposing factors include chronic alcoholism, adrenal gland dysfunction, hepatic insufficiency or failure,
13. Signs and symptoms of hypoglycaemia include
14. Common causes of diabetic ketoacidosis are: inadequate insulin dose,
15. The signs and symptoms of diabetic ketoacidosis include the following: diuresis, warm, dry skin, dry mucous membranes,
16. HHNK (hyperosmolar hyperglycaemic non-ketotic coma)
17. HHNK tends to develop over several days,
18. Signs and symptoms include polyuria and
19. CNS dysfunction may result in
20. Precipitating factors include the following: inadequate insulin secretion or action,

B

a) *advanced age, pre-existing cardiac or renal disease, stress, infection, trauma, burns, myocardial infarction, medication use, supplemental parenteral and enteral feedings.*

b) *and it has a high mortality rate.*

c) *blindness, kidney disease, peripheral neuropathy, autonomic neuropathy, heart disease and stroke, atherosclerosis, cardiovascular disease, or peripheral vascular disease.*

d) *blood glucose levels bellow about 4 mmol/L.*

e) *decreased use of glucose by the body cells, increased mobilization of fats from the fat storage areas, or depletion of protein in body tissues and muscle wasting.*

f) *failure to take insulin, infection, increased stress (injury), increased dietary intake, decreased metabolic rate, emotional stress, alcohol consumption, pregnancy.*

g) *glucose "spills" into the urine and the effect is dehydration.*

h) *hypoglycaemia (insulin shock), hyperglycaemia (diabetic ketoacidosis) and hyperosmolar hyperglycaemic non-ketotic coma (HHNK).*

i) *is a life threatening emergency that most often occurs in older patients with type 2 diabetes.*

j) *it is a protein that would be digested if it were consumed orally.*

k) *lethargy, confusion and coma.*

l) *malnutrition, pancreatic tumour, cancer, sepsis, hypothermia, administration of beta-blockers, salicylates in ill children, intentional overdose with insulin, oral hypoglycaemic agents or salicylates.*

m) *nervousness, trembling, irritability, psychotic behaviour, weakness and poor coordination, confusion, appearance of intoxication, weak, rapid pulse, cold, clammy skin, drowsiness, seizures, coma.*

n) *physical exertion, alcohol or drug effects, pregnancy and lactation, or decreased dietary intake.*

o) *polydipsia, orthostatic hypotension, dry mucous membranes, and tachycardia.*

p) *results in the formation of strongly acidic ketone bodies (called ketoacids).*

q) *tachycardia, thready pulse, postural hypotension, weight loss, polyuria, polydipsia, acidosis, abdominal pain, anorexia, nausea, vomiting, acetone breath odour, Kussmaul respirations, decreased level of consciousness.*

r) this acidosis, along with the usually severe dehydration can lead to death.

s) too much insulin, a delayed or missed meal, vigorous physical activity, and certain antibiotics.

t) which may result in the short term in ketoacidosis and in the long term in severe atherosclerosis.

Exercise 2
Translate the expressions. Try to explain their meanings in English.

Attributed, decreased use, resultant, storage areas, in the long term, depletion, muscle wasting, urine, ability, significant portion, shift, strongly acidic, continuous, acidosis, lifesaving, systemic disease, blindness, neuropathy, incidence, bladder and bowel control, are likely to, genetically engineered, administered by injection, self-administer, emergencies, physical exertion, pregnancy and lactation, missed meal, vigorous physical activity, predisposing factors, salicylates in ill infants, intentional overdose, appear quickly, demonstrate, trembling, irritability, combative behaviour, weakness, confusion, cold, clammy skin, drowsiness, unconsciousness, permanent brain damage, absence of or resistance to, failure, trauma, surgery, emotional stress, diuresis, dry mucous membranes, tachycardia, thready pulse, postural, breath odour, carbon dioxide level, unresponsive, drug overdose, life threatening emergency, mortality rate, precipitating factors, advanced age, burns, supplemental parenteral and enteral feedings,

Exercise 3
Answer the following questions. Prepare short talks and/or dialogues on these topics.

1. What are the effects of decreased insulin levels?
2. What are long-term complications of diabetes mellitus?
3. Explain the term diabetic emergencies.
4. Predisposing factors, signs and symptoms of hypoglycaemia.
5. Predisposing factors, signs and symptoms of diabetic ketoacidosis.
6. Predisposing factors, signs and symptoms of HHNK (hyperosmolar hyperglycaemic non-ketotic coma).

Vocabulary 5

Fill in the meanings in your mother language:

abdominal /æbˈdɒm.ɪ.nəl/
acetone /ˈæs.ɪ.təʊn/
acidic /əˈsɪd.ɪk/
acidosis /ˌæs.ɪˈdəʊ.sɪs/
action /ˈæk.ʃən/
administer /ədˈmɪn.ɪ.stər/

administration /əd.ˌmɪn.ɪˈstreɪ.ʃən/
advanced /ədˈvɑːnt st/
agent /ˈeɪ.dʒənt/
amputation /ˌæm.pjʊˈteɪ.ʃən/
anorexia /æn.əˌrek.si.ə/
appear /əˈpɪər/
assess /əˈses/
atherosclerosis /ˌæθ.ə.rəʊ.skləˈrəʊ.sɪs/
attempt /əˈtempt/
attribute /ˈæt.rɪ.bjuːt/
available /əˈveɪ.lə.blˌ/
behaviour /bɪˈheɪ.vjə/
bladder /ˈblæd.ər/
blindness /ˈblaɪnd.nəs/
bowel /ˈbaʊ.əl/
cancer /ˈkænt .sər/
carry /ˈkær.i/
clammy /ˈklæm.i/
coma /ˈkəʊ.mə/
comatose /kəʊ.məˌtəʊz/
combative /ˈkɒm.bə.tɪv/
common /ˈkɒm.ən/
confusion /kənˈfjuː.ʒən/
consciousness /ˈkɒn.ʃəs.nəs/
consumption /kənˈsʌmp .ʃən/
control /kənˈtrəʊl/
damage /ˈdæm.ɪdʒ/
dehydration /ˌdiː.haɪˈdreɪ.ʃən/
delayed /dɪˈleɪd/
demonstrate /ˈdem.ən.streɪt/
deplete /dɪˈpliːt/
depletion /dɪˈpliː.ʃən/
disease /dɪˈziːz/
diuresis /ˌdaɪ.jʊəˈriː.sɪs/
dose /dəʊs/
drowsiness /ˈdraʊ.zɪ.nəs/
emotional /ɪˈməʊ.ʃən.əl/
ensure /ɪnˈʃɔːr/
enteral /ˈen.tə.rəl/
excessive /ekˈses.ɪv/
extreme /ɪkˈstriːm/
failure /ˈfeɪ.ljə/
feeding /ˌfiː.dɪŋ/
formation /fɔːˈmeɪ.ʃən/
generalize /ˈdʒenrəˌlaɪz/
genetically /dʒəˈnet.ɪk.əl.i/
engineered /ˌen.dʒɪˈnɪərd/
heart /hɑːt/ **disease** /dɪˈziːz/
hyperglycaemia /ˌhaɪ.pə.glaɪˈsiːmi.ə/
Hyperosmolar /ˌhaɪ.pə.ɒz.
mɒ.lər/ **Hyperglycaemic** /ˌhaɪ.
pə.glaɪ.ˈsiː.mɪk/ **Nonketotic** /
ˌnɒn.ke.tɒt.ɪk/ **Coma** /ˈkəʊmə/
hypotension /ˌhaɪ.pəʊˈten.ʃən/
hypothermia /ˌhaɪ.pəʊ ˈθɜː.mi.ə/
incidence /ˈɪnt .sɪ.dənts/
infusion /ɪnˈfjuː.ʒən/
injury /ˈɪn.dʒər.i/
insufficiency /ˌin.sə.ˈfiʃ.ən.siː/
intentional /ɪnˈten.ʃən.əl/
intermediate /ˌɪn.təˈmiː.di.ət/
intoxication /ɪnˌtɒk.sɪˈkeɪ.ʃən/
involuntary /ɪnˈvɒləntərɪ/
ketoacid /kiː.təʊ.æ.sɪd/
ketoacidosis /ˈkiː.təʊˌæ.ɪˈdəʊ.sɪs/
ketone /ˈkiː.təʊn/ **body** /ˈbɒd.i/
Kussmaul /kö s.məʊl/
respiration /ˌrespəˈreɪʃən/
lactation /lækˈteɪ.ʃən/
lethargy /ˈləθ.ə.dʒɪ/
life-threatening /ˈlaɪfˌθret.ən.ɪŋ/
lifesaving /ˈlaɪfˌseɪ.vɪŋ/
like /laɪk/
long /ˌlɒŋ/ **-acting** /ækt.ɪŋ/
markedly /ˈmɑː.kɪd.li/
medication /ˌmed.ɪˈkeɪ.ʃən/
missed /mɪsd/
mobilization /ˌməʊ.bɪ.laɪˈzeɪ.ʃən/
molecule /ˈmɒl.ɪ.kjuːl/
mortality /mɔːˈtæl.ə.ti/ **rate** /reɪt/
mucous membrane /
ˌmjuː.kəsˈmem.breɪn/
muscle /ˈmʌs.əl/ **wasting** /weɪst.ɪŋ/
nausea /ˈnɔː.zi.ə/
neuropathy /njʊˈrɒp.ə.θɪ/
obesity /əʊ ˈbiː.sɪ.ti/
odour /ˈəʊ.dər/
onset /ˈɒnˌset/
orally /ˈɔː.rə.li/
orthostatic /ˌɔː.θəˈstæt.ɪk/

overdose /ˈəʊ.və.dəʊs/
parenteral /pəˈren.tə.rəl/
permanent /ˈpɜː.mə.nənt/
physical /ˈfɪz.ɪ.kəl/
postural /ˈpɒs.tʃə.rəl/
hypotension /ˌhaɪ.pəʊˈten.ʃən/
precipitating /prɪˈsɪp.ɪ.teɪt.ɪŋ/
pregnancy /ˈpreg.nən.si/
preparation /ˌprepəˈreɪʃən/
production /prəˈdʌk.ʃən/
provide /prəˈvaɪd/
psychotic /saɪˈkɒt.ɪk/
raise /reɪz/
rapid /ˈræp.ɪd/
reabsorb /riː.əbˈzɔːb/
reach /riːtʃ/
related /rɪˈleɪ.tɪd/
requirement /rɪˈkwaɪə.mənt/
resultant /rɪˈzʌl.tənt/
rise /raɪz/
salicylate /səˈlɪs.ə.leɪt/
salt /sɒlt/
seizure /ˈsiː.ʒə/
self-administer /self.ədˈmɪn.ɪ.stər/
sepsis /ˈsep.sɪs/
shift /ʃɪft/
short /ʃɔːt/ **-term** /tɜːm/
significant /sɪgˈnɪf.ɪ.kənt/
spill /spɪl/
stage /steɪdʒ/
stomach /ˈstʌm.ək/
stroke /strəʊk/
supplemental /ˌsʌp.lɪˈmen.təl/
surgery /ˈsɜː.dʒər.i/
suspected /səˈspek.tɪd/
tachycardia /ˌtæk.ɪˈkɑː.di.ə/
thready /ˈθred.i/ **pulse** /pʌls/
thus /ðʌs/
toward /tʊˈwɔːrd/
trembling /ˈtrem.bl̩.ɪŋ/
tumour /ˈtjuː.mər/
unconsciousness /ʌnˈkɒn.ʃəs.nəs/
undiagnosed /ʌnˈdaɪ.əg.nəʊzd/
unresponsive /ˌʌn.rɪˈspɒn.sɪv/
unusual /ʌnˈjuːʒʊəl/
urine /ˈjʊə.rɪn/
vigorous /ˈvɪg.ər.əs/
voluntary /ˈvɒl.ən.tər.i/
vomit /ˈvɒm.ɪt/
weakness /ˈwiːk.nəs/
weight /weɪt/ **loss** /lɒs/

Solution to Exercise 1
1e, 2t, 3g, 4p, 5r, 6c, 7j, 8h, 9d, 10n, 11s, 12l, 13m, 14f, 15q, 16i, 17b, 18o, 19k, 20a

Unit 6 - Female reproductive system. Pregnancy. Growth and development review.

Organs of the female reproductive system

The female reproductive organs include the **ovaries, fallopian tubes, uterus, vagina, external genital organs and mammary glands.**

Specialized structures of pregnancy

Placenta

The placenta is a **disc-like organ** composed and **interlocking foetal and maternal tissues.** It is the organ of **exchange** between the mother and the foetus and is responsible for the following five functions:

- **Transfer of gases.** The diffusion of **oxygen and carbon dioxide** through the **placental membrane** is **similar** to that occurs in the **lungs.**
- **Transport of nutrients.** Other **metabolic substrates** required by the foetus **diffuse into foetal blood** in the same manner as oxygen.

Diffusion also transports other substrates, including **fatty acids, potassium, sodium and chloride**. The placenta also actively **absorbs** some **nutrients** from **maternal blood.**

- **Excretion of wastes**. Waste products, such as urea, uric acid and creatinine, **diffuse** from foetal blood **into maternal blood.** They are excreted with the waste products of the mother.
- **Hormone production**. The **placenta** becomes a **temporary endocrine gland**, secreting **oestrogen and progesterone. By the third month** of foetal development **the corpus luteum** on the ovary is **no longer needed** to sustain the pregnancy. Oestrogen, progesterone, and other hormones **maintain the uterine lining**, **prevent** the occurrence of **menses**, and **stimulate changes** in the pregnant woman's **breasts, vagina, cervix, and pelvis** that prepare her body for **delivery and lactation**.
- **Formation of a barrier**. The placenta forms a **barrier against some harmful substances** and chemicals in the mother's circulation. It does not fully protect the foetus. Certain **medications** easily **cross the placenta,** including **steroids, narcotics, anaesthetics, and some antibiotics**.

Umbilical cord

Deoxygenated blood flows **from the foetus to the placenta** through the **umbilical arteries. Oxygenated blood** returns through the **umbilical vein**. This system is **independent** of and separated from the maternal circulation. **At birth** the various **arteriovenous shunts close** in most infants.

Amniotic sac and amniotic fluid

The **amniotic sac is a fluid-filled cavity** that completely surrounds and **protects the embryo. Amniotic fluid** originates from several foetal sources including foetal **urine** and **secretions from the respiratory tract, skin, and amniotic membranes.** The **rupture** of the amniotic membranes produces the **watery discharge** at the time of delivery.

Adjustments of the infant at birth

Birth results in the infant's loss of the placental connection with the mother, which results in the **loss of metabolic support**. After a normal delivery by a mother who is not depressed with anaesthetics, a newborn usually begins to **breath spontaneously**. This occurs when the **chest exits the birth canal** or with some **external stimulation**. These powerful first breaths **open the alveoli,** which allows **further respirations** to occur with much less effort. **Blood flow** through the **placenta ceases at birth.** As a result of the changes in pressure, the **arteriovenous shunts close** normally within a few hours after birth.

Foetal growth and development

The developing **ovum** is called an **embryo** during the **first 8 weeks** of pregnancy, and from 8 weeks **until birth** it is **called a foetus.** The period during which the foetus grows and develops within the uterus is known as **gestation.** Gestation usually **averages 40 weeks** and is divided into 90-day periods called **trimesters. Conception** occurs about **14 days after** the first day of the last **menstrual period**; thus the obstetrician can calculate foetal development as well as the estimated delivery date.

First lunar month

- Foundations form for the **nervous system, genitourinary system, skin, bones and lungs.**
- Buds of **arms and legs** begin to form.
- **Rudiments of eyes, ears, and nose** appear.

Second lunar month

- The head is disproportionately large because of **brain development.**
- **Gender** differentiation begins.
- The centres of **bones** begin to **ossify.**

Third lunar month

- **Fingers and toes** are distinct.
- The **placenta is complete.**
- **Foetal circulation is complete.**

Fourth lunar month

- **Gender** is differentiated.
- Rudimentary **kidneys secrete urine.**
- **Heartbeat** is present.
- **Nasal septum and palate** close.

Fifth lunar month

- Foetal **movements** are felt by the mother.
- **Heart sounds** are perceptible with a fetoscope.

Sixth lunar month

- The **skin** appears **wrinkled.**
- **Eyebrows** and **fingernails** develop.

Seventh lunar month

- The **skin is red.**
- The **pupillary membrane disappears** from the eyes.
- If born, the **infant cries and breathes** but frequently dies.

Eight lunar month

- The **foetus is viable** if born.
- The **eyelids** open.
- **Fingerprints** are set.

- Vigorous foetal **movement** occurs.

Ninth lunar month

- The **face and body** have a loose, **wrinkled appearance** because of subcutaneous fat deposits.
- **Amniotic fluid decreases** somewhat.

Tenth lunar month

- **Skin is smooth.**
- **Eyes** are uniformly **slate coloured.**
- The bones of the **skull are ossified** and nearly together at sutures.

Growth and development review

Children have unique anatomical, physiological and psychological characteristics that change during their development.

Newborn (first few hours of life)

The method most commonly used to **evaluate** the newborn is the **Apgar score.** It routinely is assessed at **1 and 5 min of age**. The Apgar evaluates **appearance, pulse rate, grimace, activity, and respirations.** A score of 7 to 10 is considered normal.

Neonate (first 28 days of life)

Although crying is common in the neonate, the crying gradually decreases throughout infancy. **Persistent crying** may indicate physiological **distress. Illnesses** that may be encountered in this age group are those that cause **respiratory problems, jaundice, vomiting, fever, sepsis, meningitis, and problems of prematurity.**

Infant (1-12 months)

By 12 months of age the development of mature nerves is nearly complete, and, along with muscle strength, enables many infants to **stand and walk** with little or no assistance.

Common **illnesses** typically affect the respiratory, gastrointestinal and central nervous system and manifest as **respiratory distress; nausea, vomiting and diarrhoea with dehydration; and seizures respectively.**

Other illnesses that may be encountered in this age group include **sepsis, meningitis, and sudden unexpected death in infancy.**

In addition, the older infant may experience **bronchiolitis, croup, foreign body airway obstruction, and physical injury from sexual abuse, neglect, falls, and motor vehicle crashes.**

Toddler (1-3 years)

By age 2, much of the **nervous system is fully developed** and **basic motor skills** (e.g. **balance and walking)** and **fine motor skills** (e.g. stacking building blocks) become visible. In addition, most children are capable of controlling **bladder and bowel** function. Basic **language skills** are mastered by age of 3.

Illnesses in this age group may cause **respiratory distress,**

vomiting and diarrhoea with dehydration, febrile seizures, sepsis, and meningitis. Toddlers are prone to **falls**. Physical injuries also occur from **poisoning** from accidental ingestions, **physical/ sexual abuse, drowning, and motor vehicles crashes.**

Preschool (3-5 years)

During the preschool years, children experience **advances in gross and fine motor skills** and develop **peer relationships** with other children. Their **play** involves acting out fantasies or using **imagination** for new situations; all of which can lead to **problem-solving skills and cognitive development.**

Preschoolers are more likely to experience injuries from **thermal burns** and are also more likely to be victims of **submersion incidents or drowning.**

School age (6-12 years)

Two key areas of development during the school-age years include an increased ability to **concentrate and learn** quickly and the **onset of puberty**. As a rule, **self-concept, moral traits and behaviour** begin to emerge. Most illnesses in school-age children are caused by **viral infection**. Injuries become more common and include **injuries from bicycle crashes, fractures from falls, and sport-related injuries.**

Adolescent (13-18 years)

During adolescence, the **final phase in growth and development** occurs. Also, in adolescence, a person reaches **reproductive maturity**. The development of **secondary sex characteristics** in both sexes heralds a final period of rapid growth. Most teenagers begin to experiment with different **identities** as they begin to develop their **personality** into that of an adult. They may experiment with **alcohol** or other **drugs, sex**, and **extreme forms of behaviour**.

Exercise 1

Match the column A with the column B. Try to learn the expressions and/or sentences by heart.

A

1. The female reproductive organs include
2. The placenta is a disc-like organ
3. The diffusion of oxygen and carbon dioxide
4. Other metabolic substrates required by the foetus
5. The placenta also actively absorbs
6. Waste products, such as urea, uric acid and creatinine,
7. The placenta becomes a temporary endocrine gland,
8. Oestrogen, progesterone, and other hormones maintain the uterine lining, prevent the occurrence of menses,
9. Certain medications easily cross the placenta,
10. Deoxygenated blood flows from the foetus to the placenta through the umbilical arteries,

11. The amniotic sac is a fluid-filled cavity
12. Amniotic fluid originates from several foetal sources including
13. Birth results in the infant's loss of the placental connection with the mother,
14. The powerful first breaths open the alveoli,
15. Blood flow through the placenta ceases at birth,
16. The developing ovum is called an embryo during the first 8 weeks of pregnancy,
17. Gestation usually averages 40 weeks
18. Conception occurs about 14 days
19. The Apgar score evaluates
20. Illnesses that may be encountered in neonates (first 28 days of life) are
21. By 12 months of age the development of mature nerves is nearly complete,
22. Common illnesses manifest as respiratory distress, nausea, vomiting and diarrhoea with dehydration, and seizures,
23. The older infant may experience bronchiolitis,
24. By age 2, much of the nervous system is fully developed
25. Most children are capable of
26. Illnesses in this age group may cause

a) after the first day of the last menstrual period.
b) and basic motor skills (e.g. balance and walking) and fine motor skills (e.g. stacking building blocks) become visible.
c) and from 8 weeks until birth it is called a foetus.
d) and is divided into 90-day periods called trimesters.
e) and stimulate changes in the pregnant woman's breasts, vagina, cervix, and pelvis that prepare her body for delivery and lactation.
f) and, along with muscle strength, enables many infants to stand and walk.
g) appearance, pulse rate, grimace, activity, and respirations.
h) respiratory distress, vomiting and diarrhoea with dehydration, febrile seizures, sepsis, and meningitis.
i) controlling bladder and bowel function and basic language skills are mastered by age of 3.
j) croup, foreign body airway obstruction, and physical injury from sexual abuse, neglect, falls, and motor vehicle crashes.
k) diffuse from foetal blood into maternal blood and are excreted with the waste products of the mother.
l) diffuse into foetal blood in the same manner as oxygen.

B

m) *including steroids, narcotics, anaesthetics, and some antibiotics.*

n) *foetal urine and secretions from the respiratory tract, skin, and amniotic membranes.*

o) *of exchange between the mother and the foetus.*

p) *other illnesses that may be encountered include sepsis, meningitis, and sudden unexpected death in infancy.*

q) *oxygenated blood returns through the umbilical vein.*

r) *secreting oestrogen and progesterone.*

s) *some nutrients from maternal blood.*

t) *that completely surrounds and protects the embryo.*

u) *the arteriovenous shunts close normally within a few hours after birth.*

v) *the ovaries, fallopian tubes, uterus, vagina, external genital organs and mammary glands.*

w) *those that cause respiratory problems, jaundice, vomiting, fever, sepsis, meningitis, and problems of prematurity.*

x) *through the placental membrane is similar to that occurs in the lungs.*

y) *which allows further respirations to occur with much less effort.*

z) *which results in the loss of metabolic support.*

Exercise 2

Translate the expressions. Try to explain their meanings in English.

Ovaries, fallopian tubes, uterus, mammary glands, placenta, interlocking, exchange, transfer of gases, placental membrane, metabolic substrates, diffuse, excretion of wastes, urea, uric acid, temporary, corpus luteum, sustain, uterine lining, occurrence, cervix, delivery and lactation, harmful substances, cross, umbilical cord, independent of, separated from, arteriovenous shunts, surrounds, rupture, watery discharge, adjustments, loss of the placental connection, breath spontaneously, external stimulation, alveoli, ceases, foetus, gestation, averages, conception, obstetrician, foundations, genitourinary system, rudiments, gender differentiation, ossify, secrete urine, heartbeat, nasal septum and palate, perceptible, eyebrows, fingernails, pupillary membrane, disappears, viable, eyelids, movement, wrinkled appearance, subcutaneous deposits, amniotic fluid, skull, ossified, sutures, review, evaluate, Apgar score, assessed, grimace, persistent, encountered, jaundice, prematurity, mature, muscle strength, enables, assistance, manifest, diarrhoea, sudden unexpected death in infancy, bronchiolitis, croup, foreign body, airway obstruction, abuse, neglect, motor vehicle crashes, toddler, motor skills, balance, visible, capable of, bladder and bowel, mastered, distress, prone to, poisoning, accidental ingestions, drowning, advances, peer relationships, imagination, problem-solving, cognitive, burns, onset, self-concept, behaviour, emerge, adolescence, heralds, personality.

Exercise 3
Answer the following questions. Prepare short talks and/or dialogues on these topics.

1. Give the names of organs of the female reproductive system.
2. What are the five functions of the placenta?
3. What are the roles of umbilical cord, amniotic sac and amniotic fluid?
4. Talk about the adjustments of the infant at birth.
5. Describe foetal growth and development.
6. Talk about the growth and development of newborns, neonates, infants and toddlers.
7. Talk about preschool children, the development during the school-age years and the growth and development during adolescence.

Vocabulary 6

Fill in the meanings in your mother language:

abuse /ə'bjuːz/
accidental /ˌæk.sɪ'den.təl/
act /ækt/ **out** /aʊt/
adjustment /ə'dʒʌst.mənt/
adolescence /ˌæd.ə'les.əns/
adolescent /ˌæd.ə'les.ənt/
advance /əd'vɑːns/
airway /'eə.weɪ/
alveolus /ˌæl.vi'əʊ.ləs/ pl **alveoli**
amniotic /ˌæm.ni'ɒt.ɪk/
membrane /'mem.breɪn/
amniotic /ˌæm.ni'ɒt.ɪk/ **sac** /sæk/
anaesthetic /ˌæn.əs'θet.ɪk/
Apgar /'æpgɑː/ **score** /skɔːr/
appearance /ə'pɪə.rənt s/
arteriovenous /ɑː.tɪə.ri.əʊ'viː.nəs/ **shunt** /ʃʌnt/
as /əz/ **a rule** /ruːl/
assistance /ə'sɪs.tənt s/
average /'æv.ər.ɪdʒ/
barrier /'bær.i.ər/
bone /bəʊn/
breast /brest/
breath /breθ/
breathe /briːð/
bronchiolitis /'brɒŋ.ki.ə'la.ɪ.tɪs/
bud /bʌd/
building /'bɪl.dɪŋ/ **blocks** /blɒks/
calculate /'kælk.jʊˌleɪt/
cavity /'kæv.ə.ti/
cease /siːs/
cervix /'sɜː.vɪks/ pl
cervices /'sɜː.vɪs.iːz/
chest /tʃest/
chloride /'klɔː.raɪd/
cognitive /'kɒg.nɪ.tɪv/
commonly /'kɒ.mən.lɪ/
complete /kəm'pliːt/
concentrate /'kɒnt .sən.treɪt/
conception /kən'sep.ʃən/
corpus /'kɔː.pəs/ **luteum** /luː.tiː.əm/
crash /kræʃ/
creatinine /kri'æt.ɪ.niːn/
cross /krɒs/
croup /kruːp/
cry /kraɪ/
delivery /dɪ'lɪv.ər.i/
deposit /dɪ'pɒz.ɪt/
depressed /dɪ'prest/
diarrhoea /ˌdaɪ.ə'riː.ə/

differentiation /ˌdɪf.ər.en.ʃiˈeɪ.ʃən/
diffusion /dɪˈfjuː.ʒən/
disappear /ˌdɪs.əˈpɪər/
disc /dɪsk/ **-like** /laɪk/
discharge /dɪsˈtʃɑːdʒ/
disproportionately /ˌdɪs.
prəˈpɔː.ʃən.ət.li/
distinct /dɪˈstɪŋkt/
distress /dɪˈstres/
drowning /ˈdraʊn.ɪŋ/
effort /ˈef.ət/
embryo /ˈem.bri.əʊ/ pl **embryos**
emerge /ɪˈmɜːdʒ/
encounter /ɪnˈkaʊn.tə/
estimated /ˈes.tɪ.meɪt.ɪd/
evaluate /ɪˈvæl.ju.eɪt/
excretion /ɪkˈskriː.ʃən/
experience /ɪkˈspɪə.ri.ənt s/
experiment /ɪkˈsper.ɪ.mənt/
eyebrow /ˈaɪ.braʊ/
eyelid /ˈaɪ.lɪd/
fallopian tube /fəˌləʊ.pi.ənˈtjuːb/
febrile /ˈfiː.braɪl/ **seizure** /ˈsiː.ʒə/
female /ˈfiː.meɪl/
fetoscope /ˈfiːtəʊˌskəʊp/
fever /ˈfiː.vər/
final /ˈfaɪ.nəl/
fine /faɪn/
fingernail /ˈfɪŋ.gə.neɪl/
fingerprint /ˈfɪŋ.gə.prɪnt/
foetal /ˈfiː.təl/
foetus /ˈfiː.təs/
foreign /ˈfɒr.ən/ **body** /ˈbɒd.i/
foundation /faʊnˈdeɪ.ʃən/
fracture /ˈfræk.tʃə/
genital /ˈdʒen.ɪ.təl/
genitourinary /ˌdʒen.ɪ.təʊˈjʊə.rɪ.nər.i/
gestation /dʒesˈteɪ.ʃən/
gradually /ˈgrædʒ.ʊ.li/
grimace /ˈgrɪ.məs/
gross /grəʊs/
harmful /ˈhɑːm.fəl/
herald /ˈher.əld/
identity /aɪˈden.tɪ.ti/
illness /ˈɪl.nəs/
imagination /ɪˌmædʒ.ɪˈneɪ.ʃən/
incident /ˈɪn.sɪ.dənt/
independent /ˌɪn.dɪˈpen.dənt/
infancy /ˈɪn.fənt .si/
infant /ˈɪn.fənt/
ingestion /ɪnˈdʒest.ʃən/
interlock /ˌɪn.təˈlɒk/
involve /ɪnˈvɒlv/
jaundice /ˈdʒɔːn.dɪs/
lining /ˈlaɪn.ɪŋ/
loose /luːs/
lunar /ˈluː.nər/ **month** /mʌnθ/
lung /lʌŋ/
mammary /ˈmæm.ər.i/ **gland** /glænd/
manifest /ˈmæn.ɪ.fest/
master /ˈmɑː.stər/
maternal /məˈtɜː.nəl/
mature /məˈtjʊər/
maturity /məˈtjʊə.rɪ.ti/
meningitis /ˌmen.ɪnˈdʒaɪ.tɪs/
menses /ˈment.siːz/
narcotic /nɑːˈkɒt.ɪk/
nasal /ˈneɪ.zəl/ **septum** /ˈsep.təm/
neglect /nɪˈglekt/
neonate /ˈniː.əʊ.neɪt/
newborn /ˈnjuː.bɔːn/
obstetrician /ˌɒb.stəˈtrɪʃ.ən/
obstruction /əbˈstrʌk.ʃən/
occurrence /əˈkʌr.ənt s/
ossify /ˈɒs.ɪ.faɪ/
ovum /ˈəuvəm/ pl **ova**
oxygenate /ˈɒk.sɪ.dʒə.neɪt/
palate /ˈpæl.ət/
peer /pɪər/
pelvis /ˈpel.vɪs/
perceptible /pəˈsep.tə.bl̩/
persistent /pəˈsɪs.tənt/
personality /ˌpɜː.sənˈæl.ə.ti/
phase /feɪz/
physiological /ˌfɪz.i.əˈlɒdʒ.ɪ.kəl/
placenta /pləˈsen.tə/
poisoning /ˈpɔɪ.zən.ɪŋ/
powerful /ˈpaʊə.fəl/
prematurity /ˌpriː.mə.ˈtjʊə.rə.ti/
preschool /priːˈskuːl/

prone /prəʊn/
psychological /ˌsaɪkəˈlɒdʒ.ɪ.kəl/
puberty /ˈpjuː.bə.ti/
pupillary /pjuː.pɪl.ər.i/
relationship /rɪˈleɪ.ʃən.ʃɪp/
reproductive /ˌriː.prəˈdʌk.tɪv/
respectively /rɪˈspek.tɪv.li/
respiratory /rɪˈspɪr.ə.tər.i/
routinely /ruˈtin.li/
rudimentary /ˌruː.dɪˈmen.tər.i/
rudiments /ˈruː.dɪ.mənts/
rupture /ˈrʌp.tʃər/
score /skɔː/
self-concept /self.kɒn.sept/
set /set/
sexual /ˈsek.sjʊəl/
skill /skɪl/
skin /skɪn/
skull /skʌl/
slate /sleɪt/
smooth /smuːð/
solve /sɒlv/
somewhat /ˈsʌm.wɒt/
spontaneously /spɒnˈteɪ.ni.ə.sli/
stack /stæk/
steroids /ˈste.rɔɪds/
strength /streŋθ/
structure /ˈstrʌk.tʃər/
subcutaneous /ˌsʌb.kjʊˈteɪ.ni.əs/
submersion /səbˈmɜː.ʃən/
substrate /ˈsʌb.streɪt/
sudden /ˈsʌd.ən/ **unexpected** /ˌʌn.ɪkˈspek.tɪd/ **death** /deθ/ **in infancy** /ˈɪnfən.sɪ /
support /səˈpɔːt/
surround /səˈraʊnd/
sustain /səˈsteɪn/
suture /ˈsuː.tʃər/
temporary /ˈtem.pər.ər.i/
throughout /θruːˈaʊt/
toddler /ˈtɒd.lər/
toe /təʊ/
trait /treɪt/
trimester /trɪˈmes.tər/
umbilical cord /ʌmˈbɪl.ɪ.kəlˌkɔːd/
urea /jʊəˈriː.ə/
uric acid /ˈjʊər.ɪkˈæs.ɪd/
uterine /ˈjuː.tər.aɪn/
uterus /ˈjuː.tər.əs/ pl **uteri**
vagina /vəˈdʒaɪ.nə/
viable /ˈvaɪ.ə.bl̩/
victim /ˈvɪk.tɪm/
visible /ˈvɪz.ɪ.bl̩/
watery /ˈwɔː.təri/
wrinkle /ˈrɪŋ.kl̩/

Solution to Exercise 1
1v, 2o, 3x, 4l, 5s, 6k, 7r, 8e, 9m, 10q, 11t, 12n, 13z, 14y, 15u, 16c, 17d, 18a, 19g, 20w, 21f, 22p, 23j, 24b, 25i, 26h

Unit 7 - Care of older patients 1

Physiological changes of ageing

The ageing process affects all body systems. However the effects on specific organ systems particularly relevant to the older adult occur in the **respiratory, cardiovascular, renal, nervous, and musculoskeletal systems.**

Respiratory system changes

Respiratory function in the older adult generally **declines** as the lung tissue ages. **With ageing**, the chest wall becomes stiffer as the bony **thorax** becomes **more rigid**. Changes lead to an **increase in residual volume** and a **decrease in vital capacity**. Other factors that affect the respiratory system are the **loss of cilia** in the airways and a **diminished cough reflex** and impaired **gag reflex** which impair the bodily defence against inhaled bacteria. The decline in these defence mechanisms makes infectious **pulmonary diseases** of the older adult more common and makes these infections more difficult to resolve.

Cardiovascular system changes

Cardiac function declines with age as a result of physiological changes and the high incidence of **atherosclerotic coronary heart disease**. Myocardial hypertrophy, coronary artery disease and haemodynamic changes predispose the older patient to **dysrhythmias**, **heart failure**, and **sudden cardiac arrest** when the cardiovascular system is placed under unexpected stress.

Renal system changes

Structural and functional changes in the kidneys occur during the ageing process. The steady **decline in kidney function** places the older patient at greater risk for **renal failure** from **trauma, obstruction, infection, and vascular occlusion**. Decreases in kidney function and loss of muscle and body water make the older patient more susceptible to **electrolyte disturbances** and more likely to experience problems with **medications or drugs.**

Nervous system changes

Although it was long thought that mental dysfunction in the older patient was caused solely by senility, it is now well known that **intellectual functioning deteriorates selectively** and may result from many **organic causes**. Some gradual changes in the patient's nervous system can result in **decreased visual acuity** and **auditory keenness** and changes in **sleep pattern**. Toxic or metabolic factors that can affect mental functioning include the use of **medications; electrolyte imbalances; hypoglycaemia; acidosis; alkalosis; hypoxia; liver; kidney and lung failure; pneumonia; congestive heart failure; cardiac dysrhythmias; infection; and the development of benign or malignant tumours.**

Musculoskeletal system changes

As the body ages, **muscles shrink**, **muscles and ligaments calcify**, and **intervertebral discs** become **thin**. **Osteoporosis** is common (especially in women). These musculoskeletal changes result in a **decrease** in total **muscle mass**, a **decrease in height**, **widening and weakening** of certain **bones**, and a **posture** that impairs mobility and **alters the balance** of the body. As a result, falls are common. Moreover, the **falls** often are associated with significant morbidity and mortality.

Other physiological changes

Other **physiological changes** that occur with ageing include changes in **body mass** and total **body water,** a **decreased ability** to maintain internal **homoeostasis**, a decrease in the function of **immunological** mechanisms, **nutritional disorders**, and **decreases** in **hearing** and **visual** acuity.

The ability of the body to maintain normal **temperature** declines over time. Because of this, the older patient is at greater risk for cold- and heat-related conditions. These include **hypothermia, heat exhaustion, and hyperthermia.**

Ageing causes a decrease in primary **antibody response**. These physiological changes increase the risk of **infection, autoimmune** disorders, and perhaps **cancer**. In addition, infections may not produce the usual signs and symptoms.

Older patients often have more than one disease and disability and signs/symptoms such as a **change in habits, rectal bleeding, malaise, fatigue, weight loss and anorexia** may result from a variety of conditions.

Many older patients consume **less than the minimum daily requirement of most vitamins,** which may be a result of loneliness and depression, decreased sensitivity to taste, decreased appetite, financial difficulties, physical infirmity, decreased vision, or a combination of these elements.

All of these elements may act to reduce the motivation to shop for and prepare fresh food. Other factors associated with **poor nutrition** are **poor dentition** and **reduced mastication**, as well as decreased intestinal secretions that **reduce absorption.**

Communication with older patients

Questioning a patient who is fatigued or easily distracted may lengthen the interview process. You should use the following techniques when communicating with older patients:

- Always **identify yourself**.
- **Speak at eye level** to ensure that the patient can see you.
- **Locate** a **hearing aid, spectacles and dentures**.
- **Turn on lights.**
- **Speak slowly**, distinctly and respectfully.
- Use the patient's **surname**.
- **Listen** closely.
- **Be patient.**
- Preserve **dignity**.
- Use **gentleness**.

Dementia

Dementia is a slow, progressive **loss of awareness of time and place** with an **inability to learn** new things or **recall recent events**. Dementia is often a result of **brain disease** caused by **strokes, genetic or viral** factors, and **Alzheimer's disease**, and is generally considered **irreversible**. Sudden outburst of **embarrassing conduct** may be the first clear signs of dementia and some patients eventually regress to a "second childhood".

Alzheimer's disease

Alzheimer's disease is a condition in which **nerve cells in the cerebral cortex die** and the brain substance shrinks. The disease does not cause death directly; patients ultimately stop eating and become malnourished **and immobilized** and are prone to concurrent infections. The cause of Alzheimer's disease is still not fully understood; **possible causes** include abnormalities in **glutamate metabolism**, chronic **infection**, toxic **poisoning by metals**, **reduction in brain chemicals**, and **genetics**.

Early symptoms mainly are related to **memory loss.** As the disease progresses, **agitation**, **violence** and **impairment of abstract thinking** occur; **judgement** and **cognitive abilities** begin to interfere with work and social relations. Once the patient is **bedridden**, skin breakdown due to **pressure sores, feeding** problems, and **pneumonia** often shorten the patient's life. Management mainly consists of **nursing** and social care for the patient and relatives.

The seven warning signs of Alzheimer's disease

- Asking **the same questions** over and over again.
- **Repeating** the same story, word for word, again and again.
- **Forgetting** how to cook, or how to make repairs, or how to play cards – **activities** that were previously done with ease and regularity.
- Loosing one's ability to pay bills.
- Getting **lost in familiar surroundings**, or **misplacing** household **objects**.
- **Neglecting to bathe** or wearing the same clothes over and over again, while insisting that they have taken a bath or that their clothes are still clean.
- **Relying on someone else**, such as a spouse, to make decisions or answer questions they previously would have handled themselves.

Parkinson's disease

Parkinson's disease is a brain disorder caused by **degeneration** of and **damage** to the part of the **brain** producing dopamine which causes **dopamine shortage** direct effects on smooth muscle contraction. This causes **tremor, joint rigidity, and slow movement**. Characteristic signs of Parkinson's disease are **trembling**, (usually beginning in one hand, arm, or leg), a **rigid posture**, **slow movements**, and a **shuffling**, unbalanced **walk**. If left untreated, the disease progresses over 10 to 15 years to severe weakness and **incapacity**.

Exercise 1
Match the column A with the column B. Try to learn the expressions and/or sentences by heart.

A

1. The ageing process affects
2. Respiratory system changes
3. The loss of cilia in the airways and a diminished cough reflex and impaired gag reflex

4. Myocardial hypertrophy, coronary artery disease and haemodynamic changes
5. The steady decline in kidney function places the older patient at greater risk for
6. Gradual changes in the patient's nervous system can result in
7. Toxic or metabolic factors that can affect mental functioning include the use of medications; electrolyte imbalances; hypoglycaemia; acidosis; alkalosis;
8. As the body ages,
9. Other physiological changes that occur with ageing include changes in body mass and total body water, a decreased ability to maintain internal
10. The older patient is at greater risk for
11. Older patients often have more than one disease and disability and signs/symptoms
12. Factors associated with poor nutrition
13. You should use the following techniques when communicating with older patients:
14. Dementia is a slow, progressive loss of awareness of time and place
15. Dementia is often a result of brain disease caused by
16. Alzheimer's disease is a condition
17. Possible causes of Alzheimer's disease include
18. As the disease progresses, agitation, violence and impairment of abstract thinking occur;
19. Once the patient is bedridden, skin breakdown due to
20. The warning signs of Alzheimer's disease are: asking the same questions, repeating the same story,
21. Parkinson's disease is a brain disorder caused by degeneration of
22. Characteristic signs of Parkinson's disease

B

a) *abnormalities in glutamate metabolism, chronic infection, toxic poisoning by metals, reduction in brain chemicals, and genetics.*

b) *always identify yourself, speak slowly, distinctly and respectfully and locate a hearing aid, spectacles and dentures.*

c) *and damage to the part of the brain producing dopamine, which causes direct effects on smooth muscle contraction.*

d) *and judgement and cognitive abilities begin to interfere with work and social relations.*

e) *are poor dentition and reduced mastication,*

as well as decreased intestinal secretions that reduce absorption.

f) *are trembling, a rigid posture, slow movements, and a shuffling, unbalanced walk.*

g) *decreased visual acuity and auditory keenness and changes in sleep pattern.*

h) *forgetting activities that were previously done with ease, getting lost in familiar surroundings, or misplacing household objects.*

i) *homoeostasis, a decrease in the function of immunological mechanisms, nutritional disorders, and decreases in hearing and visual acuity.*

j) *hypothermia, heat exhaustion, and hyperthermia.*

k) *hypoxia; liver; kidney and lung failure; pneumonia; congestive heart failure; cardiac dysrhythmias; infection; and the development of benign or malignant tumours.*

l) *impair the bodily defence against inhaled bacteria.*

m) *in which nerve cells in the cerebral cortex die and the brain substance shrinks.*

n) *lead to an increase in residual volume and a decrease in vital capacity.*

o) *muscles shrink, muscles and ligaments calcify, and intervertebral discs become thin.*

p) *predispose the older patient to dysrhythmias, heart failure, and sudden cardiac arrest.*

q) *pressure sores, feeding problems, and pneumonia often shorten the patient's life.*

r) *renal failure from trauma, obstruction, infection, and vascular occlusion.*

s) *strokes, genetic or viral factors, and Alzheimer's disease, and is generally considered irreversible.*

t) *such as a change in habits, rectal bleeding, malaise, fatigue, weight loss and anorexia may result from a variety of conditions.*

u) *the respiratory, cardiovascular, renal, nervous, and musculoskeletal systems.*

v) *with an inability to learn new things or recall recent events.*

Exercise 2

Translate the expressions. Try to explain their meanings in English.

Ageing, declines, increase, residual volume, decrease in, vital capacity, diminished, gag reflex, impair the bodily defence, resolve, incidence, myocardial hypertrophy, coronary artery disease, predispose, cardiac arrest, renal failure, vascular occlusion, susceptible to, electrolyte disturbances, deteriorates, selectively, organic causes, visual acuity, auditory keenness, sleep pattern, imbalances, congestive heart failure, benign or malignant tumours, muscles and ligaments calcify, thin intervertebral discs, posture, impairs mobility, alters the balance, morbidity and mortality, heat exhaustion, body response, in addition, disability, change in habits, rectal bleeding, malaise, fatigue, daily requirement, decreased sensitivity to taste, poor dentition, reduced mastication, easily distracted, identify yourself, hearing aid, spectacles, dentures, awareness of time and place, recall recent events, strokes, irreversible, outburst of embarrassing conduct, regress, cerebral cortex, malnourished, immobilized, prone to, concurrent, poisoning by metals, memory loss, agitation, violence, impairment of judgement, cognitive abilities, interfere with, bedridden, pressure sores, nursing, dopamine shortage, smooth muscle contraction, tremor, joint rigidity, trembling, rigid posture, shuffling, unbalanced walk, untreated, incapacity, warning signs, familiar surroundings, misplacing objects, insisting, relying on, handled.

Exercise 3
Answer the following questions. Prepare short talks and/or dialogues on these topics.

1. Talk about physiological changes of ageing (respiratory system, cardiovascular system, renal system, nervous system, musculoskeletal system)
2. Talk about other physiological changes.
3. How to communicate with older patients?
4. What is the cause of Alzheimer's disease?
5. What are the seven warning signs of Alzheimer's disease?
6. Describe Parkinson's disease.

Vocabulary 7

Fill in the meanings in your mother language:

acuity /ə'kjuː.ə.ti/
ageing /'eɪ.dʒɪŋ/
agitation /ˌædʒ.ɪ'teɪ.ʃən/
alkalosis /ˌælkə'ləʊ.sɪs/
Alzheimer's disease /
'ɔltsˌhaɪ.mərz.dɪˌziz/
antibody /'æn.tiˌbɒd.i/
atherosclerosis /ɑrˌtɪər
i oʊ sklə'roʊ sɪs/
auditory /'ɔː.dɪ.tər.i/
autoimmune /ˌɔː.təʊ.ɪ'mjuːn/
awareness /ə'weə.nəs/
bathe /beɪð/
bedridden /'bed.rɪ.dən/
benign /bɪ'naɪn/
bleeding /'bliː.dɪŋ/
bowel /'baʊ.əl/ **habits** /'hæb.ɪts/
calcify /'kæl.sɪ.faɪ/
cardiac /'kɑː.di.æk/ **arrest** /ə'rest/
cardiovascular /ˌkɑː.di.əʊ'væs.kjʊ.lər/
childhood /'tʃaɪld.hʊd/
cilium /'sɪl.i.əm/ pl **cilia** /'sɪl.i.ə/
combination /ˌkɒm.bɪ'neɪ.ʃən/
concurrent /kən'kʌr.ənt/
congestive /kən'dʒes.tɪv/ **heart** /
hɑːt/ **failure** /'feɪ.ljər/
consume /kən'sjuːm/
cough /kɒf/
defence /dɪ'fens/

degeneration /dɪˌdʒen.əˈreɪ.ʃən/
dementia /dɪˈmen.ʃə/
dentition /denˈtɪʃ.ən/
dentures /ˈden.tʃəz/
deteriorate /dɪˈtɪə.ri.ə.reɪt/
dignity /ˈdɪg.nɪ.ti/
disability /ˌdɪs.əˈbɪl.ɪ.ti/
distinctly /dɪˈstɪŋkt.li/
distracted /dɪˈstræk.tɪd/
disturbance /dɪˈstɜː.bəns/
dysrhythmia /dɪsˈrɪð.mi.ə/
embarrassing /ɪmˈbær.ə.sɪŋ/
familiar /fəˈmɪl.i.ər/ **with** /wɪð/
gag /gæg/ **reflex** /ˈriː.fleks/
genetics /dʒəˈnet.ɪks/
gentleness /ˈdʒen.tlˌ.nəs/
glutamate /ˈgluː.tə.meɪt/
gradual /ˈgræd.jʊ.əl/
handle /ˈhæn.dlˌ/
hearing /ˈhɪə.rɪŋ/ **aid** /eɪd/
heart /hɑːt/ **failure** /ˈfeɪ.ljər/
heat /hiːt/ **exhaustion** /ɪgˈzɔːs.tʃən/
household /ˈhaʊs.həʊld/
hyperthermia /ˌhaɪ.pəˈθɜː.mɪ.ə/
hypertrophy /haɪˈpɜː.trə.fi/
impaired /ɪmˈpeəd/
impairment /imˈpeərˌmənt/
inability /ˌɪn.əˈbɪl.ɪ.ti/
incapacity /ˌɪn.kəˈpæs.ə.ti/
infirmity /ɪnˈfɜː.mə.ti/
inhale /ɪnˈheɪl/
insist /ɪnˈsɪst/
intervertebral /ˌɪn.tɜːrˈvɜː.tɪ.brəl/ **disc** /dɪsk/
intestinal /ˌin.ˈtes.tin.əl/
irreversible /ˌɪr.ɪˈvɜː.sɪ.bl̩/
joint /dʒɔɪnt/
judgement /ˈdʒʌdʒ.mənt/
keenness /ˈkiːn.nəs/
lengthen /ˈleŋk .θən/
ligament /ˈlɪg.ə.mənt/
loneliness /ˈləʊn.li.nəs/
malnourished /ˌmælˈnʌr.ɪʃt/
malaise /mælˈeɪz/
malignant /məˈlɪg.nənt/
mastication /ˌmæs.tikˈei.ʃən/
metal /ˈmet.əl/ **alloy** /ˈæl.ɔɪ/
metal /ˈmet.əl/
misplace /ˌmɪsˈpleɪs/
mobility /məʊˈbɪl.ɪ.tɪ/
morbidity /ˌmɔːˈbɪd.ɪ.ti/
nursing /ˈnɜː.sɪŋ/
occlusion /əˈkluː.ʒən/
osteoporosis /ˌɒs.ti.əʊ.pəˈrəʊ.sɪs/
outburst /ˈaʊt.bɜːst/
Parkinson's /ˈpɑː.kɪn.sənz/ **disease** /dɪˈziːz/
particularly /pəˈtɪk.jʊ.lə.li/
patient /ˈpeɪ.ʃənt/
pneumonia /njuːˈməʊ.ni.ə/
posture /ˈpɒs.tʃər/
previously /ˈpriː.vi.əs.li/
progress /ˈprəʊ.gres/
recall / rɪˈkɔːl/
recent /ˈriː.sənt/
rectal /ˈrek.təl/
relevant /ˈrel.ə.vənt/
rely /rɪˈlaɪ/ **on** /ɒn/
renal /ˈriː.nəl/
repeat /rɪˈpiːt/
residual /rɪˈzɪd.ju.əl/
resolve /rɪˈzɒlv/
respectfully /rɪˈspekt.fəl.i/
rigid /ˈrɪdʒ.ɪd/
rigidity /rɪˈdʒɪd.ɪ.ti/
selectively /ˌsɪl.ekˈtɪv.ɪ.ti/
senility /sɪˈnɪl.ɪ.ti/
shortage /ˈʃɔː.tɪdʒ/
shorten /ˈʃɔː.tən/
shrink /ʃrɪŋk/
shuffle /ˈʃʌf.l̩/
sign /saɪn/
sleep /sliːp/ **pattern** /ˈpæt.ən/
solely /ˈsəʊl.lɪ/
sore /sɔːr/
spectacle /ˈspek.tɪ.kl̩/
spouse /spaʊs/
steady /ˈsted.i/
stiff /stɪf/
surroundings /səˈraʊn.dɪŋz/

susceptible /sə'sep.tɪ.bl̩/
thorax /'θɔː.ræks/
thought /θɔːt/
trauma /'trɔː.mə/
tremor /'trem.ər/
turn /tɜːn/ **on** /ɒn/
ultimately /'ʌl.tɪ.mət.li/
unbalanced /ʌn'bæl.ənst/
unexpected /ˌʌn.ɪk'spek.tɪd/
untreated /ʌn'triː.tɪd/
variety /və'raɪə.ti/
violence /'vaɪə.ləns/
visual /'vɪʒ.u.əl/ **acuity** /ə'kjuː.ə.ti/
vital /'vaɪ.təl/ **capacity** /kə'pæs.ə.ti/
weaken /'wiː.kən/
weakness /'wiːk.nəs/
wearing /'weə.rɪŋ/
widen /'waɪ.dən/

Solution to Exercise 1
1u, 2n, 3l, 4p, 5r, 6g, 7k, 8o, 9i, 10j, 11t, 12e, 13b, 14v, 15s, 16m, 17a, 18d, 19q, 20h, 21c, 22f

Unit 8 - Care of older patients 2

Two common endocrine disorders often are seen in patients; diabetes and thyroid disease.

Diabetes

Type 2 (**non-insulin-depended**) diabetes is most common in older patients and more common when the person is **overweight**. The following are associated risk factors for complications related to diabetes:

- decreased **ability to care for self**
- **living alone**
- **concurrent illnesses**
- decline in **renal function**
- **polydrug** use

A combination of **dietary measures, weight reduction**, and **oral hypoglycaemic** agents can usually keep type 2 diabetes under control. In most cases, insulin injections are not required. However, if poorly controlled, diabetes can lead to **complications** such as **retinopathy, peripheral neuropathy** (ulcers on the feet are common), and **kidney damage**.

Diabetic patients also have a risk for **atherosclerosis, hypertension**, and other **cardiovascular disorders**, and for **cataracts**. The patient may complain of profound **thirst** and frequent **urination**, leading to **dehydration** and **electrolyte loss**. Predisposing factors to coma include infection, **non-concordance** with **medications**, polydrug use (**polypharmacy**), **pancreatitis, stroke, hypothermia, heat stroke, and myocardial infarction**.

Gastrointestinal haemorrhage

Signs and symptoms of gastrointestinal bleeding include **vomiting of blood** or **coffee-ground emesis**; **blood-tinged** stools or **black**, tarry **stools**; and **weakness, syncope** or **pain**. The older the patient, the higher the risk of death, due to the following:

- Older patients are less able to **compensate for acute blood loss**.
- They are **less likely to feel symptoms** and therefore seek treatment at later stages of disease.

- They are more likely to be **taking aspirin or non-steroidal anti-inflammatory drugs**, which places them at higher risk for **ulcer** disease and bleeding.
- They are at higher risk for **colon cancer, intestinal vascular abnormalities, and diverticulitis.**
- They are more likely to be on **blood-thinning medications**.

Obstruction

Bowel obstruction generally occurs in patients with prior **abdominal surgeries or hernias** and also in those with **colonic cancer**. Most complain of **constipation**, abdominal **cramping** and an **inability to pass wind**; other signs and symptoms can include protracted **vomiting** of food or **bile** and vomiting of **faecal material.**

Problems with continence

Some factors associated with **continence** are affected by age and include a decrease in **bladder capacity**, **involuntary** bladder **contractions**, **decreased ability to postpone voiding**, and **medications** that can affect bladder and bowel control. Urinary incontinence can vary in severity. It can be only mild incontinence or it can be total incontinence, with complete **loss of bladder control**. **Bowel incontinence** in the older patient usually is the result of faecal impaction, which occurs when faeces lodged in the rectum **irritate and inflame the lining**. If incontinence is chronic, it can lead to **skin irritation**, tissue breakdown and **urinary tract infection**. Patients with mild cases often wear **absorptive undergarments** to relieve discomfort and embarrassment.

Problems with elimination

Causes of difficulty in urination usually result from **enlargement of the prostate** (in men), urinary tract **infection**, **urethral strictures,** and acute or chronic **renal failure**. Difficulty in bowel elimination is often associated with **diverticular disease, constipation and colorectal cancer.** Problems with elimination can cause great **pain and anxiety** for older patients. These conditions call for further evaluation to identify the cause and select the appropriate therapy.

Pressure ulcers

Pressure ulcers (also known as **decubitus** ulcer) are common in older patients and often develop on the skin of patients who are **bedridden or immobile**. Most pressure ulcers occur in the lower **legs, back, and buttocks**, and over the **sacrum**. They often affect **victims of stroke** or other illnesses that result in a loss or change in the **sensation of pain**. Skin exposure to **moisture**, poor nutrition, and **friction** or shear also may be factors for developing pressure ulcers; other causes include **vascular and metabolic disorders**, **trauma** and **cancer**. They generally start as **red, painful areas** that become purple before the skin breaks down, and then further develop into **open sores**. Pressure ulcers should be covered with **sterile dressing** using aseptic technique. The patient must be referred to further appropriate care.

Osteoarthritis

It is a degenerative condition which results from **cartilage loss and wear and tear on the joints**. The condition leads to pain, stiffness, and sometimes loss of function of the affected joint.

Osteoporosis

Osteoporosis is a natural part of ageing; it especially is common in older **women after menopause,** due to a decrease in the hormone oestrogen that helps maintain bone mass. The **loss of bone density** causes bone to become **brittle**; consequently, they can **fracture easily** and this is often the first sign of osteoporosis. Typical sites for fractures are just above the **wrist**, at t**he head of the femur,** and at one or several **vertebrae** (often a spontaneous fracture).

Problems with vision

Vision impairments can severely limit daily activities with a loss of independence in older patients. The following are some effects of ageing on vision:

- **reading** difficulties
- poor **depth perception**
- poor **adjustment** of the eyes to variations in **distance**
- altered **colour perception**
- **sensitivity** to light
- decreased visual **acuity**

Two common eye conditions that develop with age are cataracts and glaucoma. A **cataract** is a loss of transparency of the lens of the eye. A cataract never causes full blindness, yet **clarity and detail of an image** progressively are lost. **Surgery** to remove the cataract is a **common** procedure. **Glaucoma** is a condition in which **intraocular pressure increases**, causing damage to the **optic nerve.** The result is nerve fibre **destruction** and partial or full loss of peripheral and central vision. Symptoms of **acute** glaucoma include dull, severe, **aching pain** in and above the eye; **fogginess** of vision; and the perception of "rainbow rings" **(halos) around lights at night**. If detected early, the condition can be treated with oral medications and **eye drops** to relieve pressure.

Problems with hearing

Not all older patients have **hearing loss,** though overall hearing tends to decrease with age. This results from degeneration of the hearing mechanism. Certain **drugs, tumours**, and some viral **infections** also can cause hearing problems. Hearing loss can interfere with the ability to **perceive speech** and it can limit the ability to **communicate**. **Hearing aid devices and surgical implants** sometimes can restore or improve hearing. **Tinnitus** can occur as a symptom of many ear disorders.

The noise in the ear (e.g. **ringing, buzzing or whistling**) sometimes may change in nature and intensity.

Problems with speech

Common problems with speech are associated with difficulty in **word retrieval**, decreased **fluency** of speech, **slowed rate** of speech and changes in voice quality. These disorders may occur from damage to the language **centres of the brain** (usually as a result of **stroke, head injury or brain tumour**), degenerative changes in the nervous system, hearing loss, disorders of the **larynx**, and **poor-fitting dentures.**

Exercise 1
Match the column A with the column B. Try to learn the expressions and/or sentences by heart.

A

1. Two common endocrine disorders often seen in older patients
2. The following are associated risk factors for complications related to diabetes:
3. If poorly controlled, diabetes can lead to
4. Diabetic patients also have a risk for
5. The patient may complain of profound thirst and frequent urination,
6. Signs and symptoms of gastrointestinal bleeding include
7. They are less likely to feel symptoms
8. Bowel obstruction generally occurs in patients
9. Most complain of constipation, abdominal cramping and an inability to pass wind;
10. Some factors associated with continence are affected by age and include
11. If incontinence is chronic,
12. Causes of difficulty in urination usually result from
13. Difficulty in bowel elimination is often associated
14. Pressure ulcers (also known as decubitus ulcer) often develop
15. Pressure ulcers generally start as red, painful areas,
16. Osteoarthritis results from
17. Osteoporosis is
18. The loss of bone density causes bone to become brittle;
19. Typical sites for fractures are just above
20. The following are some effects of ageing on vision:
21. A cataract is a loss of transparency of the lens of the eye;
22. Symptoms of acute glaucoma
23. Overall hearing tends to decrease with age;
24. Tinnitus (e.g. ringing, buzzing or whistling)
25. Common problems with speech are associated with
26. These disorders may occur from damage to the language centres of the brain,

B

a) *a decrease in bladder capacity, involuntary bladder contractions, decreased ability to postpone voiding, and medications that can affect bladder and bowel control.*
b) *and therefore seek treatment at later stages of disease.*
c) *are diabetes and thyroid disease.*
d) *atherosclerosis, hypertension, and other cardiovascular disorders, and for cataracts.*
e) *can occur as a symptom of many ear disorders.*
f) *cartilage loss and wear and tear on the joints.*
g) *certain drugs, tumours, and some viral infections also can cause hearing problems.*
h) *common in older women after menopause.*
i) *complications such as retinopathy, peripheral neuropathy, and kidney damage.*
j) *consequently, they can fracture easily.*
k) *decreased ability to care for self, concurrent illnesses, decline in renal function and polydrug use.*
l) *degenerative changes in the nervous system, hearing loss, disorders of the larynx, and poor-fitting dentures.*
m) *difficulty in word retrieval, decreased fluency of speech, slowed rate of speech and changes in voice quality.*
n) *enlargement of the prostate, urinary tract infection, urethral strictures, and acute or chronic renal failure.*
o) *glaucoma is a condition in which intraocular pressure increases, causing damage to the optic nerve.*
p) *include dull, severe, aching pain in and above the eye; fogginess of vision; and the perception of "rainbow rings" around lights at night.*
q) *it can lead to skin irritation, tissue breakdown and urinary tract infection.*
r) *leading to dehydration and electrolyte loss.*
s) *on the skin of patients who are bedridden or immobile; most pressure ulcers occur in the lower legs, back, and buttocks.,*
t) *other signs and symptoms can include protracted vomiting of food or bile and vomiting of faecal material.*
u) *reading difficulties, poor depth perception, poor adjustment of the eyes to variations in distance, altered colour perception, sensitivity to light, decreased visual acuity.*
v) *the skin breaks down, and then further develop into open sores.*
w) *the wrist, at the head of the femur, and at one or*

several vertebrae (often a spontaneous fracture).

x) *vomiting of blood or coffee-ground emesis; blood-tinged stools or black, tarry stools; and weakness, syncope or pain.*

y) *with diverticular disease, constipation and colorectal cancer.*

z) *with prior abdominal surgeries or hernias and also in those with colonic cancer.*

Exercise 2
Translate the expressions. Try to explain their meanings in English.

Ability to care for self, concurrent, poorly controlled, retinopathy, neuropathy, cataracts, profound thirst, non-concordance with medications, coffee-ground emesis, blood-tinged stools, syncope, compensate for, more likely, colon cancer, diverticulitis, blood-thinning medications, surgeries or hernias, constipation, cramping, inability to pass wind, protracted vomiting, affected, involuntary bladder contraction, postpone voiding, irritate and inflame the lining, irritation, tissue breakdown, absorptive undergarments, enlargement, urethral strictures, diverticular disease, constipation, evaluation, pressure ulcers, bedridden, buttocks, sacrum, victims of stroke, sensation of pain, exposure to moisture, friction, painful areas, open sores, sterile dressing, referred to, degenerative condition, stiffness, bone density, brittle, consequently, wrist, at the head of the femur, vertebrae, depth perception, poor adjustment, distance, colour perception, sensitivity, transparency, lens, blindness, clarity, image, intraocular pressure, partial or full loss, dull, severe pain, fogginess, "rainbow rings", eye drops, relieve pressure, hearing loss, interfere with, perceive speech, surgical implants, tinnitus, nature and intensity, word retrieval, decreased fluency, language centres, poor-fitting dentures.

Exercise 3
Answer the following questions. Prepare short talks and/or dialogues on these topics.

1. What conditions are associated risk factors for complications related to diabetes?
2. Describe gastrointestinal problems (haemorrhage, obstruction, problems with continence and elimination).
3. What are causes of osteoarthritis and osteoporosis?
4. Describe problems with vision, problems with hearing and problems with speech.

Vocabulary 8

Fill in the meanings in your mother language:

absorptive /əbˈzɔːp.tɪv/
aching /eɪk.ɪŋ/ **pain** /peɪn/
anti-inflammatory / æn.tɪ.ɪnˈflæm.ə.tər.i/

anxiety /æŋˈzaɪ.ə.ti/
appetite /ˈæp.ɪ.taɪt/
aseptic /ˌeɪˈsep.tɪk/
associated /əˈsəʊ.si.eɪ.tɪd/
back /bæk/
blood /blʌd/ **-thinning** /θɪn.ɪŋ/
blood /blʌd/ **-tinged** /tɪndʒd/
body /ˈbɒd.i/ **mass** /mæs/
brittle /ˈbrɪt.l̩/
buttock /ˈbʌt.ək/
buzz /bʌz/
care /keər/ **for self** /self/
cartilage /ˈkɑː.təl.ɪdʒ/
cataract /ˈkæt.ə.rækt/
clarity /ˈklær.ɪ.ti/
closely /ˈkləʊ.sli/
coffee /ˈkɒf.i/ **-ground** /graʊnd/
colonic /kəˈlɑn.ɪk/
colorectal /kəʊ.ləʊˈrek.təl/
compensate /ˈkɒm.pən.seɪt/
consequently /ˈkɒnt.sɪ.kwənt.lɪ/
constipation /ˌkɒnt.stɪˈpeɪ.ʃən/
continence /ˈkɑːn.t̬ən.əns/
continue /kənˈtɪn.juː/
coronary /ˈkɒr.ən.ər.i/ **artery** /ˈɑːtərɪ/
cumulative /ˈkjuː.mjʊ.lə.tɪv/
decubitus /dɪˈkjuː.bit.əs/
degenerative /dɪˈdʒen.ər.ə.tɪv/
density /dent.sɪ.ti/
depth /depθ/
destruction /dɪˈstrʌk.ʃən/
detect /dɪˈtekt/
device /dɪˈvaɪs/
discomfort /dɪˈskʌm.fət/
distance /ˈdɪs.tənt s/
diverticulitis /ˌdaɪ.vəˌtɪk.jʊˈlaɪ.tɪs/
dressing /ˈdres.ɪŋ/
drug /drʌg/
dull /dʌl/
element /ˈel.ɪ.mənt/
elimination /ɪˌlɪm.ɪˈneɪ.ʃən/
embarrassment /ɪmˈbær.əs.mənt/
emesis /eˈmɪ.sɪs/
enlargement /ɪnˈlɑːdʒ.mənt/
event /ɪˈvent/
eye /aɪ/ **drops** /drɒps/
faecal /ˈfiː.kəl/
faeces /ˈfiː.siːz/
femur /ˈfiːmə/
finally /ˈfaɪ.nə.li/
fluency /ˈfluː.ən.si/
fogginess /ˈfɒg.ɪ.nəs/
frequent /ˈfriː.kwənt/
friction /ˈfrɪk.ʃən/
full /fʊl/
glaucoma /glɔːˈkəʊmə/
haemorrhage /ˈhem.ər.ɪdʒ/
halo /ˈheɪ.ləʊ/
hazardous /ˈhæz.ə.dəs/
hearing /ˈhɪə.rɪŋ/ **loss** /lɒs/
hernia /ˈhɜː.ni.ə/
hypertension /ˌhaɪ.pəˈten.tʃən/
image /ˈɪm.ɪdʒ/
immobile /ɪˈməʊ.baɪl/
immobilize /ɪˈməʊ.bəl.aɪz/
immunological /ˌɪm.jʊ.nəʊ.ˈlodʒ.ɪ.kəl/
impaction /ɪmˈpæk.ʃən/
impair /ɪmˈpeər/
implant /ɪmˈplɑːnt/
incontinence /ɪnˈkɒn.tɪ.nəns/
inflamed /ɪnˈfleɪmd/
interfere /ˌɪn.təˈfɪər/
intraocular /ˌɪn.trəˈɒk.jʊ.lər/
irritate /ˈɪr.ɪ.teɪt/
irritation /ˌɪr.ɪˈteɪ.ʃən/
larynx /ˈlær.ɪŋks/ pl **larynges**
lens /lenz/
limit /ˈlɪm.ɪt/
lodge /lɒdʒ/
make /meɪk/ **up** /ʌp/ **for** /fɔːr/
memory /ˈmem.ər.i/ **loss** /lɒs/
menopause /ˈmen.ə.pɔːz/
metabolic /ˌmet.əˈbɒl.ɪk/ **rate** /reɪt/
mild /maɪld/
moisture /ˈmɔɪs.tʃər/
motility /ˌməʊ.ˈtil.i.ˈtiː/
natural /ˈnætʃ.ər.əl/
nature /ˈneɪ.tʃə/
nerve /nɜːv/ **fibre** /ˈfaɪ.bər/
neurological /ˌnjʊə.rəˈlɒdʒ.ɪ.kəl/

noise /nɔɪz/
non-steroidal /ˌnɒnˈste.rɔɪd.əl/
optic /ˈɒp.tɪk/
osteoarthritis /ˌɒs.ti.əʊ.ɑːˈθraɪ.tɪs/
overall /ˌəʊ.vəˈrɔːl/
pancreatitis /ˌpæŋ.krɪ.əˈtaɪ.tɪs/
partial /ˈpɑː.ʃəl/
pass /pɑːs/ **wind** /wɪnd/
perception /pəˈsep.ʃən/
polydrug /ˈpɒl.i.drʌg/
polypharmacy /ˈpɒl.i.ˈfɑː.mə.si/
poor-fitting /pɔːrˈfɪt.ɪŋ/
postpone /pəʊstˈpəʊn/
prescribe /prɪˈskraɪb/
preserve /prɪˈzɜːv/
pressure /ˈpreʃ.ə/ **ulcer** /ˈʌl.sər/
primary /ˈpraɪ.mə.ri/
prior /ˈpraɪə/ **to** /tʊ/
procedure /prəˈsiːdʒə/
profound /prəˈfaʊnd/
prostate (gland) /ˈprɒs.teɪtˌglænd/
protracted /prəʊˈtrækt.ɪd/
purple /ˈpɜː.plˌ/
quality /kwɒ.lɪ.tɪ/
quarter /ˈkwɔː.tər/
rainbow /ˈreɪn.bəʊ/
reduction /rɪˈdʌk.ʃən/
refer /rɪˈfɜːr/ **to** /tʊ/
regress /rɪˈgres/
relative /ˈrel.ə.tɪv/
relieve /rɪˈliːv/
remove /rɪˈmuːv/
renal /ˈriː.nəl/ **failure** /ˈfeɪ.ljər/
repair /rɪˈpeə/
report /rəˈpoːt/
restore /rɪˈstɔːr/
retinopathy /ˌret.ɪnˈɒp.ə.θi/
retrieval /rɪˈtriː.vəl/
ring /rɪŋ/
ringing /rɪŋ.ɪŋ/
sacrum /ˈseɪ.krəm/
seek /siːk/ **(sought, sought)**
select /sɪˈlekt/
severe /sɪˈvɪər/
severely /sɪˈvɪə.li/
severity /sɪˈver.ɪ.ti/
shear /ˈʃɪə.r/
speech /spiːtʃ/
spontaneous /spɒnˈteɪ.ni.əs/
stiffness /ˈstɪf.nəs/
stool /stuːl/
stricture /ˈstrɪk.tʃər/
surgical /ˈsɜː.dʒɪ.kəl/
tarry /ˈtær.i/
taste /teɪst/
therapy /ˈθer.ə.pi/
tinnitus /ˈtɪn.ɪ.təs/
toxic /ˈtɒk.sɪk/
transparency /trænˈspær.ən.si/
ulcer /ˈʌl.sər/
undergarment /ˈʌn.dəˌgɑː.mənt/
urethral /jʊəˈriː.θrəl/
urinary /ˈjʊə.rɪ.nər.i/
urination /ˌjʊə.rɪˈneɪ.ʃən/
variation /ˌveə.riˈeɪ.ʃən/
vascular /ˈvæs.kjʊ.lər/
vertebra /ˈvɜː.tɪ.brə/ pl **vertebrae**
voice /vɔɪs/
void /vɔɪd/
warning /ˈwɔː.nɪŋ/ **sign** /saɪn/
wear /weə/ **and tear** /tɪə/
whistle /ˈwɪs.l̩/
wound /wuːnd/
wrist /rɪst/

Solution to Exercise 1
1c, 2k, 3i, 4d, 5r, 6x, 7b, 8z, 9t, 10a, 11q, 12n, 13y, 14s, 15v, 16f, 17h, 18j, 19w, 20u, 21o, 22p, 23g, 24e, 25m, 26l

Unit 9 - Care of older patients 3

Older patients are at increased risk for **adverse drug reactions**. Age-related changes that affect absorption include **increased gastric pH** and **decreased gastrointestinal motility**. Drug-induced metabolic changes are especially significant in the elderly; this is because they often take **several different drugs** for multiple diseases and conditions, which further increases their risk for adverse reactions. Drugs may not produce the desired effect or may cause major drug **toxicity**. Other common reasons for drug-induced illness include **dispensing errors, non-concordance, confusion, forgetfulness, vision impairment and the self-selection** of drugs. In addition, older adults commonly have several prescriptions from more than one physician; or take prescribed medications along with **over-the-counter drugs** that may have **synergistic** or **cumulative** effects. Finally, changes in habits regarding **alcohol, diet and exercise** also can affect drug metabolism.

Substance abuse

Substance abuse involving alcohol and other drugs is more common in the older population than might be expected. Individuals often have a **history** of alcohol and other drug abuse. Substance abuse often is attributed to **severe stress** which may result from life changes, changes in health or appearance, loss of employment, loss of life partner, illness, malnutrition, loneliness, loss of independent living arrangements, and others. Ingestion of even small amounts of alcohol by the older patient can cause intoxication.

Signs of alcohol abuse:

Anorexia, confusion, denial, frequent falling, hostility, insomnia, mood swings

Other drug abuse:

Altered level of consciousness, falling, hallucinations, memory changes, orthostatic hypotension, poor coordination, restlessness, weight loss

Hypothermia

The signs and **symptoms** may include an **altered mental state, slurred speech, ataxia and dysrhythmias**. In severe cases, coma without signs of life may be present. An older patient may develop hypothermia while **indoors**. This is due in part to the following characteristics of older adults:

- They are **less able to make up for environmental heat loss**.
- They have a **decreased ability to sense changes** in temperature.
- They have **less** total **body water** to store heat.
- They are **less likely** to develop tachycardia to **increase cardiac output** in response to cold stress.
- They have a **decreased ability to shiver** to increase body heat.

The following are other **medical causes** of hypothermia in older patients: arthritis, drug overdose, hepatic failure, hypoglycaemia, infection, Parkinson's disease, stroke, thyroid disease, uraemia.

Hyperthermia

Hyperthermia is less common, yet hyperthermia carries a **significant mortality** rate. The condition most likely results from exposure to high temperatures. These temperatures most likely continue for several days (e.g. **during a heat wave**). Hyperthermia also may result from medical conditions. Hyperthermic illness may present as **heat cramps, heat exhaustion or heat stroke**.

Behavioural and psychiatric disorders

In addition to the neurological disorders such as dementia and Alzheimer's disease, depression and suicide are common in older patients. **Depression** is a serious illness that calls for specialist evaluation. In the older patient, depression can result from physiological and psychological causes and various personality disorders. The **signs and symptoms** of depression vary by individual. They may include the following: decreased libido, deep feelings of worthlessness and guilt, extreme isolation, feelings of hopelessness, irritability, loss of appetite, loss of energy (fatigue), recurrent thoughts of death, significant weight loss, sleeplessness, suicide attempts.

Common causes of depression in the older patient:

Physical: dehydration, electrolyte imbalance, fever, hyponatraemia, hypoxia, medications, metabolic disturbance, organic brain disease, reduced cardiac output, thyroid disease

Psychological: fear of dying, financial insecurity, loss of a spouse, loss of independence, significant illness.

Signs and symptoms of elder abuse and neglect:

Physical abuse

- **Bruises, black eyes, lacerations** and **rope marks**
- Bone **fractures**, skull fractures
- Open **wounds**, untreated injuries in **various stages of healing**
- **Sprains, dislocations**, and **internal injuries/bleeding**
- Physical signs of being subjected to **punishment**, and signs of being **restrained**
- An elder's sudden **change in behaviour**
- An elder's **report of being hit, slapped, kicked or mistreated**

Emotional or psychological abuse

- Being emotionally **upset or agitated**
- Being **extremely withdrawn** and non-communicative or non-responsive
- Unusual **behaviour** usually being attributed to dementia (e.g. **sucking, biting or rocking**)

- An elder's **report** of being verbally or emotionally **mistreated**

Neglect and self-neglect

- **Dehydration, malnutrition**, untreated or improperly attended **medical conditions**, and poor personal **hygiene**
- Hazardous or unsafe **living conditions** (lack of heat or running water)
- Unsanitary or unclean living quarters (e.g. animal/insect **infestation**, no functioning **toilet** and faecal/urine **smell**)
- Inappropriate and/or inadequate **clothing**, lack of the necessary **medical aids (eyeglasses, hearing aids, and dentures)**
- Grossly **inadequate housing** or homelessness
- An elder's report of being mistreated

Exercise 1
Match the column A with the column B. Try to learn the expressions and/ or sentences by heart.

A

1. Age-related changes that affect absorption
2. The elderly often take several different drugs for multiple diseases and conditions,
3. Other common reasons for drug-induced illness include
4. Older adults take prescribed medications along with over-the-counter drugs
5. Signs of alcohol abuse are
6. Signs of other drug abuse include altered
7. The signs and symptoms of hypothermia may
8. Older adults have a decreased ability to sense changes in temperature
9. They have less total body water to store heat
10. The following are other medical causes of hypothermia in older patients:
11. Hyperthermia results from exposure to high temperatures which
12. Hyperthermic illness may present
13. The signs and symptoms of depression may include the following:
14. Common physical causes of depression in the older patient are
15. Common psychological causes of depression in the older patient are
16. Signs and symptoms of physical abuse and neglect include:
17. Signs and symptoms of emotional or psychological abuse and neglect include:
18. Signs and symptoms of neglect and self-neglect are dehydration, malnutrition, untreated or improperly attended medical conditions,

lack of the necessary medical aids (eyeglasses, hearing aids, and dentures),

B

a) *an elder's report of being verbally or emotionally mistreated, being emotionally upset or agitated, being non-communicative or non-responsive, sucking, biting or rocking.*

b) *and are less able to make up for environmental heat loss.*

c) *and have a decreased ability to shiver to increase body heat.*

d) *anorexia, confusion, denial, frequent falling, hostility, insomnia, or mood swings.*

e) *arthritis, drug overdose, hepatic failure, hypoglycaemia, infection, Parkinson's disease, stroke, thyroid disease, uraemia.*

f) *as heat cramps, heat exhaustion or heat stroke.*

g) *bruises, black eyes, lacerations, fractures, open wounds, untreated injuries in various stages of healing, sprains, dislocations, internal injuries/bleeding, and an elder's report of being hit, slapped, kicked or mistreated.*

h) *continue for several days (e.g. during a heat wave).*

i) *dehydration, electrolyte imbalance, fever, hyponatraemia, hypoxia, medications, metabolic disturbance, organic brain disease, reduced cardiac output, and thyroid disease.*

j) *dispensing errors, non-concordance, confusion, forgetfulness, vision impairment and the self-selection of drugs.*

k) *extreme isolation, feelings of hopelessness, irritability, loss of appetite, fatigue, sleeplessness, and suicide attempts.*

l) *fear of dying, financial insecurity, loss of a spouse, loss of independence, significant illness.*

m) *include an altered mental state, slurred speech, ataxia and dysrhythmias.*

n) *include increased gastric pH and decreased gastrointestinal motility.*

o) *level of consciousness, falling, hallucinations, memory changes, orthostatic hypotension, poor coordination, restlessness, and weight loss.*

p) *poor personal hygiene, lack of heat or running water, animal/insect infestation, no functioning toilet and faecal/urine smell, inadequate clothing, and grossly inadequate housing or homelessness.*

q) *that may have synergistic or cumulative effects.*

r) *which further increases their risk for adverse reactions.*

Exercise 2
Translate the expressions. Try to explain their meanings in English.

Adverse, motility, drug-induced, multiple diseases, desired effect, dispensing errors, non-concordance, confusion, forgetfulness, vision impairment, physician, prescriptions, over-the-counter drugs, synergistic or cumulative, abuse, attributed, arrangements, ingestion, confusion, denial, hostility, insomnia, mood swings, orthostatic hypotension, restlessness, altered mental state, slurred speech, ataxia, indoors, make up for, ability to sense, shiver, uraemia, mortality rate, heat wave, medical conditions, heat cramps, heat exhaustion, heat stroke, behavioural, personality disorders, feelings of worthlessness and guilt, hopelessness, recurrent thoughts, suicide attempts, hyponatraemia, fear, neglect, bruises, lacerations, untreated injuries, stages of healing, sprains, dislocations, punishment, restrained, hit, slapped, kicked, mistreated, upset or agitated, extremely withdrawn, non-responsive, sucking, biting or rocking, lack of heat or running water, inadequate clothing, medical aids, eyeglasses, hearing aids, dentures.

Exercise 3
Answer the following questions. Prepare short talks and/or dialogues on these topics.

1. What are the reasons for drug-induced illness?
2. What are the signs of alcohol and other drug abuse?
3. What are the dangers of hypothermia and hyperthermia in elderly people?
4. Talk about behavioural and psychiatric disorders in elderly people.
5. What are the signs and symptoms of elder abuse and neglect?

Vocabulary 9

Fill in the meanings in your mother language:

adverse /ˈæd.vɜːs/
agitated /ˈædʒ.ɪ.teɪ.tɪd/
arrangement /əˈreɪndʒ.mənt/
arthritis /ɑːˈθraɪ.tɪs/
ataxia /əˈtæk.si.ə/
attend /əˈtend/
biting /ˈbaɪ.tɪŋ/
black /blæk/ **eye** /aɪ/
bruise /bruːz/
clothing /ˈkləʊ.ðɪŋ/
communicative /kəˈmjuː.nɪ.kə.tɪv/
cramp /kræmp/
denial /dɪˈnaɪ.əl/
depression /dɪˈpreʃ.ən/
desired /dɪˈzaɪəd/
dislocation /ˌdis.loʊˈkeiˌʃən/
dispensing /dɪˈspens.ɪŋ/
dying /ˈdaɪ.ɪŋ/
error /ˈer.ər/
evaluation /ɪˌvæl.juˈeɪ.ʃən/
exposure /ɪkˈspəʊ.ʒər/
eyeglasses /ˈaɪˌglɑː.sɪz/
fear /fɪə/
feeling /ˈfiː.lɪŋ/
forgetfulness /fəˈget.fʊl.nɪs/
grossly /ˈgrəʊs.li/
guilt /gɪlt/
habits /ˈhæb.ɪts/

healing /hiːlɪŋ/
heat /hiːt/ **wave** /weɪv/
heat /hiːt/ **stroke** /strəʊk/
hepatic /hepˈæt.ɪk/
hit /hɪt/ **(hit, hit)**
homelessness /ˈhəʊm.ləs.nəs/
hopelessness /ˈhəʊp.ləs.nəs/
hostility /hɒsˈtɪl.ɪ.ti/
hygiene /ˈhaɪ.dʒiːn/
improperly /ɪmˈprɒp.ər.li/
inappropriate /ˌɪn.əˈprəʊ.pri.ət/
independence /ˌɪndɪˈpendəns/
indoors /ˌɪnˈdɔːz/
induce /ɪnˈdjuːs/
infestation /ˌɪn.fesˈteɪ.ʃən/
insect /ˈɪn.sekt/
insecurity /ˌɪn.sɪˈkjʊə.rɪ.ti/
insomnia /ɪnˈsɒm.ni.ə/
isolation /ˌaɪ.səl.eɪ.ʃən/
kick /kɪk/
laceration /ˌlæs.ərˈeɪ.ʃən/
lack /læk/
libido /lɪˈbiː.dəʊ/
likely /ˈlaɪ.kli/
living /ˈlɪvɪŋ/ **conditions** /kənˈdɪʃ.əns/
mark /mɑːk/
mistreat /ˌmɪsˈtriːt/
mood /muːd/ **swing** /swɪŋ/
non /ˌnɒn/ **-concordance** /kənˈkɔː.dəns/
over-the-counter /ˌəʊ.və.ðəˈkaʊn.tər/
personality /ˌpɜː.sənˈæl.ə.ti/
disorder /dɪˈsɔː.dər/
physician /fɪˈzɪʃ.ən/
prescription /prɪˈskrɪp.ʃən/
punishment /ˈpʌn.ɪʃ.mənt/
recurrent /rɪˈkʌr.ənt/
responsive /rɪˈspɒn.sɪv/
restlessness /ˈrest.ləs.nəs/
rock /rɒk/
rope /rəʊp/
running /ˈrʌn.ɪŋ/ **water** /ˈwɔː.tər/
sense /sens/
shiver /ˈʃɪv.ər/
slap /slæp/
sleeplessness /ˈsliːp.ləs.nəs/
slurred /ˈslɜːd/
smell /smel/
sprain /spreɪn/
suck /sʌk/
suicide /ˈsuː.ɪ.saɪd/ **attempt** /əˈtempt/
synergistic /sɪn.əˈdʒɪs.tɪk/
unclean /ʌnˈkliːn/
unsafe /ʌnˈseɪf/
unsanitary /ˌʌnˈsæn.ɪ.tər.i/
upset /ʌpˈset/
uraemia /jʊəˈriː.mɪ.ə/
withdrawn /wɪðˈdrɔːn/
worthlessness /ˈwɜːθ.ləs.nəs/

Solution to Exercise 1
1n, 2r, 3j, 4q, 5d, 6o, 7m, 8b, 9c, 10e, 11h, 12f, 13k, 14i, 15l, 16g, 17a, 18p

Unit 10 - Physical well-being. Nutrition 1

Wellness components

Wellness has two main aspects: physical well-being and mental and emotional health. Several factors play a major role in maintaining **physical health**. These factors include **good nutrition, physical fitness, ample sleep,** and the **prevention of disease and injury**.

Nutrition

Nutrients are foods that hold the **elements** necessary for **body function**. The **six categories** of nutrients are **carbohydrates, fats, proteins, vitamins, minerals, and water.**

Carbohydrates are derived primarily from **plant** foods. The only important source of **animal**

carbohydrates is **lactose** (milk sugar). Plants store carbohydrates as **starch**.

All **dietary fats** contain a mixture of saturated and unsaturated **fatty acids. Saturated** fats are found mainly in meat and dairy products and in some vegetable fats. **Unsaturated** fats are **subdivided** further into polyunsaturated and monounsaturated fats. **Polyunsaturated** fats are found in **safflower, corn, soybeans, and cottonseed oils and in some fish**. Omega-3 fatty acids are found mainly in cold-water fish such as tuna, salmon, and mackerel. **Monounsaturated** fats are liquid **vegetable oils** such as olive oil. Like polyunsaturated fats, these may also decrease blood cholesterol levels. **Trans fats** are **unsaturated** fatty acids formed when vegetable **oils** are **processed** and made more **solid** or into a more **stable** liquid. Trans fats are present in a wide range of foods, such as **baked** goods and **fried** foods and some **margarine** products. Trans fats also occur naturally in low amounts in meat and dairy products. **Cholesterol** is present in all foods of **animal origin** and is concentrated heavily in **fat and in poultry skin**. Cholesterol is a **white, waxy substance** found in **every cell** and is **needed** by the body for normal functioning. Not all cholesterol is harmful; an adequate amount of cholesterol is needed for body functions. Cholesterol is manufactured **in the liver** and is carried through the **bloodstream**. Adding cholesterol to the diet can **raise blood cholesterol** levels and increase the risk of **heart disease and stroke**.

Proteins are made of **hydrogen, oxygen, carbon, and nitrogen** (and most contain **sulphur and phosphorus**). Proteins are vital to building body tissue during **growth, maintenance, and repair.** When proteins are digested, they **break down** into **amino acids** (classified as essential or non-essential). **Essential** amino acids are needed for body growth and cellular life and must be obtained in food because they **are not made in the body**. **Non-essential** amino acids are not needed for body health and growth and **can be made** in the body. Proteins that contain all the essential amino acids are **complete** proteins and are found in **meats and dairy** products. Proteins that are **missing** one or more essential amino acids are **incomplete** proteins (e.g. those in **grains and vegetables**). Proteins can be used as a source of energy but should **be spared** for their more important role in body health.

Vitamins are **organic** substances that are present in minute amounts in foods. Because vitamins are **crucial for metabolism** and **cannot be made** in adequate amounts by the body, they must be gained through **food or vitamin supplements**. Vitamins are water-soluble or fat-soluble. Vitamins **C and B** complex are **water-soluble** vitamins and cannot be stored in the body, so these must **come from the daily diet. Fat-soluble** vitamins (vitamins **A, D, E, and K**) can be **stored** in the body, so a daily dietary intake of these vitamins is not required.

Minerals are **inorganic** elements that occur naturally **in the earth** and play a key role in biochemical reactions in the body. Minerals include **calcium, chromium, iron, magnesium, selenium, and zinc**, and like vitamins, minerals **come from the diet**. Diseases caused by vitamin deficiency include **scurvy, rickets, or beriberi**. Making proper food choices can help to prevent them.

Water is the most important nutrient because **cellular function** depends on a fluid environment. Water composes **50–60% of the total body weight.** (Infants have the greatest percentage of body water; older adults have the least.) Water is obtained through consumption of **liquids and fresh fruits and vegetables**.

Exercise 1
Match the column A with the column B. Try to learn the expressions and/or sentences by heart.

A

1. Wellness has two main aspects:
2. Several factors play a major role in maintaining physical health:
3. The six categories of nutrients are
4. Saturated fats are found mainly
5. Unsaturated fats are subdivided further
6. Polyunsaturated fats are found in
7. Omega-3 fatty acids are
8. Monounsaturated fats are
9. Trans fats are unsaturated fatty acids formed when vegetable oils
10. Trans fats are present in
11. Cholesterol is present in all foods of animal origin
12. Cholesterol is manufactured
13. Adding cholesterol to the diet can
14. Proteins are made of
15. Proteins are vital to
16. When proteins are digested, they
17. Essential amino acids are needed for body growth and cellular life
18. Proteins that contain all the essential amino acids are
19. Proteins that are missing one or more essential amino acids
20. Vitamins are organic substances that are crucial for metabolism and cannot be made by the body,
21. Vitamins C and B complex are water-soluble vitamins and
22. Fat-soluble vitamins (vitamins A, D, E, and K) can be stored in the body
23. Minerals, inorganic elements that occur naturally in the earth
24. Diseases caused by vitamin deficiency
25. Water which composes 50–60% of the total body weight

B

a) *and is concentrated heavily in fat and in poultry skin.*
b) *and must be obtained in food because they are not made in the body.*
c) *are incomplete proteins (e.g. those in grains and vegetables).*
d) *are processed and made more solid or into a more stable liquid.*
e) *baked goods, fried foods and some margarine products.*
f) *break down into amino acids (classified as essential or non-essential).*
g) *building body tissue during growth, maintenance, and repair.*
h) *cannot be stored in the body, so these must come from the daily diet.*
i) *carbohydrates, fats, proteins, vitamins, minerals, and water.*
j) *complete proteins and are found in meats and dairy products.*
k) *found mainly in cold-water fish such as tuna, salmon, and mackerel.*
l) *good nutrition, physical fitness, ample sleep, and the prevention of disease and injury.*
m) *hydrogen, oxygen, carbon, and nitrogen (and most contain sulphur and phosphorus).*
n) *in meat and dairy products and in some vegetable fats.*
o) *in the liver and is carried through the bloodstream.*
p) *include calcium, chromium, iron, magnesium, selenium, and zinc, and like vitamins, minerals come from the diet.*
q) *include scurvy, rickets, or beriberi.*
r) *into polyunsaturated and monounsaturated fats.*
s) *is the most important nutrient because cellular function depends on a fluid environment.*
t) *liquid vegetable oils such as olive oil.*
u) *physical well-being and mental and emotional health.*
v) *raise blood cholesterol levels and increase the risk of heart disease and stroke.*
w) *safflower, corn, soybeans, and cottonseed oils and in some fish.*
x) *so a daily dietary intake of these vitamins is not required.*
y) *they must be gained through food or vitamin supplements.*

Exercise 2
Translate the expressions. Try to explain their meanings in English.

Well-being, derived from, plant source, starch, fatty acids, subdivided, safflower, corn, soybeans, cottonseed, processed, solid, stable liquid, trans fats, poultry skin, waxy substance, manufactured, hydrogen, oxygen, carbon, nitrogen, sulphur, phosphorus, growth, maintenance, repair, essential amino acids, obtained, complete proteins, grains, be spared, crucial, gained through, supplements, water-soluble, stored, dietary intake, required, calcium, chromium, iron, magnesium, selenium, zinc, scurvy, rickets, beriberi, choices, cellular function, fluid environment.

Exercise 3
Answer the following questions. Prepare short talks and/or dialogues on these topics.

1. What factors play a major role in maintaining physical health?
2. What are the six categories of nutrients?
3. Describe the role of carbohydrates.
4. What do you know about dietary fats?
5. Why are proteins vital to building body tissue?
6. Describe the functions of vitamins, minerals and water.

Vocabulary 10

Fill in the meanings in your mother language:

ample /ˈæm.pl̩/
beriberi /ˌber.ɪˈber.i/
cellular /ˈsel.jʊ.lər/
corn /kɔːn/
cotton /ˈkɒt.ən/ **seed** /siːd/
crucial /ˈkruː.ʃəl/
deficiency /dɪˈfɪʃ.ənt.si/
derive /dɪˈraɪv/
earth /ɜːθ/
grain /greɪn/
incomplete /ˌɪn.kəmˈpliːt/
liquid /ˈlɪk.wɪd/
maintenance /ˈmeɪn.tɪ.nəns/
miss /ˈmɪs/
origin /ˈɒr.ɪ.dʒɪn/
phosphorus /ˈfɒs.fər.əs/
process /ˈprəʊ.ses/
rickets /ˈrɪk.ɪts/
safflower /ˈsæ.flaʊər/
scurvy /ˈskɜː.vi/
solid /ˈsɒl.ɪd/
soybean /ˈsɔɪˌbiːn/
spare /speər/
stable /ˈsteɪ.bl̩/
subdivide /ˌsʌb.dɪˈvaɪd/
sulphur (S) /ˈsʌl.fər/
supplement /ˈsʌp.lɪ.mənt/
trans fats /ˈtrænz.fæts/
waxy /ˈwæk.si/
well-being /ˌwelˈbiː.ɪŋ/
wellness /ˈwel.nəs/

Solution to Exercise 1
1u, 2l. 3i, 4n, 5r, 6w, 7k, 8t, 9d, 10e, 11a, 12o, 13v, 14m, 15g, 16f, 17b, 18j, 19c, 20y, 21h, 22x, 23p, 24q, 25s

Unit 11 - Physical well-being. Nutrition 2

Fat and cholesterol control
Tips for a healthy eating plan

- Select **lean** cuts of meat, such as **loin and round cuts**, and **trim all visible fat**.
- Buy **lower-fat versions** of your favourite **dairy products**, such as **skim milk** and **skim milk–based cheeses**.
- For added flavour, use **herbs and spices in place**

of high-fat flavourings or sauces on vegetables, meats, poultry, and fish.

- **Chill** soups and stews and **skim off the fat** that collects on the surface.
- Choose **low-fat or non-fat** versions of your favourite **salad dressings**, mayonnaise, yoghurt, and sour cream.
- Use **low-fat or fat-free marinades** to tenderize and add flavour to leaner cuts of meat.

Tips to reduce saturated fats

- Use polyunsaturated or monounsaturated oil when a recipe calls for melted shortening or butter.
- Use vegetable oil margarine in place of butter or lard. Look for whipped, lower-fat tub margarine.

Tips to be fat smart

- **Saturated fats** usually are **solid at room temperature**. They mainly come from **animal foods**, such as **meat, poultry, butter, and whole milk. Coconut, palm, and palm kernel oils** are also high in saturated fat. Saturated fat is responsible for raising blood-cholesterol levels.
- **Polyunsaturated fats** usually are **liquid** at room temperature. They are found in vegetable oils. **Safflower, sunflower, corn, and soybean oils** contain the highest amounts of these polyunsaturated fats. Polyunsaturated fats can help **decrease high blood-cholesterol levels** when part of a good diet.
- **Monounsaturated** fats also are **liquid** at room temperature. They are found in vegetable oils, such as **canola and olive oil.** Monounsaturated fats can help to **decrease high blood-cholesterol levels** if they are part of a lower-fat diet.
- **Dietary cholesterol** comes only from animal sources, such as the **fat in dairy products, egg yolks, meats, poultry, and seafood.** Vegetables, fruits, and grains do not contain cholesterol.
- **Hydrogenation** is a process that **makes oil more solid** at room temperature. Hydrogenated vegetable oils give some processed foods a longer shelf life. Examples of those foods include margarine and crackers.

Free radicals and antioxidants

- Free radicals are natural **by-products of chemical reactions** in the body that can **produce cellular injury**. The build-up of these free radicals increases **with age.** The build-up is thought to be the cause of many diseases, including **heart disease, diabetes, and some cancers.** Substances that can generate free radicals can be found in **fried foods, alcohol, tobacco smoke, pesticides, and air pollution.**

- **Antioxidants** are known as **free-radical scavengers.** They are compounds that reduce the formation of free radicals or react with and **neutralize them**, making them non-toxic to cells. Antioxidants **occur naturally** in the body. They also occur naturally in certain foods such as **fruits, vegetables, and whole grains. Beta carotene (a form of vitamin A) and vitamins C and E** are popular **antioxidant supplements.** These may benefit a person's health.

The ABCs of nutrition
Vitamin A

Proper **eye function**; keeps **skin, hair**, and **nails** healthy; helps maintain healthy **gums, glands, bones, teeth**; helps ward off infection; may protect against lung cancer. **Source**: *liver, dairy products, fish, carrots, yellow squash, dark-green leafy vegetables, corn, tomatoes, papaya.*

Vitamin B_1 (thiamine)

Helps convert carbohydrates into **biological energy**; promotes proper **nerve** function. **Source**: *pork, unrefined and enriched cereals, organ meats, legumes, nuts.*

Vitamin B_2 (riboflavin)

Crucial in the production of **body energy. Source**: *milk, cheese, yoghurt, green leafy vegetables, fruits, bread, cereals, meats.*

Vitamin B_3 (niacin)

Lowers cholesterol levels in blood only in very high doses; may protect against cardiovascular disease. **Source**: *yeast, meats including liver, cereals, legumes, seeds.*

Vitamin B_6

Essential for **protein breakdown** and absorption. **Source**: *beef, poultry, fish, pork, bananas, nuts, whole grains, vegetables.*

Vitamin B_{12}

Essential for the healthy function of **nerve tissue. Source**: *meats, meat products, shellfish, fish, poultry, eggs.*

Biotin

Needed for **breakdown of glucose** (a type of sugar) and formation of certain **fatty acids** necessary for several important body functions. **Source**: *meats, poultry, fish, eggs, nuts, seeds, legumes, vegetables.*

Vitamin C (ascorbic acid)

Strengthens **blood vessel walls**; keeps **gums** healthy;

promotes **healing** of cuts and wounds. **Source**: *strawberries, citrus fruits, tomatoes, cabbage, cauliflower, broccoli, greens.*

Vitamin D

Helps build and maintain **teeth and bones**; needed for body to **absorb calcium. Source**: *egg yolks, fish and cod liver oil, fortified milk, and butter.*

Vitamin E

Helps form **red blood cells, muscle** tissue, and other tissues; may protect against heart disease. **Source**: *poultry, seafood, seeds, nuts, cooked greens, wheat germ, fortified cereals, eggs.*

Vitamin K+

Needed for normal **clotting of blood. Source**: *spinach, broccoli, Brussels sprouts, kale, turnip greens.*

Minerals

Calcium

Helps build **strong bones and teeth**; promotes proper **muscle and nerve** function; helps **blood to clot**; helps **activate enzymes** needed to convert food to energy; may protect against the development of fragile, porous bones. **Source**: *milk, cheese, yoghurt, buttermilk, other dairy products, green leafy vegetables.*

Chromium

Works **with insulin** to maintain **normal blood sugar. Source**: *whole-grain cereals, condiments (black pepper, thyme), meat products, cheeses.*

Iron

Essential to **make haemoglobin,** the **oxygen-carrying** component of red blood cells. **Source**: *red meat and liver, shellfish and fish, legumes, dried apricots, fortified breads, and cereals.*

Magnesium

Activates enzymes needed to **release energy** in body; promotes **bone growth**; needed to make **cells and genetic** material. **Source**: *green leafy vegetables, beans, nuts, fortified whole-grain cereals and breads, oysters, scallops.*

Potassium

With sodium, helps to regulate body's **fluid balance**; plays a major role in **muscle contraction, nerve conduction, beating** of the heart. **Source**: *bananas, citrus fruits, dried fruits, deep yellow vegetables, potatoes, legumes, milk, bran cereal.*

Selenium

Interacts **with vitamin E** to **prevent breakdown of cells** in body. **Source**: *organ meats, seafood, meats, cereals and grains, egg yolks, onions, garlic, mushrooms.*

Sodium

Helps maintain **body fluid balance. Source**: *salt, processed foods, foods in brine, salted chips and crackers, cured meats, soy sauce.* Sodium is so prevalent that low intake is very rare. The problem is avoiding excessive intake of sodium.

Zinc

Boosts the **immune system** and helps fight disease; **element in** more than 100 **enzymes-proteins** that are essential to **digestion** and other functions. **Source**: *red meats, some seafood, grains.*

Exercise 1
Match the column A with the column B. Try to learn the expressions and/or sentences by heart.

A

1. Select lean cuts of meat, such as
2. Buy lower-fat dairy products
3. For added flavour, use herbs and spices
4. Chill soups and stews
5. Choose low-fat or non-fat salad dressings,
6. Use vegetable oil margarine
7. Saturated fats usually are solid at room temperature; they mainly come from animal foods, such as
8. Polyunsaturated fats usually are liquid at room temperature; they are found in vegetable oils;
9. Dietary cholesterol comes only from animal sources,
10. Hydrogenated vegetable oils
11. Free radicals are natural by-products of chemical reactions in the body
12. Substances that can generate free radicals
13. Antioxidants are compounds that reduce the formation of free radicals
14. Antioxidants occur naturally in fruits, vegetables, and whole grains
15. Vitamin A keeps skin, hair, and nails healthy;
16. Vitamin B1 helps convert carbohydrates into biological energy, and vitamin B_3 lowers cholesterol levels in blood and may protect against cardiovascular disease;
17. Vitamin C strengthens
18. Vitamin D helps build and maintain
19. Vitamin E helps form red blood cells, muscle tissue, and other tissues;
20. Calcium helps build strong bones and teeth; promotes proper muscle and nerve function;
21. Chromium works with insulin
22. Iron is essential to make haemoglobin,
23. Magnesium activates enzymes needed to
24. Potassium helps to regulate body's fluid balance; plays a major role in muscle contraction, nerve conduction, and
25. Sodium helps maintain body fluid balance,

B

a) and skim off the fat that collects on the surface.
b) and use low-fat or fat-free marinades to tenderize

and add flavour to leaner cuts of meat.

c) *and vitamin A and vitamins C and E are popular antioxidant supplements.*

d) *beating of the heart; selenium interacts with vitamin E to prevent breakdown of cells in body.*

e) *blood vessel walls; keeps gums healthy; promotes healing of cuts and wounds*

f) *can be found in fried foods, alcohol, tobacco smoke, pesticides, and air pollution.*

g) *give some processed foods a longer shelf life.*

h) *helps blood to clot; helps activate enzymes needed to convert food to energy; and may protect against the development of fragile, porous bones.*

i) *in place of butter or lard.*

j) *in place of high-fat flavourings or sauces.*

k) *it helps maintain healthy gums, glands, bones, teeth; helps ward off infection.*

l) *loin and round cuts, and trim all visible fat.*

m) *may protect against heart disease; vitamin K+ is needed for normal clotting of blood.*

n) *meat, poultry, butter, and whole milk; coconut, palm, and palm kernel oils are also high in saturated fat.*

o) *or react with and neutralize them, making them non-toxic to cells.*

p) *promotes proper nerve function; vitamin* B_2 *is crucial in the production of body energy.*

q) *release energy in body; promotes bone growth; and is needed to make cells and genetic material.*

r) *safflower, sunflower, corn, and soybean oils contain the highest amounts of polyunsaturated fats.*

s) *while zinc boosts the immune system and helps fight disease.*

t) *such as skim milk and skim milk–based cheeses.*

u) *such as the fat in dairy products, egg yolks, meats, poultry, and seafood; vegetables, fruits, and grains do not contain cholesterol.*

v) *teeth and bones; it is needed for body to absorb calcium.*

w) *that can produce cellular injury; the build-up of free radicals increases with age.*

x) *the oxygen-carrying component of red blood cells.*

y) *to maintain normal blood sugar.*

z) *vitamin* B_6 *is essential for protein breakdown and absorption and vitamin* B_{12} *is essential for the healthy function of nerve tissue.*

Exercise 2

Translate the expressions. Try to explain their meanings in English.

Lean meat, loin and round cuts, trim all visible fat, skim milk–based cheeses, herbs and spices in place of high-fat flavourings, chill, skim off the fat, salad dressings, tenderize and add flavour, melted shortening, lard, whipped, tub margarine, smart, coconut, palm kernel oils, safflower, sunflower, corn, canola, egg yolks, shelf life, natural by-products, cellular injury, build-up, generate, free-radical scavengers, compounds, gums, glands, ward off, yellow squash, convert, promotes, unrefined and enriched cereals, organ meats, legumes, high doses, breakdown, seeds, blood vessel walls, healing, cabbage, cauliflower, cod liver oil, wheat germ, fortified cereals, clotting of blood, Brussels sprouts, kale, turnip greens, buttermilk, condiments, shellfish, apricots, fortified whole-grain cereals, oysters, scallops, fluid balance, muscle contraction, nerve conduction, bran cereal, organ meats, foods in brine, cured meats, prevalent.

Exercise 3
Study the following information. Ask and answer questions.

- Liver, dairy products, fish, carrots, yellow squash, dark-green leafy vegetables, corn, tomatoes, and papaya are sources of: **Vitamin A**
- Pork, unrefined and enriched cereals, organ meats, legumes, and nuts are sources of: **Vitamin B_1**
- Milk, cheese, yoghurt, green leafy vegetables, fruits, bread, cereals, and meats are sources of: **Vitamin B_2**
- Yeast, meats including liver, cereals, legumes, and seeds are sources of: **Vitamin B_3**
- Beef, poultry, fish, pork, bananas, nuts, whole grains, and vegetables are sources of: **Vitamin B_6**
- Meats, meat products, shellfish, fish, poultry, and eggs are sources of: **Vitamin B_{12}**
- Meats, poultry, fish, eggs, nuts, seeds, legumes, or vegetable are sources of: **Biotin**
- Strawberries, citrus fruits, tomatoes, cabbage, cauliflower, broccoli, or greens are sources of: **Vitamin C**
- Egg yolks, fish and cod liver oil, fortified milk, and butter are sources of: **Vitamin D**
- Poultry, seafood, seeds, nuts, cooked greens, wheat germ, fortified cereals, or eggs are sources of: **Vitamin E**
- Spinach, broccoli, Brussels sprouts, kale, turnip and greens are sources of: **Vitamin K+**
- Milk, cheese, yoghurt, buttermilk, other dairy products, or green leafy vegetables are sources of: **Calcium**
- Whole-grain cereals, condiments (black pepper, thyme), meat products, cheeses are sources of: **Chromium**

- Red meat and liver, shellfish and fish, legumes, dried apricots, fortified breads, and cereals are sources of: **Iron**
- Green leafy vegetables, beans, nuts, fortified whole-grain cereals and breads, oysters, or scallops are sources of: **Magnesium**
- Bananas, citrus fruits, dried fruits, deep yellow vegetables, potatoes, legumes, milk, or bran cereal are sources of: **Potassium**
- Organ meats, seafood, meats, cereals and grains, egg yolks, onions, garlic, or mushrooms are sources of: **Selenium**
- Salt, processed foods, foods in brine, salted chips and crackers, cured meats, soy sauce are sources of: **Sodium**
- Red meats, some seafood, grains are sources of: **Zinc**

Exercise 4
Answer the following questions. Prepare short talks and/or dialogues on these topics.

1. Give a few tips for a healthy eating plan.
2. What do you know about free radicals and antioxidants?
3. Explain the functions of vitamins A, B_1, B_2, B_3, B_6, B_{12}, C, D, K+.
4. What are their sources?
5. Talk about the importance of minerals and their sources (calcium, chromium, iron, magnesium, potassium, selenium, sodium and zinc).

Vocabulary 11

Fill in the meanings in your mother language:

apricot /ˈeɪ.prɪ.kɒt/
ascorbic acid /əˌskɔː.bɪkˈæs.ɪd/
benefit /ˈben.ɪ.fɪt/
biotin /baɪˈɒt.iːn/
boost /buːst/
bran /bræn/
brine /braɪn/
broccoli /ˈbrɒk.əl.i/
Brussels sprout /ˌbrʌs.əlz ˈspraʊt/
build-up /ˈbɪld.ʌp/
buttermilk /ˈbʌt.ə.mɪlk/
by-product /ˈbaɪˌprɒd.ʌkt/
cabbage /ˈkæb.ɪdʒ/
canola /kəˈnɒl.ə/
cauliflower /ˈkɒl.ɪˌflaʊ.ər/
cereal /ˈsɪə.ri.əl/
chromium /ˈkrəʊ.mi.əm/
clot /klɒt/
coconut /ˈkəʊ.kə.nʌt/
cod /kɒd/
condiment /ˈkɒn.dɪ.mənt/
cracker /ˈkræk.ər/
cured /kjʊəd/ **meat** /miːt/
cut /kʌt/
egg /eg/ **yolk** /jəʊk/
fight /faɪt/
flavouring /ˈfleɪ.vər.ɪŋ/
fortified /ˈfɔː.tɪˌfaɪd/
fragile /ˈfrædʒ.aɪl/
free /friː/ **radical** /ˈræd.ɪ.kəl/
garlic /ˈgɑː.lɪk/
greens /griːnz/
gum /gʌm/
hydrogenation /ˌhaɪ.drɪ.dʒəˈneɪ.ʃən/
interact /ˌɪn.təˈrækt/
iron /aɪən/
kale /keɪl/

kernel /ˈkɜː.nəl/
lard /lɑːd/
leafy /ˈliː.fi/
lean /liːn/
liver /ˈlɪv.ər/ **oil** /ɔɪl/
loin /lɔɪn/
melt /melt/
mushroom /ˈmʌʃ.ruːm/
niacin /ˈnaɪ ə sɪn/
onion /ˈʌn.jən/
oyster /ˈɔɪ.stər/
palm /pɑːm/
papaya /pəˈpaɪ.ə/
pepper /ˈpep.ər/
pesticide /ˈpes.tɪ.saɪd/
pollution /pəˈluː.ʃən/
porous /ˈpɔː.rəs/
riboflavin /ˌraɪ boʊˈfleɪ vɪn/
round /raʊnd/
scallop /ˈskɒl.əp/
scavenger /ˈskæv.ɪn.dʒər/
seed /siːd/
selenium /səˈliː.ni.əm/
shelf /ʃelf/ **life** /laɪf/
shellfish /ˈʃel.fɪʃ/
shortening /ˈʃɔː.tən.ɪŋ/
skim /skɪm/
squash /skwɒʃ/
stew /stjuː/
strengthen /ˈstreŋ.θən/
sunflower /ˈsʌnˌflaʊər/
tenderize /ˈten.dər.aɪz/
thiamine /ˈθaɪ.ə.miːn/
thyme /taɪm/
trim /trɪm/
tub /tʌb/
turnip /ˈtɜː.nɪp/
ward /wɔːd/ **off** /ɒf/
wheat /wiːt/ **germs** /dʒɜːmz/
whip /wɪp/
whole /həʊl/ **grain** /greɪn/
yeast /jiːst/
zinc /zɪŋk/

Solution to Exercise 1
1l, 2t, 3j, 4a, 5b, 6i, 7n, 8r, 9u, 10g, 11w, 12f, 13o, 14c, 15k, 16p, 17z, 18e, 19v, 20m, 21h, 22y, 23x, 24q, 25d, 26s

Unit 12 - Principles of weight control. Physical fitness.

People who are **overweight** tend to be at higher risk for developing certain illnesses, including **high blood pressure, diabetes mellitus, heart disease, and some cancers.** The tenets of weight control are to eat the **right balance** of foods **in moderation, limit fat** consumption, and **exercise** regularly. Anyone committed to weight control for a healthier life should set **realistic** goals. A healthy lifestyle is balanced with proper nutrition and exercise. A healthy diet includes a **variety** of foods that are **low in fat, saturated fat, and cholesterol,** and plenty of **grain products, vegetables, and fruit.** A diet should also be **moderate in simple sugars, salt, and sodium. Alcoholic beverages** should be avoided or consumed only in moderation.

Fat contents of various foods

- **More than 90%** fat: *whipped cream, pork sausage, cooking oils, margarine, butter, gravy, mayonnaise*
- **More than 80%** fat: *spare ribs, cream cheese, salad dressing, high-fat steaks*

(T-bone, porterhouse, tenderloin, fillet mignon)

- **More than 70% fat:** *peanuts, hot dogs, pork chops, most cheeses and nuts, sirloin steak, bacon, lamb chops*
- **More than 60% fat**: *potato crisps, regular ground beef, ham, eggs*
- **More than 50% fat**: *round steak, pot roast, creamed soup, ice cream, sweet rolls*
- **More than 40%** fat: *whole milk, cake, doughnuts, French fries*
- **More than 30%** fat: *muffins, biscuits, fruit pies, low-fat milk, cottage cheese, tuna, chicken, turkey*
- **More than 20%** fat: *lean fish, beef liver, ice milk*
- **More than 10%** fat: *bread, pretzels, whole grains, legumes*
- **Less than 10%** fat: *sherbet, non-fat milk, most fruits and vegetables, baked potatoes*

Fibre

The human body requires fibre to maintain good health and to fight disease. Fibre (found only in plant foods) may be soluble or insoluble.

Examples:

- **Soluble fibre** includes fibre obtained from *peas, beans, oats, barley, and some fruits and vegetables*. This type of fibre helps control the level of blood sugar. Soluble fibre may also lower the level of blood cholesterol.
- **Insoluble fibre** (found in whole grains and many vegetables) helps hold water in the colon and can reduce or prevent constipation. This type of fibre may also help prevent intestinal disease (e.g. haemorrhoids).

Exercise 1a
Match the column A with the column B. Try to learn the expressions and/or sentences by heart.

A

1. People who are overweight tend to be
2. The tenets of weight control are
3. A healthy diet includes a variety of foods that are low in fat, saturated fat, and cholesterol,
4. A diet should also be moderate in simple sugars, salt, and sodium;
5. Whipped cream, pork sausage, cooking oils, margarine, butter, gravy, mayonnaise all have:
6. Spare ribs, cream cheese, salad dressing, high-fat steaks (T-bone, porterhouse, tenderloin, fillet mignon) all have:
7. Peanuts, hot dogs, pork chops, most cheeses and nuts, sirloin steak, bacon, lamb chops all have:

8. Potato crisps, regular ground beef, ham, eggs all have:
9. Round steak, pot roast, creamed soup, ice cream, sweet rolls all have:
10. Whole milk, cake, doughnuts, French fries all have:
11. Muffins, biscuits, fruit pies, low-fat milk, cottage cheese, tuna, chicken, turkey all have:
12. Lean fish, beef liver, ice milk all have:
13. Bread, pretzels, whole grains, legumes all have:
14. Sherbet, non-fat milk, most fruits and vegetables, baked potatoes all have:
15. Fibre (found only in plant foods)
16. Soluble fibre includes fibre obtained from
17. Insoluble fibre (found in whole grains and many vegetables)

B

a) alcoholic beverages should be avoided or consumed only in moderation.
b) and plenty of grain products, vegetables, and fruit.
c) at higher risk for developing certain illnesses, including high blood pressure, diabetes mellitus, heart disease, and some cancers.
d) helps hold water in the colon and can reduce or prevent constipation.
e) less than 10% fat:
f) may be soluble or insoluble.
g) more than 10% fat.
h) more than 20% fat.
i) more than 30% fat.
j) more than 40% fat.
k) more than 50% fat.
l) more than 60% fat.
m) more than 70% fat.
n) more than 80% fat.
o) more than 90% fat.
p) peas, beans, oats, barley, and some fruits and vegetables.
q) to eat the right balance of foods in moderation, limit fat consumption, and exercise regularly.

Physical fitness

Physical fitness varies from person to person and may be described as a condition that helps persons look, feel, and do their best. Physical fitness is influenced by **age, sex, heredity, personal habits, exercise, and eating habits.** Being physically fit offers many **benefits**, which include the following:

- decreased **resting heart rate** and **blood pressure**
- increased **oxygen-carrying** capacity
- enhanced **quality of life**
- increased **muscle mass** and **metabolism**
- increased **resistance to injury**
- improved personal appearance and **self-image**

- maintenance of **motor skills** throughout life.

Cardiovascular endurance

A **physical examination** or **fitness assessment** should be carried out before undertaking an exercise regimen for the first time. The purpose of these assessments is to **evaluate** a person's present **physical condition** and to create baseline assessments for **weight**, including **body mass index; high blood pressure**; **heart trouble**; **arthritis** or other bone problems; **muscular**, **ligament**, or **tendon** problems; and other known or suspected diseases. These assessments help to establish a **heart-rate target zone** as well. Ideally, the heart-rate zone should be maintained during exercise for **20 minutes** to increase **cardiovascular endurance.**

Muscle strength

Another part of the fitness assessment tests muscular strength and endurance. Muscular **strength** is the ability of a muscle to **exert force for a brief period**, whilst muscle **endurance** is the ability of a muscle or a group of muscles to sustain repeated contractions or to **continue applying force** against a fixed object. The tenets of training for muscle strength and endurance should consider **isometric and isotonic** exercises, **resistance**, **repetitions**, **sets**, and **frequency**. **Isometric** exercises are those that do not result in **any movement of a joint**. These exercises do not increase muscle bulk very much. However, they do strengthen the muscle. **Isotonic** exercises move a joint through a **range of motion** against **resistance of a fixed weight**. These exercises **add muscle bulk** by creating tension within the muscle. **Resistance** refers to the amount of **weight moved or lifted** during isotonic exercises. A **repetition (rep)** refers to the full execution of an exercise **from start to finish**. A **set** is the **number of times** an exercise (rep) is done from start to finish. **Frequency** refers to **the least number** of workouts that will have a **positive effect**.

Muscular flexibility

Flexibility refers to the ability to move joints and use muscles through their **full range of motion**. A lack of normal flexibility may lead to muscle strains and other injuries. Muscular flexibility can be improved by **stretching** exercises. These exercises must be done slowly, without a bouncing motion, and the intensity should be mild. A person should **not strain or hold the breath** and should feel **no pain** or discomfort. How often these exercises are done should match an individual's specific level of activity.

The importance of sleep

Sleep plays an important role in being physically fit because it helps to **rejuvenate** a tired body. The average adult needs seven to eight hours of sleep each day. *Circadian* is Latin for 'about a day'. The **circadian rhythm** is the physiological **ebb and flow** of the body as it relates to the rotation of the earth. This timing system is based roughly on the solar day as the earth rotates in its course around the sun. For example, a person **gets hungry or tired**, energetic or moody, at fairly set times each day as the body systems change. The level of **melatonin and cortisol** affects the periods of **sleepiness and wakefulness**. Release of these hormones is stimulated by the **dark** and is suppressed by **light**. Thus when the line between night and day is disrupted on an ongoing basis, irritability, depression, and illness can result. The circadian rhythm causes the **jet lag** that occurs during air travel to a distant time zone. Studies suggest that the symptoms of jet lag may be relieved by the administration of melatonin.

Getting your Zs

Working nights, **24-hour** shifts, and **rotating shifts** can inhibit getting enough rest. The following are some helpful tips:

- Allow some time to unwind and **relax before trying to go to sleep.**
- Consider **exercise** before sleeping as a **way to reduce stress**.
- **Avoid stimulants** (e.g. caffeine in coffee, fizzy pop, tea, and chocolate) during the last few hours of your work shift.
- Eat **simple carbohydrates** (e.g. biscuits or candy bar) to **release serotonin** (a hormone that may help induce sleep).
- Keep your sleeping **area cool and dark** so that your body will think it is night-time.
- Make sure your family and friends know about your work shifts and your sleeping schedule to **minimize interruptions**.
- Try to maintain a normal period of dedicated **sleep time each day**.
- **Consult a physician** about your sleep difficulties when needed.

Exercise 1b
Match the column A with the column B. Try to learn the expressions and/or sentences by heart.

A

1. Physical fitness may be described
2. Physical fitness is influenced
3. Being physically fit offers many benefits:
4. The purpose of a physical examination or fitness assessment is to evaluate a person's present physical condition and to create baseline assessments for weight,
5. Muscular strength is the ability of a muscle to exert force for a brief period, whilst muscle endurance
6. Isometric exercises are those that do not result in any movement of a joint,

7. Isotonic exercises move a joint through a range of motion against resistance of a fixed weight,
8. Resistance refers to the amount of weight moved or lifted during isotonic exercises;
9. A set is the number of times an exercise (rep) is done from start to finish;
10. Flexibility refers to the ability to move joints and use muscles through their full range of motion;
11. Stretching exercises must be done slowly,
12. The average adult needs
13. A person gets hungry or tired, energetic or moody,
14. The level of melatonin and cortisol affects
15. The circadian rhythm causes the jet lag
16. Allow some time to
17. Avoid stimulants (e.g. caffeine in coffee, fizzy pop, tea, and chocolate)
18. Eat simple carbohydrates (e.g. biscuits or candy bar)
19. Consult a physician about

B

a) *a lack of normal flexibility may lead to muscle strains and other injuries.*

b) *a repetition (rep) refers to the full execution of an exercise from start to finish.*

c) *as a condition that helps persons look, feel, and do their best.*

d) *at fairly set times each day as the body systems change.*

e) *by age, sex, heredity, personal habits, exercise, and eating habits.*

f) *during the last few hours of your work shift.*

g) *frequency refers to the least number of workouts that will have a positive effect.*

h) *including body mass index; high blood pressure; heart trouble; arthritis or other bone problems; muscular, ligament, or tendon problems; and other known or suspected diseases.*

i) *increased resistance to injury, increased muscle mass and metabolism, and maintenance of motor skills throughout life.*

j) *is the ability of a muscle to sustain repeated contractions or to continue applying force against a fixed object.*

k) *relax before trying to go to sleep.*

l) *seven to eight hours of sleep each day.*

m) *that occurs during air travel to a distant time zone.*

n) *the periods of sleepiness and wakefulness.*

o) *they add muscle bulk by creating tension within the muscle.*

p) they do not increase muscle bulk but they do strengthen the muscle.

q) to release serotonin (a hormone that may help induce sleep).

r) without a bouncing motion, and the intensity should be mild.

s) your sleep difficulties when needed.

Exercise 2

Translate the expressions. Try to explain their meanings in English.

Tenets, right balance, in moderation, committed to, realistic goals, plenty of, avoided, consumed, whipped cream, spare ribs, porterhouse, tenderloin, fillet mignon, peanuts, chops, sirloin steak, lamb, round steak, pot roast, sweet rolls, whole milk, doughnuts, turkey, beef liver, soluble fibre, peas, beans, oats, barley, whole grains, hold water, colon, prevent constipation, intestinal disease, heredity, personal habits, resting heart rate, muscle mass, resistance, self-image, motor skills, physical examination, undertaking regimen, baseline assessments, body mass index, heart trouble, ligament, tendon, suspected, heart-rate target zone, endurance, exert force, brief period, sustain, applying force, fixed object, isometric, isotonic, repetitions, muscle bulk, range of motion, creating tension, moved or lifted, full execution, workouts, muscle strains, stretching, bouncing motion, match, rejuvenate, circadian rhythm, rotation, energetic or moody, sleepiness and wakefulness, suppressed, disrupted, jet lag, rotating shifts, inhibit, unwind, fizzy pop, minimize interruptions, consult a physician.

Exercise 3

Answer the following questions. Prepare short talks and/or dialogues on these topics.

1. What are the principles of weight control ?
2. Which foods have the highest and and lowest content of fat?
3. Why is fibre important?
4. What are the benefits of being fit?
5. Explain the term cardiovascular endurance.
6. What is the difference between muscle strength and muscle endurance?
7. How can you improve muscular flexibility?
8. Why is sleep important?
9. What do you understand by "Getting Your Zs"?

Vocabulary 12

Fill in the meanings in your mother language:

add /æd/
apply /əˈplaɪ/
assessment /əˈses.mənt/
bacon /ˈbeɪ.kən/
barley /ˈbɑː.li/
baseline /ˈbeɪsˌlaɪn/
bean /biːn/
beverage /ˈbev.ər.ɪdʒ/
biscuit /ˈbɪs.kɪt/

blood /blʌd/ **cell** /sel/
bouncing /ˈbaʊnt.sɪŋ/
brief /briːf/
candy bar /ˈkæn.di ˌbɑr/
chicken /ˈtʃɪk.ɪn/
chop /tʃɒp/
circadian /sɜːˈkeɪ.di.ən/
commit /kəˈmɪt/
consider /kənˈsɪd.ər/
cool /kuːl/
cottage /ˈkɒt.ɪdʒ/ **cheese** /tʃiːz/
course /kɔːs/
create /kriːˈeɪt/
crisp /krɪsp/
dedicated /ˈded.ɪ.keɪ.tɪd/
disrupt /dɪsˈrʌpt/
doughnut /ˈdəʊ.nʌt/
ebb /eb/
endurance /ɪnˈdjʊə.rənt s/
execution /ˌek.sɪˈkjuː.ʃən/
fibre /ˈfaɪ.bər/
fillet mignon /fɪˈleɪ.minˈjɑn/
fizzy /ˈfɪz.i/ **pop** /pɒp/
flexibility /ˌflek.sɪˈbɪl.ə.ti/
French /frentʃ/ **fries** /fraɪs/
frequency /ˈfriː.kwən.si/
goal /gəʊl/
gravy /ˈgreɪ.vi/
ground /graʊnd/ **beef** /biːf/
habit /ˈhæb.ɪt/
haemorrhoids /ˈhem.ər.ɔɪdz/
heart /hɑːt/ **rate** /reɪt/
hold /həʊld/
in moderation /ˌmɒd.ərˈeɪ.ʃən/
insoluble /ɪnˈsɒl.jʊ.blˌ/
interruption /ˌɪn.təˈrʌp.ʃən/
isometric /ˌaɪ.səʊˈmet.rɪk/
isotonic /aɪ.səʊ ˈtɒn.ɪk/
jet lag /ˈdʒet.læg/
lamb /læm/
lift /lɪft/
mass /mæs/
match /mætʃ/
melatonin /mel.əˈtəʊ.nɪn/
moody /ˈmuː.di/
motion /ˈməʊ.ʃən/
motor /ˈməʊ.tər/
muffin /ˈmʌf.ɪn/
muscle /ˈmʌs.lˌ/ **bulk** /bʌlk/
oats /əʊts/
ongoing /ˈɒŋˌgəʊ.ɪŋ/
pea /piː/
peanut /ˈpiː.nʌt/
pie /paɪ/
pork /pɔːk/
porterhouse steak /ˌpɔː.tə.haʊsˈsteɪk/
pot /pɒt/
pretzel /ˈpret.səl/
purpose /ˈpɜː.pəs/
range /reɪndʒ/
regimen /ˈredʒ.ɪ.mən/
rejuvenate /rɪˈdʒuː.vən.eɪt/
release /rəˈliːs/
repetition /ˌrepɪˈtɪ.ʃən/
resistance /rɪˈzɪs.tənt s/
roast /rəʊst/
rotation /rəʊ ˈteɪ.ʃən/
roughly /ˈrʌf.lɪ/
sausage /ˈsɒs.ɪdʒ/
schedule /ˈʃedjuːl/
self-image /self.ˈɪm.ɪdʒ/
serotonin /ˌse.rəˈtəʊ.nɪn/
set /set/
sherbet /ˈʃɜː.bət/
sleepiness /ˈsliː.pɪ.nəs/
solar /ˈsəʊ.lər/
spare ribs /ˌspeəˈrɪbz/
strain /streɪn/
stretching /stretʃ.ɪŋ/
suppress /səˈpres/
suspect /səˈspekt/
sweet /swiːt/ **roll** /rəʊl/
T-bone steak /ˌtiː.bəʊnˈsteɪk/
tenderloin /ˈten.də.lɔɪn/
tendon /ˈten.dən/
tenet /ˈten.ɪt/
tension /ˈten.ʃən/
tired /ˈtaɪəd/
tuna /ˈtjuː.nə/
turkey /ˈtɜː.ki/

undertake /ˌʌndəˈteɪk/
unwind /ʌnˈwaɪnd/
wakefulness /ˈweɪk.fəl.nəs/
weight /weɪt/
whole /həʊl/ **milk** /mɪlk/
workout /ˈwɜː.kaʊt/
zone /zəʊn/
Zs, zap /zæp/

Solution to Exercise 1a
1c, 2q, 3b, 4a, 5o, 6n, 7m, 8l, 9k, 10j, 11i, 12h, 13g, 14e, 15f, 16p, 17d

Solution to Exercise 1b
1c, 2e, 3i, 4h, 5j, 6p, 7o, 8b, 9g, 10a, 11r, 12l, 13d, 14n, 15m, 16k, 17f, 18q, 19s

Unit 13 - Disease prevention. Mental and emotional health.

Cardiovascular disease

For most people, cardiovascular disease can be altered through living a healthy life. **Boosting cardiovascular endurance** can help to prevent this disease, but other steps also are needed in the fight. These steps include the following:

- **eliminating cigarette** smoking
- **controlling high blood pressure**
- maintaining a favourable **body fat composition** through regular exercise
- maintaining a **good total cholesterol**/high-density lipoprotein ratio
- monitoring **triglyceride** levels
- **controlling diabetes**
- avoiding excessive **alcohol** intake
- eating **healthy foods**
- **reducing stress**
- obtaining **risk assessments** periodically

Cancer

The term *cancer* includes more than **100 diseases** affecting nearly every part of the body. All these diseases are potentially **life-threatening**. Most common cancers are linked to one of three environmental risk factors: **smoking**, **sunlight**, or **diet**. Dietary factors are associated with some cancers of the **gastrointestinal** tract and may be linked to others, such as cancer of the **breast, prostate, or uterus**. A lack of **dietary fibre** is believed to be a risk factor. Steps in preventing cancer include the following:

- elimination of **smoking**
- **dietary** changes
- limitation of **sun** exposure; use of sunscreen
- regular **physical examinations**
- attention to the **warning signs**
- periodic **risk** assessment.

The seven warning signs of cancer (CAUTION) as designated by the American Cancer Society

- change in **bowel or bladder habits**
- a **sore throat** that does not heal

- unusual **bleeding or discharge**
- **thickening or lump** in the breast or elsewhere
- **indigestion** or **difficulty swallowing**
- obvious **change in a wart or mole**
- **nagging cough or hoarseness**

Infectious disease

Most infectious diseases can be avoided by doing two things. The first is practising good personal **hygiene**, including hand washing. The second is following **universal precautions** and other guidelines in the workplace.

Exercise 1a
Match the column A with the column B. Try to learn the expressions and/ or sentences by heart.

A

1. Boosting cardiovascular endurance can help
2. Important steps include the following:
3. Most common cancers are linked to
4. Dietary factors are associated with some cancers of the gastrointestinal tract
5. Steps in preventing cancer include the following:
6. The seven warning signs of cancer include:
7. Most infectious diseases can be avoided by practising good personal hygiene,

B

a) *and following universal precautions and other guidelines in the workplace.*
b) *and may be linked to others, such as cancer of the breast, prostate, or uterus.*
c) *change in bowel or bladder habits, a sore throat that does not heal, unusual bleeding or discharge, thickening or lump in the breast or elsewhere, indigestion or difficulty swallowing, obvious change in a wart or mole, nagging cough or hoarseness.*
d) *controlling high blood pressure, maintaining a good total cholesterol/high-density lipoprotein ratio, and controlling diabetes.*
e) *elimination of smoking, dietary changes, limitation of sun exposure and attention to the warning signs.*
f) *smoking, sunlight, or diet.*
g) *to prevent cardiovascular disease.*

Mental and emotional health

Many factors play a role in mental and emotional health. An important factor is to be aware of **warning signs** that could signal a potential problem (e.g. signs of **substance misuse** and health disorders caused by **anxiety and stress**).

Also key to maintaining good **emotional health** is realizing the value of having personal time and being connected with **family, peers, and the community**.

Substance misuse and abuse control

The misuse and abuse of drugs and other substances may lead to **chemical dependency (addiction)**. Substance misuse or abuse control may call for professional counselling. Warning signs of addiction and addictive behaviour include the following:

- using a substance to **relieve tension**
- using an **increasing amount** of the substance
- **lying** about using the substance
- experiencing **guilt** about using the substance
- **avoiding discussion** about using the substance
- experiencing **interference with daily activities** as a result of substance abuse.

Common drugs and substances that are misused or abused are: alcohol, central nervous system **stimulants** (e.g. cocaine and amphetamines), cigarettes and other tobacco products, hallucinogens, inhalants, marijuana, narcotics and related drugs, sedative-hypnotics, tranquillizers, sedatives, appetite suppressants, laxatives, cough and cold preparations, nasal sprays and analgesics.

Smoking cessation

Cigarette smoking is a major health hazard. The health ramifications of cigarette smoking are numerous, including an increased risk of: **coronary heart** disease, **myocardial infarction**, **chronic obstructive pulmonary disease**, sudden **death**, dying from a variety of **diseases**, **miscarriage**, **premature birth**, and **birth defects.** Smokers may name many reasons for continuing to smoke, including peer pressure, relief of stress, weight control, and others. **Nicotine** is the stimulant in tobacco, but there are **other harmful chemicals** including **hydrocarbons (tar)** and **carbon monoxide**. Exposure to these chemicals is also considered a health hazard for non-smokers. Non-smokers have an increased risk of developing smoking-related illnesses through **passive smoking**. Many resources and **smoking cessation** programmes are available to those who want to quit smoking. Other methods that may be used alone or with these programmes include the use of prescription and non-prescription drugs such as **dermal patches** and **nicotine chewing gum**. These products decrease the physical effects of smoking cessation.

Body changes when you stop smoking

Within **20 minutes** of your last cigarette: pulse and blood pressure drop to normal, body temperature of hands and feet increases to normal.

Within **8 hours** of your last cigarette: carbon monoxide level in blood drops to normal, oxygen level in blood increases to normal.

Within **48 hours** of your last cigarette: chance of heart attack decreases, nerve endings begin to regenerate, ability to smell and taste is enhanced.

Within **2 weeks to 9 months** after your last cigarette: circulation improves, walking becomes easier, coughing, sinus congestion, fatigue, and shortness of breath decrease.

Within **10 years** of your last cigarette: lung cancer death rate drops, precancerous cells are replaced, risk for other cancers, such as those of the mouth, larynx, oesophagus, bladder, kidney, and pancreas, decreases.

Anxiety and stress

Anxiety can be defined as the worry or dread about future uncertainties. Stress can be positive although it is usually thought of as having a **negative effect** (e.g. **fear, depression, and guilt**).

Personal time for meditation and contemplation

Setting aside some personal time can boost mental and perhaps even physical health. This time can be spent meditating or contemplating. **Meditation** is a form of relaxation. The person may **focus on something** that holds some attraction (e.g. controlled breathing). This quiet time provides an uninterrupted period for **thoughtful introspection (contemplation)** of important things in a person's life.

Family, peer, and community connections

Belonging to a group can affect a person's motivation and performance in a positive way. These groups provide a connection with others who share similar values and interests. These bonds are healthy and raise **self-esteem** and provide a way for one to **contribute to group activities and goals**.

Freedom from prejudice

Accepting **cultural differences** gives people the chance to learn about other cultures. Such acceptance also helps them to see cultural variations in a positive light. Providing healthcare to patients of some cultures may call for special **communication skills** and may require some further education to understand the **customs and beliefs** of that culture.

Exercise 1b
Match the column A with the column B. Try to learn the expressions and/ or sentences by heart.

A

1. Be aware of warning signs that could signal a potential problem
2. The misuse and abuse of drugs and other substances
3. Warning signs of addiction and addictive behaviour include the following:
4. Common drugs and substances that are misused or abused are:

5. The health ramifications of cigarette smoking include an increased risk of:
6. Nicotine is the stimulant in tobacco, but there are other harmful chemicals
7. Non-smokers have an increased risk of developing
8. Dermal patches and nicotine chewing gum
9. When you stop smoking, within 20 minutes of your last cigarette:
10. When you stop smoking, within 48 hours of your last cigarette:
11. When you stop smoking, within 2 weeks to 9 months after your last cigarette:
12. When you stop smoking, within 10 years of your last cigarette:
13. Stress is usually thought of as having
14. Belonging to a group can affect a person's motivation and performance in a positive way, can raise self-esteem
15. Providing healthcare to patients of some cultures may call for

B

a) *a negative effect (e.g. fear, depression, and guilt).*

b) *alcohol, central nervous system stimulants, cigarettes, hallucinogens, inhalants, marijuana, narcotics, sedative-hypnotics, tranquillizers, sedatives, appetite suppressants, laxatives, cough and cold preparations, nasal sprays and analgesics.*

c) *and provide a way for one to contribute to group activities and goals.*

d) *chance of heart attack decreases, nerve endings begin to regenerate, ability to smell and taste is enhanced.*

e) *circulation improves, walking becomes easier, coughing, sinus congestion, fatigue, and shortness of breath decrease.*

f) *coronary heart disease, myocardial infarction, chronic obstructive pulmonary disease, sudden death, miscarriage, premature birth, and birth defects.*

g) *decrease the physical effects of smoking cessation.*

h) *e.g. signs of substance misuse and health disorders caused by anxiety and stress.*

i) *including hydrocarbons (tar) and carbon monoxide.*

j) *lung cancer death rate drops, precancerous cells are replaced, risk for other cancers, such as those of the mouth, larynx, oesophagus, bladder, kidney, and pancreas, decreases.*

k) *may lead to chemical dependency (addiction),*

which calls for professional counselling.

l) *pulse and blood pressure drop to normal, body temperature of hands and feet increases to normal.*

m) *smoking-related illnesses through passive smoking.*

n) *special communication skills and may require some further education to understand the customs and beliefs of that culture.*

o) *using a substance to relieve tension, using an increasing amount of the substance, and experiencing interference with daily activities.*

Exercise 2
Translate the expressions. Try to explain their meanings in English.

Altered, boosting, body fat composition, high-density, lipoprotein ratio, obtaining, affecting, uterus, sun exposure, warning signs, bowel or bladder habits, sore throat, heal, bleeding, discharge, thickening or lump, indigestion, difficulty swallowing, obvious, wart or mole, nagging cough, hoarseness, precautions, guidelines, mental and emotional health, substance misuse, realizing the value, abuse, chemical dependency, addiction, relieve tension, increasing amount, experiencing guilt, interference with daily activities, inhalants, tranquillizers, appetite suppressants, laxatives, ramifications, coronary heart disease, chronic obstructive pulmonary disease, miscarriage, premature birth, relief of stress, harmful, cessation, quit smoking, dermal patches drop to normal, ability to smell and taste, coughing, sinus congestion, shortness of breath, larynx, oesophagus, bladder, kidney, dread, fear, setting aside, boost mental health, meditation, relaxation, focus on, holds some attraction, thoughtful introspection, contemplation, motivation and performance, share interests, raise self-esteem, freedom from prejudice, acceptance, customs and beliefs.

Exercise 3
Answer the following questions. Prepare short talks and/or dialogues on these topics.

1. What to do to prevent cardiovascular disease?
2. What to do to prevent cancer?
3. What are the seven warning signs of cancer?
4. What is meant by mental and emotional health?
5. What are the warning signs of addiction?
6. Which are the common drugs and substances that are misused or abused?
7. Why is smoking cessation important?
8. Talk about body changes after you stop smoking.
9. How to prevent anxiety and stress?

Vocabulary 13

Fill in the meanings in your mother language:

acceptance /əkˈsep.tənt s/
addiction /əˈdɪk.ʃən/
addictive /əˈdɪk.tɪv/
alter /ɒl.tər/
amphetamine /æmˈfet.ə.miːn/
attention /əˈten.ʃən/
attraction /əˈtræk.ʃən/
avoid /əˈvɔɪd/
belief /bɪˈliːf/
birth /bɜːθ/
bond /bɒnd/
carbon monoxide /ˌkɑː. bən.məˈnɒk.saɪd/
cessation /sesˈeɪ.ʃən/
Chronic /ˈkrɒnɪk/ **Obstructive** / əbˈstrʌk.tɪv/ **Pulmonary** /ˈpʊl. mə.nə.ri/ **Disease** /dɪˈziːz/ **COPD**
cocaine /kəʊ ˈkeɪn/
cold /kəʊld/
composition /ˌkɒm.pəˈzɪʃ.ən/
congestion /kənˈdʒes.tʃən/
contemplation /ˌkɒn.təmˈpleɪ.ʃən/
counselling /ˈkaʊnt .səl.ɪŋ/
custom /ˈkʌs.təm/
death /deθ/ **rate** /reɪt/
dependency /dɪˈpen.dənt .si/
dermal /dɜː.məl/
drop /drɒp/
eliminate /ɪˈlɪm.ɪ.neɪt/
environmental /ɪnˌvaɪ.rən.ˈmen.təl/
favourable /ˈfeɪ.vər.ə.bl̩/
focus /ˈfəʊkəs/
freedom /ˈfriː.dəm/
guidelines /ˈgaɪdˌlaɪnz/
hallucinogen /ˌhæl.uːˈsɪn.ə.dʒən/
hazard /ˈhæz.əd/
heal /hiːl/
hoarseness /hɔː.snəs/
hydrocarbon /ˌhaɪ.drəʊ ˈkɑː.bən/
hypnotic /hɪpˈnɒt.ɪk/
indigestion /ˌɪn.dɪ.dʒes.tʃən/
inhalant /ɪnˈheɪl.ənt/
interference /ˌɪn.təˈfɪə.rənt s/
introspection /ˌɪn.trəˈspek.ʃən/
laxative /ˈlæk.sə.tɪv/
limitation /ˌlɪm.ɪˈteɪ.ʃən/
link /lɪŋk/
lipoprotein /ˌlɪp.ə .ˈprəʊ.tiːn/
lump /lʌmp/
lying /ˈlaɪ.ɪŋ/ **about** /əˈbaʊt/
marijuana /ˌmær.əˈwɑː.nə/
miscarriage /ˈmɪsˌkær.ɪdʒ/
misuse /ˌmɪsˈjuːs/
mole /məʊl/
monitor /ˈmɒn.ɪ.tər/
nag /næg/
nicotine /ˈnɪk.ə.tiːn/
oesophagus /ɪˈsɒf.ə.gəs/
patch /pætʃ/
precancerous /ˌpriːˈkænt .sər.əs/
precaution /prɪˈkɔː.ʃən/
prejudice /ˈpredʒ.ʊ.dɪs/
premature /ˈprem.ə.tʃər/
quit /kwɪt/
ramifications /ˌræm.ɪ.fɪˈkeɪ.ʃənz/
ratio /ˈreɪ.ʃi.əʊ/
regenerate /rɪˈdʒen.ər.eɪt/
regular /ˈreg.jʊ.lər/
sedative /ˈsed.ə.tɪv/
self-esteem /self.ɪˈstiːm/
set /set/ **aside** /əˈsaɪd/
share /ʃeə/
shortness /ˈʃɔːt.nəs/ **of breath** /breθ/
sore /sɔː/ **throat** /θrəʊt/
sunlight /ˈsʌn.laɪt/
sunscreen /ˈsʌn.skriːn/
suppressant /səˈpres.ənt/
tar /tɑː/
thicken /ˈθɪk.ən/
thoughtful /ˈθɔːt.fəl/
tranquillizer /ˈtræŋ.kwɪ.laɪ.zər/
triglyceride /traɪ.glɪs.ə.raɪd/
uncertainty /ʌnˈsɜː.tən.ti/
wart /wɔːt/

Solution to Exercise 1a
1g, 2d, 3f, 4b, 5e, 6c, 7a

Solution to Exercise 1b
1h, 2k, 3o, 4b, 5f, 6i, 7m, 8g, 9l, 10d, 11e, 12j, 13a, 14c, 15n

Unit 14 - Stress. Reactions to stress.

As previously stated, stress can be **positive and negative**. The responses to stress may be **physical, emotional,** or both. **Good stress (eustress)** is a positive response to stimuli and is considered **protective. Bad stress (distress)** is a **negative** response to environmental stimuli.

Phases of the stress response

The three stages of the stress response are the alarm reaction, resistance, and exhaustion.

Alarm reaction

The human body can prepare itself quickly to do battle or run from danger. This **fight-or-flight** reaction occurs when a **situation threatens** one's safety or comfort. This reaction is considered **positive.** The stress prepares individuals to **defend** themselves. The body **reacts equally** to events that are pleasant or unpleasant, dangerous or exciting, happy or sad. The purpose of the response is to rapidly achieve top physical preparedness **to cope with** the event.

The alarm reaction is set off by the **autonomic** nervous system. This reaction is coordinated by the **hypothalamus**, which triggers the **pituitary gland** to release **adrenocorticotropic** hormone into the bloodstream. This stress hormone stimulates the production of **glucose.** The hormone also increases the concentration of **nutrients** in the blood. Adrenocorticotropic hormone also activates the **adrenal glands** for an intense sympathetic **discharge of adrenaline** and **noradrenaline.** These hormones cause the **heartbeat** to increase, **blood pressure** to rise, and the **pupils** of the eyes to dilate, which improves **vision.**

Together these hormones relax the bronchial tree for **deeper breathing**, increase **blood sugar**, slow the digestive process, and **shift blood** supply to accommodate the **clotting** mechanism. The body is **ready for an emergency**. The alarm reaction takes only seconds. When the body realizes that an event is **not dangerous**, the response stops and bodily **functions return** to normal.

Resistance

The stress response raises the level of resistance to the agent that provoked it. That is, if a particular stress persists long enough, a person's reactions change.

Exhaustion

As stress continues, **coping mechanisms weaken** and resistance fails. When any reservoir of adaptive resources no longer exists, resistance to other types of stress tends to decline as well.

Factors that trigger the stress response

Each person has unique means to deal with stressful situations. Many factors can trigger the stress response. Examples include the following:

- **loss** of something that is of value
- **injury or threat** of injury
- **poor health or nutrition**
- **frustration**
- **ineffective coping** skills.

Physiological and psychological effects of stress

Anxiety is a common symptom of stress. Feeling anxious in certain situations or unusual circumstances is normal and provides a **warning system** that **protects** people from **being overwhelmed** by a sudden stimulation. Sometimes stress is not reduced by a solution to the conflict or emergency, which may lead to an **ongoing** state of **vigilance and alertness** beyond the initial event. This kind of anxiety fails to stimulate effective coping. Anxiety **interferes with thought** processes and with **relationships** and **work performance**. A person may develop problems **concentrating**, lose the ability to trust others, or become isolated or **withdrawn**. Individuals who are often exposed to stressful situations or who are unable to cope with stressful events may experience a **chronic state** of anxiety. This state may lead to **physical, emotional, cognitive, and behavioural effects**.

Warning signs and symptoms of stress

Physical: cardiac rhythm disturbances, chest pain, difficulty breathing, nausea, profuse sweating, sleep disturbances, vomiting.

Emotional: anger, denial, fear, feeling of being overwhelmed, inappropriate emotions, panic reactions.

Cognitive: confusion, decreased level of awareness, difficulty making decisions, disorientation, distressing dreams, memory problems, poor concentration.

Behavioural: changes in eating habits, crying spells, excessive silence, hyperactivity, increased alcohol consumption, increased smoking, withdrawal.

Exercise 1a

Match the column A with the column B. Try to learn the expressions and/or sentences by heart.

A

1. Good stress (eustress) is a positive response to stimuli and is considered protective;
2. The three stages of the stress response are:
3. The fight-or-flight reaction occurs when
4. The purpose of the response is to rapidly achieve
5. This reaction is coordinated by the hypothalamus,
6. This stress hormone stimulates the production of glucose;

7. Adrenocorticotropic hormone also activates the adrenal glands
8. These hormones cause the heartbeat to increase,
9. Together these hormones relax the bronchial tree for deeper breathing, increase blood sugar,
10. When the body realizes that an event is not dangerous,
11. If a particular stress persists long enough,
12. As stress continues,
13. Examples of factors that can trigger the stress response include the following:
14. Feeling anxious in certain situations or unusual circumstances is normal
15. Anxiety interferes with thought processes
16. Individuals who are often exposed to stressful situations
17. Physical signs and symptoms of stress may be manifested as:
18. Emotional signs and symptoms of stress are:
19. Cognitive signs and symptoms of stress may be:
20. Behavioural signs and symptoms of stress can include:

B

a) *a situation threatens one's safety or comfort.*

b) *and provides a warning system that protects people from being overwhelmed by a sudden stimulation.*

c) *and with relationships and work performance.*

d) *anger, denial, fear, feeling of being overwhelmed, inappropriate emotions, and panic reactions.*

e) *bad stress (distress) is a negative response to environmental stimuli.*

f) *blood pressure to rise, and the pupils of the eyes to dilate.*

g) *cardiac rhythm disturbances, chest pain, difficulty breathing, nausea, profuse sweating, sleep disturbances, or vomiting.*

h) *changes in eating habits, crying spells, excessive silence, hyperactivity, increased alcohol consumption, increased smoking or withdrawal.*

i) *confusion, decreased level of awareness, difficulty making decisions, disorientation, distressing dreams, memory problems, as well as poor concentration.*

j) *coping mechanisms weaken and resistance fails.*

k) *for an intense sympathetic discharge of adrenaline and noradrenaline.*

l) *loss of something that is of value, injury or threat of injury, poor health or nutrition, frustration, ineffective coping skills.*

m) *or who are unable to cope with stressful events may experience a chronic state of anxiety.*
n) *slow the digestive process, and shift blood supply to accommodate the clotting mechanism.*
o) *the alarm reaction, resistance, and exhaustion.*
p) *the hormone also increases the concentration of nutrients in the blood.*
q) *the response stops and bodily functions return to normal.*
r) *the stress response raises the level of resistance to the agent that provoked it.*
s) *top physical preparedness to cope with the event.*
t) *which triggers the pituitary gland to release adrenocorticotropic hormone into the bloodstream.*

Reactions to stress

Adaptation is a process that involves learning ways to deal with stressful situations. **Defence mechanisms** are adaptive functions that assist a person to adjust to stressful situations. **Denial** is a defence mechanism that might be used to separate a person from the event. **Coping** is an active process of confronting. Coping involves gathering information to change or adjust to a new situation. People may also use harmful or **negative coping mechanisms**. An individual may become withdrawn or use alcohol or other drugs. Some may have angry outbursts towards family members and co-workers whilst others become silent. These negative coping mechanisms should be seen as signs that an individual is having trouble dealing with stress. **Burnout** can be the result of cumulative stress. Burnout is defined by physical and emotional exhaustion and negative attitudes. It can develop when one is exposed to chronic stress that cannot be managed with usual coping mechanisms. **Problem-solving** involves analysing a problem and finding options to deal with the issue. Problem-solving allows a person to identify the problem clearly and come up with a course of action. **Mastery** refers to the ability to see many options and solutions for problematic situations. Mastery results from extensive experience and the use of effective coping mechanisms with situations that are similar.

Stress management techniques

To manage stress well, a person must recognize the early warning signs of anxiety. Some of the **physical effects of anxiety** include the following: heart palpitations, difficult or rapid breathing, dry mouth, chest tightness or pain, anorexia (lack of appetite), nausea, vomiting, diarrhoea, abdominal cramps, flatulence, 'butterflies', flushing, diaphoresis (profuse sweating), body temperature fluctuation, urgency and frequency in urination, dysmenorrhoea (painful menstruation), decreased sexual drive or performance, aching muscles, joints. Physical effects that may **not be as noticeable** include the following: increased blood pressure and heart rate, blood shunting (diversion of the flow) to muscles, increased blood glucose levels, increased adrenaline production by adrenal glands, reduced gastrointestinal peristalsis, pupillary dilation.

If signs and symptoms of stress-related illness appear, the person should seek appropriate medical or psychological help. **Methods** one may initially use to **manage stress** include reframing, controlled breathing, progressive relaxation, and guided imagery. **Reframing** involves first looking at the situation from a different emotional viewpoint and then placing it in a different frame that fits the facts of another situation equally well. This acts to change the meaning of the situation. **Controlled breathing** is a natural stress-control technique whereby a person concentrates on depth and rate of breathing to achieve a calming effect. **Progressive relaxation** is a stress-reduction strategy in which the person systematically tightens and relaxes particular muscle groups (from head to toe or toe to head). **Guided imagery** is used with meditation. Another person familiar with the technique acts as a guide during a stress response. The person experiencing stress can then focus on an image that helps relieve stress.

Other ways to fight stress include **being aware of personal limitations**, **peer counselling**, and **group discussions**. **Proper diet, sleep,** and **rest** also help to relieve stress. In addition, pursuing positive activities can balance work and recreation.

Exercise 1b
Match the column A with the column B. Try to learn the expressions and/ or sentences by heart.

A

1. Defence mechanisms are adaptive functions
2. Denial is a defence mechanism
3. Coping involves gathering information
4. Negative coping mechanisms should be seen
5. Burnout can develop when one is exposed to
6. Problem-solving allows a person
7. Mastery refers to the ability to see
8. Physical effects of anxiety include the following:
9. Methods one may initially use to manage stress include
10. Reframing involves first looking at the situation from a different emotional viewpoint
11. Controlled breathing is a natural stress-control technique
12. Progressive relaxation is a stress-reduction strategy
13. Guided imagery is used with meditation; another person acts as a guide

14. Other ways to fight stress include

B

a) *and the person experiencing stress can focus on an image that helps relieve stress.*
b) *and then placing it in a different frame; this acts to change the meaning of the situation.*
c) *as signs that an individual is having trouble dealing with stress.*
d) *being aware of personal limitations, peer counselling, and group discussions.*
e) *chronic stress that cannot be managed with usual coping mechanisms.*
f) *heart palpitations, difficult or rapid breathing, chest tightness or pain, anorexia, nausea, vomiting, diarrhoea, abdominal cramps, flatulence, flushing, or diaphoresis.*
g) *in which the person systematically tightens and relaxes particular muscle groups (from head to toe or toe to head).*
h) *many options and solutions for problematic situations.*
i) *reframing, controlled breathing, progressive relaxation, and guided imagery.*
j) *that assist a person to adjust to stressful situations.*
k) *that might be used to separate a person from the event.*
l) *to change or adjust to a new situation.*
m) *to identify the problem clearly and come up with a course of action.*
n) *whereby a person concentrates on depth and rate of breathing to achieve a calming effect.*

Exercise 2
Translate the expressions. Try to explain their meanings in English.

As previously stated, eustress, distress, do battle or run from danger, fight-or-flight reaction, threatens, defend, equally, exciting, preparedness, cope with, set off, triggers, pituitary gland, adrenal glands, discharge, heartbeat, pupils dilate, bronchial tree, shift blood supply, clotting mechanism, realizes that, persists, exhaustion, weaken, reservoir, adaptive resources, decline, deal with, ineffective, coping skills, being overwhelmed, solution to the conflict, ongoing, vigilance and alertness, interferes with, thought processes, ability to trust, withdrawn, cognitive, behavioural, profuse sweating, anger, denial, inappropriate, confusion, awareness, distressing dreams, memory, eating habits, crying spells, silence, adaptation, defence mechanisms, adjust to, denial, separate, coping, gathering information, harmful, withdrawn, angry outbursts, burnout, cumulative, exhaustion, attitudes, problem-solving, course of action, mastery, options, solutions, manage stress, recognize, palpitations, chest tightness, cramps, flatulence, 'butterflies', flushing, diaphoresis, profuse sweating, fluctuation, urgency in urination, dysmenorrhoea, sexual drive, aching muscles, noticeable, diversion, flow, adrenal glands, pupillary dilation, initially, reframing, progressive relaxation, guided imagery, viewpoint, change the meaning, depth and rate, calming effect, progressive relaxation, tightens and relaxes, guided imagery, relieve stress, aware, peer counselling, pursuing.

Exercise 3
Answer the following questions. Prepare short talks and/or dialogues on these topics.

1. What is the difference between eustress and distress?
2. Which are the three phases of the stress response?
3. Describe alarm reaction, resistance and exhaustion.
4. Which factors trigger the stress response?
5. Describe physiological and psychological effects of stress.
6. Characterise warning signs and symptoms of stress.
7. Characterise reactions to stress (adaptation, defence mechanisms, denial, coping, problem-solving, mastery).
8. Describe physical effects of anxiety.
9. Describe methods used to manage stress (reframing, controlled breathing, progressive relaxation, and guided imagery).

Vocabulary 14

Fill in the meanings in your mother language:

accommodate /ə'kɒm.ə.deɪt/
adaptation /ˌæd.əp'teɪ.ʃən/
adaptive /ə'dæp.tɪv/
adjust /ə'dʒʌst/
adrenal gland /ə'driː.nəl.glænd/
adrenocorticotropic /əˌdriː.nəʊˌkɔː.tɪ.kəʊ'trɒf.ɪk/ **ACTH**
alarm /ə'lɑːm/
alertness /ə'lɜːt.nəs/
analyse /'æn.əl.aɪz/
anger /'æŋ.gər/
aware /ə'weər/
behavioural /bɪ'heɪ.vjə.rəl/
blood /blʌd/ **supply** /sə'plaɪ/
bronchial /'brɒŋ.ki.əl/ **tree** /triː/
burnout /'bɜːn.aʊt/
butterfly /'bʌt.ə.flaɪ/ **(have butterflies in one's stomach)**
calming /kɑːm.ɪŋ/
circumstance /'sɜː.kəm.stɑːnt s/
clotting /'klɑt̬.ɪŋ/
comfort /'kʌm.fət/
confront /kən'frʌnt/
cope /kəʊp/ **with** /wɪð/
crying /'kraɪ.ɪŋ/
deal /dɪəl/ **with** /wɪð/
diaphoresis /ˌdaɪ.ə.fə'riː.sɪs/
digestive /da ɪ'dʒes.tɪv/
dilation /daɪ'leɪ.ʃən/
diversion /da ɪ'vɜː.ʃən/
dream /driːm/
dysmenorrhoea /ˌdɪs.men.ə'riə/

eustress /juːˈstres/
exhaustion /ɪgˈzɔːs.tʃən/
exposed /ɪkˈspəʊzd/
extensive /ɪkˈstent .sɪv/
fail /feɪl/
fight or flight /ˌfaɪt.ɔː.ˈflaɪt/
fit /fɪt/
flatulence /ˈflæt.jʊ.lənts/
fluctuation /ˌflʌk.tjuˈeɪ.ʃən/
flush /flʌʃ/
frame /freɪm/
frustration /frʌsˈtreɪ.ʃən/
gather /ˈgæð.ər/
guide /gaɪd/
hyperactivity /ˌhaɪ.pərˈækˈtɪv.ɪ.ti/
imagery /ˈɪm.ɪ.dʒər.i/
ineffective /ˌɪn.ɪˈfek.tɪv/
issue /ˈɪʃ.uː/
loss /lɒs/
manage /ˈmæn.ɪdʒ/
mastery /ˈmɑː.stər.i/
meaning /ˈmiː.nɪŋ/
means /miːnz/
memory /ˈmem.ər.i/
muscle /ˈmʌs.l̩/
noticeable /ˈnəʊ.tɪ.sə.bl̩/
option /ˈɒp.ʃən/
overwhelm /ˌəʊ.vəˈwelm/
palpitations /ˌpæl.pɪˈteɪ.ʃənz/
particular /pəˈtɪk.jʊ.lər/
performance /pəˈfɔː.məns/
persist /pəˈsɪst/
preparedness /prɪˈpeəd.nəs/
profuse /prəˈfjuːs/
protective /prəˈtek.tɪv/
provoke /prəˈvəʊk/
pupil /ˈpjuː.pəl/
pursue /pəˈsjuː/
realize /ˈrɪə.laɪz/
recognize /ˈrek.əg.naɪz/
relax /rɪˈlæks/
reservoir /ˈrez.ə.vwɑːr/
resource /rɪˈzɔːs/
safety /ˈseɪftɪ/
set /set/ **off** /ɒf/
silence /ˈsaɪ.lənts/
silent /ˈsaɪ.lənt/
spell /spel/
sudden /ˈsʌd.ən/
sweating /swet.ɪŋ/
threat /θret/
threaten /ˈθret.ən/
tighten /ˈtaɪ.tən/
tightness /ˈtaɪt.nəs/
trust /trʌst/
urgency /ˈɜː.dʒənt .si/
viewpoint /vjuː.pɔɪnt/
vigilance /ˈvɪdʒ.ɪ.lənt s/
withdrawal /wɪðˈdrɔː.əl/

Solution to Exercise 1a
1e, 2o, 3a, 4s, 5t, 6p, 7k, 8f, 9n, 10q, 11r, 12j, 13l, 14b, 15c, 16m, 17g, 18d, 19i, 20h

Solution to Exercise 1b
1j, 2k, 3l, 4c, 5e, 6m, 7h, 8f, 9i, 10b, 11n, 12g, 13a, 14d

Chapter II
Human nutrition and prevention of food-borne diseases

Unit 1 - Human nutrition. Human gastrointestinal tract 1

Nutrition is the study of the relationship between **food and drink** in their **relationship** to **health or disease**, especially in determining an **optimal diet** for purposes of **health, weight loss, body building**, or other purposes. It is practised by nutritionists.

Nutrition and health

Nutrition is a cornerstone that affects and defines the health of all people. There exists a large category of disease which are thought to be caused, at least in part, by malnutrition, or the lack of proper nutrition. These include:

- **heart disease**
- some **cancers**
- **diabetes**
- **beriberi**
- **rickets**
- **scurvy**
- **vitamin deficiency disease**
- **kwashiorkor and marasmus**
- **pellagra**
- **poor immune function**, potentially leading to a wide range of other illnesses.

Additionally, several diseases directly or indirectly are impacted by diet, and require very close attention to the nutrient content of food. These include:

- **metabolic or nutritionally related** disease such as **diabetes** or **endemic goitre.**
- various **eating disorders** such as **binge eating, anorexia nervosa, or bulimia.**

Metabolism and food intake

Metabolism

Metabolism is the biochemical **transformation of energy and matter** within the body. Most commonly, this refers to the **digestion of food**, and to the **disposal of wastes.** Each living cell has a metabolism **(cell metabolism)** as well as multicellular organisms like plants, animals and humans have a "**total**" **metabolism** that can differ from that of the individual cells. The metabolic pathways form a two-part process:

- **Catabolism** – when the body uses food for energy. Catabolism is **destructive** metabolism; **larger organic molecules** are broken down **into smaller constituents.** This usually occurs with the **release of energy** (usually as ATP).
- **Anabolism** – when the body uses food to **build or mend cells**. Anabolism is **constructive** metabolism; small precursor **molecules are assembled into larger organic molecules**. This always **requires the input of energy** (often as ATP).

The halt of metabolism in a living organism is usually defined as **its death.** Some organisms can reduce their metabolism to almost zero for certain periods of time. **Spores of fungi can survive** thousands of years in that state. But every life form is bound to have metabolism at some point of its life cycle, with the possible **exception of viruses**, which **use their hosts metabolism**.

Autotrophic nutrition

Green plants, algae, and some **bacteria** are **autotrophs** ("**self-feeders**"). Most of them use the energy of **sunlight** to assemble **inorganic precursors**, chiefly **carbon dioxide and water**, into the array of organic macromolecules of which they are made. The process is **photosynthesis**. Photosynthesis makes the ATP needed for the anabolic reactions in the cell.

Heterotrophic nutrition

All other organisms, including ourselves, are **heterotrophs**. We secure all our energy **from organic molecules** taken in from **our surroundings** ("food"). Although heterotrophs may feed partially or exclusively on other heterotrophs, all the food molecules come ultimately from autotrophs.

Heterotrophs degrade some of the organic molecules that take in (catabolism) to make the ATP for synthesizing the others into the macromolecules of which they are made (anabolism). **Humans** are heterotrophs. We are totally **dependent on** ingested preformed **organic molecules as the building blocks** to meet our anabolic needs.

The steps

- **Ingestion**: taking food within the body
- **Digestion**: the enzyme-catalysed hydrolysis of

polysaccharides (e.g. starch) **to sugars**
proteins to **amino acids**
fats to **fatty acids and glycerol**
nucleic acids to **nucleotides**

- **Absorption** into the body and transport to the cells)

Exercise 1a

Match the column A with the column B. Try to learn the expressions and/or sentences by heart.

A

1. Nutrition is the study of the relationship between food and drink in their relationship to health or disease,
2. Diseases caused by the lack of proper nutrition include:
3. Several diseases impacted by diet, include:
4. Metabolism is the biochemical transformation of energy and matter within the body
5. Catabolism is destructive metabolism;
6. Anabolism is constructive metabolism;
7. Spores of fungi can reduce their metabolism
8. Viruses
9. Green plants, algae, and some bacteria are autotrophs; they use the energy of sunlight

10. Humans are heterotrophs, they are totally dependent on
11. Digestion means the enzyme-catalysed hydrolysis of

B

a) *determining an optimal diet for purposes of health, weight loss, body building, or other purposes.*
b) *diabetes or endemic goitre and eating disorders such as binge eating, anorexia nervosa, or bulimia.*
c) *heart disease, some cancers, diabetes, beriberi, rickets, scurvy, vitamin deficiency disease, kwashiorkor and marasmus, pellagra and poor immune function.*
d) *i.e. the digestion of food, and to the disposal of wastes.*
e) *ingested preformed organic molecules as the building blocks to meet their anabolic needs.*
f) *larger organic molecules are broken down into smaller constituents; this usually occurs with the release of energy.*
g) *polysaccharides to sugars, proteins to amino acids, fats to fatty acids and glycerol, and nucleic acids to nucleotides.*
h) *small precursor molecules are assembled into larger organic molecules; this always requires the input of energy.*
i) *to almost zero for certain periods of time; they can survive thousands of years in that state.*
j) *to assemble carbon dioxide and water into the array of organic macromolecules in the process called photosynthesis.*
k) *use their hosts metabolism.*

Human gastrointestinal tract

Humans (and most animals) digest all their food extracellularly; that is, outside of cells. **Digestive enzymes** are secreted from cells lining the inner surfaces of various **exocrine glands**. The enzymes hydrolyse **the macromolecules** in food into **small, soluble molecules** that can be **absorbed** into cells.

Ingestion

Food placed in the mouth is

- **ground** into finer particles by **the teeth,**
- **moistened** and lubricated by **saliva** (secreted by three pairs of **salivary glands**)
- small amounts of starch are digested by the **amylase** present in saliva
- the resulting bolus of **food is swallowed** into the **pharynx**, then **oesophagus** and
- carried by **peristalsis** to the **stomach**

The stomach

The wall of the stomach is lined with millions of **gastric glands**, which together secrete 400-800 ml of **gastric juice** at each meal. Three kinds of cells are found in the gastric glands:

- parietal cells
- "chief" cells
- mucus-secreting cells

Parietal cells secrete

- **hydrochloric acid** (HCL)
- **intrinsic factor** is a protein that binds ingested vitamin B_{12} and enables it to be absorbed by the intestine. A **deficiency** of intrinsic factor causes **pernicious anaemia**.

Chief cells

The "chief" cells synthesize and secrete **pepsinogen**, the precursor to the proteolytic **enzyme pepsin**. Its action **breaks long polypeptide chains** into shorter lengths. Secretion by the gastric glands is stimulated by the **hormone gastrin**. Gastrin is released by endocrine cells in the stomach in response to the arrival of food.

Absorption in the stomach

Very little occurs. However, some water, certain ions, and such drugs as **aspirin** and **ethanol** are absorbed from the stomach into the blood (accounting for the quick relief of a headache after swallowing aspirin and the rapid appearance of ethanol in the blood after drinking alcohol). As the **contents** of the stomach become thoroughly **liquefied,** they **pass into the duodenum**, the first segment (about 10 inches long) of the **small intestine**.

Two ducts enter the duodenum:

- one draining the **gall bladder** and hence the **liver**
- the other draining the exocrine portion of the **pancreas.**

The liver

The **liver secretes bile**. Between meals it **accumulates** in the **gall bladder**. **When food**, especially when it contains fat, **enters the duodenum**, the release of the hormone cholecystokinin (CCK) stimulates the **gall bladder to contract** and **discharge its bile** into the duodenum.

Bile contains:

- **Bile acids**. These amphiphilic steroids emulsify ingested fat. The hydrophobic portion of the steroid dissolves in the fat while the negatively charged side chain interacts with water molecules. The mutual repulsion of these negatively charged droplets keeps them from coalescing. Thus large **globules of fat** (liquid at body temperature) **are emulsified into tiny droplets** that can be more easily digested and absorbed.
- **Bile pigments.** These are the products of the **breakdown of haemoglobin** removed

by the liver from old red body cells. The brownish colour of the bile pigments imparts the characteristic brown colour of the faeces.

The **capillary beds of most tissues** drain **into veins** that lead directly **back to the heart.** But blood draining **the intestines** is an **exception**. The veins draining the intestine **lead to** a second set of capillary beds in **the liver**. Here the liver **removes many of the materials that were absorbed by the intestine:**

- **Glucose** is removed and converted into **glycogen**.
- **Other monosaccharides** are removed and converted into **glucose**.
- Excess **amino acids are removed** and deaminated.

The **amino group** is converted into **urea**.

The **residue** can then enter the pathways of cellular respiration and be **oxidized for energy**.

- Many non-nutritive molecules, such as **ingested drugs**, are removed by the **liver** and, often, **detoxified**.

The liver serves as a gatekeeper **between the intestines** and the **general circulation**. It screens blood reaching it in the **hepatic portal system** so that its composition when it leaves will be close to normal for the body. Furthermore, this homoeostatic **mechanism** works both ways. When, for example, the **concentration of glucose** in the blood drops between meals, the liver releases more to the blood by

- **converting its glycogen** stores to glucose (glycogenolysis)
- **converting certain amino acids** into glucose (gluconeogenesis)

The pancreas

The pancreas consists of **clusters of endocrine cells** (the **islets of Langerhans**) and **exocrine cells** whose secretions drain into the duodenum.

Pancreatic fluid contains:

- **Sodium bicarbonate**. This **neutralizes the acidity** of the fluid arriving from the stomach.
- **Pancreatic amylase**. This enzyme hydrolyses **starch** into a mixture of **maltose and glucose**.
- **Pancreatic lipase**. This enzyme **hydrolyses** ingested **fats** into a mixture of **fatty acids and monoglycerides**. Its action is enhanced by the detergent effect of bile.
- **4 "zymogens "** - proteins that are precursors to active proteases. These are immediately converted into the active **proteolytic enzymes.**

- **Nucleases**. These hydrolyse ingested **nucleic acids** (RNA and DNA) into their component **nucleotides.**

The secretion of **pancreatic fluid** is controlled by two hormones:

- **Secretin**, which mainly affects the **release of sodium bicarbonate**
- **Cholecystokinin** (CCK), which stimulates the **release of the digestive enzymes.**

Exercise 1b
Match the column A with the column B. Try to learn the expressions and/or sentences by heart.

A

1. Digestive enzymes hydrolyse the macromolecules in food
2. Food placed in the mouth is ground by the teeth, moistened by saliva, small amounts of starch are digested by the amylase,
3. As the contents of the stomach become thoroughly liquefied,
4. Two ducts enter the duodenum:
5. The liver secretes bile;
6. When food enters the duodenum,
7. Bile contains bile acids which emulsify ingested fat into tiny droplets
8. The capillary beds of most tissues drain into veins that lead directly back to the heart, but he veins draining the intestine
9. Many non-nutritive molecules, such as ingested drugs,
10. The liver screens blood reaching it in the hepatic portal system
11. When the concentration of glucose in the blood
12. The pancreas consists of clusters of endocrine cells (the islets of Langerhans)
13. Pancreatic fluid contains:

B

a) and bile pigments which are the products of the breakdown of haemoglobin.
b) and exocrine cells whose secretions drain into the duodenum.
c) and the resulting food is swallowed into the pharynx, then oesophagus and carried by peristalsis to the stomach.
d) are removed by the liver and, often, detoxified.
e) between meals it accumulates in the gall bladder.
f) drops between meals, the liver releases more to the blood.
g) into small, soluble molecules that can be absorbed into cells.
h) lead to a second set of capillary beds in the liver and many of the materials

that were absorbed by the intestine are removed here.

i) *one draining the gall bladder and hence the liver, the other draining the exocrine portion of the pancreas.*

j) *so that its composition when it leaves will be close to normal for the body.*

k) *sodium bicarbonate, pancreatic amylase, pancreatic lipase, 4 "zymogens" and nucleases.*

l) *the gall bladder contracts to discharge its bile into the duodenum.*

m) *they pass into the duodenum, the first segment of the small intestine.*

Exercise 2
Translate the expressions. Try to explain their meanings in English.

Relationship, body building, lack of, proper nutrition, rickets, scurvy, vitamin deficiency, kwashiorkor, marasmus, pellagra, impacted, close attention, endemic goitre, binge eating, transformation of energy and matter, disposal of wastes, differ from, destructive, constituents, release of energy, build or mend cells, assembled, input, halt, fungi, survive, life cycle, algae, array, ingestion, digestion, cells lining, the inner surfaces, exocrine glands, hydrolyse, ground, moistened, salivary glands, swallowed, oesophagus, parietal cells, hydrochloric acid, binds, pernicious anaemia, precursor, breaks long polypeptide chains, endocrine cells, accounting for, quick relief, appearance, contents, pass into the duodenum, small intestine, gall bladder, draining, pancreas, accumulates, contract, discharge, bile acids, emulsify, dissolves, negatively charged, interacts with, mutual repulsion, droplets, globules, pigments, faeces, capillary beds, tissues, drain, converted, urea, residue, cellular respiration, hepatic portal system, islets of Langerhans, sodium bicarbonate, pancreatic amylase, pancreatic lipase, detergent effect of bile, precursors, nucleic acids (RNA and DNA).

Exercise 3
Answer the following questions. Prepare short talks and/or dialogues on these topics.

1. Give the names of diseases which are thought to be caused by malnutrition.
2. Give the names of diseases which are directly or indirectly impacted by diet.
3. Characterise metabolism (catabolism and anabolism).
4. Explain the terms autotrophic and heterotrophic nutrition.
5. Digestion of polysaccharides, proteins, fats, and nucleic acids.
6. What are the parts of human gastrointestinal tract?
7. What are the functions of the mouth?
8. What are the functions of the stomach?
9. What are the functions of the liver?

10. What are the functions of the pancreas?

Vocabulary 1

Fill in the meanings in your mother language:

absorption /əb'sɔ:pʃən/
account /ə'kaʊnt/ **for** /fə/
accumulate /ə'kju:mjʊˌleɪt/
additionally /ə'dɪʃənəli/
alga /'ælgə/ **algae** /'ældʒi:/
amphiphilic /ˌæm fə'fɪl ɪk/
anabolism /ə'næbəˌlɪzəm/
array /ə'reɪ/
assemble /ə'sembəl/
autotroph /'ɔ təˌtrɒf/
bile /baɪl/ **pigment** /'pɪgmənt]/
binge /bɪndʒ/ **eating** /i:tɪŋ/
bolus /bəʊ.ləs/
bound /baʊnd/
capillary /kə'pɪl.ər.i/ **bed** /bed/
catabolism /kə'tæbəˌlɪzəm/
catalyse /'kætəˌlaɪz/
charged /'tʃɑ:dʒd/
chief /tʃi:f/
chiefly /'tʃi:flɪ/
cholecystokinin /ˌkɒlɪˌsɪstə'kaɪnɪn/
cluster /'klʌstə/
coalesce /ˌkəʊə'lɛs/
composition /ˌkɒmpə'zɪʃən/
constituent /kən'stɪtjʊənt/
convert /'kɒn vɜrt/
cornerstone /'kɔ:nəˌstəʊn/
deaminate /di:'æmɪˌneɪt/
degrade /dɪ'greɪd/
destructive /dɪ'strʌktɪv/
detergent /dɪ'tɜ:dʒənt/
determine /dɪ'tɜ:m.ɪn/
detoxify /di:'tɒksɪˌfaɪ/
differ /'dɪfə/
digestion /dɪ'dʒestʃən/
discharge /dɪs'tʃɑ:dʒ/
disposal /dɪ'spəʊzəl/
drain /dreɪn/
droplet /'drɒplɪt/
duct /dʌkt/
duodenum /ˌdju:əʊ'di:nəm/
endemic /en'demɪk/
enzyme /'enzaɪm/
exception /ɪk'sɛpʃən/
exocrine /'ɛksəʊˌkraɪn/ **gland** /glænd/
extracellularly /ˌɛkstrə'sɛljʊlə/
fungus /'fʌŋgəs/ pl **fungi**
gall /gɔ:l/ **bladder** /blædə/
gastric /'gæstrɪk/
gastrin /'gæstrɪn/
gatekeeper /'geɪtˌki:pə/
globule /'glɒbju:l/
gluconenolysis /ˌglu:kəʊˌni:əʊ'l ə sɪs/
gluconeogenesis /ˌglu:kəʊˌni:əʊ' dʒɛnɪsɪs/
goitre /'gɔɪ.tər/
ground /graʊnd/
halt /hɔ:lt/
hence /hens/
heterotrophic /ˌhɛtərəʊ'trɒfɪk/
hydrolysis /haɪ'drɒlɪsɪs/
hydrolyze /'haɪ drəˌlaɪz/
hydrophobic /ˌhaɪdrə'fəʊbɪk/
impact /'ɪm.pækt/
impart /ɪm'pɑ:t/
ingestion /ɪn'dʒestʃən/
inorganic /ˌɪnɔ:'gænɪk/
input /'ɪnˌpʊt/
interact/ˌɪntər'ækt/
ion /'aɪən/
kwashiorkor /ˌkwæʃɪ'ɔ:kə/
lining /'laɪnɪŋ/
liquefy /'lɪkwɪˌfaɪ/
lubricate /'lu:brɪˌkeɪt/
marasmus /mə'ræzməs/
mend /mend/
mixture /'mɪkstʃə/
moisten /'mɔɪsən/
monoglyceride /ˌmɒn ə'glɪs əˌraɪd/
mucus /'mju:kəs/
multicellular /ˌmʌl ti'sɛl jə lər/
mutual /'mju:tʃʊəl/

nuclease /ˈnjuːklɪˌeɪz/
nucleic /nuˈkli ɪk/ **acid** /ˈæs ɪd/
nucleotide /ˈnjuːklɪəˌtaɪd/
oesophagus /iːˈsɒfəgəs/
pancreatic/ˌpæŋkrɪˈætɪk/
lipase /ˈlaɪpeɪs/
parietal /pəˈraɪɪtəl/
pathway /ˈpɑːθˌweɪ/
pepsin /ˈpɛpsɪn/
pepsinogen /pɛpˈsɪnədʒən/
pharynx /ˈfærɪŋks/
photosynthesis /ˌfəʊtəʊˈsɪnθɪsɪs/
polypeptide /ˌpɒlɪˈpɛptaɪd/
chain /tʃeɪn/
portal /ˈpɔːtəl/
portion /ˈpɔːʃən/
precursor /prɪˈkɜːsə/
protease /ˈprəʊtɪˌeɪs/
proteolytic /ˌprəʊtɪˈɒlɪtɪk/
purpose /ˈpɜːpəs/
relationship /rɪˈleɪʃənʃɪp/
release /rɪˈliːs/
relief /rɪˈliːf/
remove /rɪˈmuːv/
repulsion /rɪˈpʌlʃən/
residue /rezɪˌdjuː/
saliva /səˈlaɪvə/
salivary gland /səˈlaɪvərɪ glænd/
screen /skriːn/
scurvy /ˈskɜːvɪ/
secret /ˈsi krɪt/
secretin /sɪˈkriːtɪn/
segment /ˈsɛgmənt/
set /set/
soluble /ˈsɒljʊbəl/
spore /spɔː/
surroundings /səˈraʊndɪŋz/
swallow /ˈswɒləʊ/
synthesize /ˈsɪnθɪˌsaɪz/
take /teɪk/ **in** /ɪn/
total /ˈtəʊtəl/
transport /ˈtrænsˌpɔːt/
ultimately /ˈʌltɪmɪtlɪ/
urea /ˈjʊərɪə/
waste /weɪst/
zymogen /ˈzaɪməʊˌdʒɛn/

Solution to Exercise 1a
1a, 2c, 3b, 4d, 5f, 6h, 7i, 8k, 9j, 10e, 11g

Solution to Exercise 1b
1g, 2c, 3m, 4i, 5e, 6l, 7a, 8h, 9d, 10j, 11f, 12b, 13k

Unit 2 - Human gastrointestinal tract 2. Foods composition.

The small intestine

The small intestine consists of three parts:

- **Duodenum**
- **Jejunum**
- **Ileum**

Digestion within the small intestine produces a **mixture of disaccharides, peptides, fatty acids, and monoglycerides.** The final digestion and absorption of these substances occurs in the **villi,** which line the inner surface of the **small intestine.**

The crypts at the base of the villi contain **stem cells** that continuously **divide by mitosis** producing:

- more **stem cells**
- cells that migrate up the surface of the villus while differentiating into columnar **epithelian cells** (the majority). They are responsible for digestion and absorption.
- **goblet** cells, which secrete mucus;

- **endocrine** cells, which secret a variety of hormones;
- **paneth** cells, which secrete antimicrobial peptides that sterilize the content of the intestine.

All of these cells replace older **cells** that continuously **die by apoptosis**. The **villi increase the surface area of the small intestine** to many times what it would be if it were simply a tube with smooth walls. In addition, the apical (exposed) surface of the epithelial cells of each villus is covered with **micro-villi** (also know as brush border). Thanks largely to these, the total surface area of the intestine is almost 200 square meters.

Incorporated in the **plasma membrane** of the micro villi are a number of **enzymes** that complete digestion:

- **aminopeptidases**
- **disaccharidases.** These enzymes convert disaccharidases into their **monosaccharides** subunits:

maltase hydrolyses **maltose** into **glucose**
sucrase hydrolyses sucrose (common table sugar) into glucose and fructose
lactase hydrolyses **lactose** (milk sugar) into **glucose and galactose**
fructose simply diffuses into the villi, but both glucose and galactose are absorbed by active transport.

- **fatty acids and monoglycerides.** These become resynthesized into fats as they enter the cells of the villus. The resulting small droplets of fat are then discharged by exocytosis into the lymph vessels, called lacteals, draining the villi.

The large intestine

The large intestine consists of three parts:

- **colon** – the biggest part
- **caecum** with appendix
- **rectum**

The large intestine receives the liquid residue after digestion and absorption are complete. This **residue** consists mostly of water as well as materials (e.g. cellulose) that were not digested. **It nourishes** a large population of **bacteria** (the contents of the small intestine are normally sterile). Most of these bacteria (of which one common species is *E. Coli*) are **harmless**. And some are actually **helpful**, for example, by synthesizing vitamin K. Bacteria flourish to such an extent that as much as 50% of the dry weight of the **faeces** may **consist of bacterial cells**. Re-absorption **of water** is the chief function of the large intestine. The large amounts of water secreted into the stomach and small intestine by the various digestive glands must be reclaimed to avoid dehydration. **If the large intestine becomes irritated**, it may discharge its contents before water re-absorption is complete causing **diarrhoea**. On the other hand, **if the colon retains its contents** too long, the faecal matter becomes dried out and compressed into hard masses causing **constipation**.

Enzymes

Enzyme (from Greek: in ferment) is a **protein**, or assemblage of protein molecules, which **facilitates** (and/or accelerates) a **biochemical reaction**. Many chemical reactions occur within cells; but without enzymes, most of them would happen too slowly to sustain life. Enzymes are essential to living organisms, and a **malfunction** of even a single enzyme out of approximately 2,000 present in our bodies can lead to **severe or lethal illness**. An example of a disease caused by an enzyme malfunction in humans is **phenylketonuria** (PKU). But not all enzymes are in living things. Enzymes are also used in everyday products such as washing detergents, where they speed up chemical reactions involved in cleaning the clothes (for example, breaking down blood stains).

Exercise 1a
Match the column A with the column B. Try to learn the expressions and/ or sentences by heart.

A

1. The small intestine consists of three parts:
2. The final digestion and absorption of a mixture of disaccharides, peptides, fatty acids, and monoglycerides
3. Stem cells that continuously divide by mitosis producing:
4. The villi increase the surface area of the small intestine;
5. Incorporated in the plasma membrane of the micro-villi are a number of enzymes that complete digestion:
6. The large intestine consists of three parts:
7. The large intestine receives the liquid residue
8. This residue consists mostly of water
9. It nourishes a large population of bacteria
10. Bacteria flourish to such an extent that
11. Re-absorption of water
12. If the large intestine becomes irritated, it may discharge its contents
13. If the colon retains its contents too long, the faecal matter
14. Enzyme is a protein
15. Enzymes are essential to living organisms, and a malfunction
16. Enzymes are also used in everyday products such as washing detergents,

B

a) *after digestion and absorption are complete.*
b) *aminopeptidases, disaccharidases and fatty acids and monoglycerides.*

c) *as much as 50% of the dry weight of the faeces may consist of bacterial cells.*
d) *as well as materials that were not digested.*
e) *becomes dried out and compressed into hard masses causing constipation.*
f) *before water re-absorption is complete causing diarrhoea.*
g) *can lead to severe or lethal illness.*
h) *colon, caecum and rectum.*
i) *duodenum, jejunum and ileum.*
j) *each villus is covered with micro-villi; the total surface area of the intestine is almost 200 square meters.*
k) *is the chief function of the large intestine.*
l) *more stem cells, columnar epithelian cells, goblet cells, endocrine cells, and paneth cells.*
m) *most of which are harmless and some are actually helpful.*
n) *occurs in the villi, which line the inner surface of the small intestine.*
o) *where they speed up chemical reactions involved in cleaning the clothes.*
p) *which facilitates (and/ or accelerates) a biochemical reaction.*

Foods composition

Nutrition is the process of **consuming**, **absorbing**, and **using nutrients** needed by the body for **growth**, **development**, and **maintenance of life**. To receive adequate, appropriate nutrition, people need to consume a **healthy diet**, which consists of a variety of **nutrients** (the chemical substances in foods that nourish the body). A healthy nutritionally adequate diet enables people to maintain a desirable **body weight** and composition (the **percentage of fat and muscle** in the body) and to perform their daily **physical and mental activities**.

The human diet must provide:

- **calories**; enough to meet daily energy needs. Nutritionists, when describing the energy content of food, typically refer to calories. The **energy content** of **fat is 9 kcal/g**, of **protein and carbohydrates 4 kcal/g**.
- **amino acids**. There are **nine "essential"** amino acids that we need for protein synthesis and that we **cannot synthesize** from other precursors.
- **fatty acids**. There are **three "essential"** fatty acids that we cannot synthesize from other precursors.
- **vitamins**. **A dozen,** or so, small organic molecules that we cannot synthesize from other precursors in our diet.
- **minerals**. Inorganic ions. We probably need **18 different ones**: a few like calcium in relatively

large amounts; most, like zinc, in "trace" amounts.

Foods consumed in the daily diet contain as many as 100,000 substances. But only 300 are classified as nutrients, and only **45** are classified as **essential nutrients.** However, food contains many other useful components, including some **fibres** (such as **cellulose, pectins,** and **stabilizers**), which improve the production, processing, storage, and packaging of foods. **Spices, flavours, substances** that add **odour or colour, phytochemicals** (substances in plants that have biologic activity in animals), and many **other natural products** improve the appearance, taste, and stability of food.

Healthy eating pyramid

The healthy eating pyramid sits on a foundation of **daily exercise**, and **weight control**. These two related elements strongly influence our chances of staying healthy. They also affect what and how we eat and how our food affects us. The other bricks of the Healthy eating pyramid include:

- **whole grain foods** (at most meals). The body needs **carbohydrates** mainly **for energy**. The best sources of carbohydrates are whole grains such as **oatmeal, whole wheat bread**, and **brown rice**. They deliver the outer (**bran**) and inner (**germ**) layers along with energy-rich **starch**. The body can't digest whole grains as quickly as it can highly processed carbohydrates such as white flour. This **keeps blood sugar and insulin levels** from rising, then falling, too quickly. Better control of blood sugar and insulin can keep hunger at bay and may prevent the development of diabetes (type 2).
- **plant oils**. Surprised that the Healthy eating pyramid puts some fats near the base, indicating they are okay to eat? Although this recommendation seems to go against conventional wisdom, it's exactly in line with the evidence and with common eating habits. Note, though, that it **specifically** mentions **plant oils**, not all types of fat. Good sources of healthy unsaturated fats include **olive, canola, soy, corn, sunflower, peanut**, and other vegetable oils, as well as **fatty fish** such as **salmon**. These healthy fats not only improve cholesterol levels (when eaten in place of highly processed carbohydrates) but can also **protect the heart** from sudden and potentially deadly rhythm problems.
- **vegetables** (in abundance) and **fruits** (2 to 3 times). A diet rich in fruits and vegetables can **decrease**

the chances of having a **heart attack or stroke**; protect against a variety of **cancers**; lower **blood pressure**; help us to avoid the painful intestinal ailment called **diverticulitis**; guard against **cataract** and macular degeneration, the major cause of **vision loss** among people over age 65; and add variety to our diet and wake up our palate.

- **nuts and legumes** (1 to 3 times). Nuts and legumes are excellent sources of **protein, fibre, vitamins, and minerals**. Legumes include **black beans, navy beans, garbanzos**, and other beans that are usually sold dried. Many kinds of nuts contain healthy fats – **almonds, walnuts, pecans, peanuts, hazelnuts, and pistachios** - and they are good for our heart.
- **fish, poultry and eggs** (0 to 2 times). These are important sources of protein. A wealth of research suggests that **eating fish** can reduce the risk of heart disease. **Chicken and turkey** are also good sources of protein and can be low in saturated fat. **Eggs**, which have long been demonized because they contain fairly high levels of cholesterol, aren't as bad as they're cracked up to be. In fact, an egg is a much better breakfast than a doughnut cooked in oil rich in trans fats or a bagel made from refined flour.
- **dairy or calcium supplement** (1 to 2 times). **Building bone** and keeping it strong takes calcium, vitamin D, exercise, and a whole lot more. Dairy products have traditionally been main source of calcium. But there are other healthy ways to get calcium than from milk and cheese, which can contain a lot of saturated fat. Three glasses of whole milk, for example, contains as much saturated fat as 13 strips of cooked bacon. If we enjoy dairy foods, it is better to stick with **no-fat or low-fat products**. If we don't like dairy products, calcium supplements offer an easy and inexpensive way to get your daily calcium.
- **red meat and butter (use sparingly)**: These sit at the top of the Healthy eating pyramid because they contain lots of saturated fat. If we eat red meat everyday, switching to fish or chicken several times a week can improve cholesterol levels. So can switching from butter to olive oil.
- **white rice, white bread, potatoes, pasta, and sweets (use sparingly)**: They can cause fast and furious

increases in blood sugar that can lead to weight gain, diabetes, heart disease, and other chronic disorders. **Whole-grain carbohydrates cause slower, steadier increases in blood sugar** that doesn't overwhelm the body's ability to handle this much needed but potentially dangerous nutrient.

- **multiple vitamin: a daily multivitamin, multi-mineral supplement** offers a kind of nutritional backup. While it can't in any way replace healthy eating, or make up for unhealthy eating, it can fill in the nutrient holes that may sometimes affect even the most careful eaters. We don't need an expensive name brand or designer vitamin. A standard, store-brand, RDA-level one is fine.
- **alcohol** (in moderation): Scores of studies suggest that having an alcoholic drink a day lowers the risk of heart disease. **Moderation is clearly important**, since alcohol has risks as well as benefits. For men, a good balance point is 1 to 2 drinks a day. For women, it's at most one drink a day.

Exercise 1b
Match the column A with the column B. Try to learn the expressions and/ or sentences by heart.

A

1. Nutrition is the process of consuming, absorbing, and using nutrients
2. A healthy nutritionally adequate diet enables people
3. The human diet must provide:
4. Food contains many other useful components,
5. Spices, flavours, substances that add odour or colour, phytochemicals
6. The best sources of carbohydrates are
7. The body can't digest whole grains as quickly as it can highly processed carbohydrates such as white flour,
8. Good sources of healthy unsaturated fats include
9. These healthy fats not only improve cholesterol levels
10. A diet rich in fruits and vegetables can decrease the chance
11. Nuts and legumes are excellent sources
12. Many kinds of nuts (almonds, walnuts, pecans, peanuts, hazelnuts, and pistachios)
13. Eating fish can reduce the risk of heart disease;
14. Dairy products have traditionally been main source of calcium

15. Red meat and butter
16. White rice, white bread, potatoes, pasta, and sweets
17. A daily multivitamin, multi-mineral supplement
18. Having an alcoholic drink a day

B

a) *and many other natural products improve the appearance, taste, and stability of food.*
b) *but can also protect the heart from sudden and potentially deadly rhythm problems.*
c) *but there are other healthy ways to get calcium than from milk and cheese, which can contain a lot of saturated fat.*
d) *calories, amino acids, fatty acids, vitamins and minerals.*
e) *can cause fast increases in blood sugar that can lead to weight gain, diabetes, heart disease, and other chronic disorders.*
f) *chicken and turkey are also good sources of protein and can be low in saturated fat.*
g) *contain healthy fats and they are good for our heart.*
h) *contain lots of saturated fat.*
i) *lowers the risk of heart disease.*
j) *needed by the body for growth, development, and maintenance of life.*
k) *of having a heart attack or stroke; protect against a variety of cancers; lower blood pressure; help us to avoid diverticulitis; and guard against cataract and macular degeneration.*
l) *of protein, fibre, vitamins, and minerals.*
m) *offers a kind of nutritional backup.*
n) *olive, canola, soy, corn, sunflower, peanut, and other vegetable oils, as well as fatty fish such as salmon.*
o) *to maintain a desirable body weight and composition (the percentage of fat and muscle in the body).*
p) *which improve the production, processing, storage, and packaging of foods.*
q) *which keeps blood sugar and insulin levels from rising, then falling, too quickly.*
r) *whole grains such as oatmeal, whole wheat bread, and brown rice.*

Exercise 2

Translate the expressions. Try to explain their meanings in English.

Small intestine, duodenum, jejunum, iIleum, villi, stem cells, mitosis, migrate, differentiating, columnar epithelian cells, goblet cells, paneth cells, apoptosis, apical, border, incorporated, convert, diffuses, lymph vessels, colon, caecum, rectum, common species, harmless, flourish, extent, re-absorption, reclaimed, irritated, diarrhoea, retains, compressed, constipation, assemblage, facilitates, accelerates, sustain life, lethal illness, speed up, blood stains, composition, maintenance of life, nourish, enables, desirable, essential, precursors, dozen, trace amounts, fibres, processing, storage, spices, flavours, odour, natural products, foundation, whole grain, oatmeal, whole wheat, bran, germ, starch, rising, recommendation, evidence, canola, corn, sunflower, peanut, salmon, potentially, deadly, abundance, decrease, heart attack, stroke, intestinal ailment, guard against, nuts and legumes, almonds, walnuts, pecans, peanuts, hazelnuts, pistachios, poultry, doughnut, bagel, supplement, building bone, strips of bacon, stick with, sparingly, switching to, overwhelm, handle, replace, in moderation, scores.

Exercise 3
Answer the following questions. Prepare short talks and/or dialogues on these topics.

1. Describe the structure and function of the small intestine.
2. Describe the structure and function of the large intestine.
3. Why are enzymes essential to living organisms?
4. Characterise the process of nutrition.
5. What must human diet provide?
6. Explain the items in healthy eating pyramid.
7. Describe the use of whole grain foods, plant oils and vegetables.
8. Describe the use of nuts and legumes, vitamins, and minerals.
9. Describe the use of fish, poultry, eggs and dairy or calcium supplement.
10. Describe the use of red meat and butter, white rice, white bread, potatoes, pasta, and sweets.

Vocabulary 2

Fill in the meanings in your mother language:

abundance /əˈbʌndəns/
accelerate /əkˈseləreɪt/
actually /ˈæktʃuəli/
add /æd/
affect /əˈfekt/
ailment /ˈeɪlmənt/
almond /ˈɑːmənd/
aminopeptidase /əˌmiː.nəʊˈpɛptɪˌdeɪs/
anti- /ˌæntiˈ/
apical /ˈæpɪkəl/
apoptosis /ˌæpəpˈtəʊsɪs/
appearance /əˈpɪə.rənt s/
appendix /əˈpendɪks/
appropriate /əˈprəʊ.pri.ət/
assemblage /əˈsem.blɪdʒ/
at /ət/ **most** /məʊst/
backup /ˈbæk.ʌp/
bacon /ˈbeɪ.kən/
bagel /ˈbeɪgəl/
base /beɪs/
border /ˈbɔːdər/
bran /bræn/
brand /brænd/ **name** /neɪm/
brand /brænd/

brick /brɪk/
brush /brʌʃ/
calcium /ˈkæl.si.əm/
canola /kəˈnɒl.ə/
cataract /ˈkæt.ə.rækt/
cecum /ˈsiː.kəm/
cellulose /ˈseljələʊs/
collumn /ˈkɒləm/
colon /ˈkəʊ.lɒn/
common /ˈkɒmən/
compress /kəmˈpres/
constipation /ˌkɒnstɪˈpeɪʃən/
consuming /ˈkənˌsjuː.mɪŋ/
content /ˈkɒntent/
conventional /kənˈvent.ʃən.əl/
crack /kræk/ **up** /ʌp/
dairy /ˈdeə.ri/
deadly /ˈdedli/
degeneration /dɪˌdʒen.əˈreɪ.ʃən/
demonize /ˈdiː.mə.naɪz/
designer /dɪˈzaɪnər/
desirable /dɪˈzaɪə.rə.bl̩/
diarrhoea /ˌdaɪəˈrɪə/
diffuse /dɪˈfjuːz/
disaccharide /daɪˈsæk.ə.raɪd/
diverticulitis /ˌdaɪ.vəˌtɪk.jʊˈlaɪ.tɪs/
doughnut /ˈdəʊ.nʌt/
dozen /ˈdʌzən/
enable /ɪˈneɪ.bl̩/
epithelium /ˌɛpɪˈθiːlɪəm/
evidence /ˈev.ɪ.dəns/
exocytosis /ˌɛksəʊsaɪˈtəʊsɪs/
exposed /ɪkˈspəʊzd/
extent /ɪkˈstent/
facilitate /fəˈsɪlɪteɪt/
fibre /ˈfaɪbər/
fill /fɪl/ **in** /ɪn/
flavour /ˈfleɪ.vər/
flour /ˈflaʊə/
flourish /ˈflʌrɪʃ/
foundation /faʊnˈdeɪ.ʃən/
furious /ˈfjʊəriəs/
garbanzo /gɑːˈbænzəʊ/
germ /dʒɜːm/
goblet /ˈgɒb.lət/
grain /greɪn/
guard /gɑːd/ **against** /əˈgenst/
habit /ˈhæb.ɪt/
handle /ˈhæn.dl̩/
happen /ˈhæpən/
harmless /ˈhɑːmləs/
hazelnut /ˈheɪzəlˌnʌt/
heart /hɑːt/ **attack** /əˈtæk/
helpful /ˈhelpfəl/
hole /həʊl/
in line /laɪn/ **with**
in moderation /ˌmɒd.ərˈeɪ.ʃən/
inexpensive /ˌɪnɪkˈspensɪv/
inner /ˈɪn.ər/
involved /ɪnˈvɒlvd/
irritated /ˈɪrɪteɪtɪd/
keep /kiːp/ **at** /æt/ **bay** /beɪ/
keep /kiːp/ **from** /frɒm/
lactase /ˈlækteɪs/
lacteal /ˈlæk.ti.əl/
large /lɑːdʒ/ **intestine** /ɪnˈtestɪn/
layer /ˈleɪ.ə/
lethal /ˈliːθəl/
lower /ˈləʊ.ə/
lymph /lɪmf/ **vessel** /ˈvesəl/
macula /ˌmæk.jʊ.lə/
maintenance /ˈmeɪn.tɪ.nəns/
maltase /ˈmɔl.teɪs/
matter /ˈmætər/
meet /miːt/ **the needs** /niːdz/
microbe /ˈmaɪ.krəʊb/
migrate /maɪˈgreɪt/
mitosis /maɪˈtəʊ.sɪs/
navy /ˈneɪvi/ **bean** /biːn/
nourish /ˈnʌrɪʃ/
oatmeal /ˈəʊtmiːl/
odour /ˈəʊ.dər/
outer /ˈaʊ.tər/
overwhelm /ˌəʊ.vəˈwelm/
packaging /ˈpækɪdʒɪŋ/
palate /ˈpæl.ət/
paneth /pæn.ət/
peanut /ˈpiː.nʌt/
pecan /ˈpiːkən/
pectin /ˈpɛktɪn/

peptidase /pɛptɪˌdeɪs/
peptide /ˈpep.taɪd/
percentage /pəˈsen.tɪdʒ/
perform /pəˈfɔːm/
phenylketonuria /ˌfiːnaɪlˌkiːtəˈnjʊərɪə/
phytochemical /ˌfaɪtəʊˈkɛmɪkəl/
pistachio /pɪˈstɑːʃɪˌəʊ/
plant /plɑːnt/ **oil** /ɔɪl/
precursor /ˌpriːˈkɜː.sər/
processing /ˈprəʊsesɪŋ/
protect /prəˈtekt/
pyramid /ˈpɪrəmɪd/
reclaim /rɪˈkleɪm/
recommendation /ˌrek.ə.menˈdeɪ.ʃən/
rectum /ˈrektəm/
refer /rɪˈfɜːr/
refined /rɪˈfaɪnd/
research /rɪˈsɜːtʃ/
retain /rɪˈteɪn/
rhythm /ˈrɪðəm/
salmon /ˈsæm.ən/
sparingly /ˈspeərɪŋli/
species /ˈspiːʃiːz/
speed /spiːd/ **up** /ʌp/
spice /spaɪs/
square /skweər/ **meter** /ˈmiːtər/
stability /stəˈbɪl.ɪ.ti/
stabilizer /ˈsteɪbɪˌlaɪzə/
stain /steɪn/
starch /stɑːtʃ/
stem /stem/ **cell** /sel/
stick /stɪk/
storage /ˈstɔː.rɪdʒ/
store /stɔːr/
strip /strɪp/
stroke /strəʊk/
substance /ˈsʌb.stəns/
sucrase /ˈsuːkreɪz/
sunflower /ˈsʌnˌflaʊər/
sustain /səˈsteɪn/
switch /swɪtʃ/
taste /teɪst/
trace /treɪs/ **element** /ˈel.ɪ.mənt/
trans fats /ˈtrænz.fæts/
turkey /ˈtɜː.ki/
walnut /ˈwɔːlˌnʌt/
wealth of /welθ/
weight /weɪt/ **gain** /geɪn/
whole /həʊl/ **milk** /mɪlk/
whole /həʊl/ **wheat** /wiːt/
wisdom /ˈwɪz.dəm/
zinc /zɪŋk/

Solution to Exercise 1a
1i, 2n, 3l, 4j, 5b, 6h, 7a, 8d, 9m, 10c, 11k, 12f, 13e, 14p, 15g, 16o

Solution to Exercise 1b
1j, 2o, 3d, 4p, 5a, 6r, 7q, 8n, 9b, 10k, 11l, 12g, 13f, 14c, 15h, 16e, 17m, 18i

Unit 3 - The importance of whole grains and dietary fibre. Diabetes mellitus.

Cereals are the most important **source of dietary fibre.** The fibre in cereals is located mainly in the outer layers of the kernel, particularly in the **bran. Rye** is of special importance in contributing dietary fibre, because it is generally consumed as **whole grain product**, and has a high dietary fibre content in the starchy endosperm. Improved diet can help unlock the door to good health. People who lead a healthy lifestyle also pay attention to their nutritional habits. Good nutrition means adequately nourishing the body by **choosing** a variety of **foods low in fat, salt and sugar** and **high in carbohydrates**, especially **starch and dietary fibre.** Mortality is significantly lower in people consuming whole grain products.

In today's world people are increasingly aware of what they eat. As the level of education and the overall well-being of people increase, public awareness of the relationship between diet and health also grows. **Knowledge of the nutritional content of foods increases** among ordinary people. This leads to improved attitudes towards healthier eating habits. It can be expected that in the future people will make food choices based on what is beneficial for their health and well-being. **Whole grains** are universally **recommended** as an integral part of the diet. Whole grains are an important source of nutrients that are in short supply in our diet, including **digestible carbohydrates, dietary fibre, resistant starch, trace minerals, certain vitamins**, and other compounds of interest in disease prevention, including **phyto-oesterogens and antioxidants**.

Physiological effects of the dietary fibre complex

- **teeth** – requires more **chewing**. Increases the secretion of **saliva**. Protects **against dental caries**. Keeps **gums healthy**.
- **stomach** – increases the secretion of saliva and **gastric juice**. Decreases the rate of evacuation of stomach contents into small intestine – prolongs the feeling of satiety. Enhances satiety – **prevents overeating and weight gain**.
- **digestive tract** – **shortens** intestinal **transit time**. Dilutes harmful substances. Beneficial for the **bacterial population** in the **large intestine**. Interrupts the enteropathic circulation of oestrogens, **reducing oestrogen levels**. **Prevents constipation**. Decreases risk of breast and colon cancer. **Alters bile acid metabolism** in the gut in a favourable way.
- **cardiovascular system** – **inhibits the absorption of** dietary **cholesterol**. **Increases** the release of **bile acids** into the intestine. **Influences** the plasma triglyceride levels and **blood clotting properties**. **Lowers blood cholesterol** levels. **Decreases** the risk of **heart disease and gallstones**.
- **blood glucose** – slows down the absorption of carbohydrates. Stabilizes blood glucose levels, especially in diabetic individuals.

Carbohydrates

Carbohydrates are a relatively basic class of chemical compound. They are **primary biological means of storing or consuming energy;** other forms being via fat and protein. Relatively **complex** carbohydrates are known as **polysaccharides.**

Pure carbohydrates contain **carbon, hydrogen, and oxygen atoms**. However, many important carbohydrates deviate from this.

Sometimes compounds containing **other elements** are also counted as carbohydrates, such as **chitin,** which **contains nitrogen**. Strictly speaking, carbohydrates are not necessary for human nutrition because **proteins can be converted to carbohydrates** – the traditional diet of some people consists of nearly zero percent carbohydrate, and they are perfectly healthy. However, they require (relatively) less water to digest than proteins or fats, and are an important source of energy.

The **simplest** carbohydrates are **monosaccharides**. Other carbohydrates are composed of **monosaccharide units**, and **break down under hydrolysis**. These may be classified as **disaccharides, oligosaccharides**, or **polysaccharides**, depending on whether they have **two, several, or many** mono-glyceride units.

Monosaccharides

Monosaccharides may be divided into **aldoses** and **ketoses**.

Disaccharides

The most common disaccharides are **sucrose** (cane or beet sugar), **lactose** (milk sugar) and **maltose**.

Polysaccharides

Polysaccharides are relatively complex unsweetened carbohydrates. Polysaccharides are polymers made up of many **monosaccharides joined together**. They are therefore **very large**, often branched, **molecules**. Properties include insolubility in water and not forming crystals. The most common polysaccharides include:

- **starches** – are polymers of glucose. Starches are insoluble in water. **Potato, rice, wheat, and maize** are major sources of starch in human diet.
- **glycogen** – is the **storage form of glucose** in animals. It is a branched polymer of glucose. Glycogen can be broken down to form substrates for respiration, through the process of **glycogenolysis**.
- **cellulose** – the structural components of plants are formed primarily from cellulose. Wood is largely cellulose and lignin, while paper and cotton are nearly pure cellulose.

Exercise 1a
Match the column A with the column B. Try to learn the expressions and/or sentences by heart.

A

1. Cereals are
2. Rye is of special importance in contributing dietary fibre,
3. Good nutrition means adequately nourishing the body
4. Whole grains are an important source of nutrients that are in short supply

in our diet, including digestible carbohydrates,
5. The dietary fibre requires
6. The dietary fibre increases
7. The dietary fibre shortens
8. The dietary fibre lowers blood cholesterol levels, influences blood clotting properties,
9. Carbohydrates are a relatively basic class of chemical compound;
10. Pure carbohydrates contain
11. Monosaccharides
12. Disaccharides
13. Polysaccharides are polymers made up of many
14. The most common polysaccharides include:

B

a) and decreases the risk of heart disease and gallstones.
b) are sucrose (cane or beet sugar), lactose (milk sugar) and maltose.
c) because it is generally consumed as whole grain product.
d) by choosing a variety of foods low in fat, salt and sugar and high in carbohydrates, especially starch and dietary fibre.
e) carbon, hydrogen, and oxygen atoms and other elements such as chitin, which contains nitrogen.
f) dietary fibre, resistant starch, trace minerals, certain vitamins, and other compounds including phyto-oesterogens and antioxidants.
g) intestinal transit time, is beneficial for the bacterial population in the large intestine and prevents constipation.
h) may be divided into aldoses and ketoses.
i) monosaccharides joined together; they are therefore very large, often branched, molecules.
j) more chewing, increases the secretion of saliva, protects against dental caries and keeps gums healthy.
k) starches, glycogen, cellulose.
l) the most important source of dietary fibre.
m) the secretion of saliva and gastric juice and prevents overeating and weight gain.
n) they are primary biological means of storing or consuming energy.

Diabetes mellitus

Diabetes mellitus is a name for any condition that is characterized by **chronic hyperglycaemia** and **disturbances of carbohydrate, protein and fat metabolism.** There are several types of the disease of variable aetiology. Sensible treatment of diabetes depends almost entirely on **blood glucose testing**, since grossly observable signs and symptoms almost never appear immediately and urine tests only summarize high blood glucose levels since the last urination. Long-term diabetes mellitus can have detrimental effects on numerous organs of the body, micro-vascular or macro-vascular damage. This can lead to the **chronic complications** of diabetes mellitus. They include:

- proliferative **retinopathy** that can lead to **blindness**;
- **peripheral neuropathy** can lead to **foot ulcers** leading to necrosis and infection (**gangrene**), eventually requiring amputation;
- **nephropathy** can cause chronic **renal failure** requiring dialysis or transplantation.
- **ischemic heart disease**, **stroke** and **neuropathy** are other possible complications.

There are several types of diabetes mellitus:

- **type 1**, most commonly first diagnosed **in children and adolescents**, an **autoimmune disorder** in which the body's own immune system **attacks** the hormone producing **beta cells of the islets of Langerhans in the pancreas**, preventing it from producing enough (or any) insulin. The autoimmune attack is generally **triggered by an infection**. Some types of **poisons** work by selectively destroying the beta cells, producing Type 1 diabetes. **Pancreatic trauma or tumour** can do so as well. Early **symptoms** of Type 1 diabetes are often **polyuria** (frequent urination) and **polydipsia** (increased thirst and concomitant increased fluid intake). There may also be **weight loss** despite normal or increased eating, increased appetite, and unreduceable **fatigue**. Type 1 is almost always treated with **insulin injections**, usually utilizing intensive insulinotherapy.
- **type 2**, in which the body's **cells become resistant to insulin,** eventually, the amount of **insulin is insufficient** to cause enough absorption of blood glucose, resulting in **hyperglycaemia** and finally in glucose being dumped by the kidneys into the urine. Type 2 often develops **later in life,** and is often accompanied by **obesity**. There is a strong **genetic** connection to Type 2 diabetes. Relatives with Type 2 are a considerable risk factor. **Dangerous** signs to watch out for include the **smell of acetone** on the patient's breath (a sign of **ketoacidosis**). **Kussmaul breathing** (**rapid, deep** breathing), and any **altered state of consciousness** or **arousal** (hostility and mania are both

possible, as is confusion), the worst form of which is the so-called "**diabetic coma**". Early **symptoms** are **polyuria**, **nausea**, **vomiting** and **abdominal pain**, with **lethargy** and **somnolence** a later development, progressing to **unconsciousness** and **coma** if untreated. Type 2 can be treated with drugs, diet and exercise.

- **type 3**, **all other specific forms**, caused by: genetic defects in beta cells, genetically related insulin resistance, diseases of the pancreas, hormonal defects, chemicals or drugs.
- **type 4** or **gestational** diabetes mellitus appears in about 2-5% of all pregnancies. About 20-50% of these women go on to develop Type 2 diabetes.

Diabetes insipidus

Diabetes insipidus (DI) is a disease characterized by **excretion** of large amounts of dilute **urine**, which disrupts the body's **water regulation**. This is a different disease from diabetes mellitus. Diabetes insipidus is often called "water diabetes" to set it apart from diabetes mellitus or sugar diabetes. The cause and treatment are not the same as for diabetes mellitus. Patients with diabetes insipidus show **most of the symptoms of diabetes mellitus** – they have to urinate often, get very thirsty and hungry, and feel weak. However, they do not have hyperglycaemia (elevated blood glucose). DI occurs when system for regulating the kidney's handling of fluids is disrupted. There are four types of DI:

- **central** DI. Damage to the **pituitary gland** can be caused by different **diseases** as well as by **head injuries**, **neurosurgery**, or **genetic disorders**. To treat the resulting anti-diuretic hormone (ADH) deficiency, a **synthetic hormone** called desmopressin can be taken by an **injection, a nasal spray, or a pill.** While taking desmopressin, you should drink fluids or water only when you are thirsty and not at other times. This is because the drug prevents water excretion and water can build up now that your kidneys are making less urine and are less responsive to changes in body fluids.
- **nephrogenic** DI. The **kidneys'** ability to **respond to ADH** can **be impaired by drugs and by chronic disorders** including polycystic kidney disease, sickle cell disease, kidney failure, partial blockage of the ureters, and inherited genetic disorders. Sometimes, the cause of nephrogenic DI is never discovered.

- **dipsogenic** DI. A third type of DI is caused by a defect in or **damage to the thirst mechanism,** which is located in the **hypothalamus**. This defect results in an abnormal increase in thirst and fluid intake that suppresses ADH secretion and increases urine output. This fluid "overload" can lead to **water intoxication**, a condition which **lowers the concentration of sodium in the blood** and can seriously damage the brain.
- **gestational** DI. A fourth type of DI occurs only **during pregnancy**. Gestational DI occurs when **an enzyme made by the placenta destroys ADH in the mother.** The placenta is the system of blood vessels and other tissue that develops in the foetus. The placenta allows exchange of nutrients and waste products between mother and foetus.

Exercise 1b
Match the column A with the column B. Try to learn the expressions and/or sentences by heart.

A

1. Diabetes mellitus is a name for any condition
2. Sensible treatment of diabetes depends almost entirely on blood glucose testing,
3. Long-term diabetes mellitus
4. Chronic complications of diabetes mellitus include:
5. Diabetes mellitus Type 1
6. The body 's own immune system attacks the hormone producing beta cells of the islets of Langerhans in the pancreas,
7. Early symptoms are often
8. Type 2, in which the body 's cells become resistant to insulin, eventually, the amount of insulin is insufficient resulting in hyperglycaemia
9. Dangerous signs to watch out for include the smell of acetone on the patient's breath (a sign of ketoacidosis), Kussmaul breathing (rapid, deep breathing),
10. Early symptoms are polyuria, nausea, vomiting and abdominal pain,
11. Diabetes insipidus is a disease characterized
12. Patients with diabetes insipidus show most of the symptoms of diabetes mellitus:
13. There are four types of diabetes insipidus:
14. Damage to the pituitary gland can be caused by
15. To treat the resulting anti-diuretic hormone (ADH) deficiency,
16. In nephrogenic DI the kidneys' ability to respond to ADH can be impaired

17. A third type of DI is caused by a defect in the thirst mechanism which
18. This fluid "overload" can lead to water intoxication,
19. Gestational DI occurs when

B

a) *a condition which lowers the concentration of sodium in the blood and can seriously damage the brain.*
b) *a synthetic hormone called desmopressin can be taken by an injection, a nasal spray, or a pill.*
c) *an enzyme made by the placenta destroys antidiuretic hormone in the mother.*
d) *and any altered state of consciousness or arousal, the worst form of which is the so-called diabetic coma.*
e) *and finally in glucose being dumped by the kidneys into the urine.*
f) *by drugs and by chronic disorders including polycystic kidney disease, sickle cell disease, kidney failure, partial blockage of the ureters, and inherited genetic disorders.*
g) *by excretion of large amounts of dilute urine, which disrupts the body's water regulation.*
h) *can have detrimental effects on numerous organs of the body, micro-vascular or macro-vascular damage.*
i) *central, nephrogenic, dipsogenic and gestational.*
j) *different diseases as well as by head injuries, neurosurgery, or genetic disorders.*
k) *is first diagnosed in children and adolescents.*
l) *polyuria and polydipsia, weight loss and fatigue.*
m) *preventing it from producing enough (or any) insulin.*
n) *proliferative retinopathy, peripheral neuropathy, nephropathy, ischemic heart disease and stroke.*
o) *results in an abnormal increase in thirst and fluid intake that suppresses ADH secretion and increases urine output.*
p) *since grossly observable signs and symptoms almost never appear immediately.*
q) *that is characterized by chronic hyperglycaemia and disturbances of carbohydrate, protein and fat metabolism.*
r) *they have to urinate often, get very thirsty and hungry, and feel weak but they do not have hyperglycaemia.*
s) *with lethargy and somnolence, a later development, progressing to unconsciousness and coma if untreated.*

Exercise 2
Translate the expressions. Try to explain their meanings in English.

Kernel, bran, starchy, endosperm, pay attention, nutritional habits, mortality, is aware of, ordinary people, attitudes, eating habits, integral part, short supply, compounds, chewing, dental caries, gums, the rate of, evacuation, feeling of satiety, intestinal, transit time, dilutes, interrupts, colon cancer, favourable, inhibits the absorption, the release of, influences blood clotting, decreases the risk, storing or consuming energy, deviate, counted as, converted, break down, under hydrolysis, be classified as, cane or beet sugar, branched, insolubility, storage form, condition, disturbances, aetiology, sensible, treatment, grossly observable, summarize, urination, detrimental, effects, proliferative retinopathy, blindness, neuropathy, ulcers, nephropathy, renal failure, triggered, poisons, trauma, tumour, polyuria, polydipsia, weight loss, fatigue, utilizing, resistant, insufficient, dumped, considerable, rapid, deep, altered state of consciousness, arousal, hostility, confusion, vomiting, abdominal pain, somnolence, pregnancies, diabetes insipidus, excretion, dilute urine, set apart from, handling of fluids, pituitary gland, neurosurgery, genetic disorders, less responsive to, impaired, sickle cell disease, partial blockage, ureters, inherited, fluid intake, overload, intoxication, placenta, foetus.

Exercise 3
Answer the following questions. Prepare short talks and/or dialogues on these topics.

1. Why is knowledge of the nutritional content of foods important?
2. Why are whole grains recommended?
3. Talk about physiological effects of the dietary fibre complex.
4. Talk about carbohydrates as a basic class of chemical compound.
5. Talk about diabetes mellitus and its chronic complications.
6. Symptoms of Type 1 diabetes.
7. Type 2, dangerous signs to watch out for.
8. Characterize diabetes insipidus.
9. Types of diabetes insipidus.

Vocabulary 3

Fill in the meanings in your mother language:
acetone /ˈæs.ɪ.təʊn/
adequate /ˈædɪkwət/
adolescent /ˌæd.əˈles.ənt/
aetiology /ˌiː.tiˈɒl.ə.dʒi/
aldose /ˈældəʊs/
alter /ɒl.tər/
amputation /ˌæm.pjʊˈteɪ.ʃən/
antidiuretic /æntiˌdaɪ.jʊˈret.ɪk/ **hormone** /ˈhɔːməʊn/
arousal /əˈraʊzəl/
attitude /ˈæt.ɪ.tjuːd/
autoimmune /ˌɔː.təʊ.ɪˈmjuːn/

aware /ə'weər/
beet /bi:t/ **sugar** /'ʃʊgə/
beta /'bi:.tə/ **cell** /sel/
blindness /'blaɪnd.nəs/
blockage /'blɒk.ɪdʒ/
branch /brɑ:ntʃ/
carbon /'kɑ:.bən/
chitin /'kaɪ.tɪn/
clotting /'klɑt̬.ɪŋ/
coma /'kəʊ.mə/
complex /'kɒm.pleks/
compound /'kɒm.paʊnd/
concomitant /kən'kɒm.ɪ.tənt/
condition /kən'dɪʃən/
confusion /kən'fju:.ʒən/
consciousness /'kɒn.ʃəs.nəs/
considerable /kən'sɪd.ər.ə.bl̩/
contribute /kən'trɪb.ju:t/
cotton /'kɒt.ən/
count /kaʊnt/
crystal /'krɪstəl/
damage /'dæm.ɪdʒ/
deficiency /dɪ'fɪʃ.ənt.si/
desmopressin /də smɒ'prɛsɪn/
despite /dɪ'spaɪt/
detrimental /ˌdet.rɪ'men.təl/
deviate /'di:vieɪt/
diabetes /ˌdaɪə'bi:.ti:z/ **insipidus** /ɪn'sɪpɪd.əs/ **dipsogenic** /ˌdɪpsəʊ'dʒɛnɪk/
dialysis /daɪ'æl.ə.sɪs/
digestible /daɪ'dʒes.tə.bl̩/
dilute /daɪ'lu:t/
disorder /dɪ'sɔ:.dər/
disrupt /dɪs'rʌpt/
disturbance /dɪ'stɜ:.bəns/
dump /dʌmp/
education /ˌedʒʊ'keɪʃən/
endosperm /'en.dəʊ.spɜ:m/
enteropathic /'entərə'pæθɪk/
entirely /ɪn'taɪə.li/
estrogen /'i:.strə.dʒən/
evacuation /ɪˌvækju'eɪʃən/
exchange /ɪks'tʃeɪndʒ/
excretion /ɪk'skri:.ʃən/
fatigue /fə'ti:g/
favourable /'feɪ.vər.ə.bl̩/
feeling /'fi:.lɪŋ/
form /fɔ:m/
gallstone /'gɔ:l.stəʊn/
gangrene /'gæŋ.gri:n/
gestational /dʒes'teɪ.ʃən.əl/
glycogenolysis /ˌglaɪ.kə.dʒɪ'nɒ.lɪ.sɪs/
grossly /'grəʊs.li/
gum /gʌm/
handling /'hænd.lɪŋ/
harmful /'hɑ:m.fəl/
hostility /hɒs'tɪl.ɪ.ti/
hydrogen /'haɪ.drɪ.dʒən/
hyperglycaemia /ˌhaɪ.pə.glaɪ'si:mi.ə/
hypothalamus /ˌhaɪ.pəʊ'θæl.ə.məs/
immediately /ɪ'mi:.di.ət.li/
impaired /ɪm'peəd/
individual /ˌɪn.dɪ'vɪd.ju.əl/
inherit /ɪn'her.ɪt/
inhibit /ɪn'hɪb.ɪt/
insolubility /ɪnˌsɒl.jʊ'bɪl.ɪ.ti/
insufficient /ˌɪn.sə'fɪʃ.ənt/
integral /'ɪn tɪ grəl/
interrupt /ˌɪn.tə'rʌpt/
intoxication /ɪnˌtɒk.sɪ'keɪ.ʃən/
kernel /'kɜ:.nəl/
ketoacidosis /'ki:.təʊˌæ.ɪ'dəʊ.sɪs/
ketose /'ki:təʊz/
Kussmaul /kö s.məʊl/ **respiration** /ˌrespə'reɪʃən/
lethargy /'ləθ.ə.dʒɪ/
lignin /'lɪgnɪn/
macrovascular /'mækrəʊ.væskjʊlə/
maltose /'mɔ:ltəʊz/
means /mi:nz/
microvascular /ˌmaɪ.krəʊ'væs.kjə.lər/
molecule /'mɒl.ɪ.kju:l/
mortality /mɔ:'tæl.ə.ti/
nasal /'neɪ.zəl/ **spray** /spreɪ/
necrosis /'nek.rəʊ.sɪs/
nephrogenic /nef.rəˌdʒen.ɪk/ **diabetes** /ˌdaɪə'bi:.ti:z/ **insipidus** /ɪn'sɪpɪd.əs/
nephropathy /nɪ'frɒp.ə.θi/
neuropathy /njʊ'rɒp.ə.θɪ/

neurosurgery /ˌnjʊə.rəʊˈsɜː.dʒər.i/
nitrogen /ˈnaɪ.trə.dʒən/
observable /əbˈzɜːvəbəl/
oligosaccharide/ˌɒlɪgəʊˈsækəˌraɪd/
ordinary /ˈɔːdənrɪ/
overall /ˌəʊ.vəˈrɔːl/
overload /ˌəʊ.vəˈləʊd/
oxygen /ˈɒk.sɪ.dʒən/
pancreas /ˈpæŋ.kri.əs/
partial /ˈpɑː.ʃəl/
peripheral /pəˈrɪfərəl/
phyto-oesterogen /ˌfaɪtəʊˈiːstrədʒən/
pill /pɪl/
placenta /pləˈsen.tə/
plasma /ˈplæz.mə/
poison /ˈpɔɪ.zən/
polycystic /ˌpɒl.ɪˈsɪs.tɪk/ **kidney** / ˈkɪd.ni/ **disease** /dɪˈziːz/
polydipsia /ˌpɒl.ɪˈdɪp.sɪ.ə/
polymer /ˈpɒl.ɪ.mər/
polyuria /ˌpɒl.ɪˈjʊə.rɪ.ə/
pregnancy /ˈpreg.nən.si/
primary /ˈpraɪ.mə.ri/
proliferative /prəˈlɪf.ər.ə.tɪv/
prolong /prəʊˈlɒŋ/
pure /pjʊər/
reduce /rɪˈdjuːs/
relative /ˈrel.ə.tɪv/
renal /ˈriː.nəl/ **failure** /ˈfeɪ.ljə/
require /rɪˈkwaɪər/
resistant /rɪˈzɪs.tənt/
responsive /rɪˈspɒn.sɪv/
retinopathy /ˌret.ɪnˈɒp.ə.θi/
satiety /səˈtaɪə.ti/
selectively /ˌsɪl.ekˈtɪv.ɪ.ti/
sensible /ˈsensɪbl/
seriously /ˈsɪərɪəslɪ/
set /set/ **apart** /əˈpɑːt/
sickle /ˈsɪk.l̩/ **cell** /sel/ **disease** /dɪˈziːz/
slow /sləʊ/ **down** /daʊn/
smell /smel/
somnolence /ˈsɒm.nəl.əns/
strictly /ˈstrɪktli/
sucrose /ˈsuː.krəʊz/
summarize /ˈsʌm.ər.aɪz/
supply /səˈplaɪ/
transplantation /ˌtrɒæn.splaːnˈtei.ʃən/
trigger /ˈtrɪg.ər/
triglyceride /traɪ.glɪs.ə.raɪd/
tumour /ˈtjuː.mər/
ulcer /ˈʌl.sər/
unconsciousness /ʌnˈkɒn.ʃəs.nəs/
universal /ˌjuːnɪˈvɜːsəl/
unlock /ʌnˈlɒk/
untreated /ʌnˈtriː.tɪd/
ureter /jʊəˈriː.tər/
urination /ˌjʊə.rɪˈneɪ.ʃən/
urine /ˈjʊə.rɪn/
utilize /ˈjuː.tɪ.laɪz/
variable /ˈveə.ri.ə.bl̩/
waste /weɪst/
watch /wɒtʃ/ **out** /aʊt/
zero /ˈzɪərəʊ/

Solution to Exercise 1a
1l, 2c, 3d, 4f, 5j, 6m, 7g, 8a, 9n, 10e, 11h, 12b, 13i, 14k

Solution to Exercise 1b
1q, 2p, 3h, 4n, 5k, 6m, 7l, 8e, 9d, 10s, 11g, 12r, 13i, 14j, 15b, 16f, 17o, 18a, 19c

Unit 4 - Proteins. Fats.

Proteins are a primary **constituent of living things** and also **nutrient sources** for organisms that do not produce their own energy from sunlight. Proteins provide most of the molecular machinery of cells. Proteins **differ from carbohydrates** chiefly in that they contain much **nitrogen** and a little bit of **sulphur**, besides **carbon, oxygen and nitrogen**.

Each protein molecule is a branched **chain of polymer of amino acids** that fold into unique **3-dimensional structures**. The shape into which a protein naturally folds is known as its **native state**, which is determined by its sequence of amino acids. In terms of human nutritional needs proteins come in two forms:

- **complete proteins** contain **all nine** of the amino acids that **humans cannot make** themselves
- **incomplete** proteins **lack** or contain only a very small proportion of **one or more.**

Our bodies can **make use of all the amino acids** they extract from food for synthesizing **new proteins**, but the inessential ones themselves need not be supplied by the diet, because **our cells can make them ourselves**. When protein is listed in a nutrition label it only refers to the amount of complete proteins in the food, though the food may be very strong in a subset of the essential amino acids. **Animal-derived foods contain all of those amino acids**, while **plants are typically stronger in some acids than others.**

All nine essential amino acids must be **part of one diet in order to survive** and are needed in a **fixed ratio**. A shortage of any one of these amino acids will constrain the body's ability to make the proteins it needs to function. Different foods contain different ratios of the essential amino acids. **By mixing foods** that are rich in some amino acids with foods that are rich in others, one can acquire all the needed **amino acids in sufficient quantities**. Omnivores typically eat a sufficient variety of foods that this is not an issue, however, **vegetarians** and especially vegans should be careful to eat **appropriate combinations** of foods (e.g. nuts and green vegetables) so as to get all the essential amino acids in sufficient quantities that the body may **produce all the proteins** that it needs.

Protein deficiency

Protein deficiency can lead to symptoms such as **fatigue, insulin resistance, hair loss, loss of hair pigment, loss of muscle mass, low body temperature, and hormonal irregularities**. Severe protein deficiency is fatal.

Excess protein

Excess protein can cause problems as well, such as causing **the immune system to overreact, liver dysfunction from increased toxic residues, possibly bone loss due to increased acidity in the blood.** Proteins can often figure in **allergies** and allergic reactions to certain foods. This is because the structure of each form of protein is slightly different, and some may trigger a **response from the immune system** while others are perfectly safe. Many people are allergic to **casein**, the protein **in milk**; **gluten**, the protein **in wheat** and other grains; the particular proteins found in **peanuts**; or those in **shellfish** or other sea-foods. It is extremely unusual for the same person to adversely react to more than two different types of proteins.

Exercise 1a
Match the column A with the column B. Try to learn the expressions and/ or sentences by heart.

A

1. Proteins are a primary constituent of living things and also nutrient sources for organisms
2. Proteins differ from carbohydrates chiefly
3. In terms of human nutritional needs proteins come in two forms:
4. The inessential amino acids
5. Animal-derived foods contain all of those amino acids,
6. All nine essential amino acids must be
7. By mixing foods that are rich in some amino acids with foods that are rich in others,
8. Vegetarians and especially vegans should be careful to eat appropriate combinations of foods
9. Protein deficiency can lead to symptoms such as
10. Excess protein can cause problems as well, such as
11. Many people are allergic to casein, the protein in milk; gluten, the protein in wheat and other grains;

B

a) *causing the immune system to overreact, liver dysfunction from increased toxic residues, and possibly bone loss due to increased acidity in the blood.*
b) *complete proteins contain all nine of the amino acids that humans cannot make themselves; incomplete proteins lack one or more amino acids.*
c) *fatigue, insulin resistance, hair loss, loss of hair pigment, loss of muscle mass, low body temperature, and hormonal irregularities.*
d) *in that they contain much nitrogen and a little bit of sulphur, besides carbon, oxygen and nitrogen.*
e) *need not be supplied by the diet, because our cells can make them ourselves.*
f) *one can acquire all the needed amino acids in sufficient quantities.*
g) *part of one diet in order to survive and are needed in a fixed ratio.*
h) *so as to get all the essential amino acids in sufficient quantities that the body may produce all the proteins that it needs.*
i) *that do not produce their own energy from sunlight.*
j) *the particular proteins found in peanuts; or those in shellfish or other sea-foods.*
k) *while plants are typically stronger in some acids that others.*

Fats

Fat is a generic term for a class of **lipids**. Fats are produced by **organic processes in animals and plants.** All fats are **insoluble in water** and have a density significantly below that of water (i.e. they **float on water.**) Fats that are liquid at **room temperature** are often referred to as **oil.** Most fats are composed primarily of triglycerides. Ingested fats provide the precursors from which **we synthesize our own fat** as well as **cholesterol** and various **phospholipids.** Fat provides our most concentrated form of energy. Its **energy content** (9kcal/gram) is over twice as great as carbohydrates and proteins (4kcal/gram). Humans can synthesize fat from carbohydrates. However, **three essential fatty acids cannot be synthesized** this way and must be incorporated in the diet. All are unsaturated; that is, have double bonds. These are: **linoleic acid, linolenic acid and arachidonic acid.**

Types of fats:

- **saturated.** Predominantly saturated fats **(solid** at room temperature) include all **animal** fats (e.g. **milk fat, lard, tallow**), as well as **palm oil, coconut oil, cocoa fat** and **hydrogenated vegetable oil** (shortening).
- **mono-unsaturated.** Examples are **olive, peanut, and rapeseed** (canola) oil.
- **polyunsaturated.** Examples: **corn, soy-bean, cotton-seed, sunflower, and safflower oils.**
- **trans fats.** Have been partially hydrogenated.
- **omega-3 fats.** Fish oils are a rich source of omega-3 fatty acids.

Products with a lot of **saturated** fats tend to be **solid at room temperature,** while products containing **unsaturated** fats tend to be **liquid** at room temperature. Different varieties of fat have seen, and indeed still see, much use as **lubricants**, although recently various synthetic substances and petroleum derivatives have taken over in most industrial applications. **In cooking**, products with a **high fat content** are often used as **enhancers of taste,** for example **butter, milk, cheese** and other dairy products. **Another use** of fat in cooking is as heat conductor in **frying.** Fat is one of the three main classes of food and the most concentrated form of metabolic energy available to humans. **Vitamins A, D and E are fat-soluble** and occur only in conjunction with fats. Fats are **sources of essential fatty acids**, an important dietary requirement. They also serve as **energy stores** for the body. Fats are **broken down** in the body to **release glycerol and free fatty acids.** The **glycerol** can be **converted to glucose by the liver** and thus used as a source of energy. The **fatty acids** are a good **source of energy** for many **tissues**, especially heart and skeletal muscle.

All varieties of fat have an extraordinary energy content. Fat acts as an energy reserve, and is **stored in fatty tissue**, normally located **subcutaneously** or surrounding organs. Fatty tissue consists of **fat cells**, designed to store energy in the form of fat. Energy is stored as fatty tissue when the nutrition/energy content of the blood remains higher than is consumed by muscular and other activity. When the **energy content in the blood lessens**, the **fatty tissue reacts by releasing a corresponding amount of energy from the fat cells**. This activity is **controlled by insulin** and other hormones in the body. Adipose, or fatty, tissue is the human body's means of **storing metabolic energy over extended periods of time**. In the modern world, excess fatty tissue on a human is often considered an aesthetic and medical problem. Fat, depending on the age and culture, is considered at once a sign of wealth, power, prestige, gluttony and sloth.

Exercise 1b
Match the column A with the column B. Try to learn the expressions and/or sentences by heart.

A

1. Fats are produced
2. Fats that are liquid at room temperature
3. Ingested fats provide the precursors from which
4. Humans can synthesize fat from carbohydrates,
5. Saturated fats (solid at room temperature)
6. Examples of mono-unsaturated fats
7. Examples of polyunsaturated fats are
8. Products with a lot of saturated fats tend to be solid at room temperature,
9. In cooking, products with a high fat content
10. Fat is one of the three main classes of food
11. Vitamins A, D and E are fat-soluble
12. Fats are broken down in the body
13. The glycerol can be converted
14. Fat acts as an energy reserve, and is stored in fatty tissue,
15. When the energy content in the blood lessens,

B

a) *and occur only in conjunction with fats.*
b) *and the most concentrated form of metabolic energy available to humans.*
c) *are often referred to as oil.*
d) *are often used as enhancers of taste, for example butter, milk, cheese and other dairy products.*
e) *are olive, peanut, and rapeseed (canola) oil.*
f) *by organic processes in animals and plants.*

g) *corn, soy-bean, cotton-seed, sunflower, and safflower oils.*

h) *however, three essential fatty acids cannot be synthesized this way and must be incorporated in the diet.*

i) *include all animal fats (e.g. milk fat, lard, tallow), as well as palm oil, coconut oil, cocoa fat and hydrogenated vegetable oil (shortening).*

j) *normally located subcutaneously or surrounding organs.*

k) *the fatty tissue reacts by releasing a corresponding amount of energy from the fat cells.*

l) *to glucose by the liver and thus used as a source of energy.*

m) *to release glycerol and free fatty acids.*

n) *we synthesize our own fat as well as cholesterol and various phospholipids.*

o) *while products containing unsaturated fats tend to be liquid at room temperature.*

Exercise 2

Translate the expressions. Try to explain their meanings in English.

Constituent, differ from, sulphur, carbon, nitrogen, unbranched chain, determined, sequence, contain, proportion, inessential, supplied, listed, subset, ratio, shortage, constrain, sufficient, omnivores, deficiency, fatigue, muscle mass, irregularities, excess, overreact, toxic residues, casein, gluten, adversely, generic term, density, float, liquid, ingested, precursors, phospholipids, incorporated, double bonds, predominantly, solid, lard, tallow, peanut, rapeseed, cotton-seed, sunflower, safflower, unsaturated, lubricants, derivatives, enhancers of taste, heat conductor, in conjunction with, energy stores, converted to glucose, extraordinary, subcutaneously, fatty tissue, consumed, lessens, corresponding, amount, extended periods of time.

Exercise 3

Answer the following questions. Prepare short talks and/or dialogues on these topics.

1. How do proteins differ from carbohydrates?
2. What is the difference between complete and incomplete proteins?
3. Characterize essential amino acids and the inessential ones.
4. Why should we be careful to eat appropriate combinations of foods?
5. What are the dangers of protein deficiency and excess protein?
6. Give characteristics of fats.
7. What types of fats do you know?
8. What is the use of fats in cooking?
9. Talk about fats as energy stores for the body.

Vocabulary 4

adipose /'æd.ɪ.pəʊz/
adversely /'æd.vɜː.sli/
aesthetic /es'θetɪk/
arachidonic /ˌær ə'kɪd.ə.nɪk/
acid /'æsɪd/
besides /bɪ'saɪdz/
bond /bɒnd/
casein /'keɪsɪɪn/
coconut /'kəʊ.kə.nʌt/
conductor /kən'dʌk.tər/
conjunction /kən'dʒʌŋk.ʃən/
constraint /kən'streɪnt/
contain /kən'teɪn/
corresponding /ˌkɒrɪ'spɒndɪŋ/
cotton /'kɒtən/ **seed** /siːd/
derivative /dɪ'rɪv.ə.tɪv/
dimensional /daɪ.men.ʃən.əl/
double /'dʌb.lˌ/
enhancer /ɪn'hɑːnsər/
excess /ek'ses/
extended /ɪk'sten.dɪd/
extraordinary /ɪk'strɔːdənrɪ/
figure /'fɪgər/
fixed /fɪkst/
float /fləʊt/
fold /fəʊld/
frying /fraɪɪŋ/
generic /dʒə'ner.ɪk/
gluten /'gluː.tən/
gluttony /'glʌtəni/
hydrogenate /'haɪdrədʒɪˌneɪt/
incomplete /ˌɪn.kəm'pliːt/
incorporate /ɪn'kɔː.pər.eɪt/
insoluble /ɪn'sɒl.jʊ.blˌ/
irregularity /ɪˌreg.jə'lær.ə.ti/
issue /'ɪʃ.uː/
lard /lɑːd/
lessen /'les.ən/
lubricant /'luːbrɪkənt/
machinery /mə'ʃiː.nə.ri/
mass /mæs/
muscle /mʌsəl/
native /'neɪtɪv/
omnivore /'ɒm.nɪ.vɔːr/
overreact /ˌəʊvəri'ækt/
palm /pɑːm/ **oil** /ɔɪl /
perfectly /'pɜːfɪktli/
petroleum /pə'trəʊ.li.əm/
phospholipid /ˌfɒsfə'lɪpɪd/
predominantly /prɪ'dɒm ə nənt.li/
prestige /pres'tiːʒ/
proportion /prə'pɔː.ʃən/
quantity /'kwɒn.tɪ.ti/
rapeseed /'reɪpˌsiːd/
ratio /'reɪ.ʃi.əʊ/
referred /rɪ'fɜːd/ **to** /tə/
safe /seɪf/
safflower /'sæ.flaʊər/
seafood /'siːˌfuːd/
sequence /'siː.kwəns/
shape /ʃeɪp/
shellfish /'ʃel.fɪʃ/
shortage /'ʃɔː.tɪdʒ/
shortening /'ʃɔː.tən.ɪŋ/
significantly /sɪg'nɪf.ɪ.kənt.li/
skeletal /'skel.ɪ.təl/
sloth /sləʊθ/
subcutaneous /ˌsʌb.kjʊ'teɪ.ni.əs/
subset /'sʌb.set/
sufficient /sə'fɪʃ.ənt/
sulphur /'sʌlfər/
sunlight /'sʌn.laɪt/
tallow /'tæl.əʊ/
tend /tend/ **to** /tə/
twice /twaɪs/
unique /juː'niːk/
unusual /ʌn'juːʒʊəl/

Solution to Exercise 1a
1i, 2d, 3b, 4e, 5k, 6g,
7f, 8h, 9c, 10a, 11j

Solution to Exercise 1b
1f, 2c, 3n, 4h, 5i, 6e, 7g, 8o, 9d,
10b, 11a, 12m, 13l, 14j, 15k

Unit 5 - Vitamins 1

All **natural vitamins** are organic food substances found only in living things, that is, **plants and animals**. With few exceptions the body cannot manufacture or synthesize vitamins. They **must be supplied in the diet** or in dietary supplements. Vitamins are **essential** to the normal functioning of our bodies. They are necessary for our **growth, vitality, and general well-being**. A lot of people think vitamins can replace food. They cannot. In fact, vitamins **cannot be assimilated without ingesting food**. That is why we suggest taking them with a meal. Vitamins help **regulate metabolism**, help **convert fat and carbohydrates into energy**, and assist in forming **bone and tissue.** Vitamins can be divided into two groups:

- **fat-soluble**, which include: Vitamin **A, D, E and K**
- **water-soluble**, which include: Vitamins of **B complex, Biotin, Vitamin C**

Vitamin A (Retinol)

- **Function**: precursor to retinal problems, the prosthetic group of all four of the **light absorbing pigments in the eye**
- **Sources: cream, butter, fish liver oils, eggs. Carrots** and some other vegetables provide beta-carotene, which the liver can convert into vitamin A
- **Deficiency**: night-blindness
- **Excess**: stored in the liver but can be toxic in large doses, especially in children. Even in adults the range between too little and too much is narrow; ingesting vitamin A in amounts not much greater than the recommended dietary allowance (RDA) leads to an **increase in bone fractures** later in life. High doses taken early in pregnancy have been linked to a greater risk of **birth defects**.

Vitamin A (retinol) is fat-soluble and is found mainly in **fish liver oils, liver, egg yolks, butter, and cream.** Primary, vitamin A deficiency is usually caused by prolonged **dietary deprivation**. It is endemic in areas, such as **southern and eastern Asia,** where rice, devoid of carotene, is the staple. Secondary vitamin A deficiency may be due to **inadequate conversion of carotene to vitamin A** or to interference with absorption, storage, or transport of vitamin A. **Interference with absorption or storage** is likely in **celiac disease, sprue, cystic fibrosis, pancreatic disease, duodenal bypass, congenital partial obstruction of the jejunum, obstruction of the bile ducts, giardiasis, and cirrhosis.** Vitamin A deficiency is **common** in protein-energy **malnutrition (marasmus or kwashiorkor)**, principally because the diet is deficient but also because vitamin A storage and transport are defective.

Symptoms and signs

The severity of the effects of vitamin A deficiency is inversely related to age. **Growth retardation** is a common sign in children. Inadequate intake or utilization of vitamin A can cause impaired dark adaptation and **night-blindness**; **xerosis of the conjunctiva and cornea; xerophthalmia and keratomalacia; keratinization of lung, GI tract, and urinary tract** epithelia; increased **susceptibility to infections;** and sometimes death.

Vitamin A toxicity

Excessive intake of vitamin A may cause acute or chronic toxicity. **Acute toxicity in children** manifests as **increased intra-cranial pressure and vomiting,** which may lead to death unless ingestion is discontinued. After **discontinuation, recovery** is spontaneous, with no residual damage. Although carotene is metabolised in the body to vitamin A at a slow rate, **excessive ingestion of carotene** does not cause vitamin A toxicity but produces **carotenemia**. This condition is usually asymptomatic but may lead to carotenosis, in which the **skin** (but not the sclera) becomes **deep yellow**, especially on the palms and soles. Carotenosis may also occur in **diabetes mellitus, myxedema, and anorexia nervosa**, possibly from a further reduction in the rate of conversion of carotene to vitamin A.

Exercise 1a

Match the column A with the column B. Try to learn the expressions and/or sentences by heart.

A

1. All natural vitamins are organic food substances
2. Vitamins are necessary for
3. Vitamins cannot be assimilated
4. Vitamins help regulate metabolism,
5. Vitamins can be divided into two groups:
6. Sources of vitamin A are
7. Vitamin A deficiency
8. A deficiency may be due to
9. Interference with absorption or storage is likely in
10. Vitamin A deficiency is common in
11. Inadequate intake or utilization of vitamin A can cause impaired dark adaptation and night-blindness; xerosis of the conjunctiva and cornea; xerophthalmia and keratomalacia;
12. Excessive intake of vitamin A manifests as increased intra-cranial pressure and vomiting,
13. After discontinuation,
14. Excessive ingestion of carotene
15. Carotenosis may also occur

B

a) (fat-soluble, i.e. vitamin A, D, E and K) and water-soluble, i.e. vitamins of B complex, biotin, vitamin C).
b) celiac disease, sprue, cystic fibrosis, pancreatic disease, duodenal bypass, congenital partial obstruction of the jejunum, obstruction of the bile ducts, giardiasis, and cirrhosis.
c) cream, butter, fish liver oils, eggs and carrots.
d) found only in living things, that is, plants and animals.
e) help convert fat and carbohydrates into energy, and assist in forming bone and tissue.
f) in diabetes mellitus, myxedema, and anorexia nervosa.
g) inadequate conversion of carotene to vitamin A or to interference with absorption, storage, or transport of vitamin A.
h) is usually caused by prolonged dietary deprivation.
i) keratinization of lung, GI tract, and urinary tract epithelia; increased susceptibility to infections; and sometimes death.
j) may lead to carotenosis, in which the skin becomes deep yellow, especially on the palms and soles.
k) our growth, vitality, and general well-being.
l) protein-energy malnutrition (marasmus or kwashiorkor).
m) recovery is spontaneous, with no residual damage.
n) which may lead to death unless ingestion is discontinued.
o) without ingesting food.

Vitamin D (Calciferol)

- **Functions**: **absorption of calcium** from the intestine and bone formation.
- **Sources**: synthesized when **ultraviolet light** strikes the skin. Present in fish **liver oils, butter, and steroid-containing foods** irradiated with ultraviolet light.
- **Deficiency**: **rickets** in children; **osteomalacia (softening of the bones)** in adults
- **Excess**: This fat-soluble vitamin is dangerous in very **high doses**, especially in infants, causing excessive calcium deposits and **mental retardation.**

Vitamin D is a **pro-hormone** with several **active metabolites** that act as **hormones.** The main function of vitamin D hormone is to **increase calcium absorption** from the intestine and promote normal **bone formation** and mineralization.

Vitamin D deficiency and dependency

Inadequate exposure to sunlight and **low dietary intake** are usually necessary for development of clinical vitamin D deficiency. Metabolic bone disease resulting from vitamin D deficiency is called **rickets** in children and **osteomalacia** in adults. These diseases result from common pathogenic factors but differ in their clinical and pathogenic expression because of the **differences between growing and mature bones.**

Rickets

Rickets is a vitamin deficiency disease of **infancy and early childhood** caused by **lack of vitamin D**. Rickets causes **soft bones**. Some people who do not get enough sun exposure, milk products, or green vegetables may develop the disease, although it is rare today. Rickets can also be caused by some other kidney and liver diseases. Rickets **causes bone pain, slowed growth** in children, **dental problems, muscle loss** and increased risk of the treatment of **fractures**.

Treatment involves increasing dietary **intake of calcium, phosphate and vitamin D.** Exposure to **sunshine, cod liver oil, halibut liver oil, and viosterol** are all sources of vitamin D.

Osteomalacia

Maternal osteomalacia can lead to **metaphyseal lesions** and **tetany** in the **newborn**. Young infants are restless and sleep poorly. They have **reduced mineralization of the skull** (craniotabes), away from the sutures. In older infants, **sitting and crawling are delayed as is fontanelle closure**. In children aged 1 to 4 years, **epiphyseal cartilages** at the lower ends of the **radius, ulna, tibia, and fibula enlarge; kyphoscoliosis develops**, and **walking is delayed**. In older children and adolescents walking is **painful**. In **adults**, demineralization (osteomalacia) occurs, particularly in the spine, pelvis, and lower extremities. As the **bones soften,** weight may cause bowing of the long bones, vertical **shortening of the vertebrae,** and flattening of the pelvic bones, which narrows the pelvic outlet.

Vitamin D toxicity

The first symptoms are **anorexia, nausea, and vomiting,** followed by **polyuria, polydipsia, weakness, nervousness, and pruritus.** A history of excessive vitamin D intake is critical for differentiating this condition from all other hypercalcemic states. Vitamin D toxicity **occurs** commonly during the **treatment** of **hypoparathyroidism** and with the misguided use of megavitamins.

Exercise 1b
Match the column A with the column B. Try to learn the expressions and/or sentences by heart.

A

1. Function of vitamin D (Calciferol) is

2. Vitamin D is present in
3. Inadequate exposure to sunlight and low dietary intake
4. Metabolic bone disease resulting from vitamin D deficiency
5. Rickets is a vitamin deficiency disease
6. Rickets causes bone pain, slowed growth in children,
7. Treatment involves
8. Maternal osteomalacia can lead
9. In older infants, sitting and crawling are delayed
10. In children aged 1 to 4 years, epiphyseal cartilages at the lower ends of the radius, ulna, tibia, and fibula enlarge;
11. As the bones soften, weight may cause bowing of the long bones,
12. The first symptoms of vitamin D toxicity
13. Vitamin D toxicity occurs commonly

B

a) absorption of calcium from the intestine and bone formation.

b) are anorexia, nausea, and vomiting, followed by polyuria, polydipsia, weakness, nervousness, and pruritus.

c) are usually necessary for development of clinical vitamin D deficiency.

d) as is fontanelle closure.

e) dental problems, muscle loss and increased risk of the treatment of fractures.

f) during the treatment of hypoparathyroidism and with the misguided use of mega-vitamins.

g) fish liver oils, butter, and steroid-containing foods irradiated with ultraviolet light.

h) increasing dietary intake of calcium, phosphate and vitamin D.

i) is called rickets in children and osteomalacia in adults.

j) kyphoscoliosis develops, and walking is delayed and painful.

k) of infancy and early childhood caused by lack of vitamin D.

l) to metaphyseal lesions and tetany in the newborn.

m) vertical shortening of the vertebrae, and flattening of the pelvic bones, which narrows the pelvic outlet.

Exercise 2

Translate the expressions. Try to explain their meanings in English.

Natural vitamins, living things, growth, assimilated, convert, soluble, precursor, retinal, fish liver oils, recommended dietary allowance, linked to, deprivation, endemic, devoid, staple, interference with, storage, celiac disease, sprue, cystic fibrosis, pancreatic disease, duodenal bypass, congenital partial obstruction, jejunum, bile ducts, giardiasis, cirrhosis, marasmus, kwashiorkor, severity, inversely related, retardation, blindness, xerosis, conjunctiva, cornea, susceptibility, toxicity, intra-cranial pressure, discontinuation, recovery, slow rate, excessive ingestion, sclera, palms, soles, myxedema, strikes, irradiated, ultraviolet, high doses, excessive calcium deposits, mental retardation, bone formation, growing, mature, infancy, early childhood, slowed growth, muscle loss, intake of calcium, phosphate and vitamin D, liver oil, metaphyseal lesions, tetany, restless, sleep poorly, craniotabes, sitting and crawling, delayed, fontanelle closure, radius, ulna, tibia, and fibula enlarge, kyphoscoliosis develops, walking is painful, demineralization (osteomalacia), spine, pelvis, lower extremities, bowing of the long bones, vertical shortening of the vertebrae, flattening of the pelvic bones, vitamin D toxicity, anorexia, nausea, and vomiting, polyuria, polydipsia, weakness, nervousness, pruritus, excessive intake, occurs, commonly, treatment of hypoparathyroidism.

Exercise 3
Answer the following questions. Prepare short talks and/or dialogues on these topics.

1. Fat-soluble and water-soluble vitamins
2. Vitamin A (function, sources, deficiency, excess)
3. In which diseases is interference with absorption or storage of vitamin A likely?
4. What are the consequences of excessive intake of vitamin A?
5. Characterise vitamin D (functions, sources, deficiency, excess).
6. Talk about vitamin D deficiency and dependency.
7. What is the difference between rickets and osteomalacia?
8. What are the symptoms of vitamin D toxicity?

Vocabulary 5

Fill in the meanings in your mother language:

assimilate /əˈsɪmɪleɪt/
asymptomatic /əˌsɪmp.təˈmæt.ɪk/
bile /baɪl/ **duct** /dʌkt/
biotin /baɪˈɒt.iːn/
bow /ˈbəʊɪŋ/
bypass /ˈbaɪ.pɑːs/
carotene /ˈkærəˌtiːn/
carotenemia /kəˈrɒtɪˌˈniːmiə/
carotenosis, /kəˈrɒtɪˌnəʊ.sɪs/
cartilage /ˈkɑː.təl.ɪdʒ/
celiac disease /ˈsiː.liː.æk.dɪˌziːz/
cirrhosis /sɪˈrəʊ.sɪs/
closure /ˈkləʊ.ʒə/
cod /kɒd/
congenital /kənˈdʒen.ɪ.təl/
conjunctiva /ˌkɒn.dʒʌŋkˈtaɪ.və/ pl **conjunctivae**
conversion /kənˈvɜː.ʃən/
cornea /ˈkɔːnɪə/ pl **corneae**
craniotabes /ˈkreɪnɪəˈteɪbiːz/
crawl /krɔːl/

cystic fibrosis /ˌsɪs.tɪk.faɪˈbrəʊ.sɪs/
defective /dɪˈfek.tɪv/
deficient /dɪˈfɪʃənt/
dependency /dɪˈpen.dənt .si/
deposit /dɪˈpɒz.ɪt/
deprivation /ˌdep.rɪˈveɪ.ʃən/
devoid /dɪˈvɔɪd/
differentiate /ˌdɪfəˈrenʃieɪt/
discontinue /ˌdɪs.kənˈtɪn.juː/
duodenal /ˌdjuː.əˈdiːˌnəl/
egg /eg/ **yolk** /jəʊk/
epiphyseal /ˌep.ɪˈfɪz.i.əl/
excessive /ekˈses.ɪv/
exposure /ɪkˈspəʊ.ʒər/
expression /ɪkˈspreʃ.ən/
extremity /ɪkˈstrem.ɪ.ti/
fibula /ˈfɪb.jʊ.lə/ pl **fibulae**
fontanelle /ˌfɒn.təˈnel/
general /ˈdʒen.ər.əl/
giardiasis /ˌdʒaɪɑːˈdaɪəsɪs/
halibut /ˈhæl.ɪ.bət/
hypercalcemic /ˌhaɪ pər kælˈsi mik/
hypoparathyroidism /ˌhaɪ.
pəʊˌpær.əˈθaɪ.rɔɪd.ɪsm/
interference /ˌɪn.təˈfɪə.rənt s/
intracranial /ˌɪn.trəˈkraɪ.ni.əl/
inversely /ɪnˈvɜːs.li/
irradiate /ɪˈreɪ.di.eɪt/
keratinization /kɪˈrætɪˌnəˈzeɪ ʃən/
keratomalacia /kɪˈrætɪməˈleɪʃɪə/
kyphoscoliosis /ˌkaɪ
foʊˌskoʊ liˈoʊ sɪs/
lesion /ˈliː.ʒən/
loss /lɒs/
manifest /ˈmæn.ɪ.fest/
manufacture /ˌmæn.jʊˈfæk.t ʃər/
maternal /məˈtɜː.nəl/
megavitamin /ˈmɛg əˌvaɪ tə mɪn/
metabolite /məˈtæb.əl.aɪt/
metaphyseal /ˌmɛt əˈfɪz i
əl/ **fracture** ˈ/fræktʃə/
misguided /mɪsˈgaɪdɪd/
myxedema /ˌmɪk sɪˈdi mə/
newborn /ˈnjuː.bɔːn/
night /naɪt/ **-blindness** /ˈblaɪnd.nəs/
obstruction /əbˈstrʌk.ʃən/
osteomalacia /ˌɒstɪəʊməˈleɪʃɪə/
outlet /ˈaʊt.let/
palm /pɑːm/
pathogenic /ˌpæθ.əˈdʒen.ɪk/
pelvic /ˈpel.vɪk/
pelvis /ˈpel.vɪs/
phosphate /ˈfɒs.feɪt/
promote /ˈprɒs.θə.tɪk/
prosthetic /ˈprɒs.θiː.sɪs/
pruritus /prʊəˈraɪ.təs/
radius /ˈreɪ.di.əs/
range /reɪndʒ/
related /rɪˈleɪ.tɪd/
replace /rɪˈpleɪs/
residual /rɪˈzɪd.ju.əl/
restless /ˈrest .ləs/
retardation /ˌriː.tɑːˈdeɪ.ʃən/
retinal /ˈret.ɪ.nəl/
retinol /ˈrɛtɪˌnɒl/
rickets /ˈrɪk.ɪts/
sclera /ˈsklɪə.rə/
severity /sɪˈver.ɪ.ti/
skull /skʌl/
sole /səʊl/
spine /spaɪn/
spontaneous /spɒnˈteɪ.ni.əs/
sprue /spruː/
staple /ˈsteɪpl/
strike /straɪk/ **(struck, struck)**
sunshine /ˈsʌnʃaɪn/
susceptibility /səˌsep.tɪˈbɪl.ɪ.ti/
suture /ˈsuː.tʃər/
tetany /ˈtet.ən.i/
tibia /ˈtɪb.i.ə/ pl **tibiae**
toxicity /tɒkˈsɪs.ɪ.ti/
treatment /ˈtriːt.mənt/
ulna /ˈʌl.nə/
ultraviolet /ˌʌltrəˈvaɪəlɪt/
utilization /ˌju.t̬ əl.əˈzeɪ.ʃən/
vertebra /ˈvɜː.tɪ.brə/ pl **vertebrae**
viosterol /vaɪˈɒs təˌrɔl/
vitality /vaɪˈtæləti/
xerophthalmia /ˌzɪərɒfˈθælmɪə/
xerosis /zɪˈrəʊsɪs/

Solution to Exercise 1a
1d, 2k, 3o, 4e, 5a, 6e, 7h, 8g, 9b, 10l, 11i, 12n, 13m, 14j, 15f

Solution to Exercise 1b
1a, 2g, 3c, 4i, 5k, 6e, 7h, 8l, 9d, 10j. 11m, 12b, 13f

Unit 6 - Vitamins 2

Vitamin E (tocopherol)

- **Function**: acts as a reducing agent in cells.
- **Sources**: egg yolk, salad greens, vegetable oils.
- **Deficiency**: anaemia, damage to the retinas.
- **Excess**: high doses may be toxic in infants.

The diseases caused by vitamin E deficiency vary widely according to species. The deficiency may cause **disorders of reproduction**; **abnormalities of muscle, liver, bone marrow, and brain function**; **haemolysis of RBCs; defective embryo-genesis;** and **exudative diathesis,** a disorder of capillary permeability. **Skeletal muscle dystrophy** may occur, and in certain species, is accompanied by **cardiomyopathy**.

Vitamin E deficiency

In humans, the main manifestation of vitamin E deficiency are:

- mild **haemolytic anaemia**
- **spinocerebral disease**

Aetiology

The smaller and more premature the infant, the greater the degree of deficiency. Vitamin E deficiency in **premature infants** persists during the first few weeks of life and can be attributed to **limited placental transfer** of vitamin E, low tissue levels at **birth**, relative **dietary deficiency in infancy**, **intestinal malabsorption**, and **rapid growth**. As the **digestive system matures**, vitamin E absorption improves, and blood **vitamin E levels rise**. In children and adults, malabsorption generally underlies vitamin E deficiency. **Genetic** abnormality in the transport of vitamin E can also play a role.

Vitamin K

- **Function**: needed for the synthesis of blood clotting factors.
- **Sources**: spinach and other green leafy vegetables, synthesized by intestinal bacteria.
- **Deficiency**: slow clotting of blood.
- **Excess**: high doses may be toxic in infants.

Vitamin K deficiency

Haemorrhagic **disease of the newborn,** caused by vitamin K deficiency, generally occurs 1 to 7 days post-partum and may be manifested by **cutaneous, GI, intra-thoracic, or, in the worst cases, intra-cranial bleeding**. Late haemorrhagic disease, which has the same clinical manifestations, occurs 1 to 3 months post-partum. It is usually associated with **malabsorption or liver disease**. Vitamin K deficiency in breastfed infants remains a major worldwide cause of infant morbidity and mortality.

In healthy adults, primary vitamin K deficiency is uncommon. **Adults** are **protected** from a lack of vitamin K because vitamin K is widely distributed in **plant and animal tissues**. However, vitamin K deficiency can occur in adults with **marginal dietary intake** if they undergo trauma, extensive **surgery**, or long-term **parenteral nutrition** with or without treatment with broad-spectrum **antibiotics**. Persons with **biliary obstruction, malabsorption, or parenchymal liver disease** also have a higher risk of vitamin K deficiency; those who ingest certain **drugs**, including **anticonvulsants, anticoagulants, certain antibiotics, salicylates**, and mega-doses of vitamin A or E are vulnerable to vitamin K-related haemorrhagic disease.

Symptoms and signs

Bleeding is the major manifestation whether the cause is inadequate dietary intake or antagonism of vitamin K by drugs. Easy **bruisability** and **mucosal bleeding** (especially **epistaxis, GI haemorrhage, menorrhagia, and hematuria)** occur in vitamin K deficiency. **Oozing of blood** from **puncture sites of incisions** may occur after trauma, and **life-threatening intra-cranial haemorrhage** can occur in **infants**. In obstructive jaundice, haemorrhage may begin as slow **ooze** from a **surgical wound, the gums, the nose, or GI mucosa**, or it may be massive into the GI tract.

Exercise 1a
Match the column A with the column B. Try to learn the expressions and/or sentences by heart.

A

1. The deficiency of vitamin E may cause
2. The main manifestation of vitamin E deficiency are:
3. Vitamin E deficiency in premature infants can be attributed to
4. Haemorrhagic disease of the newborn, caused by vitamin K deficiency,
5. Late haemorrhagic disease,
6. Vitamin K deficiency can occur in adults
7. Persons with biliary obstruction, malabsorption, or parenchymal liver disease
8. Those who ingest certain drugs, including anticonvulsants, anticoagulants, certain antibiotics, salicylates,
9. Easy bruisability and mucosal bleeding (especially epistaxis, GI haemorrhage, menorrhagia, and hematuria)

10. Oozing of blood from puncture sites of incisions may occur after trauma,
11. In obstructive jaundice, haemorrhage may begin as

B

a) also have a higher risk of vitamin K deficiency.
b) and life-threatening intra-cranial haemorrhage can occur in infants.
c) and mega-doses of vitamin A or E are vulnerable to vitamin K-related haemorrhagic disease.
d) disorders of reproduction; abnormalities of muscle, liver, bone marrow, and brain function; haemolysis of RBCs; defective embryogenesis; and exudative diathesis.
e) is usually associated with malabsorption or liver disease.
f) limited placental transfer of vitamin E, low tissue levels at birth, relative dietary deficiency in infancy, intestinal malabsorption, and rapid growth.
g) may be manifested by cutaneous, GI, intra-thoracic, or intra-cranial bleeding.
h) mild haemolytic anaemia and spinocerebral disease.
i) occur in vitamin K deficiency.
j) slow ooze from a surgical wound, the gums, the nose, or GI mucosa, or it may be massive into the GI tract.
k) with marginal dietary intake if they undergo trauma, extensive surgery, or long-term parenteral nutrition with or without treatment with broad-spectrum antibiotics.

Vitamin B_3 (Niacin/Nicotinic acid)

- **Function**: this member of the B vitamins group is a precursor of NAD and NADP.
- **Sources**: meat, yeast, milk, enriched bread and breakfast cereals
- **Deficiency**: pellagra (producing skin lesions); a risk where corn is the staple carbohydrate.
- **Excess**: accidental ingestion of very high doses produces brief illness, but niacin is water-soluble and any excess is quickly excreted.

Niacin deficiency

Severe deficiencies are the principal **causes of pellagra.** Primary deficiency usually occurs in areas where **maize** (Indian corn) forms a **major part of the diet.** Bound niacin, found in maize, is not assimilated in the intestinal tract unless it has been previously **treated with alkalis**, as in the preparation of **tortillas**. Amino acid imbalance may also contribute to deficiency, since pellagra is common in India among persons who eat **millet with high leucine content**. Secondary deficiency occurs in **diarrhoeas, cirrhosis, and alcoholism** as well as after extensive postoperative use of **nutrient infusions lacking vitamins.**

Symptoms and signs

Pellagra is characterized by **cutaneous, mucous membrane, CNS, and GI symptoms.** The complete **syndrome** of advanced deficiency includes symmetric photosensitive **rash, scarlet stomatitis, glossitis, diarrhoea, and mental aberrations.** Symptoms may appear alone or in combination.

Four types of **cutaneous lesions** are recognized:

- **acute** lesions consisting in **erythema**, followed by **vesiculation**, **bullae**, **crusting**, and **desquamation**.
- **intertrigo**, also acute, characterized by **redness, maceration, abrasion** and secondary infection
- **chronic hypertrophy**, in which **skin** is **thickened, inelastic, fissured,** and deeply **pigmented** over pressure points
- **chronic atrophic lesions**, with **dry, scaly, inelastic** skin too large for the part it covers (seen in older pellagrins)

Mucous membrane symptoms primarily affect the **mouth** but may also affect the **vagina and urethra. Scarlet glossitis and stomatitis** are characteristic of acute deficiency. As the lesion progresses, the tongue and oral mucous membranes become **bright scarlet,** followed by a **sore mouth**, increased **salivation**, and **oedema of the tongue**. **Ulcerations** may appear under the tongue, on the **mucosa** of the **lower lip**, and opposite the **molar teeth**. **GI symptoms** include **burning** of the **mouth, pharynx, and oesophagus** and **abdominal discomfort** and **distension**. Later, nausea, vomiting and diarrhoea may occur. Diarrhoea, often bloody is serious. **CNS symptoms** include:

- **organic psychosis**, characterized by **memory impairment, disorientation, confusion, and confabulation** (excitement, depression, mania, and delirium predominate in some patients; in others, the reaction is paranoid)
- **encephalopathic syndrome,** characterized by **clouding of consciousness. cogwheel rigidity** of the extremities, and **uncontrollable sucking** and **grasping reflexes**. Differentiating these CNS changes from those in thiamine deficiency is difficult.

Niacin deficiency must be **distinguished** from other causes of **stomatitis, glossitis, diarrhoea, and dementia**. Diagnosis is easy when the clinical findings include skin and mouth lesions, diarrhoea, delirium, and dementia.

Vitamin B_5 (Pantothenic acid)

- **Function**: "anti-stress vitamin," essential component of coenzyme A, important in the secretion of hormones.
- **Sources**: peas and beans (except green beans), lean meat, poultry, fish, and whole-grain cereals.
- **Deficiency**: **fatigue, headaches, nausea, tingling in the hands, depression, muscle weakness**. Pathogenic acid deficiency is rarely observed in humans.
- **Excess**: sensitivity to the teeth, diarrhoea.

Vitamin B_6 (Pyridoxine)

- **Function**: important in blood, CNS, and skin metabolism, necessary for maintaining of healthy **immune system** functions, for **protecting the heart from cholesterol deposits**, and for **preventing kidney stone** formation; responsible for the manufacture of hormones, red blood cells, neurotransmitters, enzymes, and prostaglandins.
- **Sources**: potatoes, bread, meat, fish, eggs, beans, bananas, nuts and seeds.
- **Deficiency**: rare
- **Excess**: irreversible neurological damage.

Primary deficiency is rare, because most foods contain vitamin B_6. Secondary deficiency may result from malabsorption, alcoholism, oral contraceptive use, chemical inactivation by drugs, excessive loss, and increased metabolic activity.

Vitamin B_7 or vitamin H (biotin)

- **Function**: necessary for the metabolism of fats, carbohydrates and amino acids.
- **Sources:** brewer's yeasts, eggs, liver, kidney, nuts, legumes.
- **Deficiency**: **hair loss**, dry, scaly skin, cracking in the corners of the mouth (called **cheilitis**), swollen and painful tongue that is magenta in colour (**glossitis**), **dry eyes, loss of appetite, fatigue, insomnia, and depression.**
- **Excess**: none identified

Vitamin B_9 (folic acid/folacin)

- **Function:** synthesis of purines and pyrimidines.
- **Sources**: green leafy vegetables, but destroyed by cooking

- **Deficiency**: **anaemia, birth defects**, women who expect to become pregnant should be extra careful that they receive adequate amounts.
- **Excess**: water-soluble and any excess easily excreted

Vitamin B_{12} (cobalamin)

- **Function**: needed for DNA synthesis, helps maintain healthy nerve cells and red blood cells.
- **Sources**: fish, poultry, liver, eggs, milk; needs intrinsic factor to be absorbed
- **Deficiency**: **pernicious anaemia;** caused by lack of intrinsic factor or a vegan diet
- **Excess**: none identified.

Exercise 1b
Match the column A with the column B. Try to learn the expressions and/or sentences by heart.

A

1. Severe niacin deficiencies
2. Primary deficiency usually occurs in areas
3. Bound niacin, found in maize, is not assimilated in the intestinal tract
4. Secondary deficiency occurs in diarrhoeas, cirrhosis, and alcoholism
5. Pellagra is characterized by
6. The complete syndrome of advanced deficiency includes
7. Acute lesions consist in
8. Intertrigo is characterized by
9. In chronic hypertrophy,
10. In chronic atrophic lesions
11. Mucous membrane symptoms primarily affect
12. As the lesion progresses, the tongue and oral mucous membranes
13. GI symptoms include
14. CNS symptoms include:
15. Encephalopathic syndrome, is characterized by
16. Niacin deficiency must be distinguished
17. Deficiency of vitamin B_5 causes
18. Vitamin B_5 is important in blood, CNS, and skin metabolism, necessary for maintaining of healthy immune system functions,
19. Secondary deficiency of vitamin B_6 (Pyridoxine) may result from
20. Deficiency of vitamin B_7 or vitamin H causes
21. Deficiency of vitamin B_9 (folic acid/folacin)
22. Deficiency of vitamin B_{12}

B

a) *are the principal causes of pellagra.*
b) *as well as after extensive postoperative use of nutrient infusions lacking vitamins.*
c) *become bright scarlet, followed by a sore mouth, increased salivation, and oedema of the tongue and*

ulcerations may appear under the tongue.

d) *burning of the mouth, pharynx, and oesophagus and abdominal discomfort and distension, later, nausea, vomiting and diarrhoea may occur.*

e) *causes pernicious anaemia.*

f) *causes anaemia, and birth defects.*

g) *clouding of consciousness, cogwheel rigidity of the extremities, and uncontrollable sucking and grasping reflexes.*

h) *cutaneous, mucous membrane, CNS, and GI symptoms.*

i) *erythema, followed by vesiculation, bullae, crusting, and desquamation.*

j) *fatigue, headaches, nausea, tingling in the hands, depression, muscle weakness.*

k) *for protecting the heart from cholesterol deposits, and for preventing kidney stone formation; is responsible for the manufacture of hormones, red blood cells, neurotransmitters, enzymes, and prostaglandins.*

l) *from other causes of stomatitis, glossitis, diarrhoea, and dementia.*

m) *hair loss, dry, scaly skin, cracking in the corners of the mouth (called cheilitis), swollen and painful tongue that is magenta in colour (glossitis), dry eyes, loss of appetite, fatigue, insomnia, and depression.*

n) *malabsorption, alcoholism, oral contraceptive use, chemical inactivation by drugs, excessive loss, and increased metabolic activity.*

o) *organic psychosis, characterized by memory impairment, disorientation, confusion, and confabulation.*

p) *redness, maceration, abrasion and secondary infection.*

q) *skin is thickened, inelastic, fissured, and deeply pigmented over pressure points.*

r) *symmetric photosensitive rash, scarlet stomatitis, glossitis, diarrhoea, and mental aberrations.*

s) *the mouth but may also affect the vagina and urethra.*

t) *the skin is dry, scaly, inelastic and too large for the part it covers.*

u) *unless it has been previously treated with alkalis, as in the preparation of tortillas.*

v) *where maize forms a major part of the diet.*

Exercise 2

Translate the expressions. Try to explain their meanings in English.

Species, disorders, reproduction, bone marrow, haemolysis, embryogenesis, exudative diathesis, capillary permeability, muscle dystrophy, haemolytic anaemia, spinocerebral disease, aetiology, premature infants, persists, attributed, limited, placental transfer, intestinal malabsorption, matures, improves, underlies, blood clotting, haemorrhagic disease, cutaneous, intra-thoracic, intra-cranial, post-partum, breastfed infants, marginal, biliary obstruction, parenchymal, liver disease, anticonvulsants, anticoagulants, bruisability, mucosal bleeding, epistaxis, menorrhagia, hematuria, oozing, puncture, incisions, surgical wound, precursor, enriched bread, staple, accidental ingestion, principal causes, maize, bound, assimilated, tortillas, imbalance, millet, leucine content, nutrient infusions, cutaneous, mucous membrane, advanced deficiency, rash, scarlet stomatitis, glossitis, mental aberrations, cutaneous lesions, recognized erythema, vesiculation, bullae, crusting, desquamation, intertrigo, maceration, abrasion, hypertrophy, thickened, inelastic, fissured, atrophic, scaly, inelastic, urethra, scarlet glossitis, stomatitis, salivation, ulcerations, mucosa, molar teeth, burning, oesophagus, discomfort, distension, psychosis, impairment, confusion, confabulation, excitement, clouding, cogwheel rigidity, fatigue, tingling, muscle weakness, sensitivity deposits, prostaglandins, irreversible, oral contraceptive, scaly skin, cracking, in the corners, cheilitis, glossitis, fatigue, insomnia, pernicious anaemia.

Exercise 3
Answer the following questions. Prepare short talks and/or dialogues on these topics.

1. Talk about vitamin E (function, sources, deficiency, excess).
2. Talk about vitamin K (function, sources, deficiency, excess).
3. Vitamin K deficiency symptoms and signs
4. Vitamin B_3 (function, sources, deficiency, excess)
5. What are the principal causes of pellagra?
6. What are the symptoms and signs of pellagra (mouth, gastrointestinal system, central nervous system)?
7. What are the symptoms and signs of vitamin B_5 deficiency?
8. What are the symptoms and signs of vitamin B_6 excess?
9. What are the symptoms and signs of vitamin B_7 deficiency?
10. Vitamin B_9 and vitamin B_{12} (function, sources, deficiency, excess)

Vocabulary 6

Fill in the meanings in your mother language:

abdominal /æbˈdɒm.ɪ.nəl/
aberration /ˌæb.əˈreɪ.ʃən/
abnormality /ˌæb.nɔːˈmæl.ə.ti/
abrasion /əˈbreɪ.ʒən/
accidental /ˌæk.sɪˈden.təl/

advanced /əd'vɑːnt st/
alkali /'ælkəˌlaɪ/
anaemia /ə'niːmɪə/
antagonism /æn'tæg.ə.nɪ.zəm/
anticoagulant /ˌæn.ti.kəʊ'æg.jʊ.lənt/
anticonvulsant /ˌæn.ti.kən'vʌl.sənt/
attribute /ə'trɪbjuːt/
atrophic /'æ trə fik/
biliary /'bɪl.i.ər.i/
bind /baɪnd/ **(bound, bound)**
bloody /'blʌd.i/
bone /bəʊn/ **marrow** /'mær.əʊ/
brewer's /'bruːər/ **yeast** /jiːst/
brief /briːf/
bright /braɪt/
bruisability /bruz.ə'bɪl ɪ ti/
bulla /'bʊl.ə/ pl **bullae** /bʊl.iː/
burn /bɜːn/
capillary /kə'pɪl.ər.i/
cardiomyopathy /ˌkɑːr.diə.maɪ'ɒp.ə.θi/
central /'sen.trəl/ **nervous** /'nɜː.
vəs/ **system** /'sɪstəm/ **CNS**
cheilitis /kaɪ'laɪ tɪs/
cloud /klaʊd/
cobalamin /koʊ'bæl ə mɪn/
coenzyme /koʊ'en.zaɪm/
cogwheel /'kɒg.wiːl/
confabulation /kən'fæb jəˌleɪ ʃən/
contraceptive /ˌkɒn.trə'sep.tɪv/
corn /kɔːn/
corner /'kɔː.nər/
cracking /'kræk.ɪŋ/
crust /krʌst/
cutaneous /kjuː'teɪ.ni.əs/
delirium /dɪ'lɪr.i.əm/
desquamation /'dɛs kwəˌmeɪ ʃən/
diathesis /daɪ'æθ ə sɪs/
discomfort /dɪ'skʌm.fət/
disease /dɪ'ziːz/
distension /dɪ'sten.ʃən/
dystrophy /dɪs.trə.fi/
embryogenesis /ˌɛmbrɪɒ'dʒɛn ə sɪs/
encephalopathic /ɛnˌsɛfə'lɒpəθɪk/
epistaxis /ˌe.pɪ.'stæk.sɪs/
erythema /ˌer.ɪ'θiː.mə/
excitement /ɪk'saɪt.mənt/
excrete /ɪk'skriːt/
extensive /ɪk'stent.sɪv/
exudative /ɪg'zu də tɪv/
fissure /'fɪʃ.ər/
folacin /'fɒl ə sɪn/
folic acid /ˌfəʊ.lɪk'æs.ɪd/
gastrointestinal /ˌgæs.
trəʊˌɪn.tes'taɪ.nəl/ **GI**
glossitis /glɒ'saɪ tɪs/
grasp /grɑːsp/
haemolysis /hiː'mɒ.lɪ.sɪs/
haemolytic /ˌhiː.mə'lɪ.tɪk/
hematuria /ˌhi mə'tʊər i ə/
hemorrhagic /'hɛm ər ɪdʒik/
hypertrophy /haɪ'pɜː.trə.fi/
imbalance /ˌɪm'bæl.ənt s/
impairment /im'peərˌmənt/
incision /ɪn'sɪʒ.ən/
inelastic /ˌɪn.ɪ'læs.tɪk/
infancy /'ɪn.fənt.si/
infusion /ɪn'fjuː.ʒən/
insomnia /ɪn'sɒm.ni.ə/
intertrigo /ˌɪntə'traɪgəʊ/
intrathoracic /ˌɪn.trə.θɔː'ræs.ɪk/
intrinsic /ɪn'trɪn.sɪk/
irreversible /ˌɪr.ɪ'vɜː.sɪ.bl̩/
jaundice /'dʒɔːn.dɪs/
kidney /'kɪd.ni/ **stone** /stəʊn/
leafy /'liː.fi/
leucine /'lu sin/
life-threatening /'laɪfˌθret.ən.ɪŋ/
lip /lɪp/
maceration /ˌmæsər'eɪʃən/
magenta /mə'dʒen.tə/
maize /meɪz/
mania /'meɪ.ni.ə/
marginal /'mɑːdʒɪnəl/
massive /'mæsɪv/
megadose /'mɛgəˌdəʊs/
menorrhagia /ˌmɛnɔː'reɪdʒɪə/
millet /'mɪlɪt/
molar /'məʊ.lər/
morbidity /ˌmɔː'bɪd.ɪ.ti/
mucosa /mjuː'kəʊ.sə/

mucous membrane /ˌmjuː.kəsˈmem.breɪn/
neurotransmitter /ˌnjʊə.rəʊ.trænzˈmɪt.ər/
niacin /ˈnaɪə.sɪn/
nicotinic /ˈnɪk.ə.tiːn.ɪk/ **acid** /ˈæsɪd/
oedema /ɪˈdiː.mə/
oozing /uːz,ɪŋ/
opposite /ˈɒp.ə.zɪt/
pantothenic /ˌpæntəˈθɛnɪk/
acid /ˈæsɪd/
paranoid /ˈpær.ən.ɔɪd/
parenchyma /pəˈrɛŋ.kə.mə/
parenteral /pəˈren.tə.rəl/
pellagra /pəˈleɪgrə/
permeability /ˌpɜː.mi.əˈbɪl.ɪ.ti/
persist /pəˈsɪst/
photosensitive /ˌfəʊ.təʊˈsen.sɪ.tɪv/
postoperative /ˌpəʊstˈɒp.ər.ə.tɪv/
postpartum /ˌpəʊstˈpɑː.təm/
predominate /prɪˈdɒm.ɪ.neɪt/
premature /ˈprem.ə.tʃər/
pressure /ˈpreʃ.ə/ **point** /ˈpɔɪnt/
principal /ˈprɪnt .sɪ.pəl/
prostaglandin /ˌprɒstəˈglændɪn/
psychosis /saɪˈkəʊ.sɪs/
puncture /ˈpʌŋk.tʃə/
purine /ˈpjʊəriːn/
pyridoxine /ˌpɪrɪˈdɒksiːn/
pyrimidine /paɪˈrɪmɪˌdiːn/
rash /ræʃ/
red /red/ **blood** /blʌd/ **cell** /sel/ **RBC**
reproduction /ˌriː.prəˈdʌk.ʃən/
rigidity /rɪˈdʒɪd.ɪ.ti/
salicylate /səˈlɪs.ə.leɪt/
salivation /ˈsæl.ɪ.veɪ.ʃən/
scaly /ˈskeɪ.li/
scarlet /ˈskɑːlət/
sensitivity /ˌsent .sɪˈtɪv.ɪ.ti/
serious /ˈsɪə.ri.əs/
sore /sɔːr/
spinocerebral /spaɪnəˈserəbrəl/
stomatitis /ˌstoʊ məˈtaɪ tɪs/
suck /sʌk/
surgery /ˈsɜː.dʒər.i/
swollen /ˈswəʊlən/
symmetric /sɪˈmetrɪk/
thiamine /ˈθaɪ.ə.miːn/
thicken /ˈθɪk.ən/
tingling /ˈtɪŋ.gl.ɪŋ/
tongue /tʌŋ/
tortilla /tɔːˈtiːə/
trauma /ˈtrɔː.mə/
ulceration /ˌʌl.sərˈeɪ.ʃən/
uncommon /ʌnˈkɒm.ən/
underlie /ˌʌn.dəˈlaɪ/
urethra /jʊəˈriː.θrə/
vagina /vəˈdʒaɪ.nə/
vesiculation /vəˈsɪk jəˌleɪ ʃən/
vulnerable /ˈvʌl.nər.ə.bl̩/
weakness /ˈwiːk.nəs/
worldwide /ˌwɜːldˈwaɪd/
wound /wuːnd/

Solution to Exercise 1a
1d, 2h, 3f, 4g, 5e, 6k,
7a, 8c, 9i, 10b, 11j

Solution to Exercise 1b
1a, 2v, 3u, 4b, 5h, 6r, 7i, 8p, 9q,
10t, 11s, 12c, 13d, 14o, 15g, 16l,
17j, 18k, 19n, 20m, 21f, 22e

Unit 7 - Vitamins 3. Minerals 1.

Vitamin C (ascorbic acid)

- **Functions**: antioxidant; co-enzyme in the synthesis of collagen; immune system function; helps maintain capillaries, bones and teeth and aids in the absorption of iron.
- **Sources**: citrus fruits, green peppers, tomatoes; destroyed by cooking.
- **Deficiency**: scurvy

Vitamin C is **essential for collagen formation** and helps maintain the **integrity** of substances of mesenchymal origin, such as **connective tissue, osteiod tissue, and dentine**. It is essential for **wound healing** and **facilitates recovery** from burns.

Vitamin C deficiency

Severe deficiency results in **scurvy**, an acute or chronic disease characterized by haemorrhagic **manifestations** and **abnormal osteoid and dentine** formation. Scurvy leads to the formation of **livid spots** on the skin, **spongy gums** and **bleeding** from almost all mucous membranes. The spots are most abundant on the thighs and legs, and a person with the ailment looks pale, feels depressed, and is partially immobilized.

Symptoms include:

- **weakness**
- **joint pain**
- black-and-blue **marks** on the skin
- **gum disease**
- **corkscrew hairs**

It takes about **three months** of vitamin C **deprivation** to begin inducing the symptoms of scurvy. **Untreated scurvy** is always **fatal**, but since all that is required for full recovery is the resumption of normal vitamin C intake, death by scurvy is rare in modern times.

In adults, primary deficiency is usually due to **food idiosyncrasies** or **improper diet. Deficiencies** occur in GI disease, especially when the patient is on an "**ulcer diet**". **Pregnancy, lactation**, and **thyrotoxicosis** increase vitamin C requirements; acute and chronic **inflammatory diseases, surgery, and burns** can significantly **increase requirements.**

Vitamin C toxicity

Most nutritionists believe that huge doses of vitamin C do not decrease the incidence or severity of the common cold or influence the progress of malignant disease or atherosclerosis. These **mega-doses** acidify the urine; they may cause diarrhoea, predispose to urinary calculi and promote iron overload.

Exercise 1a

Match the column A with the column B. Try to learn the expressions and/or sentences by heart.

A

1. Vitamin C is an antioxidant; serves as a co-enzyme in the synthesis of collagen;
2. Vitamin C is essential for collagen formation
3. It is essential for wound healing
4. Vitamin C deficiency results in scurvy, an acute or chronic disease characterized by
5. Scurvy leads to the formation of
6. Symptoms of scurvy include:
7. It takes about three months of vitamin C deprivation
8. Pregnancy, lactation, and thyrotoxicosis

9. Acute and chronic inflammatory diseases,

B

a) and facilitates recovery from burns.
b) and helps maintain the integrity of connective tissue, osteiod tissue, and dentine.
c) has immune system function; helps maintain capillaries, bones and teeth and aids in the absorption of iron.
d) haemorrhagic manifestations and abnormal osteoid and dentine formation.
e) increase vitamin C requirements.
f) livid spots on the skin, spongy gums and bleeding from almost all mucous membranes.
g) surgery, and burns can significantly increase requirements.
h) to begin inducing the symptoms of scurvy.
i) weakness, joint pain, black-and-blue marks on the skin, gum disease, corkscrew hairs.

Minerals 1

Vitamins cannot be assimilated without the aid of minerals. And though the body can manufacture a few vitamins, it **cannot manufacture a single mineral**. All tissues and internal fluids of our body contain varying quantities of minerals. Minerals are **constituents of the bones, teeth, soft tissue, muscle, blood, and nerve cells.** They are vital to overall mental and physical well-being.

Minerals act as **catalysts** for many biological reactions within the body, including **muscle response**, the transmission of messages through the **nervous system**, the production of **hormones**, **digestion**, and the **utilization of nutrients** in foods. **Some minerals** are needed in such vanishingly **small amounts** that it is practically impossible to prepare a diet that does not include them. However, **totally synthetic diets** are now available for intravenous feeding of people who cannot eat. This so-called total parenteral nutrition has revealed, unexpectedly, some additional trace element needs; chromium and molybdenum.

Minerals can be divided into two groups:

- **Macro-elements**: inorganic nutrients needed in relatively **high daily amounts** (i.e. more than 100 mg per day) – e.g. **Ca, P, Mg, Na, K, Cl, S.**
- **Micro-elements** = trace elements: a group of chemical elements that are needed in **minute quantities** for the proper growth, development, and physiology of an organism – e.g. **Fe, I, F, Zn, Cu, Mn, Cr, Se, Co, Mo.**

Calcium (Ca)

- **Functions**: essential for **blood clotting, intracellular signalling, muscle contraction**, used for **building bones and teeth** and in maintaining bone strength.
- **Sources**: dairy products, vegetables, legumes, fish, seafood, meat, eggs.
- **Deficiency**: osteoporosis.
- **Excess**: some mineral imbalances such as zinc, but combined with a magnesium deficiency it may cause kidney stones.

Calcium is essential to **almost every function** in the body. For most of these only **trace amounts** are needed. However, large amounts of calcium are needed to make bone (which is 18% calcium), so **substantial amounts** are needed in the diet, especially during **infancy, childhood, and pregnancy**. A **temporary deficit** in the amount of calcium in the diet can be compensated for by its **removal from** the huge reserves in **bone.** Ageing **humans** lose calcium from their bones so that in time they become **fragile**, a condition known as **osteoporosis**.

Avoiding osteoporosis

- If you are **older than 50 years**, your **recommended daily allowance** (RDA) of **1200 mg of calcium,** preferably in a soluble form (milk, milk products, or supplements containing calcium gluconate or calcium lactate.
- **Exercise**. It might help develop bone mass and even if it doesn't, it will be rewarding in other ways.
- For women **after menopause**, treatment with **oestrogen** seems to be an effective way to avoid osteoporosis.

Phosphorus (P)

- **Functions**: important element in **cell protoplasm** and **nervous tissue**, role in biological molecules such as **DNA and RNA** where it forms part of those molecules' molecular backbones. Living cells also utilize inorganic phosphorus to store and transport cellular energy via ATP. With Ca used for **building bones and teeth** and in maintaining bone strength.
- **Sources**: meat, poultry and fish, eggs, seeds, milk, carbonated soft drinks, broccoli, apples, carrots, asparagus, bran, brewer's yeast and corn.
- **Deficiency: painful bones**, irregular breathing, **fatigue, anxiety, numbness, skin**

sensitivity and changes in body weight.

- **Excess**: harmful as it can **interfere with calcium absorption.**

Calcium and phosphorus are important minerals. They maintain good **teeth and bones** and keep **muscles and nerves** working properly. Healthy **kidneys** help **control** the amount of **calcium and phosphorus in the blood**. When the kidneys are not working properly, they cannot remove enough phosphorus from the blood. When the calcium and phosphorus are not **balanced** and within good levels, bone disease can develop. **High phosphorus levels** cause blood **calcium levels to drop.** When phosphorus levels are high a message is sent to the bones (by a hormone) telling them to release calcium and "bind" the phosphorus, that is, remove the phosphorus from the blood. **Bones become brittle** due to the loss of calcium.

Deficiency symptoms may result in **itching (arms, legs, back, chest)**, **red eyes**, continuous **bone pain** (especially **hips, knees, ankles and heels**), **bones** that **break** easily and **blood vessels become clogge**d with calcium that should be in the bones. This can cause **sores** that won't heal, **strokes, and heart attacks**.

Exercise 1b

Match the column A with the column B. Try to learn the expressions and/or sentences by heart.

A

1. Vitamins cannot be assimilated
2. The body can manufacture a few vitamins,
3. Minerals are constituents of
4. Minerals act as catalysts for many biological reactions within the body, including
5. Minerals can be divided into two groups:
6. Calcium is essential for
7. Substantial amounts of calcium are needed in the diet,
8. Ageing humans lose calcium from their bones
9. If you are older than 50 years, your recommended daily allowance is 1, 200 mg of calcium
10. Phosphorus is important element
11. Sources of phosphorus are
12. Calcium and phosphorus are important minerals;
13. Healthy kidneys help control
14. When the calcium and phosphorus
15. High phosphorus levels cause blood calcium levels to drop
16. Deficiency symptoms may result in itching (arms, legs, back, chest), red eyes, continuous bone

pain (especially hips, knees, ankles and heels),

B

a) *and bones become brittle due to the loss of calcium.*

b) *are not balanced and within good levels, bone disease can develop.*

c) *blood clotting, intracellular signalling, muscle contraction, and is used for building bones and teeth and in maintaining bone strength.*

d) *bones that break easily and blood vessels become clogged with calcium that should be in the bones.*

e) *but it cannot manufacture a single mineral.*

f) *especially during infancy, childhood, and pregnancy.*

g) *in a soluble form (milk, milk products), or supplements.*

h) *in cell protoplasm and nervous tissue.*

i) *macro-elements e.g. Ca, P, Mg, Na, K, Cl, S and micro-elements e.g. Fe, I, F, Zn, Cu, Mn, Cr, Se, Co, Mo.*

j) *meat, poultry and fish, eggs, seeds, milk, carbonated soft drinks, broccoli, apples, carrots, asparagus, bran, brewer's yeast and corn.*

k) *muscle response, the transmission of messages through the nervous system, the production of hormones, digestion, and the utilization of nutrients in foods.*

l) *so that in time they become fragile, a condition known as osteoporosis.*

m) *the amount of calcium and phosphorus in the blood.*

n) *the bones, teeth, soft tissue, muscle, blood, and nerve cells.*

o) *they maintain good teeth and bones and keep muscles and nerves working properly.*

p) *without the aid of minerals.*

Magnesium (Mg)

- **Functions:** helps with **formation of bone and teeth** and assists the **absorption of calcium and potassium**, used to **relax the muscles**, necessary for cellular metabolism, regulating the neuromuscular **activity of heart**, assists in controlling **blood pressure,** assists the **parathyroid gland** to **process vitamin D.**
- **Sources:** dairy products, fish, meat and seafood, legumes, apples, apricots, avocados, bananas, whole grain cereals, nuts, dark green vegetables, and cocoa.
- **Deficiency**: **neuromuscular** manifestations, **personality changes**, **cardiovascular** problems, **insomnia**, **poor memory, painful periods, depression, hypertension and confusion**.
- **Excess**: in severe cases by people with kidney

or heart problems lead to coma and death.

Magnesium plays an important role in regulating the neuromuscular activity of the heart; maintains normal **heart rhythm**; necessary for **proper calcium and vitamin C metabolism;** converts **blood sugar into energy**. **Deficiency** symptoms may result in calcium depletion, **heart spasms, nervousness, muscular excitability**, **confusion**; **kidney stones**.

Sodium (Na)

- **Functions**: **electrolyte** in the body and is required in the **manufacture of hydrochloric acid in the stomach.**
- **Sources**: table salt, anchovies, bacon, carrot, spinach, root celery, eggs.
- **Deficiency**: rare; nausea, dizziness, poor concentration and muscle weakness.
- **Excess**: **high blood pressure**, **loss of calcium** from our body.

Sodium ions (Na^+) play a diverse role in many **physiological processes**. Excitable cells, for example, rely on the entry of Na^+ to cause a depolarization. Sodium chloride (better known as common **salt**) is most common compound of sodium. Therefore, deficiency symptoms are not known.

Potassium (K)

- **Functions**: electrolyte in the body, necessary for **growth, building muscles**, transmission of nerve impulses, **heart activity**.
- **Sources**: fruit, vegetables as well as whole grains, citrus fruit, molasses, fish and unprocessed meats.
- **Deficiency: fatigue, cramping legs, muscle weakness, slow reflexes, acne, dry skin, mood changes, irregular heartbeat**.
- **Excess:** heart and kidney failure.

Potassium works with sodium to regulate the body's **waste balance** and normalize heart rhythms; **aids in clear thinking** by sending **oxygen to the brain**; **preserves proper alkalinity** of body fluids; stimulates the kidneys to **eliminate poisonous body wastes;** assists in reducing high blood pressure; promotes healthy skin. **Deficiency** symptoms may result in poor reflexes, nervous disorders, respiratory failure, cardiac arrest, and muscle damage.

Chloride (Cl)

- **Function**: works with potassium and sodium, the two electrolytes, to **control the flow of fluid in blood vessels and tissues**, as well as **regulating acidity** in the body, and also forms

part of hydrochloric acid in the stomach.

- **Sources**: table salt as well as kelp, olives, tomatoes, celery.
- **Deficiency**: extremely rare; may cause excessive loss of potassium in the urine, weakness and lowered blood pressure.
- **Excess**: a high concentration of chloride in the body may result in **fluid retention**, but sodium is normally the culprit for the retention.

Sulphur (S)

- **Functions**: **essential element of protein, biotin** as well as **vitamin B_1; part** of the chemical **structure of the amino acids** methionine, cysteine, taurine and glutathione; **needed in the synthesis of collagen**, which is needed for good **skin integrity**; **detoxify** the body, assists the immune system and **fight the effects of ageing**, as well as age related illness such as **arthritis**.
- **Sources**: eggs, garlic, lettuce, cabbage and Brussels sprouts.
- **Deficiency:** only really happen if a diet is deprived of protein, or a poorly planned vegan diet.
- **Excess**: none identified

Exercise 1c
Match the column A with the column B. Try to learn the expressions and/ or sentences by heart.

A

1. Magnesium helps with formation of bone and teeth
2. Magnesium is necessary for cellular metabolism, regulates the neuromuscular activity of heart,
3. Sources of magnesium are
4. Magnesium plays an important role in regulating the neuromuscular activity of the heart;
5. Deficiency symptoms may result in
6. Sources of sodium are
7. Sodium ions (Na^+) play a diverse role
8. Sodium chloride (better known as common salt)
9. Potassium is necessary for growth, building muscles,
10. Sources of potassium are
11. Symptoms of potassium deficiency are
12. Potassium works with sodium to regulate the body's waste balance;
13. Potassium preserves proper alkalinity of body fluids; stimulates the kidneys to eliminate poisonous body wastes;
14. Potassium deficiency symptoms may result

15. Chloride works with potassium and sodium to control the flow of fluid in blood vessels and tissues,
16. A high concentration of chloride in the body
17. Sulphur is essential element of
18. Sulphur is part of the chemical structure of the amino acids methionine, cysteine, taurine and glutathione;
19. Sulphur is needed for good skin integrity; assists the immune system and fights the effects
20. Sources of sulphur are

B

a) *and assists the absorption of calcium and potassium.*
b) *and is needed in the synthesis of collagen.*
c) *as well as regulating acidity in the body, and also forms part of hydrochloric acid in the stomach.*
d) *assists in controlling blood pressure, and assists the parathyroid gland to process vitamin D.*
e) *assists in reducing high blood pressure and promotes healthy skin.*
f) *calcium depletion, heart spasms, nervousness, muscular excitability, confusion or kidney stones.*
g) *dairy products, fish, meat and seafood, legumes, apples, apricots, avocados, bananas, whole grain cereals, nuts, dark green vegetables, and cocoa.*
h) *eggs, garlic, lettuce, cabbage and Brussels sprouts.*
i) *fatigue, cramping legs, muscle weakness, slow reflexes, acne, dry skin, mood changes, and irregular heartbeat.*
j) *fruit, vegetables, whole grains, citrus fruit, molasses, fish and unprocessed meats.*
k) *in many physiological processes.*
l) *in poor reflexes, nervous disorders, respiratory failure, cardiac arrest, and muscle damage.*
m) *is compound of sodium.*
n) *maintains normal heart rhythm; is necessary for proper calcium and vitamin C metabolism and converts blood sugar into energy.*
o) *may result in fluid retention, but sodium is normally the culprit for the retention.*
p) *normalizes heart rhythms and aids in clear thinking by sending oxygen to the brain.*
q) *of ageing, as well as age related illness such as arthritis.*
r) *protein, biotin as well as vitamin* B_1.
s) *table salt, anchovies, bacon, carrot, spinach, root celery and eggs.*
t) *transmission of nerve impulses, and heart activity.*

Exercise 2

Translate the expressions. Try to explain their meanings in English.

Integrity, origin, connective tissue, wound healing, facilitates, recovery, osteoid, dentine, livid spots, spongy gums, abundant, ailment, marks, deprivation, untreated, fatal, recovery, resumption, idiosyncrasies, lactation, thyrotoxicosis, surgery, huge doses, incidence, severity, malignant, acidify, urinary calculi, overload, assimilated, manufacture, internal, contain, constituents, overall well-being, transmission of message, utilization, vanishingly small amounts, intravenous feeding, parenteral nutrition, trace element, minute quantities, blood clotting, maintaining imbalances, infancy, temporary deficit, compensated, removal, ageing, fragile, bone mass, cellular energy, carbonated soft drinks, asparagus, bran, brewer's yeast, numbness, skin sensitivity, interfere with, drop, brittle, itching, hips, heels, blood vessels, clogged, sores, parathyroid gland, manifestations, personality changes, insomnia, poor memory, painful, confusion, regulating, converts, depletion, excitability, hydrochloric acid, dizziness, muscle weakness, diverse, rely on, compound, molasses, cramping, mood changes, irregular heartbeat, eliminate poisonous body wastes, respiratory failure, flow, fluid retention, skin integrity, deprived of.

Exercise 3

Answer the following questions. Prepare short talks and/or dialogues on these topics.

1. Vitamin C (functions, sources, deficiency)
2. What are the symptoms of scurvy?
3. Which conditions increase vitamin C requirements?
4. Why are minerals important?
5. Calcium (functions, sources, deficiency, excess)
6. Avoiding osteoporosis
7. Phosphorus (functions, sources, deficiency, excess)
8. Characterise magnesium (functions, sources, deficiency, excess).
9. Characterise sodium (functions, sources, deficiency, excess).
10. Characterise potassium (functions, sources, deficiency, excess).
11. Characterise chloride (functions, sources, deficiency, excess).
12. Characterise sulphur (functions, sources, deficiency, excess).

Vocabulary 7

Fill in the meanings in your mother language:

abundant /ə'bʌn.dənt/
acidify /ə'sɪd.ɪ.faɪ/
acidity /ə'sɪdɪtɪ/
acne /'æk.ni/
act /ækt/

additional /əˈdɪʃ.ən.əl/
age /eɪdʒ/
aid /eɪd/
alkalinity /ˌæl kəˈlɪn ɪ ti/
anchovy /ˈæn.tʃə.vi/ pl **anchovies**
apricot /ˈæp rɪˌkɒt/
arm /ɑːm/
arthritis /ɑːˈθraɪ.tɪs/
asparagus /əˈspær.ə.gəs/
atherosclerosis /ˌæθ.ə.rəʊ.skləˈrəʊ.sɪs/
available /əˈveɪ.lə.blˌ/
avocado /ˌævəˈkɑːdəʊ/
backbone /ˈbæk.bəʊn/
brittle /ˈbrɪt.l̩/
Brussels sprout /ˌbrʌs.əlz ˈspraʊt/
cabbage /ˈkæb.ɪdʒ/
calcium /ˈkæl.si.əm/
gluconate /ˈglu kən eɪt/
calcium /ˈkæl.si.əm/ **lactate** /lækˈteɪt/
cardiac /ˈkɑː.di.æk/ **arrest** /əˈrest/
catalyst /ˈkætəlɪst/
catecholamine /ˌkæt ɪˈkɒl əˌmin/
celery /ˈsel.ər.i/
chest /tʃest/
chloride /ˈklɔː.raɪd/
chromium (Cr) /ˈkrəʊ.mi.əm/
clogged /klɒgd/
collagen /ˈkɒl.ə.dʒən/
compensate /ˈkɒmpənseɪt/
connective tissue /kəˌnek.tɪvˈtɪʃ.uː/
continuous /kənˈtɪn.ju.əs/
corkscrew /ˈkɔːkskruː/
cramp /kræmp/
culprit /ˈkʌl prɪt/
cysteine /ˈsɪstɪˌiːn/
decrease /dɪˈkriːs/
dentine /ˈden.tiːn/
depletion /dɪˈpliː.ʃən/
depolarization /diːˌpəʊ.lər.aɪˈzeɪ.ʃən/
diverse /daɪˈvɜːs/
drop /drɒp/
electrolyte /ɪˈlek.trə.laɪt/
excitability /ɪkˌsaɪ.təˈbɪl.ə.tɪ/
excitable /ɪkˈsaɪ.tə.bl̩/
fragile /ˈfrædʒ.aɪl/
garlic /ˈgɑː.lɪk/
glutathione /ˌgluːtəˈθaɪəʊn/
hairs /heər/
healing /hiːlɪŋ/
heartbeat /ˈhɑːt.biːt/
heel /hiːl/
huge /hjuːdʒ/
hydrochloric acid /ˌhaɪd.
rə.klɒr.ɪkˈæs.ɪd/
idiosyncrasy /ˌɪd.i.əˈsɪŋ.krə.si/
incidence /ˈɪnt .sɪ.dənts/
integrity /ɪnˈteg.rə.ti/
internal /ɪnˈtɜː.nəl/
intracellular /ˌɪn.trəˈsel.jə.lər/
intravenous /ˌɪn.trəˈviː.nəs/
itching /ˈɪtʃ.ɪŋ/
joint /dʒɔɪnt/
lactation /lækˈteɪ.ʃən/
lettuce /ˈletɪs/
livid /ˈlɪvɪd/
magnesium (Mg) /mægˈniː.zi.əm/
malignant /məˈlɪg.nənt/
manifestation /ˌmæn.ɪ.fesˈteɪ.ʃən/
mark /mɑːk/
memory /ˈmem.ər.i/
mesenchymal /ˈmɛs ɛŋ kaɪməl/
methionine /mɛˈθaɪ əˌnin/
minute /maɪˈnjuːt/
molasses /məˈlæs ɪz/
molybdenum /mɒlˈɪb.dɪ.nəm/
mood /muːd/
nervousness /ˈnɜː.vəs.nəs/
neuromuscular /ˈnjʊə.rəʊˌmʌs.kjʊ.lər/
numbness /ˈnʌm.nəs/
origin /ˈɒr.ɪ.dʒɪn/
osteiod /ˌɒs ti oʊɪd/
osteoporosis /ˌɒs.ti.əʊ.pəˈrəʊ.sɪs/
pale /peɪl/
parathyroid gland /ˌpær.
əˈθaɪ.rɔɪdˌglænd/
pepper /ˈpep.ər/
period /ˈpɪə.ri.əd/
personality /ˌpɜː.sənˈæl.ə.ti/
phosphorus (P) /ˈfɒs.fər.əs/
poisonous /ˈpɔɪ.zən.əs/

potassium (K) /pə'tæs.i.əm/
process /'prəʊ.ses/
protoplasm /'prəʊ.tə.plæz.əm/
recovery /rɪ'kʌv.ər.i/
relax /rɪ'læks/
rely /rɪ'laɪ/ **on** /ɒn/
removal /rɪ'mu:.vəl/
resumption /rɪ'zʌmʃən/
retention /rɪ'ten.ʃən/
reveal /rɪ'vi:l/
reward /rɪ'wɔ:d/
root /ru:t/
signal /'sɪg.nəl/
sodium (Na) /'səʊ.di.əm/
spasm /'spæz.əm/
spongy /'spʌnðʒi/
spot /spɒt/
strength /streŋθ/
taurine /'tɔr aɪn/
temporary /'tem.pər.ər.i/
thigh /θaɪ/
thyrotoxicosis /θaɪ.rəʊ.tɒk.sɪ.kəʊ.sɪs/
unexpected /ˌʌn.ɪk'spek.tɪd/
urinary /'jʊə.rɪ.nər.i/ **calculus** /'kæl.kjʊ.ləs/ pl **calculi**
vanish /'væn.ɪ.ʃ/
vital /'vaɪ.təl/

Solution to Exercise 1a
1c, 2b, 3a, 4d, 5f, 6i, 7h, 8e, 9g

Solution to Exercise 1b
1p, 2a, 3n, 4k, 5i, 6c, 7f, 8l, 9g, 10h, 11j, 12o, 13m, 14b, 15a, 16d

Solution to Exercise 1c
1a, 2d, 3g, 4n, 5f, 6s, 7k, 8m, 9t, 10j, 11i, 12p, 13e, 14l, 15c, 16o, 17r, 18b, 19q, 20h

Unit 8 - Minerals 2

Iron (Fe)

- **Functions**: **necessary for** production of **haemoglobin** and **myoglobin**, also for **oxygenation of red blood cells**, a healthy **immune** system and for **energy** production.
- **Sources**: **Heme iron** (present in red blood cells and muscles) found in meat, poultry and fish – is readily absorbed; **Non-heme iron** – with the absorption more influenced by other dietary factors, are present in cereals, fruits, grains, beans and vegetables.
- **Deficiency**: anaemia, and red blood cells that have a low haemoglobin concentration.
- **Excess:** high iron content in the body has been linked to cancer and heart disease.

Iron is incorporated in a number of **body constituents**, notably cytochromes, myoglobin and haemoglobin. Not surprisingly, an iron deficiency shows up first as **anaemia.** In developed countries iron deficiency is the most common mineral deficiency. It is particularly common among **women** because of the loss of blood during **menstruation** and the need for extra iron during **pregnancy and breast-feeding. Marginal iron intake** is so **widespread** that some nutritionists want to have iron added to common foods like bread and cereals, just as some vitamins now are. However, excess iron in the body also leads to problems, and this has made the proposal controversial.

Iodine (I)

- **Functions**: production of hormones by the **thyroid gland**, which are needed to help form **bones**, keeping **skin, nails, hair and teeth** in prime condition; iodine is necessary for stabilizing **body weigh**t as well as controlling **cholesterol levels**; helpful in **preventing cancer of the breast and womb**.
- **Sources**: eggs, milk, sea fish and seafood, sea vegetables.
- **Deficiency**: constipation, obesity, weakness, mental slowness and problems; goiter.
- **Excess**: also goiter.

A **goitre is a swelling in the neck** due to an enlarged thyroid gland. The most common cause for goitre in the world is iodine deficiency. Iodine is necessary for the synthesis of the **thyroid hormones**. Goitre was previously common in many areas that were deficient in iodine in the soil. The condition now is practically absent in **affluent nations**, where table salt is supplemented with iodine. There are fears by some health workers that a resurgence of goitre might occur because of the trend to use **rock salt** (which has not been fortified with iodine) and also less salt use in general. The **use of iodized salt** (table salt to which a small amount of sodium iodine, KI, is added) has reduced the incidence of goiter in most developed countries.

Fluorine (F)

- **Functions**: constituent of **bones and teeth**, beneficial in most cases in preventing dental caries.
- **Sources**: **water, food** grown in areas where fluorine is present in the soil and water.
- **Deficiency**: none identified.
- **Excess**: stains in the teeth with mottled spots – known as **dental fluorosis**.

The value of fluoride was first recognized as a **preventive for dental caries** (cavities). Humans get most of their fluoride in **drinking water**. **Water fluoridation** has been controversial. Leaving aside the philosophical and political questions raised by proponents and opponents of fluoridation, the safety and efficacy of this public health measure has been thoroughly established.

Zinc (Zn)

- **Functions**: necessary for a **healthy immune system**, in the growth and maintenance of muscles; used in **fighting skin problems** such as **acne,**

boils and sore throats; needed for cell division, and is **needed** by the tissue of the **hair, nails and skin** to be in top form.

- **Sources**: muscle meat, poultry, fish and seafood, whole grains, nuts, seeds and brewer's yeast.
- **Deficiency:** under-performing immune system, open to infections, allergies, **night blindness, loss of smell, falling hair**, white spots under finger nails, **skin problems, sleep disturbances, fertility** in men.
- **Excess: nausea, diarrhoea, dizziness, drowsiness and hallucinations**

Zinc is incorporated in many enzymes and transcription factors. Zinc **supplements** are popular for their supposed antioxidant properties and to **hasten the recovery from colds**. Excessive intake of zinc causes a brief illness. Its most frequent cause is from ingested acidic food or drink that has been stored in galvanized **(zinc-coated) containers**.

Exercise 1a
Match the column A with the column B. Try to learn the expressions and/or sentences by heart.

A

1. Iron is necessary for production of haemoglobin and myoglobin,
2. Iron is found in meat, poultry and fish
3. Iron deficiency is particularly common among women
4. Iodine is needed for production of hormones by the thyroid gland; it
5. Iodine is necessary for stabilizing body weight as well as controlling cholesterol levels; it is
6. A goitre is a swelling in the neck due to an enlarged thyroid gland;
7. Iodine is necessary for
8. The use of iodized salt has reduced
9. Fluorine is constituent of bones and teeth, it
10. Zinc is necessary for a healthy immune system, the growth and maintenance of muscles and is
11. Zinc is needed by the tissue,
12. Deficiency of zinc causes infections, allergies, night blindness, loss of smell,
13. Excess of zinc causes
14. Zinc supplements are popular for their antioxidant properties and

B

a) *also helpful in preventing cancer of the breast and womb.*
b) *as well as in cereals, fruits, grains, beans and vegetables.*
c) *because of the loss of blood during menstruation and the need for extra*

iron during pregnancy and breast-feeding.

d) *falling hair, white spots under finger nails, skin problems, or sleep disturbances.*

e) *for oxygenation of red blood cells, a healthy immune system and for energy production.*

f) *helps to form bones, and keep skin, nails, hair and teeth in prime condition.*

g) *is beneficial in most cases in preventing dental caries.*

h) *nausea, diarrhoea, dizziness, drowsiness and hallucinations*

i) *the hair, nails and skin to be in top form.*

j) *the incidence of goiter in most developed countries.*

k) *the most common cause for goitre is iodine deficiency.*

l) *the synthesis of the thyroid hormones.*

m) *they are supposed to hasten the recovery from colds.*

n) *used in fighting skin problems such as acne, boils and sore throats.*

Copper (Cu)

- **Functions**: necessary for the **absorption and utilization of iron**; helps oxidise **vitamin C** and works with vitamin C to **form elastin and collagen**; required in the **formation of haemoglobin, red blood cells** as well as **bones**; necessary for the **manufacture of** the neurotransmitter **noradrenaline** and for the **pigmentation of hair**.
- **Sources**: whole grain, liver, molasses, and nuts.
- **Deficiency**: increased **blood fat** levels, general **weakness, impaired respiration**, **skin sores**.
- **Excess:** toxic levels will lead to diarrhoea, vomiting, liver damage as well as discolouration of the skin and hair, while mild excess will result in **fatigue**, **irritability**, **depression** and **loss of concentration** and **learning disabilities**.

Manganese (Mn)

- **Functions**: enables the body to **utilize vitamin C, B_1, biotin and choline**; used in the manufacture of **fat, sex hormones and breast milk** in females; **antioxidant** nutrient; important in the blood **breakdown of amino acids** and the production of energy; activates various **enzymes** which are important for **proper digestion** and utilization of foods; is a catalyst in the breakdown of fats and cholesterol; helps **nourish the nerves and brain**; necessary for normal skeletal development; maintains sex hormone production.

- **Sources**: nuts, avocados, eggs, brown rice, spices, whole grains, leafy greens, tea and coffee.
- **Deficiency**: rare, can include poor bone growth, problems with the disks between the vertebrae, birth defects, and problems with blood glucose levels and reduced fertility. Serious deficiency **in children** can result in **paralysis, deafness and blindness**.
- **Excess**: none identified.

Chromium (Cr)

- **Function**: works with insulin in the **metabolism of sugars** and stabilizes blood sugar levels; cleans the arteries by **reducing cholesterol** and **triglyceride levels**; helps **transport amino acids** to where the body needs them; helps **control the appetite**. Medical research has shown that persons with **low levels** of chromium in their bodies are more susceptible to having **cancer and heart problems** and becoming **diabetic**.
- **Sources**: eggs, beef, whole grains, brewer's yeast as well as molasses.
- **Deficiency**: **glucose intolerance** in diabetics; **arteriosclerosis, heart disease, depressed growth, obesity, tiredness.**
- **Excess**: rare, can include **dermatitis, gastrointestinal ulcers, liver and kidney damage.**

Selenium (Se)

- **Functions**: major **antioxidant** nutrient, protects cell membranes and prevents free radical generation thereby decreasing the risk of cancer and disease of the heart and blood vessels. Medical surveys show that increased selenium intake **decreases the risk of breast, colon, lung and prostate cancer**. Selenium also **preserves tissue elasticity**; slows down the ageing and hardening of tissues through oxidation; helps in the treatment and prevention of dandruff.
- **Sources**: Brazil nuts, whole grains, shellfish.
- **Deficiency**: **premature ageing**, heart disease, dandruff, and loose skin
- **Excess**: selenium is **toxic**, large doses can cause **hair loss, tooth decay, brittle nails, white spots, poor appetite, sour taste** in the mouth, loss of feeling in the hands and feet, change in skin pigmentation and the breath may have a garlic smell.

Cobalt (Co)

- **Functions**: part of the vitamin B_{12} molecule, **required in the manufacture of red blood cells and in preventing anaemia.**
- **Sources:** pulses and vegetables.
- **Deficiency**: none identified.
- **Excess**: may damage the heart muscles, and may cause an over-production of red blood cells or damage to the thyroid gland.

Molybdenum (Mo)

Functions: **antioxidant; component of three different enzymes**, which is involved in the metabolism of DNA and RNA – iron as well as food into energy.

Sources: milk, lima beans, spinach, liver, grain, peas and other vegetables.

Deficiency: abnormal excretion of sulphur metabolites; low uric acid concentrations, impotence in older males.

Excess: can interfere with the metabolism of copper in the body, can give symptoms of gout, and may cause diarrhoea, anaemia and slow growth.

Exercise 1b
Match the column A with the column B. Try to learn the expressions and/or sentences by heart.

A

1. Copper is necessary for the absorption and utilization of iron; helps oxidise vitamin C, is required in the formation of red blood cells
2. Toxic levels will lead to diarrhoea, vomiting, liver damage as well as discolouration of the skin and hair,
3. Manganese is used in the manufacture of
4. Manganese activates various enzymes which are important for proper digestion
5. Serious deficiency in children
6. Chromium works with insulin in the metabolism of sugars and stabilizes blood sugar levels;
7. Deficiency of chromium causes glucose intolerance in diabetics;
8. Selenium is major antioxidant nutrient, protects cell membranes and prevents free radical generation
9. Medical surveys show that increased selenium intake decreases
10. Deficiency of selenium causes premature ageing,
11. Selenium is toxic, large doses can cause hair loss, tooth decay, brittle nails, white spots, poor appetite, sour taste in the mouth,
12. Cobalt is required in the manufacture
13. Deficiency of molybdenum causes
14. Excess of molybdenum can interfere with the metabolism

B

a) *abnormal excretion of sulphur metabolites; low uric acid concentrations, and impotence in older males.*
b) *and is necessary for the manufacture of the neurotransmitter noradrenaline and for the pigmentation of hair.*
c) *and utilization of foods and helps nourish the nerves and brain.*
d) *arteriosclerosis, heart disease, depressed growth, obesity and tiredness.*
e) *can result in paralysis, deafness and blindness.*
f) *cleans the arteries by reducing cholesterol and triglyceride levels; helps transport amino acids and helps control the appetite.*
g) *fat, sex hormones and breast milk in females.*
h) *heart disease, dandruff, and loose skin.*
i) *loss of feeling in the hands and feet, change in skin pigmentation and the breath may have a garlic smell.*
j) *of copper in the body, can give symptoms of gout, and may cause diarrhoea, anaemia and slow growth.*
k) *of red blood cells and in preventing anaemia.*
l) *the risk of breast, colon, lung and prostate cancer.*
m) *thereby decreasing the risk of cancer and disease of the heart and blood vessels.*
n) *while mild excess will result in fatigue, irritability, depression and loss of concentration and learning disabilities.*

Exercise 2

Translate the expressions. Try to explain their meanings in English.

Incorporated, constituents, particularly, marginal, proposal, mental slowness, goiter, soil, affluent nations, resurgence, rock salt, fortified, in general, incidence, dental caries, mottled spots, fluorosis, recognized, preventive, proponents and opponents, efficacy, established, maintenance, fighting, boils, sore throats, brewer's yeast, night blindness, sleep disturbances, fertility, dizziness, drowsiness, hasten the recovery, zinc-coated containers, utilization, fatigue, irritability, learning disabilities, nourish, disks between the vertebrae, birth defects, deafness and blindness, medical research, gout, susceptible, tiredness, dermatitis, gastrointestinal ulcers, free radical generation, premature ageing, loss of feeling, excretion, uric acid, interfere with.

Exercise 3

Answer the following questions. Prepare short talks and/or dialogues on these topics.

1. Characterise iron (functions, sources, deficiency, excess).

2. Characterise iodine (functions, sources, deficiency, excess).
3. Characterise fluorine (functions, sources, deficiency, excess).
4. Characterise zinc (functions, sources, deficiency, excess).
5. Characterise copper (functions, sources, deficiency, excess).
6. Characterise manganese (functions, sources, deficiency, excess).
7. Characterise chromium (functions, sources, deficiency, excess).
8. Characterise selenium (functions, sources, deficiency, excess).
9. Characterise cobalt (functions, sources, deficiency, excess).
10. Characterise molybdenum (functions, sources, deficiency, excess).

Vocabulary 8

Fill in the meanings in your mother language:

affluent /ˈæflʊənt/
beef /biːf/
boil /bɔɪl/
Brazil /brəˈzɪl/ **nut** /nʌt/
breakdown /ˈbreɪk.daʊn/
cavity /ˈkæv.ə.ti/
choline /ˈkoʊ lin/
coated /ˈkoʊ tɪd/
cobalt (Co) /ˈkəʊbɔːlt/
cold /kəʊld/
component /kəmˈpəʊ.nənt/
container /kənˈteɪ.nər/
controversial /ˌkɒn.trəˈvɜː.ʃəl/
copper (Cu) /ˈkɒp.ər/
cytochrome /ˈsaɪ təˌkroʊm/
dandruff /ˈdæn.drʌf/
deafness /ˈdef.nəs/
decay /dɪˈkeɪ/
dermatitis /ˌdɜː.məˈtaɪ.təs/
disk /dɪsk/
division /dɪˈvɪʒən/
drowsiness /ˈdraʊ.zɪ.nəs/
efficacy /ˈef.ɪ.kə.si/
elasticity /ˌɪl.æsˈtɪs.ɪ.ti/
elastin /ɪˈlæstɪn/
establish /ɪˈstæb.lɪʃ/
fear /fɪə/
female /ˈfiː.meɪl/
fertility /fɜːˈtɪlɪtɪ/
fluorine (F) /ˈflʊəriːn/
fluorosis /flʊˈroʊ sɪs/
fortified /ˈfɔː.tɪˌfaɪd/
free /friː/ **radical** /ˈræd.ɪ.kəl/
galvanize /ˈgæl vəˌnaɪz/
generation /ˌdʒenəˈreɪʃən/
goiter /ˈgɔɪ tər/
gout /gaʊt/
haemoglobin /ˌhiː.məˈgləʊ.bɪn/
hallucination /həˌluː.sɪˈneɪ.ʃən/
harden /ˈhɑː.dən/
hasten /ˈheɪ.sən/
heme /him/
immune /ɪˈmjuːn/
impotence /ˈɪm.pə.təns/
iodine (I) /ˈaɪ.ə.diːn/
iron (Fe) /aɪən/
learning /ˈlɜːnɪŋ/ **disability** /ˌdɪs.əˈbɪl.ɪ.ti/
lima bean /ˈliː.mə ˌbiːn/
male /meɪl/
manganese (Mn) /ˈmæŋ.gə.niːz/
molybdenum (Mo) /mɒlˈɪb.dɪ.nəm/
mottled /ˈmɒt.lˌd/
myoglobin /ˌmaɪ.əˈgləʊ.bɪn/
noradrenaline /ˌnɔːr.əˈdrɛn.ə.lɪn/
opponent /əˈpəʊnənt/

oxygenation /ˈɒk.sɪ.dʒə.neɪ.ʃən/
paralysis /pəˈræl.ə.sɪs/
proponent /prəˈpəʊnənt/
proposal /prəˈpəʊzəl/
prostate /ˈprɒs.teɪt/
pulses /pʌlsɪz/
readily /ˈred.ɪ.li/
recognize /ˈrek.əg.naɪz/
resurgence /rɪˈsɜːdʒəns/
selenium (Se) /səˈliː.ni.əm/
sodium /ˈsəʊ.di.əm/ **iodine** /ˈaɪ.ə.diːn/
soil /sɔɪl/
sore /sɔː/ **throat** /θrəʊt/
sour /saʊər/
surprisingly /səˈpraɪ.zɪŋ.li/
survey /ˈsɜːveɪ/
susceptible /səˈsep.tɪ.bl̩/
thyroid gland /ˈθaɪə.rɔɪdˌglænd/
tired /taɪəd/
transcription /trænˈskrɪp.ʃən/
uric acid /ˈjʊər.ɪkˈæs.ɪd/
womb /wuːm/

Solution to Exercise 1a
1e, 2b, 3c, 4f, 5a, 6k, 7l, 8j, 9g, 10n, 11i, 12d, 13h, 14m

Solution to Exercise 1b
1b, 2n, 3g, 4c, 5e, 6f, 7d, 8m, 9l, 10h, 11i, 12k, 13a, 14j

Unit 9 - Nutritional and eating disorders. Risks of malnutrition.

Nutritional disorders
Malnutrition

Protein-energy malnutrition (PEM) – under-nutrition or over-nutrition – is one of the nutritional problems recognized by the WHO as public health problems in different parts of the world. PEM is characterized not only by an **energy deficit** due to a reduction in all **macro-nutrients** but also by a deficit in many **micro-nutrients** (**nutritional anaemia**, **vitamin A deficiency**, and **iodine deficiency**). Primary PEM (under-nutrition) has long been regarded as a problem of underprivileged socioeconomic groups, especially those from less developed countries.

Although **severe malnutrition** (**kwashiorkor** and/or **marasmus**) are rare except in countries hit by natural **disasters** such as **drought and war**, mild and moderate malnutrition are quite common. The prevalence of this form of malnutrition varies from 21 to 70% depending on the continent and/or country. This form of malnutrition may not be any less deleterious on the immune response than severe malnutrition, especially when it occurs in the context of **poor sanitation**, **infections**, and multiple **nutritional deficiencies**. Clinically, PEM has three forms: **dry** (thin, desiccated), **wet** (oedematous, swollen), and a **combined form** between the two extremes. The form depends on the balance of non-protein and protein sources of energy. Each of the three forms can be graded as **mild, moderate, or severe**.

The dry form, marasmus, results from **near starvation** with **deficiency** of **protein and non-protein nutrients**. The marasmic child consumes very little food – often because his mother is unable to breastfeed – and is very thin from **loss of muscle and body fat.** Marasmus is the predominant form of PEM in most developing countries. It is associated with the early abandonment or **failure of breastfeeding** and with consequent infections, most notably those causing **infantile gastroenteritis**. These infections result from improper hygiene and inadequate knowledge of infant rearing that are prevalent in the rapidly growing slums of developing countries. In marasmus, **energy intake is insufficient** for the body's requirements, and **the body draws on its own stores. Liver glycogen** is exhausted within a few hours, and **skeletal muscle protein** is then used via glucogenogenesis to maintain adequate plasma glucose. At the same time, **triglycerides in fat depots** are **broken down into free fatty acids**, which provide some energy for most tissues, but not for the nervous system. When near starvation is prolonged, **fatty acids** are incompletely oxidized **to ketone bodies**, which **can be used by the brain** and other organs for energy. Marasmic infants have **hunger, gross weight loss, growth retardation**, and **wasting of subcutaneous fat and muscle**.

The wet form is called kwashiorkor, an African word meaning "**first child-second child.**" It refers to the observation that the first child develops PEM when the **second child** is born and **replaces the first child at the breast**. The weaned child is fed a thin gruel of poor nutritional quality (compared with mother's milk) and **fails to thrive.** Kwashiorkor is less common and is usually manifested as marasmic kwashiorkor. It tends to be confined to **parts of the world** (rural Africa, the Caribbean and Pacific islands) where staple and weaning foods – such as **yam, cassava, sweet potato, and green banana – are protein deficient and excessively starchy.** Kwashiorkor is characterised by generalized **oedema**; flaky paint **dermatosis**; **thinning**, **de-colouration**, and **reddening** of the hair, **enlarged fatty liver**; and **apathy** in addition to **retarded growth.**

Starvation

Starvation is the structural and functional changes due to the **total lack of intake of energy and essential nutrients**. Starvation is the most severe form of malnutrition. It may result **from fasting, famine, anorexia nervosa, and catastrophic disease of the gastrointestinal tract, stroke, or coma.** The basic metabolic response to starvation is conservation of energy and body tissues. However, the body will mobilize its own tissues as a source of energy, which results in the **destruction of visceral organs and muscle** and in extreme **shrinkage of adipose tissue**. Total starvation is **fatal in 8 to 12 weeks.**

Symptoms and signs

Loss of organ weight is **greatest** in the **liver and intestine, moderate** in the **heart and kidneys**, and **least in nervous system. Muscle mass shrinks** and **bones protrude**. The **skin** becomes **thin, dry, inelastic, pale and cold.** The hair is dry and sparse and falls out easily. Most body systems are affected. Intellect remains clear, but **apathy and irritabilit**y are common. The patient feels weak.

Exercise 1a
Match the column A with the column B. Try to learn the expressions and/ or sentences by heart.

A

1. Protein-energy malnutrition is characterized not only by an energy deficit due to a reduction in all macro-nutrients
2. Although severe malnutrition (kwashiorkor and/ or marasmus) are rare except in countries hit by natural disasters such as drought and war,
3. Clinically, PEM has three forms: dry (thin, desiccated), wet (oedematous, swollen),
4. The dry form, marasmus, results from near starvation
5. Marasmus is associated with the early abandonment or failure of breastfeeding
6. In marasmus, energy intake is insufficient for the body's requirements
7. Liver glycogen is exhausted within a few hours, and skeletal muscle protein
8. Triglycerides in fat depots are broken down into free fatty acids,
9. Marasmic infants have hunger,
10. The wet form is called kwashiorkor,
11. The weaned child is fed a thin gruel of poor nutritional quality
12. Yam, cassava, sweet potato, and green banana
13. Kwashiorkor is characterised by generalized oedema; flaky paint dermatosis;
14. Starvation is the structural and functional changes
15. It may result from fasting, famine, anorexia nervosa,
16. The body will mobilize its own tissues as a source of energy,
17. In starvation, loss of organ weight is greatest in the liver and intestine,
18. Muscle mass shrinks and bones protrude; the skin becomes thin, dry, inelastic, pale and cold

B

a) *(compared with mother's milk) and fails to thrive.*
b) *an African word meaning "first child-second child."*
c) *and a combined form between the two extremes.*
d) *and catastrophic disease of the gastrointestinal tract, stroke, or coma.*
e) *and the body draws on its own stores.*
f) *and with consequent infections, most notably those causing infantile gastroenteritis.*
g) *are protein deficient and excessively starchy.*

h) *but also by a deficit in many micro-nutrients (nutritional anaemia, vitamin A deficiency, and iodine deficiency).*

i) *due to the total lack of intake of energy and essential nutrients.*

j) *gross weight loss, growth retardation, and wasting of subcutaneous fat and muscle.*

k) *intellect remains clear, but apathy and irritability are common.*

l) *is then used via glucogenogenesis to maintain adequate plasma glucose.*

m) *mild and moderate malnutrition are quite common.*

n) *moderate in the heart and kidneys, and least in nervous system.*

o) *thinning, de-colouration, and reddening of the hair, enlarged fatty liver; and apathy in addition to retarded growth.*

p) *which provide some energy for most tissues, but not for the nervous system.*

q) *which results in the destruction of visceral organs and muscle and in extreme shrinkage of adipose tissue.*

r) *with deficiency of protein and non-protein nutrients.*

Risks of malnutrition
Persons in the following circumstance may be at risk of malnutrition:

Infancy and childhood: Because of the **high demand** for energy and essential nutrients, infants and children are at particular risk of under-nutrition. Protein-energy malnutrition in children consuming inadequate amounts of protein, calories, and other nutrients is a particularly **severe form of under-nutrition** that **retards growth and development**. Haemorrhagic **disease of the newborn,** a life-threatening disorder, is due to **inadequate vitamin K**. **Deficiencies of iron, folic acid, vitamin C, copper, zinc, and vitamin A** may occur in inadequately fed infants and children. In **adolescence**, nutritional requirements increase because the growth rate increases. **Anorexia nervosa**, a form of starvation, may affect adolescent girls.

Pregnancy and lactation: Requirements for all nutrients are increased during pregnancy and lactation. **Aberrations of diet**, including pica (the consumption of non-nutritive substances, such as clay and charcoal), are common in pregnancy. **Anaemia** due to folic acid deficiency is common in pregnant women, especially those who have taken oral contraceptives. **Folic acid supplements** are now recommended for pregnant women to prevent neural tube defects (spina bifida) in their children. An exclusively breastfed infant can develop vitamin B_{12}

deficiency if the mother is a **vegan**. An **alcoholic mother** may have a handicapped and stunted child with **foetal alcohol syndrome**, which is due to the effects of ethanol and malnutrition of foetal development.

Old age: A diminished sense of **taste and smell,** loneliness, physical and mental **handicaps**, **immobility**, and chronic **illness** can militate against adequate dietary intake in the elderly. Absorption is reduced, possibly contributing to **iron deficiency, osteoporosis** (also related to **calcium deficiency**), and **osteomalacia** due to **lack of vitamin D** and absence of exposure to sunshine. With ageing – independent of disease or dietary deficiency – there is progressive **loss of lean body mass**, amounting to about 10 kg in men and 5 kg in women. It accounts for the decrease in BMR, total body weight, skeletal mass, and height and for the increase in mean body fat (as percentage of body weight) from about 20 to 30% in men and from 27 to 40% in women. These changes and a **reduction in physical activity** result in **lower energy and protein requirements** compared with those of younger adults.

Chronic disease: In patients with chronic disease, malabsorption states (including those resulting from surgery) tend to **impair the absorption** of fat-soluble vitamins, vitamin B_{12}, calcium, and iron. **Liver disease** impairs the storage of vitamins A and B_{12} and interferes with the metabolism of protein and energy sources. Patients with **kidney disease**, including those on dialysis, are prone to develop deficiencies of protein, iron, and vitamin D. Some patients with **cancer** and many with **AIDS** have anorexia, which complicates treatment. In patients receiving long-term **home parenteral nutrition** – most commonly after total or near-total **resection of the gut** – vitamin and trace mineral deficiencies must be especially guarded against. A physician should ensure that **biotin, vitamin K, selenium, molybdenum, manganese, and zinc** are adequately **supplied**.

Vegetarian diets: The most common form of vegetarianism is **ovo-lacto vegetarianism**, in which meat and fish are eschewed but **eggs and dairy products are eaten**. Iron deficiency is the only risk. Ovo-lacto vegetarians tends to live longer and to develop fewer chronic disabling conditions than their meat-eating peers. However, their lifestyle usually includes **regular exercise and abstention from alcohol and tobacco**, which may contribute to their **better health**. **Vegans** consume **no animal products** and are susceptible to **vitamin B_{12} deficiency**. Yeast extracts and oriental-style fermented foods provide this vitamin. Intake of calcium, iron, and zinc also tends to be low. A **fruitarian diet**, which consists solely of fruit, is deficient in protein, salt, and many micro-nutrients and is **not recommended.**

Fad diets: Many commercial diets are claimed to enhance

well-being or reduce weight. A physician should be alert to early evidence of **nutrient deficiency or toxicity** in patients adhering to them. Such diets have resulted in frank **vitamin, mineral, and protein deficiency** states and **cardiac, renal, and metabolic disorders** as well as some deaths. Very low calorie diets cannot sustain health for long. Some trace mineral supplements have induced toxicity.

Alcohol or drug dependency: Patients with alcohol or drug problems are notoriously unreliable when questioned about their eating habits, so making judicious inquiries of relatives or acquaintances may be necessary. **Addiction** leads to a **disturbance of lifestyle** in which adequate nourishment is neglected. **Absorption and metabolism** of nutrients are also **impaired**. High levels of alcohol are poisonous and can cause **tissue injury**, particularly of the **GI tract, liver, pancreas, brain, and peripheral nervous system**. Beer drinkers who continue to consume food may gain weight, but alcoholics who consume hard liquor loose weight and become undernourished. **Drug addicts** are usually **emaciated**. Alcoholism is the most common cause of thiamine deficiency and may lead to deficiencies of magnesium, zinc, and other vitamins.

Exercise 1b
Match the column A with the column B. Try to learn the expressions and/ or sentences by heart.

A

1. Because of the high demand for energy and essential nutrients,
2. Haemorrhagic disease of the newborn,
3. Deficiencies of iron, folic acid, vitamin C, copper, zinc, and vitamin A
4. In adolescence, nutritional requirements increase
5. Requirements for all nutrients
6. Anaemia due to folic acid deficiency
7. An alcoholic mother may have a handicapped and stunted child with foetal alcohol syndrome,
8. In the elderly absorption is reduced, possibly contributing to
9. These changes and a reduction in physical activity result in
10. Liver disease impairs the storage of vitamins A and B_{12} and interferes with
11. Patients with kidney disease, including those on dialysis,
12. In patients receiving long-term home parenteral nutrition, most commonly after total or near-total resection of the gut,

13. A physician should ensure that
14. The most common form of vegetarianism is ovo-lacto vegetarianism,
15. Ovo-lacto vegetarians tend to live longer
16. Their lifestyle usually includes regular exercise and abstention from alcohol and tobacco,
17. A physician should be alert to early evidence
18. Such diets have resulted in frank vitamin, mineral, and protein deficiency states
19. Addiction leads to a disturbance of lifestyle
20. High levels of alcohol are poisonous and can cause

h) *in which adequate nourishment is neglected.*
i) *in which meat and fish are eschewed but eggs and dairy products are eaten.*
j) *infants and children are at particular risk of under-nutrition.*
k) *iron deficiency, osteoporosis (also related to calcium deficiency), and osteomalacia due to lack of vitamin D and absence of exposure to sunshine.*
l) *is common in pregnant women, especially those who have taken oral contraceptives.*
m) *lower energy and protein requirements compared with those of younger adults.*
n) *may occur in inadequately fed infants and children.*
o) *of nutrient deficiency or toxicity in patients adhering to fad diets.*
p) *the metabolism of protein and energy sources.*
q) *tissue injury, particularly of the GI tract, liver, pancreas, brain, and peripheral nervous system.*
r) *vitamin and trace mineral deficiencies must be especially guarded against.*
s) *which is due to the effects of ethanol and malnutrition of foetal development.*
t) *which may contribute to their better health.*

B

a) *a life-threatening disorder, is due to inadequate vitamin K.*
b) *and cardiac, renal, and metabolic disorders as well as some deaths.*
c) *and to develop fewer chronic disabling conditions than their meat-eating peers.*
d) *are increased during pregnancy and lactation.*
e) *are prone to develop deficiencies of protein, iron, and vitamin D.*
f) *because the growth rate increases.*
g) *biotin, vitamin K, selenium, molybdenum, manganese, and zinc are adequately supplied.*

Exercise 2
Translate the expressions. Try to explain their meanings in English.

Under-nutrition, over-nutrition, recognized, regarded, kwashiorkor, marasmus, rare, disasters, drought, prevalence, deleterious, desiccated, oedematous, swollen, mild, moderate, severe, predominant, consequent, rearing, prevalent, insufficient, exhausted, fat depots, incompletely oxidized, growth retardation, wasting, subcutaneous, observation, weaned child, thin gruel, fails to thrive, protein deficient, excessively starchy, dermatosis, thinning, retarded growth, starvation, fasting, coma, conservation of energy, destruction of visceral organs, shrinkage of adipose tissue, apathy and irritability, circumstance, retards growth, development, haemorrhagic disease, newborn, life-threatening disorder, inadequately, requirements, aberrations, pica, contraceptives, folic acid, supplements, spina bifida, stunted, osteomalacia, exposure to sunshine, accounts for, requirements, compared, impair, interferes with, prone to, home parenteral nutrition, resection of the gut, guarded against, disabling conditions, contribute, susceptible to, oriental-style fermented foods, tends to, physician, be alert, evidence of, sustain health, unreliable, eating habits, disturbance of, lifestyle, poisonous, hard liquor, undernourished, drug addicts.

Exercise 3
Answer the following questions. Prepare short talks and/or dialogues on these topics.

1. What is protein-energy malnutrition (PEM)?
2. Talk about the dry form, marasmus.
3. Talk about the wet form, kwashiorkor.
4. Starvation as the most severe form of malnutrition, causes and symptoms.
5. Talk about the risks of malnutrition in infancy and childhood.
6. Talk about the risks of malnutrition in pregnancy and lactation.
7. Talk about the risks of malnutrition in elderly and chronically ill patients.
8. Dangers of malnutrition in alcohol or drug dependency.

Vocabulary 9

Fill in the meanings in your mother language:

abandonment /ə'bæn.dən.mənt/
abstention /əb'stenʃən/
adhere /əd'hɪər/
adolescence /ˌæd.ə'les.əns/
affected /ə'fekt.ɪd/
alert /ə'lɜːt/
apathy /'æpəθi/
breastfeed /'brest.fiːd/
cassava /kə'sɑː.və/
charcoal /'tʃɑːr.koʊl/
circumstance /'sɜː.kəm.stɑːnt s/
clay /kleɪ/
compare /kəm'peər/

confined /kən'faɪnd/
consequent /'kɒnsɪkwənt/
conservation /ˌkɒn.sə'veɪ.ʃən/
consume /kən'sjuːm/
context /'kɒntekst/
deficit /'def.ɪ.sɪt/
deleterious /ˌdel.ɪ'tɪə.ri.əs/
dermatosis /ˌdɜr mə'toʊ sɪs/
desiccated /'des.ɪ.keɪ.tɪd/
diminished /dɪ'mɪn.ɪ.ʃt/
disabling /dɪ'seɪ.blɪŋ/
disaster /dɪ'zɑː.stər/
draw /drɔː/
drought /draʊt/
drug /drʌg/ **addict** /'æd.ɪkt/
emaciated /ɪ'meɪ.si.eɪ.tɪd/
eschew /ɪs'tʃuː/
exclusively /ɪk'skluː.sɪv.li/
exhausted /ɪg'zɔː.stɪd/
extract /ɪk'strækt/
extreme /ɪk'striːm/
fad /fæd/
failure /'feɪ.ljə/
famine /'fæmɪn/
fast /fɑːst/
fatal /'feɪ.təl/
ferment /fə'ment/
flake /fleɪk/
foetal /'fiː.təl/ **alcohol** /'æl.kə.hɒl/ **syndrome** /'sɪn.drəʊm/
frank /fræŋk/
fruitarian /fru'tɛər i ən/
gastroenteritis /ˌgæs.trəʊˌen.tə'raɪ.tɪs/
grade /greɪd/
gross /grəʊs/
gut /gʌt/
handicap /'hændɪkæp/
hard /hɑːd/ **liquor** /'lɪkər/
hunger /'hʌŋ.gər/
immobility /ˌɪm.ə'bɪl.ə.ti/
impair /ɪm'peər/
infantile /'ɪn.fən.taɪl/
inquiry /ɪn'kwaɪə.rɪ/
interfere /ˌɪn.tə'fɪər/
irritability /ˌɪr.ɪ.tə'bɪl.ɪ.ti/
judicious /dʒuː'dɪʃəs/
ketone /'kiː.təʊn/ **body** /'bɒd.i/
loneliness /'ləʊn.li.nəs/
mild /maɪld/
militate /'mil.ɪ.teɪt/
mobilize /'məʊ.bɪ.laɪz/
moderate /'mɒd.ər.ət/
multiple /'mʌl.tɪ.pl̩/
neural /'njʊə.rəl/
notably /'nəʊ.tə.bli/
notorious /nəʊ'tɔːriəs/
oedematous /ɪ'diː.mə.təs/
overnutrition /'əʊ.vər.njuː'trɪʃ.ən/
paint /peɪnt/
particular /pə'tɪk.jʊ.lər/
peer /pɪər/
pica /'paɪ kə/
prevalence /'prevələns/
prevalent /'prev.əl.ənt/
prone /prəʊn/
protrude /prə'truːd/
rear /rɪər/
regard /rɪ'gɑːd/
requirement /rɪ'kwaɪə.mənt/
resection /rɪ'sek.ʃən/
retard /rɪ'tɑːd/
rural /'rʊərəl/
sanitation /ˌsæn.ɪ'teɪ.ʃən/
severe /sɪ'vɪər/
shrinkage /'ʃrɪŋ.kɪdʒ/
slum /slʌm/
socioeconomic /ˌsəʊ.si.əʊˌek.ə'nɒm.ɪk/
solely /'səʊl.lɪ/
sparse /spɑːs/
spina bifida /ˌspaɪ.nə'bɪf.ɪ.də/
starchy /'stɑː.tʃi/
starvation /stɑː'veɪ.ʃən/
stunt /stʌnt/
thrive /θraɪv/
tube /tjuːb/
undernutrition /ˌʌn dər nu'trɪʃ ən/
unreliable /ˌʌn.rɪ'laɪə.bl̩/
visceral /'vɪs.ər.əl/
wasting /weɪst.ɪŋ/
wean /wiːn/

World /wɜːld/ **Health** /helθ/ **Organization** /ˌɔːgənaɪˈzeɪʃən/ **WHO**

Solution to Exercise 1a
1h, 2m, 3c, 4r, 5f, 6e, 7l, 8p, 9j, 10b, 11a, 12g, 13o, 14i, 15d, 16q, 17n, 18k

Solution to Exercise 1b
1j, 2a, 3n, 4f, 5d, 6l, 7s, 8k, 9m, 10p, 11e, 12r, 13g, 14i, 15c, 16t, 17o, 18b, 19h, 20q

Unit 10 - Obesity. Eating disorders.

Another form of malnutrition, which is associated with altered immune responses, is obesity. In contrast to under-nutrition, obesity results from "**over-nutrition**" - dietary intake above the need and requirement of an individual leading to higher body weight for height. In addition to obesity, there is **malnutrition in premature infants** which results from **maternal nutritional deficiencies, hypertension, or smoking.** These infants are usually born with reduced body reserves of different nutrients and only **partially mature immune system.** As a result they ought to be monitored both nutritionally as well as for morbidity due to infection.

Traditionally, obesity has been defined as a body weight of more than 30% above ideal or desirable weight on standard height. Now, it is usually defined in terms of the **body mass index (BMI)** – **weight (in kilograms) divided by the square of the height (in meters).** The prevalence of obesity varies significantly by **sex, age, socio-economic status, and race.** In one sense, the cause of obesity is simple – **expending less energy than is consumed.** But in another sense, it is exclusive; involving the regulation of body weight, primarily body fat. How this regulation is achieved is not yet fully understood. Weight is regulated with great precision. Regulation of body weight is believed to occur not only in person of normal weight but also among many obese persons, in whom obesity is attributed to an elevation in the set point around which weight is regulated. The **determinants of obesity** can be divided into the **genetic**, the **environmental**, and the **regulatory**.

Genetic determinants: Recent discoveries have helped explain how genes may determine obesity and how they may influence the regulation of body weight. For example, mutations in the **ob gene** have led to massive obesity in mice. Cloning the ob gene led to the identification of **leptin, a protein coded by this gene;** leptin is produced **in adipose tissue cells** and acts to control body fat. The existence of leptin supports the idea that **body weight is regulated**, because **leptin serves as a signal between adipose tissue** and the areas of the **brain that control energy metabolism,** which influences body weight.

Environmental determinants: The fact that genetic influences account for only 33% of the variation in body weight means that the **environment exerts an enormous influence**. This influence is dramatically illustrated by the marked increase in the prevalence of obesity in the past decade. Socio-economic status is an important influence on obesity, particularly among women. The negative correlation between socio-economic status and obesity reflects an underlying cause. Longitudinal studies have shown that **growing up with lower socio-economic status** is a powerful **risk factor for obesity**. Socio-economic factors are major influences on both **energy intake** and **energy expenditure. A sedentary lifestyle**, so prevalent in Western societies, is another major environmental influence promoting obesity. Physical activity not only expends energy but also helps control food intake.

Regulatory determinants: **Pregnancy** is a major determinant of obesity in some women. Although most women weigh only a little bit more a year after delivery, about 15% weigh 8-10 kg more with each pregnancy.

An **increase in fat cells** and **adipose tissue mass** during **infancy and childhood** – and for some severely obese persons, even during **adulthood – predisposes to obesity**. This increase can result in five times as many fat cells in obese persons as in persons with normal weight. **Dieting reduces only fat cell size, not all fat cell number**. As a result, persons with hyper-cellular adipose tissue can reduce to a normal weight only by markedly **depleting the lipid content** of each cell. Such depletion and the associated events at the cell membrane may set a **biologic limit on their ability to lose weight** and may explain their difficulty in reducing to a normal weight. Drugs have recently been added to the list of determinants of obesity because of the increased use of pharmacotherapy. **Limiting the use of drug treatment** to prevent weight gain may present a serious therapeutic dilemma.

Endocrine factors have been traditionally viewed as important determinants of obesity. **Hyperinsulinism** from pancreatic neoplasms, **hypercortisolism** from Cushing's syndrome, the **ovarian dysfunction** of poly-cystic ovary syndrome, and **hypothyroidism** have all been implicated in some cases of obesity, but endocrine determinants affect only a very small number of obese persons.

Psychological **factors**, once viewed as important determinants of obesity, are now believed to be limited largely to **two deviant eating patterns. Binge eating disorder** is characterized by the consumption of **large amounts of food in a short time** with a subjective sense of loss of control during the binge and distress after it. Unlike patients with bulimia nervosa, these patients **do not engage in compensatory behaviours**, such as vomiting; thus their binges contribute to excessive caloric intake. Binge eating disorder is believed to occur in 10 – 20% of persons entering weight reduction programs. **The night-eating syndrome** consists of morning anorexia, evening hyperphagia, and insomnia. It occurs in about 10% of persons seeking treatment for obesity.

The symptoms and signs of obesity consist of immediate consequences of the **large adipose tissue mass**. Prominent among them is **sleep apnoea**, a seriously under-diagnosed disorder, characterized by moments during sleep when **breathing ceases**, as often as hundreds of times a night. In the obesity-**hypoventilation syndrome (pickwickian syndrome)** impairment of breathing leads to **hypercapnia**, a reduced effect of CO_2 in stimulating respiration, **hypoxia**, **cor pulmonale**, and a risk of **premature death.**

Obesity may lead to orthopaedic **disturbances** of weight-bearing and non-weight-bearing joints. **Skin disorders** are particularly common; increased sweat and skin secretions, trapped in thick folds of skin, produce a culture medium conducive to **fungal and bacterial growth** and infections. The level of general psychopathology, as assessed by psychological tests, does not differ between persons who are obese and those who are not. However, for some young women in upper and middle socio-economic groups, **psychological problems** are **linked to obesity.** The current view is that the intense prejudice and discrimination to which obese persons are subjected is the source of these problems. In addition to the eating disorders noted above, these problems include disparagement of **body image,** a condition in which persons feel that their body is grotesque and loathsome. These women believe that others view them with hostility and contempt, which makes them self-conscious and **impairs social functioning.**

Exercise 1a
Match the column A with the column B. Try to learn the expressions and/or sentences by heart.

A

1. In contrast to under-nutrition, obesity results from over-nutrition;
2. Malnutrition in premature infants
3. Obesity is usually defined in terms of the body mass index (BMI) ;
4. The cause of obesity is
5. The determinants of obesity
6. Body weight is regulated, because leptin serves as a signal between adipose tissue
7. Growing up with lower socio-economic status
8. Socio-economic factors are major influences
9. An increase in fat cells and adipose tissue mass during infancy and childhood
10. Dieting reduces only fat cell size,
11. Persons with hyper-cellular adipose tissue can reduce to
12. Hyperinsulinism from pancreatic neoplasms, hypercortisolism from Cushing's syndrome,
13. Binge eating disorder is characterized by the consumption of large amounts of food in a short time

14. Unlike patients with bulimia nervosa, patients with binge eating disorder do not engage in
15. The night-eating syndrome consists of
16. Sleep apnoea is characterized by moments during sleep
17. In the obesity-hypoventilation syndrome (pickwickian syndrome) impairment of breathing
18. Increased sweat and skin secretions
19. Psychological problems linked to obesity

B

a) a normal weight only by markedly depleting the lipid content of each cell.
b) and the areas of the brain that control energy metabolism, which influences body weight.
c) can be divided into the genetic, the environmental, and the regulatory.
d) compensatory behaviours, such as vomiting; thus their binges contribute to excessive caloric intake.
e) dietary intake above the need of an individual leading to higher body weight for height.
f) expending less energy than is consumed.
g) impair social functioning.
h) is a powerful risk factor for obesity.
i) on both energy intake and energy expenditure.
j) leads to hypercapnia, hypoxia, cor pulmonale, and a risk of premature death.
k) morning anorexia, evening hyperphagia, and insomnia.
l) not all fat cell number.
m) predisposes to obesity.
n) produce a culture medium conducive to fungal and bacterial growth and infections.
o) results from maternal nutritional deficiencies, hypertension, or smoking.
p) the ovarian dysfunction of poly-cystic ovary syndrome, and hypothyroidism have all been implicated in some cases of obesity.
q) weight (in kilograms) divided by the square of the height (in meters).
r) when breathing ceases, as often as hundreds of times a night.
s) with a subjective sense of loss of control during the binge and distress after it.

Eating disorders

Eating disorders often are **long-term illnesses** that may require long-term treatment. In addition, eating disorders frequently occur with other mental disorders such as **depression**, **substance abuse**, and **anxiety disorders**. The earlier these disorders are diagnosed and treated, the better the chances are for full recovery. This fact sheet identifies the common

signs, symptoms, and treatment for three of **the most common eating disorders**: anorexia nervosa, bulimia nervosa, and binge-eating disorder. More than 90% of those who have eating disorders are women between the ages of 12 and 25.

Anorexia nervosa

A disorder characterized by a disturbed sense of body image, a **morbid fear of obesity**, a refusal to maintain a minimally normal body weight, and, in women, amenorrhoea. The aetiology is unknown, but **social factors** appear to be important. Emphasis on the **desirability of being thin** pervades Western society, and obesity is considered unattractive, unhealthy, and undesirable. Some persons are probably **predisposed** because of undefined **psychologic, genetic, or metabolic vulnerability**. Anorexia nervosa is **rare in areas with a genuine food shortage**. About 95% of persons who have anorexia are women.

People who have anorexia develop unusual eating habits such as **avoiding food** and meals, **picking out a few foods** and eating them in **small amounts,** weighing their food, and **counting the calories** of everything they eat. Also, they may **exercise excessively.** Anorexia can **slow the heart rate** and **lower blood pressure**. Those who **use drugs** to stimulate **vomiting, bowel movements**, or **urination** are also at high risk for **heart failure**. Starvation can also lead to heart failure, as well as **damage the brain**. Anorexia may also cause **hair and nails** to grow **brittle**. Mild **anaemia, swollen joints, reduced muscle mass**, and **light-headedness** also commonly occur as a consequence of this eating disorder.

Symptoms and signs

Many persons who develop the disorder are **meticulous, compulsive, and intelligent**, with very high standards for achievement and success. The first indications of the impending disorder are **concern about body weight** and restriction of food intake. Patients usually **resist treatment**. Patients are often manipulative, lying about food intake and **concealing** behaviour, such as **induced vomiting**. Binge eating followed by induced vomiting and the use of laxatives and diuretics occurs in 50% of anorectics. Even patients who appear cachectic tend to remain very active (including pursuing **vigorous exercise** programs), are free of symptoms of nutritional deficiencies, and have **no unusual susceptibility to infections. Depression** is common.

Treatment

Treatment has two phases: **short-term intervention** to restore body weight and save life and **long-term therapy** to improve psychologic functioning and prevent relapse. The first goal for treatment is to ensure the person's physical health, which involves **restoring a healthy body weight**. Treatment usually involves **individual** psychotherapy and **family** therapy. **Behavioural therapy** also has been effective for helping a person return to healthy eating habits.

Bulimia nervosa

People who have bulimia **eat an excessive amount of food** in a single episode and almost **immediately make themselves vomit or use laxatives or diuretics** to get rid of the food in their bodies. They have an intense **fear of gaining weight**. The **acid** in vomit can **wear down** the outer layer of **the teeth, inflame** and damage the **oesophagus**, and **enlarge** the **glands** near the cheeks (giving the appearance of **swollen cheeks**). Damage to the **stomach** can also occur from frequent vomiting. **Irregular heartbeats, heart failure, and death** can occur from chemical imbalances and the **loss of important minerals** such as potassium. **Peptic ulcers, pancreatitis,** and long-term **constipation** are also consequences of bulimia. Unless malnutrition is severe, any **substance abuse problems** are usually treated first. The next goal of treatment is to reduce or eliminate the person's binge eating and purging behaviour.

Binge-eating disorder

People with this recently recognized disorder have frequent episodes of **compulsive overeating**, but unlike those with bulimia, they **do not purge their bodies of food.** During these food binges, they often **eat alone and very quickly**, regardless of whether they feel hungry or full. They often **feel shame or guilt** over their actions. Unlike anorexia and bulimia, binge-eating disorder occurs almost **as often in men as in women**. Binge-eating disorder can cause **high blood pressure** and **high cholesterol** levels. Other effects of binge-eating disorder include **fatigue, joint pain, type II diabetes, gallbladder disease, and heart disease.**

Exercise 1b
Match the column A with the column B. Try to learn the expressions and/or sentences by heart.

A

1. Eating disorders frequently occur with other mental disorders
2. Anorexia nervosa is characterized by a disturbed sense of body image,
3. Some persons are probably predisposed
4. Anorexia nervosa is rare
5. People who have anorexia develop unusual eating habits such as
6. Those who use drugs to stimulate
7. Mild anaemia, swollen joints, reduced muscle mass, and light-headedness
8. The first indications of the impending disorder are
9. Patients are often manipulative, lying about food intake
10. Even patients who appear cachectic tend to remain very active,

11. The first goal for treatment is to ensure the person's physical health,
12. People who have bulimia eat an excessive amount of food in a single episode and almost immediately
13. The acid in vomit can wear down the outer layer of the teeth,
14. Irregular heartbeats, heart failure, and death can occur from chemical imbalances
15. Peptic ulcers, pancreatitis, and long-term constipation
16. People with binge-eating disorder have frequent episodes of compulsive overeating,
17. Unlike anorexia and bulimia,
18. Binge-eating disorder can cause high blood pressure and high cholesterol levels;

B

a) *a morbid fear of obesity, a refusal to maintain a minimally normal body weight, and, in women, amenorrhoea.*
b) *also commonly occur as a consequence of this eating disorder.*
c) *and concealing behaviour, such as induced vomiting.*
d) *and the loss of important minerals such as potassium.*
e) *are also consequences of bulimia.*
f) *are free of symptoms of nutritional deficiencies, and have no unusual susceptibility to infections.*
g) *avoiding food and meals, picking out a few foods and eating them in small amounts, weighing their food, and counting the calories of everything they eat.*
h) *because of undefined psychologic, genetic, or metabolic vulnerability.*
i) *binge-eating disorder occurs almost as often in men as in women.*
j) *but unlike those with bulimia, they do not purge their bodies of food.*
k) *concern about body weight and restriction of food intake.*
l) *in areas with a genuine food shortage.*
m) *inflame and damage the oesophagus, and enlarge the glands near the cheeks.*
n) *make themselves vomit or use laxatives of diuretics to get rid of the food in their bodies.*
o) *other effects include fatigue, joint pain, type II diabetes, gallbladder disease, and heart disease.*
p) *such as depression, substance abuse, and anxiety disorders.*
q) *vomiting, bowel movements, or urination are also at high risk for heart failure.*
r) *which involves restoring a healthy body weight.*

Exercise 2
Translate the expressions. Try to explain their meanings in English.

Altered immune responses, premature infants, morbidity, desirable, divided by, prevalence, expending, achieved, precision, attributed to, elevation, discoveries, genes, adipose tissue, supports, account for, exerts, marked increase, correlation, underlying cause, longitudinal studies, growing up, expenditure, sedentary lifestyle, promoting, after delivery, predisposes to, depleting, determinants, affect, deviant eating patterns, binge eating disorder, distress, compensatory behaviours, hyperphagia, insomnia, seeking treatment, consequences, prominent, sleep apnoea, weight-bearing joints, fungal and bacterial growth, current view, prejudice, hostility and contempt, mental disorders, substance abuse, anxiety disorders, recovery, body image, morbid fear, refusal, amenorrhoea, aetiology, desirability, predisposed, vulnerability, genuine, food shortage, picking out, counting the calories, exercise excessively, bowel movements, urination, brittle hair and nails, swollen joints, light-headedness, compulsive, achievement, success, impending disorder, concern about, restriction, resist treatment, concealing behaviour, pursuing, vigorous exercise, susceptibility, intervention, prevent relapse, make themselves vomit, use laxatives of diuretics, get rid of, wear down the teeth, inflame the oesophagus, enlarge the glands, peptic ulcers, pancreatitis, constipation, binge eating, purging behaviour, feel shame or guilt, fatigue.

Exercise 3
Answer the following questions. Prepare short talks and/or dialogues on these topics.

1. Obesity as a form of malnutrition.
2. Genetic determinants of obesity.
3. Environmental determinants of obesity.
4. Regulatory determinants of obesity (nutrition during infancy and childhood, pregnancy, endocrine factors)
5. Describe binge eating disorder.
6. Describe anorexia nervosa (characteristics, symptoms and signs, treatment).
7. What is the difference between bulimia nervosa and binge-eating disorder?

Vocabulary 10

Fill in the meanings in your mother language:

abuse /əˈbjuːz/
achievement /əˈtʃiːv.mənt/
adulthood /ˈæd.ʌlt.hʊd/
amenorrhoea /eɪˌmɛn əˈri ə/
anorexia nervosa /æn.əˌrek.si.ə.nəˈvəʊ.sə/
anxiety /æŋˈzaɪ.ə.ti/
disorder /dɪˈsɔː.dər/
avoid /əˈvɔɪd/

bear /beə/ **weight** /weɪt/
behavioural /bɪˈheɪ.vjə.rəl/
binge /bɪndʒ/
bowel /ˈbaʊ.əl/ **movement** /ˈmuːv.mənt/
bulimia /bjuːˈlɪmɪə/
nervosa /nɜːˈvəʊsə/
cachectic /kəˈkɛk.tik/
cachexia /kəˈkɛk si ə/
cease /siːs/
cloning /ˈkloʊ.nɪŋ/
code /kəʊd/
compensatory /ˌkɒm.pənˈseɪt.ə ri/
compulsive /kəmˈpʌl.sɪv/
conceal /kənˈsiːl/
conducive /kənˈdjuːsɪv/
consequence /ˈkɒn.sɪ.kwəns/
contempt /kənˈtempt/
cor pulmonale /ˈkɔr ˌpʊl məˈnæl i/
correlation /ˌkɒrəˈleɪʃən/
current /ˈkʌr.ənt/
Cushing's /ˈkʌʃ.ɪŋz/
syndrome /ˈsɪndrəʊm/
deplete /dɪˈpliːt/
determinant /dɪˈtɜː.mɪ.nənt/
deviant /ˈdiːviənt/
dilemma /daɪˈlem.ə/
discovery /dɪˈskʌvəri/
discrimination /dɪˌskrɪm.ɪˈneɪ.ʃən/
disparagement /dɪˈspær ɪdʒ mənt/
distress /dɪˈstres/
diuretic /ˌdaɪ.jʊə ˈret.ɪk/
divide /dɪˈvaɪd/
dysfunction /dɪsˈfʌŋk.ʃən/
eating /iː.tɪŋ/ **disorder** /dɪˈsɔː.dər/
elevation /ˌel.ɪˈveɪ.ʃən/
emphasis /ˈem.fə.sɪs/
engage /ɪnˈgeɪdʒ/
enlarge /ɪnˈlɑːdʒ/
enormous /ɪˈnɔːməs/
environment /ɪnˈvaɪə .rən .mənt/
exclusive /ɪkˈskluː.sɪv/
exert /ɪgˈzɜːt/
expenditure /ɪkˈspendɪtʃər/
fungal /ˈfʌŋ.gəl/
genuine /ˈdʒɛn jʊ ɪn/
get /get/ **rid** /rɪd/ **of** /əv/
gland /glænd/
goal /gəʊl/
guilt /gɪlt/
hypercapnia /ˌhaɪ.pə.kæp.niə/
hypercellular /ˌhaɪ pərˈseljələr/
hypercortisolism /ˌhaɪ pərˈkɔr təˌsɔˌlɪz əm/
hyperinsulinism /ˌhaɪ pərˈɪn sə lɪˌnɪz əm/
hyperphagia /ˌhaɪ pərˈfeɪ dʒi ə/
hypothyroidism /ˌhaɪ pəˈθaɪ rɔɪˌdɪz əm/
hypoventilation /ˌhaɪ. pəʊˌven.tɪˈleɪ.ʃən/
hypoxia /haɪˈpɒk.sɪə/
image /ˈɪm.ɪdʒ/
impending /ɪmˈpen.dɪŋ/
induce /ɪnˈdjuːs/
inflame /ɪnˈfleɪm/
influence /ˈɪn.flʊ.əns/
intervention /ˌɪn.təˈven.ʃən/
laxative /ˈlæk.sə.tɪv/
leptin /ˈlɛp tɪn/
lie /laɪ/
light-headedness /ˌlaɪtˈhed.ɪd.nəs/
lipid /ˈlɪp.ɪd/
loathsome /ˈləʊð.səm/
longitudinal /ˌlɒn.dʒɪˈtjuː.dɪ.nəl/
manipulative /məˈnɪp jəˌleɪ tɪv/
markedly /ˈmɑː.kɪd.li/
mature /məˈtjʊər/
meticulous /məˈtɪk.jʊ.ləs/
mice /maɪs/
morbid /ˈmɔː.bɪd/
mutation /mjuːˈteɪ.ʃən/
neoplasm /ˈniː.ə.plæz.əm/
ob gene /dʒiːn/
ought /ɔːt/
ovarian /əʊˈveə.ri.ən/
ovary /ˈəʊ.vər.i/
overeat /ˌoʊ vərˈit/
pancreatitis /ˌpæŋ.krɪ.əˈtaɪ.tɪs/
partially /ˈpɑː.ʃəl.i/

peptic /'pep.tɪk/ **ulcer** /'ʌl.sər/
pervade /pər'veɪd/
pharmacotherapy / ˌfɑr mə koʊ'θɛr ə pi/
pick /pɪk/ **out** /aʊt/
pickwickian /pɪk'wɪk i ən/ **syndrome** /'sɪn droʊm/
polycystic /ˌpɒlɪ'sɪstɪk/ **ovary** / 'əʊvərɪ/ **syndrome** /'sɪndrəʊm/
powerful /'paʊə.fəl/
precision /prɪ'sɪʒən/
predispose /ˌpriː.dɪ'spəʊz/
prejudice /'predʒ.ʊ.dɪs/
primarily /praɪ'mer.ɪ.li/
prominent /'prɒm.ɪ.nənt/
promote /prə'məʊt/
psychopathology /ˌsaɪ. kəʊ.pə'θɒl.ə.dʒi/
purge /pɜːdʒ/
pursue /pə'sjuː/
race /reɪs/
reflect /rɪ'flekt/
refusal /rɪ'fjuː.zəl/
regulator /'reg.jʊ.leɪ.tər/
relapse /rɪ'læps/
restriction /rɪ'strɪk.ʃən/
sedentary /'sed.ən.tər.i/
self-conscious /self.kɒn.ʃəs/
shame /ʃeɪm/
sheet /ʃiːt/
sleep /sliːp/ **apnoea** /'æp.ni.ə/
square /skweər/
sweat /swet/
syndrome /'sɪn.drəʊm/
trapped /træpd/
undefined /ˌʌn dɪ'faɪnd/
underdiagnose /'ʌndə'daɪəgnəʊz/
vigorous /'vɪg.ər.əs/
wear /weə/ **down** /daʊn/
weigh /weɪ/

Solution to Exercise 1a
1e, 2o, 3q, 4f, 5c, 6b, 7h, 8i, 9m, 10l, 11a, 12p, 13s, 14d, 15k, 16r, 17j, 18n, 19g

Solution to Exercise 1b
1p, 2a, 3h, 4l, 5g, 6q, 7b, 8k, 9c, 10f, 11r, 12n, 13m, 14d, 15e, 16j, 17i, 18o

Unit 11 - Food-borne diseases. Biological hazards. Pathogenic bacteria 1.

Food-borne disease is caused by **contaminated foods or beverages**. More than 250 different food-borne diseases have been described. There are four types of hazards in food that can cause illness, injury and even death:

- **biological hazards** are living organisms including **bacteria, parasites, viruses, moulds, natural toxins and prions.**
- **chemical hazards** include **cleaners, sanitizers, pesticides, paints** and other chemicals that can make food dangerous to eat.
- **physical hazards** are substances that can cause choking or internal injury. These include items such as **glass, metal, wood chips, and jewellery**.
- **allergens** are substances that can cause an allergic reaction – **fish, shellfish, nuts, eggs, dairy products, sulphites, soy products, sesame seeds, wheat,** and others.

These different diseases have many **different symptoms**, so there is no syndrome that is food-borne illness. However, the microbe or toxin enters the body through the **gastrointestinal tract**, and often causes the first symptoms there, so **nausea, vomiting, abdominal cramps and diarrhoea** are common symptoms in many food-borne diseases.

We live in a microbial world, and there are many opportunities for food to become contaminated as it is produced and prepared. Many food-borne **microbes** are present in healthy **animals** (usually in their **intestines**) raised for food. **Meat and poultry carcasses** can become contaminated during **slaughter** by contact with small amounts of intestinal contents. Similarly, fresh **fruits and vegetables** can be contaminated if they are **washed or irrigated** with water that is contaminated with **animal manure or human sewage**. Later in food processing, other food-borne microbes can be introduced from infected humans who handle the food, or by **cross contamination** from some other raw **agricultural products.**

The **spectrum** of food-borne diseases is constantly changing. A century ago, **typhoid fever, tuberculosis and cholera** were common food-borne diseases. Today food-borne infections have taken their place. **Newly recognized microbes** emerge as public health problems for several reasons: microbes can easily spread around the world, new microbes can evolve, the environment and ecology are changing, **food production practices** and **consumption habits** change, and because **laboratory tests** can now identify microbes that were previously unrecognised.

Factors of food-borne diseases prevalence

The most important factors in the prevalence of food-borne illness are the **lack of knowledge** on the part of **food handlers and consumers** and **negligence** (despite knowledge) in safe food handling. Surveys of food-borne disease outbreak worldwide have shown that most cases of food-borne disease occur as the result of an **error in handling food** during preparation, whether in **homes**, in **food service** and **catering establishments**, in the **canteens** of hospitals, schools or the military, or at **banquets** and **parties**. Most cases of food-borne disease could have been avoided – even when the original foodstuff was contaminated.

Most food-borne disease outbreaks result from food handling leading to contamination with and/or survival and growth of micro-organisms:

- **contamination with micro-organisms**:
  use of contaminated **equipment**
  contamination by infected **persons**
  use of contaminated raw **ingredients**
  cross-contamination

addition of toxic **chemicals** or use of foods containing natural toxicants
- **survival of micro-organisms**: inadequate **heating** inadequate **cooking**
- **growth of micro-organisms**: inadequate **refrigeration** inadequate **cooling** keeping food **insufficiently hot**

Improvements in standards of **personal hygiene**, the development of basic **sanitation**, safe **water supplies**, effective **vaccination** programs, food **control** infrastructure, and the increasing application of technologies such as **pasteurization** have either **eradicated** or considerably reduced many food-borne diseases (e.g. **poliomyelitis, brucellosis, cholera, typhoid and paratyphoid fevers and milk-borne salmonellosis)** in industrialized countries. Nevertheless, food-borne diseases remain a widespread **public health** problem in these countries.

The dominant problems are **salmonellosis** and **campylobacteriosis**. Industrialized countries have also been affected by a number of new or newly recognized food-borne diseases such as **listeriosis** and **enterohaemorrhagic *E. coli*** infections. Due to rigorous monitoring and to food safety and **quality controls** by large food manufacturers and retailers, the food supply is generally safe from chemicals. Nevertheless, accidental contamination or adulteration does occur. In both Europe and North America, **misidentification of mushrooms** is one of the **leading causes** of illness and death from chemical intoxicants.

Incidence of some food-borne diseases has decreased following specific prevention programs. For example, **freezing of meat** has contributed to the **decline of trichinellosis**. Most continuing outbreaks are **due to under-cooking** of **pork and game** meat. Another disease of which the incidence had decreased tremendously and which has even been eradicated in some countries is brucellosis. This success should be attributed to animal health measures and the pasteurization of milk. Unfortunately, too many cases of **brucellosis** still occur in some industrialized countries due to consumption or utilization of **raw milk or cheese made with raw milk**.

Exercise 1a
Match the column A with the column B. Try to learn the expressions and/ or sentences by heart.

A

1. Food-borne disease is caused by
2. Biological hazards are living organisms
3. Chemical hazards include
4. Physical hazards are substances that can cause choking or internal injury;

5. Allergens are substances that can cause an allergic reaction;
6. The microbe or toxin enters the body through the gastrointestinal tract,
7. Meat and poultry carcasses can become contaminated
8. Fresh fruits and vegetables can be contaminated
9. In food processing, other food-borne microbes can be introduced from infected humans
10. Microbes can easily spread around the world, new microbes can evolve,
11. Food handling leading to contamination with micro-organisms:
12. Food handling leading to survival and growth of micro-organisms:
13. Improvements in standards of personal hygiene, the development of basic sanitation, safe water supplies, effective vaccination programs, application of technologies such as pasteurization
14. The dominant problems are
15. Newly recognized food-borne diseases
16. Misidentification of mushrooms
17. Freezing of meat has contributed to the decline of trichinellosis;
18. Brucellosis still occurs in some industrialized countries

B

a) *and often causes the first symptoms there, such as nausea, vomiting, abdominal cramps and diarrhoea.*
b) *are listeriosis and enterohaemorrhagic E. coli infections.*
c) *cleaners, sanitizers, pesticides, paints and other chemicals that can make food dangerous to eat.*
d) *contaminated foods or beverages.*
e) *due to consumption or utilization of raw milk or cheese made with raw milk.*
f) *during slaughter by contact with small amounts of intestinal contents.*
g) *fish, shellfish, nuts, eggs, dairy products, sulphites, soy products, sesame seeds, wheat, and others.*
h) *have either eradicated or considerably reduced many food-borne diseases (e.g. poliomyelitis, brucellosis, cholera, typhoid and paratyphoid fevers and milk-borne salmonellosis).*
i) *if they are washed or irrigated with water that is contaminated with animal manure or human sewage.*
j) *inadequate heating, inadequate cooking, inadequate refrigeration, inadequate cooling, keeping food insufficiently hot.*

k) *including bacteria, parasites, viruses, moulds, natural toxins and prions.*
l) *is one of the leading causes of illness and death from chemical intoxicants.*
m) *most continuing outbreaks are due to under-cooking of pork and game meat.*
n) *or by cross contamination from raw agricultural products.*
o) *salmonellosis and campylobacteriosis.*
p) *the environment and ecology are changing, and food production practices and consumption habits change.*
q) *the use of contaminated equipment, contamination by infected persons, use of contaminated raw ingredients, cross-contamination, addition of toxic chemicals.*
r) *these include items such as glass, metal, wood chips, and jewellery.*

Biological hazards

Biological hazards in food can have four possible effects. They can:

- be present in food **without causing food-borne illnesses** or affecting people (i.e., inert);
- **be beneficial** in food production (e.g., yeasts);
- cause food to spoil without causing illness in humans (i.e., **food spoilage** organisms);
- be **pathogenic** (i.e., can cause illness and death).

Biological hazards are living organisms including:

- **pathogenic bacteria**
- **parasitic protozoa and helminths**
- **viruses**
- **moulds**
- natural **toxins**
- other pathogenic agents – **prions**.

Pathogenic bacteria 1

Bacteria are single-celled micro-organisms that live in **air, water, soil**, or in the **bodies of humans or animals**. Food-borne disease can occur when food or water contaminated with bacteria or their toxins is ingested.

***Escherichia coli* O157: H7**

Most illness has been associated with eating **undercooked, contaminated ground beef**. **Person-to person contact** in families and childcare centres is also an important mode of transmission. Infection can also occur after drinking **raw milk** and after swimming or drinking **sewage-contaminated water**. Bacteria in diarrhoeal stools of infected persons can be passed from one person to another if **hygiene or hand washing habits** is **inadequate**. This is particularly likely among **toddlers** who are not toilet trained. Most persons recover without antibiotics or other specific treatment in 5 – 10 days.

- **cook** all ground beef thoroughly.
- avoid spreading harmful bacteria in your kitchen. **Keep raw meat separate** from ready-to-eat foods. **Wash hands, counters, and utensils** with hot **soapy water** after they touch raw meat. Never place cooked ground beef on the unwashed plate that held raw patties.
- drink only **pasteurised milk, juice or cider**. Commercial juice with an extended shelf life that is sold at room temperature has been pasteurised although this is generally not indicated on the label.
- **wash fruits and vegetables** thoroughly, especially those that will not be cooked.
- drink municipal **water** that has been **treated with chlorine** or other effective disinfectants. Avoid swallowing lake or pool water while swimming.
- make sure that children **wash their hands** carefully with soap **after bowel movements**, and that persons wash hands after changing soiled diapers.

Salmonella spp.

The *Salmonella* germ is actually a group of bacteria that can cause diarrhoeal illness in humans. They are microscopic living creatures that **pass from faeces of people or animals to other people or animals**. Most people develop **diarrhoea, fever, and abdominal cramps**. The illness usually lasts 4 to 7 days and most persons recover without treatment. The elderly, infants, and those with impaired immune systems are more likely to have a severe illness.

Salmonella live in the intestinal tracts of **humans** and other **animals**, including **birds**. Contaminated foods usually **look and smell normal.** Contaminated foods are often of animal origin, such as **beef, poultry, milk or eggs**, but all foods, including vegetables may become contaminated. Thorough cooking kills *Salmonella.*

- **Cook poultry, ground beef, and eggs thoroughly** before eating.
- **Do not eat** or drink foods containing **raw eggs, or raw unpasteurized milk.** Note: Raw eggs may be unrecognised in some foods such as home-made **hollandaise sauce,** caesar and other **salad dressings**, **tiramisu**, home-made **ice cream**, home-made **mayonnaise**, cookie **dough**, and **frostings**.
- Be particularly **careful with foods** prepared **for infants**. Breast-feeding prevents

salmonellosis and many other health problems.

Clostridium botulinum

Clostridium botulinum is an anaerobic, Gram-positive spore-forming rod that produces a potent **neurotoxin**. The **spores are heat-resistant** and can survive in foods that are incorrectly or minimally processed. The organism and its spores are widely distributed in nature. They occur in both cultivated and forest **soils**, bottom sediments of **streams, lakes,** and **coastal waters**, and in the intestinal tracts of **fish and mammals**, and in the gills and viscera of crabs and other **shellfish. Food-borne botulism** (as **distinct** from **wound** botulism and **infant** botulism) is a severe type of **food poisoning** caused by the ingestion of foods containing the potent **neurotoxin** formed during growth of the organism. The **toxin** is heat labile and **can be destroyed if heated at 80°C for 10 minutes and longer. Sausages, meat products, canned vegetables and seafood products** have been the most frequent vehicles for human botulism. Early signs of **intoxication** consists of marked **lassitude, weakness and vertigo**, usually followed by **double vision** and progressive **difficulty in speaking and swallowing**. Difficulty in **breathing, weakness** of other muscles, **abdominal distension**, and **constipation** may also be common symptoms. Botulinal toxin has been demonstrated in a considerable variety of foods, such as **canned corn, peppers, green beans, soups, beets, asparagus, mushrooms, ripe olives, spinach, tuna fish, chicken and chicken livers and liver pâté, and luncheon meats, ham, sausage, stuffed eggplant, lobster, and smoked and salted fish.**

Staphylococcus aureus

Staphylococcus aureus is a spherical bacterium (coccus). Some strains are capable of producing a highly heat-stable protein toxin that causes illness in humans. The onset of symptoms is usually rapid and the most common **symptoms** are **nausea, vomiting, retching, abdominal cramping, and prostration**. In more severe cases, **headache, muscle cramping**, and transient changes in **blood pressure** and **pulse rate** may occur. Recovery generally takes two days.

Foods that are frequently incriminated in staphylococcal food poisoning include meat and **meat** products; **poultry and egg products**; **salads such as egg, tuna, chicken, potato, and macaroni**; bakery products such as **cream-filled pastries, cream pies, and chocolate éclairs; sandwich fillings; and milk and dairy products.** Foods that require considerable handling during preparation and that are kept at slightly elevated temperatures after preparation are frequently involved in staphylococcal food poisoning. ***Staphylococci*** are present in the **nasal passages and throats** and on the **hair and skin** of 50% or more of healthy individuals. Human intoxication is caused by ingesting enterotoxins produced in food usually because the food has not been kept **hot enough (60°C**, or above) or **cold enough (7.2°C**, or bellow).

Exercise 1b
Match the column A with the column B. Try to learn the expressions and/or sentences by heart.

A

1. Biological hazards are living organisms including:
2. Bacteria are single-celled micro-organisms that live
3. *Escherichia coli* - illness has been associated
4. Person-to person contact in families and childcare centres
5. Bacteria in diarrhoeal stools of infected persons can be passed from one person to another
6. Cook all ground beef thoroughly
7. Keep raw meat separate
8. Wash hands, counters, and utensils with hot soapy water
9. Wash fruits and vegetables thoroughly,
10. Make sure that children wash their hands
11. The *Salmonella* germ is actually a group
12. The bacteria pass from faeces of people or animals
13. Contaminated foods usually
14. Contaminated foods are often beef, poultry, milk or eggs,
15. Do not eat or drink foods
16. Raw eggs may be unrecognised in
17. *Clostridium botulinum* produces a potent neurotoxin;
18. Food-borne botulism is a severe type of food poisoning
19. The toxin can be destroyed
20. Sausages, meat products, canned vegetables and seafood products have been
21. Signs of intoxication consists of marked lassitude, weakness and vertigo,
22. Botulinal toxin has been demonstrated in
23. *Staphylococcus aureus* can produce
24. The most common symptoms are
25. Foods that are frequently incriminated in staphylococcal food poisoning include meat and meat products; poultry and egg products;
26. Staphylococci are present in the nasal passages and throats

B

a) a highly heat-stable protein toxin that causes illness in humans.
b) after they touch raw meat.
c) and drink only pasteurised milk, juice or cider.
d) and on the hair and skin of 50% or more of healthy individuals.

e) *but all foods, including vegetables may become contaminated.*
f) *canned corn, peppers, green beans, soups, beets, asparagus, mushrooms, ripe olives, spinach, tuna fish, chicken and chicken livers and liver pâté, and luncheon meats, ham, sausage, stuffed eggplant, lobster, and smoked and salted fish.*
g) *carefully with soap after bowel movements.*
h) *caused by the ingestion of foods containing the potent neurotoxin formed during growth of the organism.*
i) *containing raw eggs, or raw unpasteurized milk.*
j) *especially those that will not be cooked.*
k) *from ready-to-eat foods.*
l) *home-made hollandaise sauce, salad dressings, tiramisu, ice cream, mayonnaise, cookie dough, and frostings.*
m) *if heated at 80°C for 10 minutes and longer.*
n) *if hygiene or hand washing habits is inadequate.*
o) *in air, water, soil, or in the bodies of humans or animals.*
p) *is also an important mode of transmission*
q) *look and smell normal.*
r) *nausea, vomiting, retching, abdominal cramping, and prostration.*
s) *of bacteria that can cause diarrhoeal illness in humans.*
t) *pathogenic bacteria, parasitic protozoa and helminths, viruses, moulds, natural toxins and other pathogenic agents (prions).*
u) *salads such as egg, tuna, chicken, potato, and macaroni; bakery products such as cream-filled pastries, cream pies, and chocolate éclairs; sandwich fillings; and milk and dairy products.*
v) *the most frequent vehicles for human botulism.*
w) *the spores can survive in foods that are incorrectly or minimally processed.*
x) *to other people or animals and most people develop diarrhoea, fever, and abdominal cramps.*
y) *usually followed by double vision and progressive difficulty in speaking and swallowing.*
z) *with eating undercooked, contaminated ground beef.*

Exercise 2
Translate the expressions. Try to explain their meanings in English.

Living organisms, moulds, prions, sanitizers, pesticides, choking, internal injury, wood chips, sulphites, cramps, intestines, slaughter, irrigated, animal manure or human sewage, introduced from, agricultural products, recognized, emerge, evolve, consumption habits, identify, prevalence, negligence, handling, disease outbreak, survival and growth, equipment, ingredients, refrigeration, insufficiently hot, sanitation, water supplies, vaccination, eradicated, poliomyelitis, brucellosis, typhoid and paratyphoid fevers, salmonellosis, campylobacteriosis, listeriosis, enterohaemorrhagic *E. coli,* rigorous monitoring, retailers, adulteration, decline of, tremendously, be attributed to, inert, beneficial, spoilage, moulds, prions, ingested, parasitic protozoa, helminths, mode of transmission, sewage-contaminated water, stools, be passed, habits, toddlers, recover, avoid spreading, extended shelf life, treated with disinfectants, bowel movements, abdominal cramps, potent neurotoxin, food poisoning, lassitude, weakness and vertigo, double vision, abdominal distension, constipation, retching, cramping, prostration, transient changes, slightly elevated, nasal passages.

Exercise 3
Answer the following questions. Prepare short talks and/or dialogues on these topics.

1. Describe biological, chemical and physical hazards and the danger of allergens.
2. Common symptoms in food-borne diseases.
3. Opportunities for food to become contaminated.
4. The spectrum of food-borne diseases.
5. Factors of food-borne diseases prevalence.
6. Contamination with and survival and growth of micro-organisms.
7. Food-borne diseases, incidence and the leading causes.
8. What do you understand by biological hazards?
9. Pathogenic bacteria and possible prevention.
10. Illness associated with *Escherichia coli.*
11. Illness associated with *Salmonella spp.*
12. Illness associated with *Clostridium botulinum*
13. Illness associated with *Staphylococcus aureus*

Vocabulary 11

Fill in the meanings in your mother language:

adulteration /əˌdʌl.təˈreɪ.ʃən/
agricultural /ˌæg.rɪˈkʌl.tʃər.əl/
allergen /ˈæl.ə.dʒən/
bacteria /bækˈtɪə.ri.ə/
banquet /ˈbæŋkwɪt/
beneficial /ˌben.ɪˈfɪʃ.əl/
beverage /ˈbev.ər.ɪdʒ/
bottom /ˈbɒt.əm/
brucellosis /ˌbru səˈloʊ sɪs/
campylobacteriosis /ˌkæmpɪləʊˈbæktə.riəʊ.sɪs/
canteen /kænˈtiːn/
capable /ˈkeɪ.pə.blˌ/
carcass /ˈkɑːkəs/
catering /ˈkeɪtərɪŋ/
choke /tʃəʊk/
cholera /ˈkɒlərə/
cleaner /ˈkliː.nər/
Clostridium /klɒˈstrɪ.dɪ.əm/
botulinum /ˈbɒt.jʊ.lɪ.nəm/
coastal /ˈkəʊstəl/
coccus /ˈkɒk əs/ pl **cocci** /koksai/
contaminated /kənˈtæm.ɪ.neɪ.tɪd/

cookie /ˈkʊki/
cooking /ˈkʊkɪŋ/
cooling /kuːlɪŋ/
counter /kaʊntə/
crab /kræb/
cream /kriːm/
creature /ˈkriː.tʃər/
cross-contamination /ˌkrɒs.kən.tæm.ɪˈneɪ.ʃən/
diaper /ˈdaɪəpər/
dough /dəʊ/
dressing /ˈdres.ɪŋ/
E. coli /ˌiːˈkəʊ.laɪ/
éclair /ɪˈkleər/
eggplant /ˈegplɑːnt/
elevated /ˈel.ɪ.veɪ.tɪd/
enterohaemorrhage /ˌɛn təˈrɒˈhɛmərɪdʒ/
enterotoxin /ˌɛn tə roʊˈtɒk sɪn/
equipment /ɪˈkwɪp.mənt/
eradicate /ɪˈræd.ɪ.keɪt/
establishment /ɪˈstæb.lɪʃ.mənt/
evolve /ɪˈvɒlv/
filling /ˈfɪl.ɪŋ/
food-borne /fuːdˈbɔːrn/
foodstuff /ˈfuːdstʌf/
frosting /ˈfrɒstɪŋ/
game /geɪm/
gill /gɪl/
Gram /græm/ **-positive** /ˈpɒz.ə.tɪv/
green /griːn/ **bean** /biːn/
ground /graʊnd/ **beef** /biːf/
handler /ˈhænd.lər/
hazard /ˈhæz.əd/
heat /hiːt/ **-stable** /ˈsteɪbl/
heating /ˈhiː.tɪŋ/
helminth /ˈhɛl mɪnθ/
hollandaise /ˌhɒl.ənˈdeɪz/ **sauce** /sɔːs/
homemade /ˌhəʊmˈmeɪd/
identify /aɪˈden.tɪ.faɪ/
incorrectly /ˌɪnkərˈekt.li/
incriminate /ɪnˈkrɪmɪneɪt/
inert /ɪnˈɜːt/
infrastructure /ˈɪn.frəˌstrʌk.tʃər/
ingredient /ɪnˈgriː.di.ənt/
injury /ˈɪn.dʒər.i/
irrigate /ˈɪr.ɪ.geɪt/
labile /ˈleɪ.baɪl/
lassitude /ˈlæs.ɪ.tjuːd/
listeriosis /lɪˌstɪə.riˈəʊ.sɪs/
lobster /ˈlɒbstər/
mammal /ˈmæm.əl/
manufacturer /ˌmæn.jʊˈfæk.tʃər.ər/
manure /məˈnjʊər/
measure /ˈmeʒ.ər/
microbe /ˈmaɪ.krəʊb/
military /ˈmɪl.ɪ.tər.i/
mode /məʊd/
mould /məʊld/
mushroom /ˈmʌʃ.ruːm/
nasal /ˈneɪ.zəl/
natural /ˈnætʃ.ər.əl/
nausea /ˈnɔː.zi.ə/
negligence /ˈneg.lɪ.dʒəns/
outbreak /ˈaʊtˌbreɪk/
parasite /ˈpær.ə.saɪt/
parasitic /ˌpær.əˈsɪt.ɪk/
paratyphoid /ˌpærəˈtaɪfɔɪd/
pass /pɑːs/
passage /ˈpæs.ɪdʒ/
pasteurise /ˈpæs.tʃər.aɪz/
pasteurization /ˌpæstəraɪˈzeɪʃən/
pastry /ˈpeɪstri/
pâté /ˈpæteɪ/
patty /ˈpæti/
pesticide /ˈpes.tɪ.saɪd/
pie /paɪ/
poliomyelitis /poʊ.li.oʊ.maɪ.ə.laɪ.tɪs/
potent /ˈpəʊ.tənt/
previously /ˈpriː.vi.əs.li/
prion /ˈpraɪ.ɒn/
prostration /prɒˈstreɪ ʃən/
protozoan /ˌprəʊ.təˈzəʊ.ən/ pl **protozoa**
raise /reɪz/
raw /rɔː/
refrigeration /rɪˌfrɪdʒ.əˈreɪ.ʃən/
retailer /ˈriːteɪlər/
retch /retʃ/
rigorous /ˈrɪgərəs/

ripe /raɪp/
rod /rɒd/
salmonella /ˌsæl.mə'nel.ə/
pl **salmonellae**
salmonellosis /ˌsæl mə nl'oʊ sɪs/
salt /sɔːlt/
sanitizer /'sæn ɪˌtaɪ zər/
separate /'sep.ər.ət/
sewage /'suː.ɪdʒ/
shelf /ʃelf/ **life** /laɪf/
slaughter /'slɔːtər/
smoke /sməʊk/
soapy /'səʊpi/
soiled /sɔɪld/
spherical /'sfer.ɪ.kəl/
spoil /spɔɪl/
spoilage /'spɔɪ lɪdʒ/
spread /spred/
Staphylococcus /ˌstæf ə lə'kɒk əs/ ***aureus*** /'ɔːrɪəs/
Staphylococcus /ˌstæf ə lə'kɒk əs/
stool /stuːl/
strain /streɪn/
stream /striːm/
stuff /stʌf/
sulphite /'sʌl faɪt/
survival /sə'vaɪ.vəl/
tiramisu /ˌtɪr.ə.mɪ'suː/
toddler /'tɒd.lər/
touch /tʌtʃ/
toxin /'tɒk.sɪn/
transient /'træn.zi.ənt/
tremendously /trɪ'mendəs.li/
trichinellosis /ˌtrɪk ə'nəloʊ sɪs/
tuberculosis /tjuːˌbɜː.kjʊ'ləʊ.sɪs/
typhoid /'taɪfɔɪd/ **fever** /'fiːvər/
undercook /ˌʌn.də'kʊk/
utensil /juː'tensəl/
vaccination /ˌvæk.sɪ'neɪ.ʃən/
vehicle /'viː.ɪ.klˌ/
vertigo /'vɜː.tɪ.gəʊ/
viscera /'vɪs.ər.ə/
vomit /'vɒmɪt/
widespread /ˌwaɪd'spred/
wood /wʊd/ **chips** /tʃɪps/

Solution to Exercise 1a
1d, 2k, 3c, 4r, 5g, 6a, 7f, 8i, 9n, 10p, 11q, 12j, 13h, 14o, 15b, 16l, 17m, 18e

Solution to Exercise 1b
1t, 2o, 3z, 4p, 5n, 6c, 7k, 8b, 9j, 10g, 11s, 12x, 13q, 14e, 15i, 16l, 17w, 18h, 19m, 20w, 21y, 22f, 23a, 24r, 25u, 26d

Unit 12 - Pathogenic bacteria 2

Campylobacter jejuni

Birds carry it without becoming ill. The bacterium is fragile. It **cannot tolerate drying** and can be **killed by oxygen**. Campylobacteriosis occur much more frequently in the summer months than in winter. Many different kinds of infection can cause diarrhoea and **bloody diarrhoea**. Patients should drink plenty of fluid as long as the diarrhoea lasts. One way to become infected is to cut **poultry** meat on a cutting board, and then use the **unwashed cutting board or utensil** to prepare **vegetables** or other raw or lightly cooked foods. Many **chicken flocks** are silently infected with *Campylobacter*, that is, the chickens are infected with the organism but show **no signs of illness.** This infection is common in the developing world. Surface water and mountain streams can become contaminated from infected faeces from cows and wild birds. **Travellers** to foreign countries are also at risk for becoming infecter with *Campylobacter.*

Prevention

- Make sure that the meat is cooked throughout (no longer pink), and juices run clear, and the inside is **cooked to 77°C** for breast meat and **82°C** for thigh meat.

Yersinia enterocolitica

The major animal reservoir for *Yersinia enterocolitica* strains that cause human illness is **pigs**, but other strains are also found in many other animals including **rodents, rabbits, sheep, cattle, horses, dogs, and cats**. Children are infected more often than adults. Most infections are uncomplicated and resolve completely. Occasionally, some persons develop **joint pain**, most commonly in the knees, ankles or wrists. A skin rash may also appear on the legs and trunk.

Prevention

- After handling raw chitterlings, **clean hands and fingertips** scrupulously with soap and water **before touching infants or their toys, bottles, or pacifiers.** Some other than the food-handler should care for children while chitterlings are being prepared.
- **Prevent cross-contamination** in the kitchen
- **Dispose of animal faeces** in a sanitary manner

Listeria monocytogenes

Listeriosis is a **serious infection** caused by eating food contaminated with the bacterium *Listeria monocytogenes.* The disease affects primarily **pregnant women, newborns**, and adults with **weakened immune systems**. Infection during pregnancy can lead to **miscarriage** or **stillbirth**, **premature delivery**, or infection of the newborn. *Listeria monocytogenes* is found in soil and water. **Vegetables** can become **contaminated** from the soil or from **manure** used as fertilizer. The bacterium has been found in a variety of raw foods, such as **uncooked meats and vegetables**, as well as in processed foods that become contaminated after processing, such as soft cheeses and cold cuts at the **deli counter**. In certain ready-to-eat foods such as hot dogs and deli meats, contamination may occur after cooking but before packaging.

Prevention

- Thoroughly **cook raw food** from animal sources, such as beef, pork, or poultry.
- **Wash raw veg thoroughly** before eating.
- Keep **uncooked meats separate** from vegetables and from cooked foods and ready-to-eat foods.
- **Avoid raw milk or foods** made from unpasteurized milk.

- **Wash hands, knives, and cutting boards** after handling uncooked foods.
- **Consume** perishable and ready-to-eat foods **as soon as possible.**
- Do not eat **hot dogs, luncheon meats, or deli meats**, unless they are **reheated until steaming hot.**
- **Avoid getting fluid from hot dog packages** on other foods, utensils, and food preparation surfaces, and wash hands after handling hot dogs, luncheon meats, and deli meats.
- Do not eat soft cheeses such as **feta, Brie, and Camembert, blue-veined cheeses**, or Mexican style cheeses such as **queso blanco, queso fresco, and Panela**, unless they have labels that clearly state they are **made from pasteurised milk.**
- **Do not eat refrigerated pâtés or meat spreads.** Canned or shelf-stable pâtés and meat spreads may be eaten.
- Do not eat **refrigerated smoked seafood**, unless it is contained in a cooked dish, such as a casserole. Refrigerated smoked seafood, such as salmon, trout, whitefish, cod, tuna or mackerel, is most often labelled as "nova-style," "lox," "kippered," "smoked," or "jerky." The fish is found in the refrigerator section or sold at deli counters of grocery stores and delicatessens. **Canned or shelf-stable smoked seafood may be eaten.**

Exercise 1a
Match the column A with the column B. Try to learn the expressions and/or sentences by heart.

A

1. *Campylobacter jejuni*
2. One way to become infected is to cut poultry meat on a cutting board,
3. Many chicken flocks are silently infected with *Campylobacter*,
4. Make sure that the meat is cooked throughout (no longer pink), and juices run clear,
5. The major animal reservoir for *Yersinia enterocolitica* strains
6. Some persons develop joint pain in the knees, ankles or wrists and
7. After handling raw chitterlings, clean hands and fingertips
8. Listeriosis is a serious infection
9. Infection during pregnancy can lead to
10. In certain ready-to-eat foods such as hot dogs and deli meats,
11. Consume perishable and

12. Do not eat hot dogs, luncheon meats, or deli meats,
13. Do not eat soft cheeses such as feta, Brie, and Camembert, blue-veined cheeses, queso blanco, queso fresco, and Panela,
14. Canned or shelf-stable
15. Do not eat refrigerated smoked seafood,

B

a) a skin rash may also appear on the legs and trunk.
b) and the inside is cooked to 77°C for breast meat and 82°C for thigh meat.
c) and then use the unwashed cutting board or utensil to prepare vegetables or other raw or lightly cooked foods.
d) before touching infants or their toys, bottles, or pacifiers.
e) cannot tolerate drying and can be killed by oxygen.
f) caused by eating food contaminated with the bacterium Listeria monocytogenes.
g) contamination may occur after cooking but before packaging.
h) is pigs, rodents, rabbits, sheep, cattle, horses, dogs, and cats.
i) miscarriage or stillbirth, premature delivery, or infection of the newborn.
j) pâtés and meat spreads may be eaten.
k) ready-to-eat foods as soon as possible.
l) that is, the chickens are infected with the organism but show no signs of illness.
m) unless it is contained in a cooked dish, such as a casserole.
n) unless they are reheated until steaming hot.
o) unless they have labels that clearly state they are made from pasteurised milk.

Vibrio cholerae serogroup O1

Cholera is the name of the infection caused by *Vibrio cholerae.* Symptoms of Asiatic cholera may vary from mild, **watery diarrhoea** to acute diarrhoea, with characteristic rice water stools. Onset of the illness is usually sudden. **Abdominal cramps, nausea, vomiting, dehydration, and shock**; after severe **electrolyte loss,** death may occur. Cholera is generally a disease spread by poor sanitation. Individuals infected with cholera **require rehydration** either intravenously or orally with a **solution** containing **sodium chloride, sodium bicarbonate, potassium chloride, and dextrose (glucose**).

Vibrio cholerae serogroup Non-O1

This bacterium infects only **humans and other primates**. It causes a disease reported to be less severe than cholera. **Diarrhoea, abdominal cramps and fever** are the predominant symptoms. Consumption of raw, improperly cooked, re-contaminated **shellfish** may lead to infection. **Antibiotics such as tetracycline** shorten the severity and duration of the illness. **Septicaemia** (bacteria gaining entry into the blood stream and multiplying therein) can occur. This complication is associated with individuals with **cirrhosis** of the liver, or who are immunosuppressed but this is relatively rare.

Vibrio parahaemolyticus

Vibrio parahaemolyticus lives in brackish saltwater and causes gastrointestinal illness in humans. It is present in higher concentrations during summer. It is halophilic, or **salt-requiring organism.** When ingested *Vibrio parahaemolyticus* causes watery **diarrhoea** often with abdominal **cramping, nausea, vomiting, fever and chills**. It can also cause an **infection of the skin** when an open wound is exposed to warm saltwater. Most people become infected by eating raw or undercooked shellfish, particularly oysters.

Vibrio vulnificus

Vibrio vulnificus, a lactose-fermenting, halophilic, gram-negative, opportunistic pathogen is found in estuarine environments and associated with various **marine species** such as **plankton, shellfish** (oysters, clams, and crabs), and **finfish**. This organism causes **wound infections, gastroenteritis**, or a syndrome known as "**primary septicaemia.**" Wound infections result from containing an open wound or by lacerating part of the body on coral, fish, etc., followed by contamination with the organism. All individuals who consume foods contaminated with organism are susceptible to gastroenteritis. Individuals with **diabetes, cirrhosis, or leukaemia**, or those who take **immunosuppressive drugs** or steroids are particularly **susceptible to primary septicaemia**. These individuals should be strongly advised not to consume raw or inadequately cooked seafood, as should AIDS/ARC patients.

Exercise 1b
Match the column A with the column B. Try to learn the expressions and/or sentences by heart.

A

1. Cholera is the name of the infection
2. Abdominal cramps, nausea, vomiting, dehydration,
3. Individuals infected with cholera require rehydration either intravenously or orally
4. *Vibrio cholerae serogroup Non-O1* infects only humans and other primates;
5. Antibiotics such as tetracycline
6. Septicaemia (bacteria gaining entry
7. *Vibrio parahaemolyticus* causes watery diarrhoea
8. It can also cause an infection of the skin

9. *Vibrio vulnificus* is associated with
10. Wound infections result from containing an open wound
11. Individuals with diabetes, cirrhosis, or leukaemia, or those who take

B

a) *and shock; after severe electrolyte loss, death may occur.*
b) *caused by Vibrio cholerae.*
c) *immunosuppressive drugs or steroids are particularly susceptible to primary septicaemia.*
d) *it causes a disease less severe than cholera.*
e) *often with abdominal cramping, nausea, vomiting, fever and chills.*
f) *or by lacerating part of the body on coral, fish, etc., followed by contamination with the organism.*
g) *shorten the severity and duration of the illness.*
h) *into the blood stream and multiplying therein) can occur.*
i) *various marine species such as plankton, shellfish (oysters, clams, and crabs), and finfish.*
j) *when an open wound is exposed to warm saltwater.*
k) *with a solution containing sodium chloride, sodium bicarbonate, potassium chloride, and dextrose (glucose).*

Exercise 2
Translate the expressions. Try to explain their meanings in English.

Tolerate drying, cutting board, utensil, silently infected, surface water, rodents, rabbits, sheep, cattle, resolve completely, skin rash, raw chitterlings, dispose of, miscarriage or stillbirth, premature delivery, after processing, deli counter, packaging, perishable and ready-to-eat foods, reheated until steaming hot, blue-veined cheeses, canned or shelf-stable pâtés, meat spreads, sudden onset, dehydration, require rehydration, sodium chloride, sodium bicarbonate, potassium chloride, dextrose, predominant, severity and duration, septicaemia, brackish salt-water, halophilic, fever and chills, undercooked, estuarine environments, oysters, primary septicaemia, lacerating, susceptible, immunosuppressive, advised.

Exercise 3
Answer the following questions. Prepare short talks and/or dialogues on these topics.

1. *Campylobacter jejuni,* sources, prevention of infection.
2. *Yersinia enterocolitica,* sources, prevention of infection.
3. *Listeria monocytogenes,* sources, prevention of infection.

4. What do you know about pathogenic bacteria *Vibrio cholerae serogroup O1* and *Vibrio cholerae serogroup Non-O1*?
5. Where can you find pathogenic bacteria *Vibrio parahaemolyticus* and *Vibrio vulnificus?*

Vocabulary 12

Fill in the meanings in your mother language:

advised /əd'vaɪzd/
ARC/AIDS
blue-veined /veɪnd/ **cheese** /tʃiːz/
board /bɔːd/
brackish /'bræk.ɪʃ/
Brie /briː/
Camembert /'kæm.əm.beər/
Campylobacter /ˌkæmpɪləʊ'bæktə/
jejuni /dʒɪ'dʒu naɪ/
casserole /'kæsəˌrəʊl/
cattle /'kætl/
chill /tʃɪl/
chitterlings /'tʃɪtəlɪŋz/
clam /klæm/
cold /kəʊld/ **cuts** /kʌts/
coral /'kɒrəl/
deli /delɪ/ **counter** /'kaʊntə/
delicatessen /ˌdel.ɪ.kə'tes.ən/
dextrose /'dek.strəʊs/
estuarine /'ɛs tʃu əˌraɪn/
feta /'fet.ə/
finfish /'fɪnˌfɪʃ/
flock /flɒk/
Gram /græm/ **-negative** /'neg.ə.tɪv/
grocery /'grəʊsəri/
halophilic /'hæl əˌfɪlɪk/
immunosuppressive /ˌɪm.jʊ.nəʊ.sə'pres.ɪv/
improperly /ɪm'prɒp.ər.li/
jejunum /dʒɪ'dʒuːnəm/
jerky /'dʒɜːki/
kipper /'kɪpə/
lacerate /'læs.ər.eɪt/
leukaemia /luː'kiːmiə/
Listeria /lɪ'stɪər i ə/ ***monocytogenes*** /'mɒn oʊˌsaɪ tə'dʒɛns/
lox /lɒks/
marine /mə'riːn/
meat /miːt/ **spread** /spred/
miscarriage /'mɪsˌkær.ɪdʒ/
multiply /'mʌltɪplaɪ/
onset /'ɒnˌset/
opportunistic /ˌɒpə'tjuːnɪst.ɪk/
oyster /'ɔɪ.stər/
pacifier /'pæs.ɪ.faɪ.ər/
Panela /'pæn ə lə/
perishable /'perɪʃəbl/
plankton /'plæŋktən/
potasium /pə'tæsiəm/
chloride /'klɔː.raɪd/
predominant /prɪ'dɒmɪnənt/
primate /'praɪmeɪt/
queso blanco /'keso 'blaŋko/
queso fresco /'keso 'fresko/
rabbit /'ræbɪt/
rehydration /ˌriː.haɪ'dreɪ.ʃən/
reservoir /'rez.ə.vwɑːr/
resolve /rɪ'zɒlv/
rodent /'rəʊ.dənt/
scrupulous /'skruːpjələs/
septicaemia /ˌsep.tɪ'siː.mi.ə/
sheep /ʃiːp/
shelf /ʃelf/
sign /saɪn/
silent /'saɪ.lənt/
sodium /'səʊ.di.əm/
chloride /'klɔːraɪd/
sodium bicarbonate /ˌsəʊ.di.əm.baɪ'kɑː.bən.ət/
solution /sə'luː.ʃən/
stable /'steɪbəl/
steam /stiːm/
stillbirth /'stɪl.bɜːθ/
tetracycline /ˌtɛ trə'saɪ klin/

trout /traʊt/
trunk /trʌŋk/
veined /veɪnd/
Vibrio /ˈvɪb riˌoʊ/ ***cholerae*** /ˈkɒl ər i/
Vibrio /ˈvɪb riˌoʊ/ ***parahaemolyticus*** /ˌpær əˌhiːməʊˈlɪtɪkəs/
Vibrio /ˈvɪb riˌoʊ/ ***vulnificus*** /ˈvʌl nɪfɪkəs/
watery /ˈwɔː.təri/
whitefish /ˈʰwaɪtˌfɪʃ/
Yersinia /*ˈyɜːsinjə*/ ***enterocolitica*** / ˌɛn tə roʊ kəˈlɪt ɪkə/

Solution to Exercise 1a
1e, 2c, 3l, 4b, 5h, 6a, 7d, 8f, 9i, 10g, 11k, 12o, 13n, 14j, 15m

Solution to Exercise 1b
1b, 2a, 3k, 4d, 5g, 6h, 7e, 8j, 9i, 10f, 11c

Unit 13 - Pathogenic bacteria 3. Parasitic protozoa and helminths 1.

Bacillus cereus

Bacillus cereus food poisoning is the general description although two recognized types of illness are caused by two distinct metabolites. A **wide variety of foods** including meats, milk, vegetables, and fish have been associated with the diarrhoeal type of food poisoning. The **vomiting-type outbreaks** have generally been associated with **rice products**; however other starchy foods such as **potato, pasta and cheese** have also been implicated. Food mixtures such as **sauces, puddings, soups, casseroles, pastries, and salads** have frequently been incriminated in food poisoning outbreaks. Although no specific complications have been associated with the **diarrhoeal and vomiting toxins produced by *Bacillus cereus*,** other clinical manifestations of *Bacillus cereus* invasion have been observed. They include bovine mastitis, severe systemic and pyogenic infections, **gangrene**, septic **meningitis**, **cellulitis**, **panopthalmitis**, **lung abscesses**, **infant death**, and **endocarditis**.

Aeromonas hydrophilla

Aeromonas hydrophilla is a species of bacterium that is present in all **freshwater environments** and in **brackish water**. Some strains are capable of causing illness in fish and amphibians as well as in **humans** who may acquire infection through **open wounds or ingestion** of the organisms in food or water. Two distinct types of gastroenteritis have been associated with *Aeromonas hydrophilla:* a **cholera-like illness** with a watery (rice and water) diarrhoea **and a dysenteric illness** characterised by loose stools containing blood and mucus. *Aeromonas hydrophilla* has frequently been found in **fish and shellfish**. It **also** has been found in market samples of **red meats** (beef, pork, lamb) and poultry. All people are believed to be susceptible to gastroenteritis, although it is most frequently observed in **very young children.**

Plesiomonas shigelloides

Plesiomonas shigelloides has been isolated from **freshwater**,

freshwater fish and shellfish and from many types of **animals** including **cattle, goats, swine, cats, dogs, monkeys, vultures, snakes, and toads**. The organisms may be present in **unsanitary water,** which has been used as drinking water, recreational water, or water used to rinse foods that are consumed without cooking or heating. Gastroenteritis is usually a **mild self-limiting disease**. Diarrhoea is watery, non-mucoid, and non-bloody; in severe cases, diarrhoea may be greenish-yellow, foamy, and blood tinged. Most infections occur in the **summer months** and correlate with environmental contamination of freshwater (rivers, streams, ponds etc.) All people may be susceptible to infection. **Infants, children and chronically ill** people are more likely to experience protracted illness and **complications**.

Shigella spp.

Shigellosis is an infectious disease caused by a group of bacteria called *Shigella.* In some persons, especially **young children and the elderly**, the diarrhoea can be so **severe**, that the patient needs to be hospitalised. A severe infection with high fever may also be associated with seizures in children less than 2 years old. Many different kinds if diseases can cause **diarrhoea and bloody diarrhoea**.

Shigellosis can usually be treated with **antibiotics**. Unfortunately, some **bacteria** have become **resistant** to antibiotics and using antibiotics can actually make the germs more resistant in the future. Therefore, when many persons in a community are affected by shigellosis antibiotics are sometimes used selectively to treat only the more severe cases. Shigellosis is particularly common and causes recurrent problems in settings where hygiene is poor and can sometimes sweep through entire communities. Children, especially **toddlers aged 2 to 4,** are the most likely to get **shigellosis**. Many cases are related to the spread of illness in child-care settings, and many more are the result of the spread of the illness in families with small children. In the developing world, shigellosis is far more common and is present in most communities most of the time. If you are travelling to the developing world, **wash, peel, or cook raw fruit and vegetables** before eating.

Miscellaneous enterics

The enteric (intestinal) bacteria have been suspected of causing acute and chronic gastrointestinal disease. The organisms may be recovered from natural environments such as **forests and freshwater** as well as from **farm produce** (vegetables) where they reside as normal microflora. Acute gastrointestinal illness may occur more frequently in underdeveloped areas of the world. The chronic illness is **common in malnourished children living in unsanitary conditions** in tropical countries. All people may be susceptible to pathogenic forms of these bacteria.

Protracted illness is more commonly experienced by the very young.

Streptococcus spp.

Group A: one species with 40 antigenic types cause **septic sore throat** and **scarlet fever.** Sore and red throat, **pain on swallowing, tonsillitis,** high **fever, headache, nausea, vomiting, malaise, rhinorrhea;** occasionally a **rash** occurs, onset 1- 3 days, **food sources** include **milk, ice cream, eggs, steamed lobster, ground ham, potato salad, egg salad, custard, rice pudding, and shrimp salad.** In almost all cases, the foodstuffs were allowed to **stand at room temperature** for several hours between preparation and consumption.

Group D: five species may produce a clinical syndrome similar to staphylococcal intoxication. Diarrhoea, abdominal cramp, nausea, vomiting, fever, chills, dizziness in 2 – 36 hours. Food **sources** include sausage**, evaporated milk, cheese, meat croquettes, meat pie, pudding, raw milk, and pasteurised milk.**

Exercise 1a
Match the column A with the column B. Try to learn the expressions and/ or sentences by heart.

A

1. *Bacillus cereus* food poisoning is the general description
2. The vomiting-type outbreaks have generally been associated with rice products;
3. Food mixtures such as sauces, puddings, soups, casseroles, pastries, and salads
4. Clinical manifestations of *Bacillus cereus* invasion include
5. *Aeromonas hydrophilla* is a species of bacterium
6. Two distinct types of gastroenteritis have been associated with *Aeromonas hydrophilla:*
7. *Aeromonas hydrophilla* has frequently been found in fish and shellfish;
8. *Plesiomonas shigelloides* has been isolated from freshwater, freshwater fish and shellfish
9. The organisms may be present in unsanitary water, which has been used as drinking water
10. In severe cases,
11. Infants, children and chronically ill people
12. Shigellosis is an infectious disease
13. A severe infection with high fever may also be associated
14. Using antibiotics can actually make the germs
15. Shigellosis is particularly common and causes recurrent problems in settings
16. If you are travelling to the developing world,

17. The enteric (intestinal) bacteria
18. The chronic illness is common in malnourished children
19. *Streptococcus spp.*, group A
20. Food sources include milk, ice cream, eggs, steamed lobster, ground ham, potato salad, egg salad, custard, rice pudding, or shrimp salad,
21. *Streptococcus spp., group D may produce a clinical syndrome similar to staphylococcal intoxication;*
22. Using antibiotics can actually make the germs
23. Shigellosis is particularly common and causes recurrent problems in settings
24. *If you are travelling to the developing world,*

B

a) a cholera-like illness with a watery diarrhoea and a dysenteric illness characterised by loose stools containing blood and mucus.

b) although two recognized types of illness are caused by two distinct metabolites.

c) and from many types of animals including cattle, goats, swine, cats, dogs, monkeys, vultures, snakes, and toads.

d) are more likely to experience protracted illness and complications.

e) bovine mastitis, severe systemic and pyogenic infections, gangrene, septic meningitis, cellulitis, panopthalmitis, lung abscesses, infant death, and endocarditis.

f) cause septic sore throat and scarlet fever.

g) caused by a group of bacteria called Shigella.

h) diarrhoea may be greenish-yellow, foamy, and blood tinged.

i) food sources include sausage, evaporated milk, cheese, meat croquettes, meat pie, pudding, raw milk, and pasteurised milk.

j) have been suspected of causing acute and chronic gastrointestinal disease.

k) have frequently been incriminated in food poisoning outbreaks.

l) however other starchy foods such as potato, pasta and cheese have also been implicated.

m) it also has been found in market samples of red meats (beef, pork, lamb) and poultry.

n) living in unsanitary conditions in tropical countries.

o) more resistant in the future.

p) recreational water, or water used to rinse foods that are consumed without cooking or heating.

q) that is present in all freshwater environments and in brackish water.
r) wash, peel, or cook raw fruit and vegetables before eating.
s) where hygiene is poor and can sometimes sweep through entire communities.
t) which were allowed to stand at room temperature for several hours between preparation and consumption.
u) with seizures in children less than 2 years old.

Parasitic protozoa and helminths 1

Parasites may be present **in food or in water** and cause disease. Ranging in size from tiny, **single-celled organisms** (**protozoa**) to **worms (helminths)** visible to the naked eye, parasites are more and more frequently being identified as causes of food-borne illness. The illnesses they can cause range **from mild discomfort** to **debilitating illness** and possible death. Parasites are organisms that derive nourishment and protection **from other living organisms** known as **hosts**. These organisms live and reproduce within the tissues and organs of infected human and animal hosts, and are often excreted in faeces.

Guardia duodenalis (G. lamblia)

Giardia duodenalis (G. lamblia) is found in every region throughout the world and has become recognized as one of the **most common causes** of water-born (and occasionally food-borne) illness. **Those at risk include:**

- persons working in **child day-care centres** and children attending day-care centres;
- **hikers, campers** or any persons who may drink from untreated water supplies
- persons with **weakened immune systems**

Prevention

- When hiking, camping, or travelling to countries where water supply may be unsafe to drink, **avoid drinking the water or boil it** for 1 minute to kill the parasite. Drinking bottled beverages or hot coffee and tea are safe alternatives.
- **Do not swallow water** while swimming.
- **Wash, peel or cook fruits and vegetables** before eating.

Entamoeba histolytica

Amebiasis (or amoebiasis) is the name of the infection caused by *E. histolytica*. **Infections** that sometimes last for years may be accompanied by:

- **no** symptoms
- **vague** gastrointestinal **distress**
- **dysentery** (with blood and mucus)

Complications include:

- **ulcerative** and **abscess** pain
- **intestinal blockage**

Amoebiasis is transmitted by **faecal contamination** of drinking water and foods, but also by direct contacts with **dirty hands** as well as by **sexual contact**. In the majority of cases, **amoebas** remain **in the intestinal tract of the host**. The infection is "not uncommon" in the **tropics and arctics**, but also in crowded situations of poor hygiene in temperate-zone **urban environments**. It is also frequently diagnosed among **homosexual men**.

Cryptosporidium parvum

Cryptosporidium parvum is a one-celled intracellular parasite (protozoa) and a significant cause of water-borne **illness** worldwide. It is found in the intestines of many herd animals including **cows, sheep, goats, deer, and elk**. The sporocysts are resistant to most chemical disinfectants but are **susceptible to drying and the ultraviolet** portion of sunlight. Large outbreaks are associated with contaminated water supplies.

Cyclospora cayetanensis

Cases of cyclosporiasis have been reported with increased frequency from various countries since the mid 1980s, in part because of the availability of better **techniques for detecting the parasite** in stool specimens. Symptoms include watery **diarrhoea** (sometimes explosive), stomach **cramps, nausea, vomiting, muscle aches, low-grade fever, and fatigue**. Symptoms may return. Some cases are without symptoms. Persons living or travelling in developing countries may be at increased risk; but infection can be acquired worldwide.

Exercise 1b
Match the column A with the column B. Try to learn the expressions and/ or sentences by heart.

A

1. Ranging in size from tiny, single-celled organisms (protozoa) to worms (helminths) visible to the naked eye,
2. Parasites are organisms that derive nourishment and protection
3. *Giardia duodenalis (G. lamblia)* is found in every region throughout the world
4. Those at risk include:
5. When hiking, camping, or travelling to countries where water supply may be unsafe to drink,
6. Wash, peel or cook
7. Amoebiasis is transmitted by faecal contamination of drinking water and foods,
8. In the majority of cases,
9. *Cryptosporidium parvum*
10. The sporocysts are resistant to most chemical disinfectants

11. Symptoms of cyclosporiasis caused by *Cyclospora cayetanensis* include

B

a) *amoebas remain in the intestinal tract of the host.*
b) *and has become recognized as one of the most common causes of water-born (and occasionally food-borne) illness.*
c) *avoid drinking the water or boil it for 1 minute to kill the parasite.*
d) *but also by direct contacts with dirty hands as well as by sexual contact.*
e) *but are susceptible to drying and the ultraviolet portion of sunlight.*
f) *from other living organisms known as hosts.*
g) *fruits and vegetables before eating.*
h) *is found in the intestines of many herd animals including cows, sheep, goats, deer, and elk.*
i) *parasites are more and more frequently being identified as causes of food-borne illness.*
j) *persons working in child day-care centres, children attending day-care centres and persons with weakened immune systems.*
k) *watery diarrhoea (sometimes explosive), stomach cramps, nausea, vomiting, muscle aches, low-grade fever, and fatigue.*

Exercise 2
Translate the expressions. Try to explain their meanings in English.

Food poisoning, starchy foods, implicated, incriminated, poisoning outbreaks, cellulitis, panopthalmitis, endocarditis, freshwater environments, dysenteric illness, loose stools, mucus, samples, cattle, goats, swine, monkeys, vultures, snakes, toads, rinse foods, mild self-limiting disease, foamy, blood tinged, correlate with, protracted illness, seizures, become resistant, recurrent problems, sweep through entire communities, peel, miscellaneous, natural environments, reside, unsanitary conditions, protracted illness, sore throat, scarlet fever, tonsillitis, malaise, rhinorrhea, lobster, custard, shrimp salad, chills, dizziness, evaporated milk, meat croquettes, worms, naked eye, mild discomfort, debilitating illness, nourishment, protection, hosts, live and reproduce, water-borne, food-borne, attending, hikers, campers, water supply, unsafe to drink, bottled beverages, vague gastrointestinal distress, ulcerative and abscess pain, intestinal blockage, temperate-zone, urban environments, intracellular parasite, herd animals, deer, availability, detecting, muscle aches, low-grade fever, fatigue.

Exercise 3
Answer the following questions. Prepare short talks and/or dialogues on these topics.

1. Describe the dangers of *Bacillus cereus.*
2. Describe the dangers of *Aeromonas hydrophilla.*
3. Describe the dangers of *Plesiomonas shigelloides.*
4. Describe the dangers of *Shigella spp.*
5. Describe the dangers of *Streptococcus spp.*
6. Talk about *Giardia duodenalis and Entamoeba histolytica.*
7. Talk about *Cryptosporidium parvum and Cyclospora cayetanensis.*

Vocabulary 13

Fill in the meanings in your mother language:

abscess /ˈæb.ses/
ache /eɪk/
acquired /əˌkwaɪ.əd/
Aeromonas /ˌeərəməˈnæs/
hydrophilla /ˌhaɪ drəˈfɪlə/
Amebiasis /əˈmiː.bɪə.sɪs/
amoeba /əˈmiː.bə/
amphibian /æmˈfɪb.i.ən/
antigenic /ˈæn.tɪ.dʒən,ɪk/
Bacillus /bəˈsɪl.əs/ ***cereus*** /ˈsɪər i əs/
boil /bɔɪl/
bottled /ˈbɒt.l̩d/
bovine /ˈbəʊvaɪn/
camper /ˈkæm.pər/
cellulitis /ˈsel.jʊ.laɪ.tɪs/
correlate /ˈkɒrɪˌleɪt/
croquette /krəˈket/
Cryptosporidium /ˌkrɪptəʊspɔːˈrɪdɪəm/
parvum /ˈpɑr vəm/
custard /ˈkʌstəd/
Cyclospora /ˌsaɪ kləˈspɔr ə/
cayetanensis /kaɪˈɛtə.nən.sɪs/
cyclosporiasis /ˌsaɪ kləˈspɔ raɪ ə sɪs/
debilitating /dɪˈbɪl.ɪ.teɪt.ɪŋ/
deer /dɪər/
derive /dɪˈraɪv/
distinct /dɪˈstɪŋkt/
dysentery /ˈdɪs.ənˌter.i/
elk /elk/
endocarditis /ˌen.dəʊ.kɑːdˈaɪ.tɪs/
Entamoeba /ˌɛn təˈmi bə/
histolytica /hɪˈstɒl.ɪ.tɪkə/
enteric /ɛnˈtɛr ɪk/
explosive /ɪkˈspləʊ.sɪv/
foamy /ˈfəʊ.mi/
freshwater /ˈfreʃˌwɔːtər/
Giardia /dʒiˈɑr di ə/ **duodenalis** /ˌdjuːəʊˈdiːnəɪlɪs/
Giardia /dʒiˈɑr di ə/
lamblia /læmbli ə/
goat /gəʊt/
herd /hɜːd/
hiker /ˈhaɪ.kər/
host /həʊst/
invasion /ɪnˈveɪ.ʒən/
lamb /læm/
loose /luːs/ **stool** /stuːl/
lung /lʌŋ/
majority /məˈdʒɒrɪtɪ/
malaise /mælˈeɪz/
mastitis /mæsˈtaɪ.tɪs/
meningitis /ˌmen.ɪnˈdʒaɪ.tɪs/
miscellaneous /ˌmɪsəlˈeɪniəs/
monkey /ˈmʌŋki/
mucoid /ˈmjuːkɔɪd/
naked /ˈneɪ.kɪd/ **eye** /aɪ/
nourishment /ˈnʌr.ɪʃ.mənt/
panopthalmitis /pænˌɒf θælˈmaɪ tɪs/
peel /piːl/
Plesiomonas /ˌpliːsiəˈmoʊ nəs/
shigelloides /ˌʃɪg əˈlɔɪdəs/

protracted /prəʊ'trækt.ɪd/
pudding /'pʊdɪŋ/
pyogenic /ˌpaɪ ə'dʒɛn ɪk/
range /reɪndʒ/
recurrent /rɪ'kʌr.ənt/
reside /rɪ'zaɪd/
rhinorrhea /ˌraɪ nə'ri ə/
rinse /rɪns/
sample /'sɑːm.pl̩/
sauce /sɔːs/
seizure /'siː.ʒə/
self-limiting /self.'lɪm.ɪ.tɪŋ/
septic /'sep.tɪk/
Shigella spp. /ʃɪ'gɛl ə/
Shigellosis /ˌʃɪg ə'loʊ sɪs/
soup /suːp/
specimen /'spes.ə.mɪn/
sporocyst /'spɔr əˌsɪst/
Streptococcus /ˌstrep.tə'kɒk.əs/
pl **streptococci** /ˌstrep.tə'kɒkaɪ/
sweep /swiːp/
swine /swaɪn/
temperate /'tempərət/ **-zone** /zəʊn/
tinged /tɪndʒd/
tiny /'taɪ.ni/
toad /təʊd/
tonsillitis /ˌtɒnsəl'aɪtɪs/
ulcerative /'ʌl.sər.ə.tɪv/
underdeveloped /ʌndədɪ'veləpt/
unsafe /ʌn'seɪf/
unsanitary /ˌʌn'sæn.ɪ.tər.i/
vague /veɪg/
vulture /'vʌltʃə/
waterborn /'wɔ tərˌbɔrn/
weaken /'wiː.kən/
worm /wɜːm/

Solution to Exercise 1a
1b, 2l, 3k, 4e, 5q, 6a, 7m, 8c, 9p, 10h, 11d, 12g, 13u, 14o, 15s, 16r, 17j, 18n, 19f, 20t, 21i

Solution to Exercise 1b
1i, 2f, 3b, 4j, 5c, 6g, 7d, 8a, 9h, 10e, 11k

Unit 14 - Parasitic protozoa and helminths 2

Anisakis simplex and related worms

Anisakiasis is most frequently diagnosed when the affected individual feels a **tingling or tickling sensation in the throat** and **coughs up** or **manually extracts** a **nematode**. In more severe cases there is acute abdominal pain, much like acute **appendicitis** accompanied by a **nauseous** feeling. With their anterior ends, the **larval nematodes** from **fish or shellfish** usually **burrow into the wall** of the **digestive tract.** Occasionally they penetrate the intestinal wall completely and are found in the body cavity. They produce a substance that attracts eosinophils and other host white blood cells to the area. The **infiltrating host cells** form a **granuloma** in the tissues surrounding the penetrated worm. In the digestive lumen, the worm can detach and reattach to other sites of the wall. Anisakids rarely reach full maturity in humans and usually are **eliminated spontaneously** from digestive tract lumen within 3 weeks of infection. In cases where the patient vomits or coughs up the worm, the disease may be diagnosed by **morphological examination** of the nematode. Other cases may require a fibre **optic device** that allows the attending physician to examine the **inside of the stomach** and the first part of the **small intestine.** These devices are equipped with a **mechanical forceps** that can be used to remove the worm.

Seafood is the principal **source** of human infections with these larval worms. These parasites are known to occur frequently in the **flesh of cod, haddock, fluke, pacific salmon, herring, flounder, and monkfish.** The disease is transmitted by raw, undercooked or insufficiently frozen fish and shellfish, and its incidence is expected to increase with the **increasing popularity of sushi and sashimi bars.** Severe cases of anisakiasis are extremely painful and require surgical intervention.

Diphyllobothrium latum

Diphyllobothriasis is the name of the disease caused by **broad fish tapeworm infections** and is characterized by **abdominal distension, flatulence,** intermittent **abdominal cramping, and diarrhoea.** *Diphyllobothrium latum* is a broad, long tapeworm, often growing to lengths between 1 and 2 m. The disease is diagnosed by finding operculate eggs (eggs with a lid) in the patient's faeces on microscopical examination. In persons that are genetically susceptible, a severe **anaemia** may develop as the result of infection. The anaemia results from the tapeworm's great requirement for an absorption of vitamin B_{12}.

Nanophyetus spp.

Nanophyetus salmicola or *N. Shikhobalowi* are the names, respectively, of the North American and Russian troglotrematoid trematodes (or flukes). These are **parasitic flatworms.** Nanophyetiasis is transmitted by the larval stage (metacercaria) of a worm that encysts in the **flesh of freshwater fishes**. In anadromous fish (migrating from salt water to fresh water for breeding), the parasite's cysts can survive the period spent at sea. **Raw, under-processed, and smoked** salmon and steel-head were implicated in the cases to date.

Eustrongylides sp.

Larval *Eustrongylides sp.* is large, bright red roundworm (nematodes). These large worms may be seen without magnification in the flesh of fish and are **normally very active after death of the fish.** They occur in freshwater fish, brackish water fish and marine fish. **The larvae** normally mature in **wading birds** such as herons, egrets, and flamingos.

***Acanthamoeba spp.* and other free living amoebae**

These organisms are ubiquitous in the environment, in **soil, water, and air.** Infections in humans are rare and are acquired through water **entering the nasal passages** (usually during swimming) and by inhalation.

Primary amoebic meningoencephalitis (PAM) occurs in persons who are generally healthy prior to infection. Central nervous system involvement arises from organisms that penetrate the nasal passages **and enter the brain.** The organisms may be isolated from spinal fluid. In untreated cases death occurs within 1 week of the onset of symptoms.

Granulomatous amoebic encephalitis (GAE) occurs in persons who are immunodeficient in some way. The **primary infection site** is thought to be in the **lungs**, and the organisms in the brain are generally associated with blood vessels, suggesting **vascular dissemination**. Foods are not analysed for these amoebae since foods are not implicated in the infection of individuals.

Ascaris lumbricoides* and *Trichuris trichiura

Humans world wide are infected with *Ascaris lumbricoides* and *Trichuris trichiura;* the eggs of these roundworms (nematode) are "sticky" and may be carried to the mouth by **hands**, other body parts, **fomites** (inanimate objects), or foods. Ascariasis (more common in North America) is also known commonly as the "large roundworm" infection and trichuriasis (more common in Europe) as "whip worm" infection. Both infections are diagnosed by finding the typical eggs in the patient's faeces, on occasion the **larval or adult worms** are found in the **faeces or throat, mouth, or nose.**

Exercise 1a
Match the column A with the column B. Try to learn the expressions and/ or sentences by heart.

A

1. Anisakiasis is most frequently diagnosed when the affected individual
2. With their anterior ends, the larval nematodes from fish or shellfish
3. The infiltrating host cells form a granuloma
4. Anisakids rarely reach full maturity in humans
5. Some cases may require a fiber optic device that allows the attending physician
6. These devices are equipped with a mechanical forceps
7. The disease is transmitted by raw, undercooked or insufficiently frozen fish and shellfish,
8. Diphyllobothriasis is the name of the disease caused by broad fish tapeworm infections
9. In persons that are genetically susceptible, a severe anaemia may develop as the result of infection
10. *Nanophyetus salmicola* or *N. Shikhobalowi*
11. *Eustrongylides sp.*
12. *Acanthamoeba spp.* and other free living amoebae
13. Humans world wide are infected with *Ascaris lumbricoides* and *Trichuris trichiura;*

B

a) and is characterized by abdominal distension, flatulence, intermittent abdominal cramping, and diarrhoea.

b) *and its incidence is expected to increase with the increasing popularity of sushi and sashimi bars.*
c) *and usually are eliminated spontaneously from digestive tract lumen within 3 weeks of infection.*
d) *are normally very active after death of the fish.*
e) *are the names, respectively, of the North American and Russian troglotrematoid trematodes (or flukes).*
f) *are ubiquitous in the environment, in soil, water, and air.*
g) *feels a tingling or tickling sensation in the throat and coughs up or manually extracts a nematode.*
h) *in the tissues surrounding the penetrated worm.*
i) *that can be used to remove the worm.*
j) *the eggs of these roundworms (nematode) are "sticky" and may be carried to the mouth by hands, other body parts, fomites (inanimate objects), or foods.*
k) *to examine the inside of the stomach and the first part of the small intestine.*
l) *usually burrow into the wall of the digestive tract.*
m) *which results from the tapeworm's great requirement for an absorption of vitamin B12.*

Parasitic protozoa and helminths
Toxoplasma gondii

Toxoplasma gondii, cause of the disease toxoplasmosis, is a single-celled microscopic parasite found **throughout the world.** These organisms can only carry out their reproductive cycle within members of the **cat family.**

People get toxoplasmosis the following ways:

- by consuming **undercooked meats**, especially **pork, lamb, or wild game**) or drinking **untreated water** (from rivers and ponds)
- **faecal-oral:** touching your hands to your mouth after gardening, handling cats, cleaning a cat's litter box
- **mother-to-foetus** (if mother is pregnant when first infected with *T. Gondii).*

Toxoplasmosis is **relatively harmless** to most people, although some may develop "**flu-like**" symptoms such as swollen lymph glands and/or muscle aches and pains. In otherwise healthy individuals, the disease is usually mild and goes away without medical treatment.

However, **dormant tissue stages** can remain in the infected individual **for life.** Persons with **weakened immune systems** such as those with HIV/AIDS infection, organ **transplant recipients**, individuals **undergoing chemotherapy**, and **infants** may develop severe toxoplasmosis.

Severe toxoplasmosis may result in **damage to the eyes or brain**. Infants becoming infected before birth can be **born retarded** or with other mental or physical problems.

Prevention

- wear **clean latex gloves** when handling raw meats
- **cook all meats** thoroughly **to 70°C**
- **wash hands, cutting boards,** and other **utensils** thoroughly with hot, soapy water after handling raw meats
- **clean cat litter boxes daily** because cat faeces more than one day old can contain mature parasites.
- wear **gloves** when you **handle garden soil or sandboxes. Cover sandboxes**. Cats may use gardens or sandboxes as litter boxes.
- **discourage cats** from **hunting and scavenging**.
- Feed cats **commercially made cat foods** or cook their food.

Trichinella spiralis

Trichinella spiralis, cause of trichinosis, is an intestinal roundworm whose larvae may **migrate from the digestive tract** and form **cysts in various muscles** of the body. People get trichinosis by consuming raw of **undercooked** meats such as pork, wild boar, bear, bobcat, cougar, fox, wolf, dog, hoarse, seal, or walrus. The illness is not spread directly from person to person.

The first **symptoms** are **nausea, diarrhoea, vomiting, fever**, and **abdominal pain**, followed by **headaches, eye swelling, aching joints and muscles, weakness**, and **itchy skin**. In severe infections, persons may experience difficulty with **coordination** and have **heart and breathing** problems. Death may occur in severe cases. Mild cases may assumed to be flu.

***Taenia saginata/Taenia solium* (Tapeworms)**

Taenia saginata (beef tapeworm) and *Taenia solium* (pork tapeworm) are parasitic worms (helminths). **Humans are the definite hosts** of both organisms. This means that the reproductive cycle and thus egg production by the organisms, occurs only within humans. The **eggs** may remain **viable in the environment** for many months. Most cases of infection with adult worms are without symptoms. Some persons may experience **abdominal pain, weight loss, digestive disturbances**, and possible **intestinal obstruction. Irritation** of the **peri-anal area** can occur, caused by worms or worm segments exiting the anus.

Cysticercosis

People get cysticercosis by consuming food or water contaminated with the eggs of *Taenia solium* (**pork tapeworm**). Worm eggs hatch and the larvae then migrate to various parts of the body and **form cysts** called cysticerci. This can be a **serious or fatal** disease if it involves organs such as the **central nervous system, heart, or eyes**. Some persons with intestinal tapeworms **may infect themselves** with eggs from their own faeces as a result of **poor personal hygiene.** Symptoms may vary depending on the organ or organ system involved. For example, an individual with cysticercosis involving the central nervous system may exhibit **neurological symptoms** such as psychiatric problems or epileptic seizures. Death is common. Symptoms may last for many years if medical treatment is not received.

Exercise 1b
Match the column A with the column B. Try to learn the expressions and/ or sentences by heart.

A

1. *Toxoplasma gondii,*
2. These organisms can only carry out their reproductive cycle
3. People get toxoplasmosis
4. Toxoplasmosis is relatively harmless to most people,
5. Persons with weakened immune systems such as those with HIV/ AIDS infection,
6. Wash hands, cutting boards, and other utensils thoroughly
7. Clean cat litter boxes daily
8. Feed cats commercially made
9. *Trichinella spiralis,* cause of trichinosis,
10. The first symptoms are nausea, diarrhoea, vomiting, fever and abdominal pain,
11. *Taenia saginata* (beef tapeworm) and *Taenia solium* (pork tapeworm)
12. The reproductive cycle and thus egg production
13. Some persons may experience abdominal pain,
14. People get cysticercosis
15. Worm eggs hatch and the larvae then migrate to various parts of the body
16. This can be a serious or fatal disease
17. An individual with cysticercosis involving the central nervous system may

B

a) although some may develop "flu-like" symptoms such as swollen lymph glands and/ or muscle aches and pains.
b) and form cysts called cysticerci.
c) are parasitic worms (helminths).
d) because cat faeces more than one day old can contain mature parasites.
e) by consuming food or water contaminated with the eggs of Taenia solium (pork tapeworm).
f) by consuming undercooked meats, by faecal-oral route or mother-to-foetus route.

g) *by the organisms, occurs only within humans.*
h) *cat foods or cook their food.*
i) *exhibit neurological symptoms such as psychiatric problems or epileptic seizures.*
j) *followed by headaches, eye swelling, aching joints and muscles, weakness, and itchy skin.*
k) *if it involves organs such as the central nervous system, heart, or eyes.*
l) *is an intestinal roundworm whose larvae may migrate from the digestive tract and form cysts in various muscles of the body.*
m) *is the cause of the disease toxoplasmosis.*
n) *organ transplant recipients, individuals undergoing chemotherapy, and infants may develop severe toxoplasmosis.*
o) *weight loss, digestive disturbances, and possible intestinal obstruction.*
p) *with hot, soapy water after handling raw meats.*
q) *within members of the cat family.*

Exercise 2
Translate the expressions. Try to explain their meanings in English.

Tingling or tickling sensation, coughs up, manually extracts, acute appendicitis, nauseous feeling, burrow into the wall, penetrate, infiltrating, host cells, granuloma tissues, surrounding, digestive lumen, detach and reattach, reach full maturity, eliminated spontaneously, morphological examination, fibre optic device, attending physician, mechanical forceps, incidence is expected to increase, surgical intervention, abdominal distension, flatulence, intermittent abdominal cramping, parasitic flatworms, under-processed, magnification, flesh of fish, nasal passages, involvement arises, spinal fluid, in untreated cases, onset of symptoms, encephalitis, vascular dissemination, fomites, single-celled, carry out reproductive cycle, wild game, untreated water, handling cats, mother-to-foetus, harmless, flu-like, swollen lymph glands, muscle aches, dormant stages, for life, transplant recipients, individuals undergoing chemotherapy, be born retarded, cutting boards, utensils, litter boxes, contain mature parasites, cover sandboxes, migrate, form cysts, eye swelling, aching joints and muscles, weakness, itchy skin, heart and breathing problems, assumed, definite hosts, remain viable, digestive disturbances, intestinal obstruction, irritation, worm eggs hatch, serious or fatal disease, epileptic seizures.

Exercise 3
Answer the following questions. Prepare short talks and/or dialogues on these topics.

1. Talk about: *Anisakis simplex and related worms, Diphyllobothrium*

latum, Nanophyetus spp. Eustrongylides sp., Ascaris lumbricoides and *Trichuris trichiura.*

2. Characterise parasitic protozoa and helminths (*Toxoplasma gondii, Trichinella spiralis, Taenia saginata, Taenia solium*)

Vocabulary 14

Fill in the meanings in your mother language:

Acanthamoeba spp /ə.keɪn.ð əˈmi bə/
aching /eɪk.ɪŋ/
amoebic /əˈmi bɪk/
anadromous /əˈnæd rə məs/
Anisakis /eɪ nɪ.seɪ ˈkɪs/
simplex /ˈsɪm plɛks/
anterior /ænˈtɪərɪə/
appendicitis /əˌpen.dɪˈsaɪ.tɪs/
Ascaris /ˈæs kə rɪs/ ***lumbricoid*** / ˈlʌm brɪˌkɔɪd/ ascariasis.
assume /əˈsjuːm/
attend /əˈtend/
boar /bɔːr/
bobcat /ˈbɑbˌkæt/
breeding /ˈbriːdɪŋ/
burrow /ˈbʌr.əʊ/
carry /ˈkær.i/ **st out** /aʊt/
cougar /ˈkuː.gər/
cough /kɒf/ **up** /ʌp/
Cysticercosis /ˌsɪs tə sərˈkoʊ sɪs/
cysticercus /ˌsɪs təˈsɜr kəs/ pl **cysticerci**
detach /dɪˈtætʃ/
Diphyllobothriasis /daɪ. fɪl.əʊ.bɒð.raɪ.ə.sɪs/
Diphyllobothrium /daɪ.fɪl. əʊ.bɒð.rː.əm/ **latum** /leɪ.təm/
discourage /dɪˈskʌr.ɪdʒ/
dissemination /dɪˌsem.əˈneɪ.ʃən/
dormant /ˈdɔr.mənt/
egret /ˈi grɪt/
encephalitis /ˌen.kef.əˈlaɪ.tɪs/
encyst /ɛnˈsɪst/
eosinophil /ˌi əˈsɪn ə fɪl/
epileptic /ˌepɪˈleptɪk/
Eustrongylides /juːstrən.dʒɪl.ɪə diːz/
exit /ˈeksɪt/
fiber /ˈfaɪbər/ **optic** /ˈɒp. tɪk/ **device** /dɪˈvaɪs/
flamingo /fləˈmɪŋgəʊ/
flatulence /ˈflæt.jʊ.lənts/
flatworm /ˈflæt.wɜːm/
flesh /fleʃ/
flounder /ˈflaʊndər/
flu-like /fluː.laɪk/
fluke /fluːk/
fomite /fəʊ.maːt/
forceps /ˈfɔː.seps/
fox /fɒks/
granuloma /græn.jəˈləʊ.mə/
granulomatous /ˌgræn jəˈloʊ mətəs/
haddock /ˈhædək/
hatch /hætʃ/
heron /ˈher.ən/
herring /ˈherɪŋ/
hunting /ˈhʌntɪŋ/
immunodeficient /ˌɪm.jəˈnɒ.dɪˈfɪʃənt/
implicate /ˈɪm.plɪ.keɪt/
inanimate /ɪˈnæn.ɪ.mət/
infiltrate /ˈɪn.fɪl.treɪt/
intermittent /ˌɪn.təˈmɪt.ənt/
involvement /ɪnˈvɒlv.mənt/
larva /ˈlɑːvə/ plural **larvae** /ˈlɑːviː/
litter box /ˈlɪtər bɒks/
lumen /ˈlu.mən/ pl **lumina**
lymph /lɪmf/ **gland** /glænd/
magnification /ˌmæg.nɪ.fɪˈkeɪ.ʃən/
maturity /məˈtjʊə.rɪ.ti/
meningoencephalitis / mɪˈnɪngə.ɛnˌsɛf əˈlaɪ tɪs/
metacercaria /ˌmɛt ə sərˈkɛər I ə/
monkfish /ˈmʌŋkˌfɪʃ/
morphological /ˌmɔː.fəˈlɒdʒ.ɪ.kəl/
Nanophyetus spp. /nəɪˈnəʊ.faɪ.iːtəs/

Nematode /'nemətəʊd/
operculum /oʊ'pɜr kjələm/
penetrate /'pen.ɪ.treɪt/
peri /'pɪər i/ **-anal** /'eɪnəl/
physician /fɪ'zɪʃ.ən/
reattach /ri ə'tætʃ/
recipient /rɪ'sɪp.i.ənt/
roundwarm /'raʊndˌwɜrm/
sandbox /'sændˌbɒks/
sashimi /sɑ'ʃi mi/
scavenge /'skævɪndʒ/
seal /si:l/
sensation /sen'seɪ.ʃən/
spinal /'spaɪ.nəl/ **fluid** /'flu:.ɪd/
steelhead /'stilˌhɛd/
sticky /'stɪk.i/
surgical /'sɜ:.dʒɪ.kəl/
sushi /'su:ʃi/
swelling /'swel.ɪŋ/
Taenia /'ti ni ə/ ***saginata***
/ seɪ dʒ ə neɪ tə/
Taenia /'ti ni ə/ ***solium*** /'soʊ li əm/
tapeworm /'teɪp.wɜ:m/
tickle /'tɪkl/
Toxoplasma /ˌtɒk sə'plæz
mə/ ***gondii*** /'gɒn di/
toxoplasmosis /ˌtɒk.səʊ.plæz'məʊ.sɪs/
trematode /'trɛm əˌtoʊd/ = fluke
Trichinella /ˌtrɪkɪ'nəl ə/
spiralis /'spaɪ rə lɪs/
trichinosis /ˌtrɪkɪ'nəʊsɪs/
Trichuris trichiura /trɪə.
kjʊ.rɪəs trɪə.kaɪ jʊræ/
Troglotrematidae /trɒg
ləʊ tri: mæt ɪ di:/
ubiquitous /ju:'bɪkwɪtəs/
vascular /'væs.kjə.lər/
viable /'vaɪ.ə.bl̩/
wade /weɪd/
walrus /'wɔ:lrəs/
whip /wɪp/ **worm** /wɜ:m/
wolf /wʊlf/

Solution to Exercise 1a
1g, 2l, 3h, 4c, 5k, 6i, 7b, 8a,
9m, 10e, 11d, 12f, 13j

Solution to Exercise 1b
1m, 2q, 3f, 4a, 5p, 6d, 7h, 8l, 9j,
10c, 11g, 12o, 13e, 14b, 15k. 16I

Unit 15 - Viruses. Moulds.

Viruses are among the smallest organisms. In order to grow and survive, they must **invade a living organism**. Viruses cannot multiply in food but can be transported in food and some can **survive freezing and normal cooking** temperatures. They can also be spread by food handlers and/or servers. The most common viruses are:

- Hepatitis A virus
- Hepatitis E virus
- Rotavirus
- Norwalk virus group
- Other viral agent

Hepatitis A virus

Hepatitis A is usually a **mild illness** characterized by **sudden onset** of **fever, malaise, nausea, anorexia**, and **abdominal discomfort**, followed in several days by **jaundice**.

Cold cuts and sandwiches, fruits and fruit juices, milk and milk products, vegetables, salads, shellfish, and iced drinks are commonly implicated in outbreaks. Water, shellfish, and salads are the most frequent sources. Contamination of foods by **infected workers** in food processing plants and restaurants is common. Outbreaks of HAV are common in **institutions**, **crowded house** projects, and **prisons** and in **military forces** in adverse situations. Many infections do not result in clinical disease, especially in children. In developing countries, the incidence of disease in adults is relatively low because of exposure to the virus in childhood. Most individuals 18 and older demonstrate an **immunity** that provides **lifelong protection** against reinfection.

Hepatitis E virus

This disease should bot be confused with hepatitis C. Symptoms include **malaise, anorexia, abdominal pain, arthralgia, and fever**. HEV is transported by the **faecal-oral route**. Water-borne and person-to-person spread have been documented. The potential exists for food-borne transmission. The disease is most often seen in **young to middle aged** adults (15 – 40 years old). **Pregnant** women appear to be exceptionally susceptible to severe disease, and excessive **mortality** has been reported in this group.

Rotaviruses

Rotaviruses are transmitted by the faecal-oral route. **Person-to-person spread** through **contaminated hands** is probably the most important means by which rota viruses are transmitted in close communities such as **paediatric and geriatric wards**, day care centres and family homes. Infected food handlers may contaminate foods that require handling and no further cooking, such as salads, fruits, and hors d'oeuvres. **Sanitary measures** adequate for bacteria and parasites seem to be ineffective in endemic control of rotavirus, as similar incidence of rotavirus infection is observed in countries with both high and low health standards.

Group A rotavirus is endemic **worldwide**. It is the leading cause of **severe diarrhoea among infants and children**, and accounts for about half of the cases requiring hospitalisation. **Group B rotavirus**, also called **adult diarrhoea rotavirus**, has caused major epidemics of severe diarrhoea affecting thousands of persons of all ages in China. **Group C** rotavirus has been associated with rare and sporadic cases of diarrhoea in children in many countries.

Humans of all ages are susceptible to rotavirus infection. Children 6 months to 2 years of age, premature infants, the elderly, and the immunocompromised are particularly prone to more severe symptoms caused by infection with group A rotavirus.

Norwalk virus

Norwalk virus and Norwalk like viruses also are referred to a '**noroviruses**'. Norwalk virus and Norwalk like viruses have been associated with outbreaks on cruise ships and in **communities**, camps, schools, institutions and families. Foods such as raw **oysters**, **cake frostings** and **salads**, as well as **drinking water**, have been implicated as a common source of viral infection in several outbreaks.

Transmission is of special concern for the **fishing industry**, since molluscan shellfish, being filter feeders, are readily contaminated with the stool-shed viruses present in human sewage.

Exercise 1a
Match the column A with the column B. Try to learn the expressions and/or sentences by heart.

A

1. In order to grow and survive, viruses
2. Some viruses can survive
3. Hepatitis A is usually a mild illness characterized
4. Cold cuts and sandwiches, fruits and fruit juices, milk and milk products, vegetables, salads, shellfish, and iced drinks
5. Outbreaks of HAV are common
6. Most individuals 18 and older demonstrate an immunity
7. Symptoms of Hepatitis E virus include
8. Pregnant women appear to be exceptionally susceptible
9. Person-to-person spread through contaminated hands is probably the most important means
10. Sanitary measures adequate for bacteria and parasites seem to be ineffective
11. Group A rotavirus
12. Children 6 months to 2 years of age, premature infants, the elderly, and the immunocompromised
13. Noroviruses have been associated with outbreaks
14. Foods such as raw oysters, cake frostings and salads, as well as drinking water,

B

a) are commonly implicated in outbreaks.

b) are particularly prone to more severe symptoms caused by infection with group A rotavirus.

c) by sudden onset of fever, malaise, nausea, anorexia, and abdominal discomfort, followed in several days by jaundice.

d) by which rotaviruses are transmitted in close communities such as paediatric and geriatric wards, day care centres and family homes.

e) freezing and normal cooking temperatures.

f) have been implicated as a common source of viral infection in several outbreaks.

g) in endemic control of rotavirus.

h) in institutions, crowded house projects, and prisons and in military forces.

i) *is the leading cause of severe diarrhoea among infants and children.*
j) *malaise, anorexia, abdominal pain, arthralgia, and fever.*
k) *must invade a living organism.*
l) *on cruise ships and in communities, camps, schools, institutions and families.*
m) *that provides lifelong protection against reinfection.*
n) *to severe disease, and excessive mortality has been reported in this group.*

Moulds

Moulds are **microscopic fungi** that live **on plant or animal** matter. Most are **filamentous** (threadlike) organisms and the production of **spores** is characteristic of fungi in general. These spores can be transported **by air, water, or insects**. Some moulds cause **allergic reactions** and respiratory problems. And a few moulds, in the right conditions, produce **'mycotoxins', poisonous substances** that that can make people sick. Moulds are composed of **long filaments** called ***hyphae***.

When mould hyphae are numerous enough to be seen by the naked eye they form a **cottony mass** called a ***mycelium***. It is the hyphae and resulting mycelia that **invade things** in our homes and cause them to **decay**.

Moulds **reproduce by *spores***. Spores are like seeds; they **germinate** to produce a **new mould colony** when they **land in a suitable place**. Unlike seeds, they are **very simple** in structure and never contain an embryo or any sort of preformed offspring. Spores are produced in a variety of ways and occur in a bewildering **array of shapes and sizes**. In spite of this diversity, spores are quite **constant in shape, colour, and form** for any given mould, and are thus very useful for mould identification. The most basic difference between spores lies in their method of **initiation**, which can be either **sexual or asexual**. Sexually initiated spores result from a matting between two **different organisms or hyphae**, whereas **asexual spores** result from a simple **internal division or external modification** of an individual hypha. For practical purposes one can learn to recognize the four kinds of **sexually determined** spores that appear in mould fungi:

- **oospores**
- **zygospores**
- **ascospores**
- **basidiospores**

Asexual spores usually occur either in **sporangia** or as **conidia**. Sporangia are modified hyphae or cells containing numerous spores. Conidia occur externally on the cells that produce them.

Aside from their role in **plant, animal, and human disease**, many moulds enter directly into human affairs, in either harmful or beneficial way. The discovery of **penicillin** by **Sir Alexander Fleming** in 1928 probably resulted in the saving of more lives than all other medical discoveries combined. Penicillin, a product of the common mould *Penicillium chrysogenum* is still one of the safest and most widely used of **antibiotics**, in spite of a more than fifty-year search for others.

The foods we eat are as nutritional to many moulds as they are to us, a fact often put to use in the preparation of food products. For example, several types of cheese, such as **Roquefort, Danish blue, Camembert, and Brie,** owe their distinctive flavour to the **presence of mould growing on them**. If the mould were absent, these cheeses would not **ripen** properly.

Yeasts, although not really moulds, are among the most important fungi in **food preparation.** Their value lies in their ability to **produce carbon dioxide** and **grain alcohol**. In **wine-making**, where the production of alcohol is valued, yeast is added to the **grape juice** to bring this about. In **bread making**, the important product is carbon dioxide, which is necessary in the **rising process**, and, again, yeast is added to the dough.

In the **production of beer**, **both alcohol and carbon dioxide,** to produce carbonation, may be necessary, although today, the carbon dioxide may be added artificially. In the Far East, a number of moulds are used in food preparation that remain unexploited in most of the world. They are used to **process** various **rice, bean and soy-bean products**.

To most of us, the **negative aspects** of moulds in foods are more noticeable than the positive. Moulds are one of the reasons food manufacturers include **preservatives** in their products. One of the most **destructive activities** of moulds in foodstuffs occurs in **stored seeds and grains**. To **guard against this**, the grain must be **dried** to very low moisture levels. Keeping grains dry in the humid tropics is particularly difficult if not, at times nearly impossible. Not only do **fungi damage the grains** or render them unpalatable, they may also **excrete** toxins – **mycotoxins** that can cause illness or even death.

Other mould-like organisms

In routine work we often encounter organisms that are **similar to moulds** but do not fit our strict definition of the term. We can put four groups of organisms into this category, bacteria, actinomycetes, yeasts, and slime moulds.

Bacteria

Bacteria represent a **very ancient group** of organisms, perhaps as old as four billion years. Colonies of bacteria are composed of **minute spore-like cells** that together form a **slimy mass**. Such colonies **never contain hyphae** and are thus easily distinguished from those of the moulds. Bacterial cells are difficult to examine, even with a good microscope, and are best seen when stained. Many bacteria are motile and swim vigorously.

Actinomycetes

These organisms are usually classified **as bacteria but have filaments like fungi,** The filaments are considerably narrower that those of moulds. Streptomyces, the only actinomycete genus commonly encountered as a 'mould', produces **grey to brightly coloured powdery colonies**, usually with a soil-like odour.

Yeasts

Yeasts are **true fungi**, but in **lacking hyphae** cannot be classed as moulds. They resemble bacteria in forming pasty or slimy colonies of spore-like cells, but differ in having these cells much larger. **Reproduction** of yeasts is usually by **budding**, a process where a smaller cell appears to **bubble** slowly out of the parent cell.

Slime moulds

Slime moulds normally **occur on logs and other natural materials** but occasionally occur in the laboratory as 'moulds'. Cellular slime moulds, the most likely to appear in the laboratory, have creeping amoeba-like cells during part of the life cycle and sporangium-like structures in another.

Exercise 1b
Match the column A with the column B. Try to learn the expressions and/ or sentences by heart.

A

1. Moulds are microscopic fungi
2. Most are filamentous (threadlike) organisms
3. A few moulds, in the right conditions, produce 'mycotoxins',
4. Moulds are composed of
5. Mould hyphae form
6. It is the hyphae and resulting mycelia that invade things
7. Moulds reproduce by *spores;*
8. In spite of diversity,
9. The most basic difference between spores lies in their method of initiation,
10. Sexually initiated spores result from a matting between two different organisms or hyphae,
11. Asexual spores usually occur either in sporangia or as conidia;
12. Penicillin, a product of the common mould *Penicillium chrysogenum* is
13. Several types of cheese, such as Roquefort, Danish blue, Camembert, and Brie,
14. The value yeasts lies in their ability
15. In wine-making, where the production of alcohol is valued,
16. In bread making, the important product is carbon dioxide,

17. In the production of beer, both alcohol and carbon dioxide,
18. Moulds are one of the reasons food manufacturers
19. One of the most destructive activities of moulds in foodstuffs
20. Not only do fungi damage the grains or render them unpalatable,
21. Colonies of bacteria are composed of
22. Yeasts resemble bacteria in forming pasty or slimy colonies of spore-like cells,
23. Reproduction of yeasts is usually by budding,
24. Slime moulds normally occur

B

a) *a cottony mass called a mycelium*
b) *a process where a smaller cell appears to bubble slowly out of the parent cell.*
c) *and the production of spores is characteristic of fungi in general.*
d) *but differ in having these cells much larger*
e) *in our homes and cause them to decay.*
f) *include preservatives in their products.*
g) *long filaments called hyphae.*
h) *minute spore-like cells that together form a slimy mass.*
i) *occurs in stored seeds and grains.*
j) *on logs and other natural materials.*
k) *owe their distinctive flavour to the presence of mould growing on them.*
l) *poisonous substances that can make people sick.*
m) *sporangia are modified hyphae or cells containing numerous spores whereas conidia occur externally on the cells that produce them.*
n) *spores are quite constant in shape, colour, and form for any given mould.*
o) *still one of the safest and most widely used of antibiotics.*
p) *that live on plant or animal matter.*
q) *they germinate to produce a new mould colony when they land in a suitable place.*
r) *they may also excrete toxins – mycotoxins that can cause illness or even death.*
s) *to produce carbon dioxide and grain alcohol.*
t) *to produce carbonation, may be necessary.*
u) *whereas asexual spores result from a simple internal division or external modification of an individual hypha.*
v) *which can be either sexual or asexual.*
w) *which is necessary in the rising process.*
x) *yeast is added to the grape juice to bring this about.*

Exercise 2
Translate the expressions. Try to explain their meanings in English.

Invade, multiply, spread, sudden onset, discomfort, jaundice, cold cuts, implicated, food processing plants, adverse, incidence, exposure, confused, arthralgia, potential, exceptionally susceptible, mortality, ineffective, accounts for, affecting, associated with, cruise ships, special concern, fungi, threadlike, insects, poisonous substances, long filament, cottony mass, germinate, mould colony, land in a suitable place, preformed offspring, diversity, initiation, matting, internal division or external modification, harmful or beneficial, medical discoveries, distinctive flavour, ripen, yeasts, rising process, include preservatives, destructive activities, guard against, moisture, unpalatable, encounter, ancient, slimy mass, stained, motile, vigorously, resemble, budding, creeping, amoeba-like, sporangium-like.

Exercise 3
Answer the following questions. Prepare short talks and/or dialogues on these topics.

1. Talk about viruses (Hepatitis A virus, Hepatitis E virus, rota-viruses, Norwalk virus).
2. What do you know about moulds?
3. Yeasts and food preparation (wine-making, bread making, production of beer).
4. Destructive activities of moulds in foodstuff.
5. Organisms that are similar to moulds.

Vocabulary 15

Fill in the meanings in your mother language:

actinomycetes /æk͵tɪn oʊ'maɪ sits/
adverse /'æd.vɜːs/
ancient /'eɪn.tʃənt/
arthralgia /aː'θræl.dʒɪ.ə/
ascospore /'æs kə͵spɔr/
aside /ə'saɪd/
basidiospore /bə'sɪd i oʊ͵spɔr/
bewildering /bɪ'wɪldərɪŋ/
bud /bʌd/
carbonation /'kɑːbəneɪʃən/
case /keɪs/
concern /kən'sɜːn/
confused /kən'fjuːzd/
cottony /'kɒtən i/
creep /kriːp/
cruise /kruːz/ **ship** /ʃɪp/
Danish /'deɪnɪʃ/ **blue** /bluː/
diversity /daɪ'vɜː.sɪ.ti/
exceptionally /ɪk'sep.ʃən.əl.i/
feeder /'fiː.dər/
filament /'fɪl.ə.mənt/
filter /'fɪltər/
force /fɔːs/
geriatric /͵dʒeri'ætrɪk/
germinate /'dʒɜːmɪneɪt/
hepatitis /͵hep.ə'taɪ.tɪs/
hors d'oeuvre /͵ɔːr'dɝːv/
hypha /'haɪfə/ (plural hyphas or **hyphae** /'haɪfiː/
in spite of /spaɪt/
ineffective /͵ɪn.ɪ'fek.tɪv/
initiation /ɪ͵nɪʃ.i'eɪ.ʃən/
insect /'ɪn.sekt/
invade /ɪn'veɪd/
log /lɒg/

mat /ˈmæt/
modification /ˌmɒd.ɪ.fɪˈkeɪ.ʃən/
moisture /ˈmɔɪs.tʃər/
mollusc /ˈmɒl əsk/
motile /ˈməʊ.taɪl/
mycelium /maɪˈsiːlɪəm/
mycotoxin /ˌmaɪkəˈtɒksɪn/
Norwalk /ˈnɔr wɔk/ **virus** /ˈvaɪ rəs/
noticeable /ˈnəʊ.tɪ.sə.bl̩/
offspring /ˈɒf.sprɪŋ/
oospore /ˈəʊəˌspɔː/
paediatric /ˌpiː.diˈæt.rɪk/
pasty /ˈpæs.ti/
Penicillium /ˌpɛnɪˈsɪlɪəm/
chrysogenum /krɪs əʊ dʒ.ɪ.nəm/
poisonous /ˈpɔɪ.zən.əs/
plant /plɑːnt/
preservative /prɪˈzɜːvətɪv/
prison /ˈprɪz.ən/
render /ˈren.dər/
resemble /rɪˈzem.bl̩/
ripen /ˈraɪpən/
rising /ˈraɪ zɪŋ/ **process** /ˈprəʊses/
Roquefort /ˈroʊk fərt/
rotavirus /ˈrəʊ.tə.ˈvaɪ.rəs/
server /ˈsɜːvər/
slime /slaɪm/
slimy /ˈslaɪmi/
sporangium /spəˈræn dʒi əm/
pl **sporangia** /spəˈræn dʒi ə/
stained /steɪnd/
survive /səˈvaɪv/
threadlike /θred.laɪk/
unexploited /ʌn ɪkˈsplɔɪ təd/
vigorously /ˈvɪg.ər.əs.li/
ward /wɔːd/
WHO, World /wɜːld/ **Health** /helθ/
Organization /ˌɔːgənaɪˈzeɪʃən/
zygospore /ˈzaɪgəʊˌspɔː/

Solution to Exercise 1a
1k, 2e, 3c, 4a, 5h, 6m, 7j, 8n, 9d, 10g, 11i, 12b, 13l, 14f

Solution to Exercise 1b
1p, 2c, 3l, 4g, 5a, 6e, 7q, 8n, 9v, 10u, 11m, 12o, 13k, 14s, 15x, 16w, 17t, 18f, 19i, 20r, 21h, 22d, 23b, 24j

Unit 16 - Natural toxins. Protoplasmic poisons.

Ciguatera fish poisoning

Ciguatera is a form of human poisoning caused by the consumption of **subtropical and tropical marine finfish**, which have **accumulated naturally occurring toxins** through their diet.

Manifestation of ciguatera in humans usually involves a combination of **gastrointestinal, neurological, and cardiovascular disorders**. Initial signs of poisoning occur within six hours after consumption of toxic fish and include **perioral numbness and tingling** (paresthesia), which may spread to the **extremities, nausea, vomiting, and diarrhoea**.

Neurological signs include intensified **paresthesia, arthralgia, myalgia, headache**, temperature sensory reversal and acute **sensitivity to temperature** extremes, **vertigo**, and **muscular weakness** to the point of **prostration**. Cardiovascular signs include **arrhythmia, bradycardia or tachycardia**, and **reduced blood pressure**. Ciguatera poisoning is usually **self-limiting.**

However, in severe cases the neurological symptoms are known to persist from weeks to months. In other cases recovered patients have experienced **recurrence** of neurological symptoms months to years after recovery. Such **relapses** are most often associated with **changes in dietary habits** or with consumption of **alcohol**.

Populations in tropical/ subtropical regions are most likely to be affected. However, the increasing per capita consumption of fishery products coupled with an increase in interregional **transportation of seafood products** has expanded the geographic range of human poisonings.

Shellfish poisoning

Shellfish poisoning is caused by a group of **toxins elaborated by planktonic algae** upon which shellfish feed. The toxins are accumulated and sometimes metabolised by the shellfish. All **shellfish** are potentially toxic; mussels, clams, cockles, scallops, and oysters.

Types of **shellfish poisoning**:

- **paralytic** shellfish poisoning
- **diarrhoeic** shellfish poisoning
- **neurotoxic** shellfish poisoning
- **amnesis** shellfish poisoning

Ingestion of contaminated shellfish results in a wide variety of symptoms, depending upon the **toxins present**, their **concentrations** in the shellfish and the **amount** of contaminated shellfish consumed. Gastrointestinal disorders, i.e., **nausea, vomiting, diarrhoea and abdominal pain** are accompanied by **chills, headache, and fever.** The neurological effects include **tingling, burning, numbness of lips, tongue and throat, muscular aches, dizziness, reversal** of the sensations of **hot and cold, drowsiness, incoherent speech, confusion, memory loss, disorientation, seizure, coma, and respiratory paralysis.**

Scombroid poisoning (also called histamine poisoning)

Scombroid poisoning is caused by the ingestion of foods that contain high levels of **histamine** and possibly other **vasoactive amines and compounds**. Histamine and other amines are formed by the **growth of certain bacteria**, either during the production of a product such as **Swiss cheese** or by **spoilage of foods** such as **fishery products**, particularly tuna or mahi mahi.

Initial symptoms include a **tingling or burning sensation in the mouth, a rash on the upper body and a drop in blood pressure.** Frequently, **headaches** and **itching** of the skin are encountered. The symptoms may progress to nausea, vomiting, and diarrhoea and may require hospitalization, particularly in the case of **elderly or impaired** patients.

Diagnosis of the illness is usually based on the patient's symptoms, time of onset, and the effect of treatment with antihistamine medication. **Neither cooking, canning, or freezing**

reduces the toxic effect. Chemical testing is the only reliable test for evaluation of a product. Fishery products that have been implicated in scombroid poisoning include the **tuna** (e.g. skipjack, and yellowfin), mahi mahi, bluefish, **sardines**, **mackerel**, amberjack, and abalone.

Other incidents of intoxication have resulted from the consumption of canned abalone-like products, canned anchovies, and fresh and frozen amberjack, bluefish sole, and scallops. In particular, **shipments of unfrozen fish** packed in refrigerated containers have posed a significant problem because of inadequate temperature control.

Tetrodotoxin

The **gonads, liver, intestines, and skin** of **pufferfish** can contain levels of tetrodotoxin sufficient to produce **rapid and violent death**. The flesh of many puffer-fish may not usually be dangerously toxic. The symptoms include **paraesthesia** in the **face and extremities**, sensations of **lightness** or **floating**, **headache, epigastric pain, nausea, diarrhoea, vomiting, reeling, difficulty in walking,** increasing **paralysis, respiratory distress, dyspnoea, cyanosis, hypotension, convulsions, mental impairment, and cardiac arrhythmia** may occur. Death usually occurs within 4 to 6 hours.

This toxicosis may be avoided by not consuming pufferfish or other animal species containing tetrodotoxin. Poisoning from tetrodotoxin is of major **public health concern** primarily in **Japan**, where 'fugu' is a traditional delicacy. It is prepared and sold in special restaurants where trained and licensed individuals **carefully remove the viscera** to reduce the danger of poisoning fish products.

Mushroom poisoning, toadstool poisoning

Mushroom poisonings are generally **acute** and are manifested by a variety of symptoms and prognoses, depending on the **amount and species consumed**. There are four categories of mushroom toxins:

- **protoplasmic poisons** (poisons that result in generalized **destruction of cells**, followed by organ failure);
- **neurotoxins** (compounds that cause **neurological symptoms** such as profuse **sweating, coma, convulsions, hallucinations, excitement, depression, spastic colon**);
- **gastrointestinal irritants** (compounds that produce rapid, transient **nausea, vomiting, abdominal cramping, and diarrhoea**); and
- **disulfiram-like** toxins. Mushrooms in this last category are generally non-toxic and produce no symptoms **unless alcohol is consumed** within 72 hours after eating them, in which

case a short-lived acute toxic syndrome is produced.

Mushroom poisonings are almost always caused by ingestion of wild mushrooms that have been collected by non-specialists. Most cases occur when **toxic species are confused with edible** species and a useful question to ask is the identity of the mushroom they thought they were picking. In the absence of a well-preserved **specimen**, the answer to this question could narrow the possible suspects considerably. Outbreaks have occurred after ingestion of **fresh, raw** mushrooms, **stir-fried** mushrooms, **home-canned** mushrooms, mushrooms **cooked in tomato sauce** (which rendered the sauce itself toxic), and mushrooms that were **blanched and frozen at home**. Cases of poisoning by home-canned and frozen mushrooms are **especially insidious** when the **preserved toadstools** are carried **to another location** and consumed at **another time**. Intoxications may occur at any time and place, with dangerous species occurring in habitat ranging from urban lawns to deep woods. Cases of mushroom poisonings generally do not resemble each other unless they are caused by the same or very closely related mushroom species.

Exercise 1a
Match the column A with the column B. Try to learn the expressions and/ or sentences by heart.

A

1. Ciguatera is a form of human poisoning caused by the consumption of subtropical and tropical marine finfish,
2. Manifestation of ciguatera in humans usually
3. Initial signs of poisoning
4. Neurological signs include intensified paraesthesia, arthralgia, myalgia, headache,
5. Cardiovascular signs include
6. Relapses are most often associated with
7. Shellfish poisoning is caused by a group of
8. Ingestion of contaminated shellfish results in a wide variety of symptoms,
9. The neurological effects include tingling, burning, numbness of lips, tongue and throat, muscular aches, dizziness,
10. Scombroid poisoning is caused by the ingestion of foods
11. Histamine and other amines are formed by the growth of certain bacteria,
12. Initial symptoms include a tingling or burning sensation in the mouth,
13. Neither cooking, canning,
14. Fishery products that have been implicated
15. Shipments of unfrozen fish packed in refrigerated containers

16. The gonads, liver, intestines, and skin of pufferfish
17. The symptoms include paraesthesia in the face and extremities, sensations of lightness or floating, headache, epigastric pain, nausea, diarrhoea, vomiting, reeling,
18. Poisoning from tetrodotoxin is of major public health concern primarily in Japan,
19. Mushroom poisonings are generally acute
20. Neurotoxins cause neurological symptoms
21. Disulfiram-like toxins
22. Most cases occur when toxic species
23. Outbreaks have occurred after ingestion of fresh, raw mushrooms, stir-fried mushrooms,

B

a) a rash on the upper body and a drop in blood pressure.

b) and are manifested by a variety of symptoms and prognoses.

c) are confused with edible species.

d) arrhythmia, bradycardia or tachycardia, and reduced blood pressure.

e) can contain levels of tetrodotoxin sufficient to produce rapid and violent death.

f) changes in dietary habits or with consumption of alcohol.

g) depending upon the toxins present, their concentrations in the shellfish and the amount of contaminated shellfish consumed.

h) difficulty in walking, increasing paralysis, respiratory distress, dyspnoea, cyanosis, hypotension, convulsions, mental impairment, and cardiac arrhythmia.

i) either during the production of a product such as Swiss cheese or by spoilage of foods such as fishery products.

j) have posed a significant problem.

k) home-canned mushrooms, and mushrooms that were blanched and frozen at home.

l) in scombroid poisoning include e.g. the tuna, sardines or mackerel.

m) include perioral numbness and tingling (paresthesia), which may spread to the extremities, nausea, vomiting, and diarrhoea.

n) involves a combination of gastrointestinal, neurological, and cardiovascular disorders.

o) or freezing reduces the toxic effect.

p) produce no symptoms unless alcohol is consumed.

q) reversal of the sensations of hot and cold, drowsiness, incoherent speech, confusion, memory loss, disorientation, seizure, coma, and respiratory paralysis.

r) *such as profuse sweating, coma, convulsions, hallucinations, excitement, depression, and spastic colon.*

s) *temperature sensory reversal and acute sensitivity to temperature extremes, vertigo, and muscular weakness.*

t) *that contain high levels of histamine and possibly other vasoactive amines and compounds.*

u) *toxins elaborated by planktonic algae upon which shellfish feed.*

v) *where 'fugu' is a traditional delicacy.*

w) *which have accumulated naturally occurring toxins through their diet.*

Protoplasmic poisons

Amatoxins

Poisoning by the amanitins is characterized by a long **latent period** (average **6-15 hours**). Symptoms appear at the end of the latent period in the form of **sudden, severe seizures of abdominal pain, persistent vomiting and watery diarrhoea, extreme thirst, and lack of urine production.** If this early phase is survived, the patient may appear to recover for a short time, but this period will generally be followed by a rapid and severe **loss of strength, prostration, and pain-caused restlessness.**

Death from **progressive and irreversible liver, kidney, cardiac, and skeletal muscle damage** may follow. Two or three days after the onset of the later phase, **jaundice, cyanosis and coldness of the skin** occur. **Death** usually follows a period of **coma** and occasionally **convulsions. If recovery occurs**, it generally requires at least a month and is accompanied by **enlargement of the liver.**

Hydrazines

There is generally a **latent period of 6-10 hours** after ingestion during which **no symptoms** are evident, followed by **sudden onset of abdominal discomfort** (a feeling of fullness), severe **headache, vomiting,** and sometimes **diarrhoea**. The toxin affects primarily the **liver**, but there are additional disturbances to **blood cells and the central nervous system**.

Orellanine

The poisoning is characterized by an extremely long **asymptomatic latent period of 3-14 days**. An intense, **burning thirst (polydipsia)** and excessive **urination (polyuria)** are the first symptoms. This may be followed by **nausea, headache, muscular pains, chills, spasms, and loss of consciousness**. In severe cases, severe renal tubular necrosis and **kidney failure** may result in **death** several weeks after poisoning. **Fatty degeneration of the liver** and severe inflammatory changes in the intestine accompany the renal damage, and recovery in less severe cases may require several months.

Neurotoxins

Poisonings by mushrooms that can cause neurological problems may be divided into three groups.

Muscarine poisoning:

Muscarine poisoning is characterized by **increased salivation, perspiration, and lacrimation**. These symptoms may be followed by **abdominal pain, severe nausea, diarrhoea, blurred vision, and laboured breathing**. Intoxication generally subsides within 2 hours.

Ibotenic acid/Muscimol poisoning

The chief symptoms are **drowsiness and dizziness** (sometime accompanied by sleep), followed by a period of **hyperactivity, excitability, illusions, and delirium**. Symptoms generally fade within a few hours. Fatalities rarely occur in adults, but in children, accidental consumption of large quantities of these mushrooms may cause convulsions, coma and other neurological problems.

Psilocybin poisoning

A number of mushrooms, when ingested, produce a syndrome **similar to alcohol intoxication** (sometimes accompanied by **hallucinations**). Onset of symptoms is usually rapid and the effects generally subside within 2 hours. Poisonings by these mushrooms are rarely fatal in adults. The most severe cases occur in small **children**, where large doses may cause the hallucinations accompanied by **fever, convulsions, coma and death**. Cases likely to be seen by the physician are **overdoses or intoxications** caused by a combination of the mushroom and some **added psychotropic substance (such as PCP).**

Gastrointestinal irritants

Poisonings caused by these mushrooms have a rapid onset. Some mushrooms may cause **vomiting and/or diarrhoea** which last for several days. **Fatalities** are relatively **rare** and are associated with **dehydration and electrolyte imbalances** caused by diarrhoea and vomiting, especially in debilitated, very young, or very old patients. Replacement of fluids and other appropriate supportive therapy will prevent death in these cases.

Disulfiram-like poisoning

A complicating factor in this type of **intoxication** is that this **species is generally considered edible** (i.e., no illness results when eaten in the absence of alcoholic beverages). **Consumption of alcoholic beverages** within 72 hours after eating it will cause **headache, nausea and vomiting, flushing, and cardiovascular disturbances** that last for 2-3 hours. All humans are susceptible to mushroom toxins. **Children** are more seriously affected and are more likely to suffer very **serious consequences** from ingestion of relatively smaller doses.

Exercise 1b
Match the column A with the column B. Try to learn the expressions and/or sentences by heart.

A

1. Symptoms of poisoning by the amanitins appear in the form of
2. This period will generally be followed
3. Death from progressive and irreversible
4. Two or three days after the onset of the later phase,
5. The toxin hydrazine affects
6. The first symptoms of orellanine poisoning are intense, burning thirst (polydipsia) and excessive urination (polyuria)
7. In severe cases, severe renal tubular necrosis
8. Muscarine poisoning is characterized by increased salivation, perspiration, and lacrimation,
9. The chief symptoms of ibotenic acid/ muscimol poisoning
10. Psilocybin poisoning can produce a syndrome
11. The most severe cases occur in small children
12. Fatalities are relatively rare and are associated with dehydration and electrolyte imbalances
13. Disulfiram-like poisoning

B

a) *and kidney failure may result in death several weeks after poisoning.*
b) *are drowsiness and dizziness, followed by a period of hyperactivity, excitability, illusions, and delirium.*
c) *by a rapid and severe loss of strength, prostration, and pain-caused restlessness.*
d) *caused by diarrhoea and vomiting, especially in debilitated, very young, or very old patients*
e) *followed by abdominal pain, severe nausea, diarrhoea, blurred vision, and laboured breathing.*
f) *jaundice, cyanosis and coldness of the skin occur.*
g) *liver, kidney, cardiac, and skeletal muscle damage may follow.*
h) *primarily the liver, but there are additional disturbances to blood cells and the central nervous system.*
i) *similar to alcohol intoxication.*
j) *sudden, severe seizures of abdominal pain, persistent vomiting and watery diarrhoea, extreme thirst, and lack of urine production*
k) *where large doses may cause the hallucinations accompanied by fever, convulsions, coma and death.*
l) *which may be followed by nausea, headache, muscular*

pains, chills, spasms, and loss of consciousness.

m) *will cause headache, nausea and vomiting, flushing, and cardiovascular disturbances*

illusions, fatalities, accidental consumption, subside, likely to be seen, electrolyte imbalances, debilitated, flushing, affected, serious consequences.

Exercise 2
Translate the expressions. Try to explain their meanings in English.

Accumulated, naturally occurring toxins, initial signs, numbness and tingling, paresthesia, arthralgia, myalgia, sensory, reversal, sensitivity, vertigo, prostration, arrhythmia, bradycardia, tachycardia, self-limiting, persist, recovered patients, experience, recurrence, relapses, dietary habits, affected, coupled with, paralytic, amnesia, burning, sensations, drowsiness, incoherent speech, confusion, memory loss, seizure, respiratory paralysis, vasoactive compounds, spoilage, rash, drop, encountered, impaired patients, canning, reliable, evaluation, implicated, incidents, shipments, gonads, flesh, paraesthesia, lightness or floating, reeling, convulsions, mental impairment, delicacy, viscera, organ failure, excitement, spastic colon, edible species, specimen, stir-fried, home-canned, blanched and frozen, insidious, resemble, latent period, restlessness, irreversible, enlargement of the liver, additional disturbances, asymptomatic, excessive urination, loss of consciousness, necrosis, kidney failure, inflammatory, salivation, perspiration, lacrimation, blurred vision, laboured breathing, drowsiness, dizziness, excitability,

Exercise 3
Answer the following questions. Prepare short talks and/or dialogues on these topics.

1. Describe ciguatera fish poisoning.
2. Describe shellfish poisoning.
3. Describe scombroid poisoning.
4. Describe tetrodotoxin poisoning.
5. Describe mushroom poisoning.
6. Characterise protoplasmic poisons (amatoxins, hydrazines, orellanine)
7. Characterise neurotoxins (muscarine, ibotenic acid/muscimol, psilocybin)
8. What is Disulfiram-like poisoning?

Vocabulary 16

Fill in the meanings in your mother language:

abalone /æb.ə.ˈləʊ.ni/
amanitin /ˌæm əˈnaɪ tən/
amatoxin /ˌæm əˈtɒk sɪn/
amberjack /ˈæm bərˌdʒæk/
amine /əˈmiːn/
amnesis /æmˈniːʒə/
antihistamine /ˌæn.tiˈhɪs.tə.miːn/
arrhythmia /əˈrɪð.mi.ə/
average /ˈæv.ər.ɪdʒ/
blanch /blɑːntʃ/
bluefish /ˈbluˌfɪʃ/

blurred /blɜːd/ **vision** /ˈvɪʒ.ən/
bradycardia /ˌbræd.ɪˈkaːdi.ə/
Ciguatera /ˌsi gwəˈtɛr ə/ **fish** /fɪʃ/
cockle /ˈkɒk.l̩/
coldness /kəʊld nəs/
convulsion /kənˈvʌl.ʃən/
couple /ˈkʌp.l/
cyanosis /ˌsaɪəˈnəʊ.sɪs/
debilitate /dɪˈbɪl.ɪ.teɪt/
delicacy /ˈdelɪkəsi/
disulfiram /ˌdaɪ.sʌlˈfɪə.
rəm/ **-ethanol** /ˈeθ.ən.ɒl/
dizziness /ˈdɪz.ɪ.nəs/
edible /ˈedɪbl/
elaborate /ɪˈlæb.ər.ət/
enlargement /ɪnˈlaːdʒ.mənt/
epigastric /ˌep.ɪˈgæs.trɪk/
evaluation /ɪˌvæl.juˈeɪ.ʃən/
evident /ˈev.ɪ.dənt/
fade /feɪd/
fatality /fəˈtæl.ə.ti/
flushing /flʌʃ.ɪŋ/
fugu /ˈfu gu/
fullness /ˈfʊl.nəs/
generalized /ˈdʒen.ə.r.ə.laɪzd/
gonad /ˈgəʊ.næd/
habitat /ˈhæbɪˌtæt/
histamine /ˈhɪs.tə.miːn/
hydrazine /ˈhaɪ drəˌzin/
ibotenic /ɪ bəʊ ten ik/ **acid** /ˈæsɪd/
illusion /ɪˈluː.ʒən/
incoherent /ˌɪn.kəʊˈhɪə.rənt/
insidious /ɪnˈsɪdiəs/
intensify /ɪnˈtensɪfaɪ/
irritant /ˈɪr.ɪ.tənt/
laboured /ˈleɪ.bəd/
lacrimation /ˌlæk.riˈmeɪ.ʃən/
latent /ˈleɪ.tənt/
lightness /ˈlaɪt nɪs/
mahi mahi /ˈmɑ hiˈmɑ hi/
medication /ˌmed.ɪˈkeɪ.ʃən/
muscarine /ˈmʌs kər ɪn/
muscimol /mus ɪ mol/
mussel /ˈmʌsəl/
myalgia /maɪˈæl.dʒi.ə/
neurotoxic /ˌnʊər oʊˈtɒk sɪk/
orellanine /əʊ.rəl əˌnin/
paralysis /pəˈræl.ə.sɪs/ pl **paralyses**
paralytic /ˌpær.əˈlɪt.ɪk/
paresthesia /ˌpær əsˈθi ʒə/
phencyklidine /fɛnˈsaɪ klɪˌdin/ **PCP**
per capita /pɜːˈkæpɪtə/
perioral /ˌper.ɪˈɔː.rəl/
perspiration /ˌpɜː.spərˈeɪ.ʃən/
pick /pɪk/
profuse /prəˈfjuːs/
progressive /prəˈgres.ɪv/
psilocybin /ˌsɪl.əˈsaɪ.bɪn/
psychotropic /saɪˈkɒˈtrɒp.ɪk/
pufferfish /pʌfə fɪʃ/
recurrence /rɪˈkʌr.əns/
reel /riːl/
relapse /rɪˈlæps/
renal /ˈriː.nəl/ **tubule** /ˈtjuː.bjuːl/
replacement /rɪˈpleɪs.mənt/
restlessness /ˈrestləs nəs/
reversal /rɪˈvɜː.səl/
scallop /ˈskæləp/
scombroid /ˈskɒm brɔɪd/
shipment /ˈʃɪpmənt/
skipjack/ˈskɪpˌdʒæk/
sole /soʊl/
subside /səbˈsaɪd/
supportive /səˈpɔː.tɪv/
suspect /səˈspekt/
tachycardia /ˌtæk.ɪˈkɑː.di.ə/
tetrodotoxin /tɛˌtroʊ dəˈtɒk sɪn/
toadstool /ˈtəʊdstuːl/
vasoactive /ˌveɪ.zəʊˈæktɪv/
yellowfin /ˈjeləʊ fɪn/

Solution to Exercise 1a
1w, 2n, 3m, 4s, 5d, 6f, 7u, 8g, 9q, 10t, 11i, 12a, 13o, 14l, 15j, 16e, 17h, 18v, 19b, 20r, 21p, 22c, 23k

Solution to Exercise 1b
1j, 2c, 3g, 4f, 5h, 6l, 7a, 8e, 9b, 10i, 11k, 12d, 13m

Unit 17 - Mycotoxins. Chemical hazards.

Mycotoxins are quite stable **chemical compounds produced by moulds**, which may **survive** various food processing activities including **baking and heat treatment**. Mycotoxins can also occur **in beer/ spirits and wine if grain or grapes are contaminated.** Mycotoxins can enter the **food chain** through **meat, eggs, milk, dairy products** if animals have eaten **contaminated animal feed. Bread** and other **grain-based products** could also contain mycotoxins if crops became contaminated in the field or during storage. Various mycotoxins are deemed to be potential carcinogens.

They can also **impair immune system** and **compromise kidney/ liver** systems. The risk to human health will depend on the type of mycotoxins, the level of exposure and the duration of exposure. Mycotoxins could also **interfere with/inhibit bacterial cultures** required for various **food-processing activities** (e.g. yoghurt, cheese making). Mycotoxin producing fungi can grow on a wide range of crops/feed including **cereal, grains, beans, peas, ground-nuts, and fruit**.

Mycotoxins produced by ***Fusarium* species** can cause a wide variety of symptoms, including haemorrhaging in the digestive tract, reproductive problems (**interfere with ovulation, conception and foetal development**), reduced food intake, **poor thrive**/ weight loss, vomiting, diarrhoea, **abortion, stillbirth and death**.

***Aspergillus* moulds** can produce a number of mycotoxins, including **alfatoxins** (these are probably **the most important mycotoxins** at global level) or **patulin** (although apples tend to be the major source, any **mouldy or rotten fruit** could contain this toxin).

Alfatoxins

The most pronounced contamination has been encountered in **tree nuts, peanuts,** and other **oilseeds**, including **corn and cotton-seed.** Alfatoxins produce **acute necrosis, cirrhosis, and carcinoma of the liver** in a number of animal species and humans may be similarly affected. Alfatoxins have been identified in corn and **corn products, peanuts and peanut products, cotton-seed, milk and tree nuts such as Brazil nuts, pecans, pistachio nuts, and walnuts**. Other grains and nuts are susceptible but less prone to contamination.

Pyrrolizidine alkaloids poisoning

Pyrrolizidine **alkaloid intoxication** is caused by consumption of plant material containing these alkaloids. The **plants** may be consumed as food, for medical purposes, or as contaminants of other agricultural crops. The alkaloids find their way into **flour** and other foods, including **milk** from cows feeding on these plants. Alkaloids have been found in the **honey** collected by bees foraging on toxic plants.

Early clinical signs include **nausea and acute upper gastric pain, acute abdominal distension** with prominent dilated veins on the abdominal wall, **fever**, and biochemical evidence of **liver dysfunction. Fever and jaundice** may be present. In some cases the lungs are affected, **pulmonary oedema** and **pleural effusion** have been observed. **Lung damage** may be prominent and has been fatal. Chronic illness from ingestion of small amounts of the alkaloids over a long period proceeds through fibrosis of the liver to **cirrhosis.**

Phytohaemogglutinin (kidney bean lectin)

Besides inducing mitosis, lectins are known for their ability to **agglutinate many mammalian red blood cells types**, alter their cell membrane transport systems, alter cell permeability to proteins, and generally **interfere with cellular metabolism.**

Phytohaemogglutinin, the presumed **toxic agent**, is found in many species of **beans**, but it is in highest concentration in red **kidney beans.** The syndrome is usually caused by the ingestion of **raw, soaked** kidney beans, either alone or in **salads or casseroles.** As few as four or five raw beans can trigger symptoms. Several outbreaks have been associated with "**slow cookers**" or **crock pots**, or in casseroles which had not reached a high **enough internal temperature** to destroy the glycoprotein lectin.

The following procedure has been recommended to render kidney, and other, beans safe for consumption:

- **soak** in water for **at least 5 hours**
- **pour away the water**
- **boil briskly** in fresh water, with occasional **stirring**, for at least **10 minutes**
- **undercooked beans** may be **more toxic** than raw beans

Grayanotoxin

Honey intoxication is caused by the consumption of honey produced from the nectar of **rhododendrons**. Generally the disease induces **dizziness, weakness, excessive perspiration, nausea, and vomiting** shortly after the toxic honey is ingested. Other symptoms that can occur are **low blood pressure** or **shock, bradyarrhythmia, sinus bradycardia, nodal rhythm, Wolf-Parkinson-White syndrome and complete atrioventricular block.**

In humans, symptoms of poisoning occur after a dose-dependent latent period and include **salivation, vomiting,** and both **circumoral and extremity paresthesia** (abnormal sensations). In severe intoxications, loss of coordination and progressive **muscular weakness** result. Grayanotoxin poisoning in humans is rare. Individuals who obtain honey from farmers who may have only a few hives are at increased risk. The pooling of massive quantities of honey during

commercial processing generally **dilutes any toxic substance.**

Other pathogenic agents

Prions are normal proteins of animal tissues that can misfold and become **infectious**: they are not cellular organisms or viruses. In their normal non-infectious state, these **proteins** may be involved **in cell-to-cell communication**. When these proteins become **abnormally shaped, i.e., infectious** prions, they are thought to come into contact with a normally shaped protein and transform that protein into the abnormally shaped prion. Prions are associated with a group of diseases called **Transmissible Spongiform Encephalopathies (TSEs)**. In humans, the illness suspected of being **food-borne** is **variant Creutzfeldt-Jacob disease.** The human disease and the cattle disease, **bovine spongiform encephalopathy (BSE)**, also known as "**mad cow**" disease, appear to be caused by the same agent.

No early acute clinical indications for TSEs have been described. After an extended period of years, these diseases result in **irreversible neurodegeneration**. Cases of vCJD usually present with **psychiatric problems**, such as **depression**. As the disease progresses, neurological signs appear **unpleasant sensations** in the limbs and/or face. There are **problems with walking and muscle coordination**. Sometimes victims become **forgetful** and experience severe problems with processing information and **speaking**. Increasingly they are unable to care for themselves until death occurs. High-risk tissues for BSE contamination induce the cattle's skull, brain, trigeminal ganglia (nerves attached to the brain), eyes, tonsils, spinal cord, dorsal root ganglia (nerves attached to the spinal cord), and the distal ileum (part of the small intestine). **Bovine meat (if free of central nervous tissue) and milk** have, to date, shown **no infectivity in test animals.**

Exercise 1a
Match the column A with the column B. Try to learn the expressions and/ or sentences by heart.

A

1. Mycotoxins are quite stable chemical compounds produced by moulds,
2. Mycotoxins can also occur
3. Bread and other grain-based products could also contain mycotoxins
4. Mycotoxins could also interfere with/inhibit bacterial cultures
5. Mycotoxin producing fungi can grow
6. Mycotoxins produced by *Fusarium* species can
7. *Aspergillus* moulds can produce
8. Any mouldy or rotten fruit
9. Alfatoxins produce
10. Alfatoxins have been identified

11. Pyrrolizidine alkaloid intoxication
12. The alkaloids find their way
13. Clinical signs include
14. Besides inducing mitosis, lectins are known for their ability to agglutinate many mammalian red blood cells types
15. Phytohaemogglutinin, the presumed toxic agent,
16. The following procedure has been recommended to render beans safe for consumption:
17. Honey intoxication with grayanotoxin
18. In humans, symptoms of poisoning occur after a dose-dependent latent period
19. The pooling of massive quantities of honey during commercial processing
20. Prions are normal proteins of animal tissues
21. Prions are associated with a group of diseases called
22. In humans, the illness suspected of being food-borne
23. The human disease and the cattle disease, bovine spongiform encephalopathy (BSE),
24. High-risk tissues for BSE contamination include

B

a) acute necrosis, cirrhosis, and carcinoma of the liver.

b) alfatoxins or patulin.

c) also known as "mad cow " disease, appear to be caused by the same agent.

d) and generally interfere with cellular metabolism.

e) and include salivation, vomiting, and both circumoral and extremity paresthesia (abnormal sensations).

f) could contain patulin.

g) generally dilutes any toxic substance.

h) if crops became contaminated in the field or during storage.

i) in beer/spirits and wine if grain or grapes are contaminated.

j) in corn products, peanut products, cotton-seed, milk and tree nuts such as Brazil nuts, pecans, pistachio nuts, and walnuts.

k) interfere with ovulation, conception and foetal development, poor thrive, abortion, stillbirth and death.

l) into flour, milk from cows feeding on these plants or honey collected by bees foraging on toxic plants.

m) is caused by consumption of plant material containing these alkaloids.

n) is caused by the consumption of honey produced from the nectar of rhododendrons.

o) is found in many species of beans, but it is in

highest concentration in red kidney beans.

p) *is variant Creutzfeldt-Jacob disease.*

q) *nausea and acute upper gastric pain, acute abdominal distension, liver dysfunction, fever and jaundice, pulmonary oedema, pleural effusion and lung damage.*

r) *on a wide range of crops/ feed including cereal, grains, beans, peas, ground-nuts, and fruit.*

s) *required for various food-processing activities (e.g. yoghurt, cheese making).*

t) *soak in water for at least 5 hours, pour away the water, boil briskly in fresh water, with occasional stirring, for at least 10 minutes.*

u) *that can misfold and become infectious: they are not cellular organisms or viruses.*

v) *the cattle's skull, brain, eyes, tonsils, spinal cord, trigeminal ganglia, dorsal root ganglia and the distal ileum.*

w) *Transmissible Spongiform Encephalopathies (TSEs).*

x) *which may survive various food processing activities including baking and heat treatment.*

Chemical hazards

Chemical contaminants in food can give rise to a number of health problems. Chemicals are divided into two primary categories: **prohibited substances** and **unavoidable poisonous** or deleterious substances (**pesticides, herbicides, growth hormones and antibiotics, additives and processing aids, lubricants, paints, cleaners and sanitizers**). Each company should make certain that none of the prohibited substances are present in ingredients or supplies.

Chemical hazards for meat and poultry

Raw materials	Pesticides, antibiotics, hormones, toxins, fertilizers, fungicides, heavy metals, PCBs.
Processing	Direct food additives-preservatives (nitrite), flavour enhancers, colour additives, indirect food additives, boiler water additives, peeling aids, defoaming agents.
Building and equipment maintenance	Lubricants, paints, coatings.
Sanitation	Pesticides, cleaners, sanitizers.
Storage and shipping	All types of chemicals, cross contamination.

Naturally occurring chemicals – contaminants

Contaminants are substances that have **not been intentionally added** to food. These substances may be present in food as a result of various stages of its production, packaging, transport or holding. They also might result from environmental contamination.

Poly-chlorinated biphenyls

Poly-chlorinated biphenyls are mixtures of individual chlorinated compounds. PCBs **do not readily break down** in the environment and thus **may remain** there for very long periods of time. PCBs also bind strongly to **soil** and are **taken up by small organisms** and fish in water and also by other **animals** that can eat these aquatic animals as food. PCBs were associated with certain kinds of cancer in humans, such as **cancer** of the **liver and biliary tract**.

3-monochloropropane diol (3-MCPD)

3-MCPD is a chemical contaminant that can form during **food processing**. Processes which were considered to be possible factors in 3-MCPD formation include:

- **Naturally** occurring levels in the raw materials
- **Storage** of **raw materials**
- Use of **chlorinated water** for washing purposes
- **Commercial** processing treatments such as **baking, evaporation, fermentation, malting, pasteurisation, roasting, smoking, spray drying, sterilization, and Ultra-High Temperature treatment**.
- **Migration** from food contact materials
- **Storage** of **prepared products**
- **Domestic** preparation including **baking, boiling, frying, grilling, and toasting.**

Dioxins

Once dioxins have entered the environment or body, they are there to stay due to their uncanny **ability to dissolve in fats** and to their rock-solid **chemical stability**. Their half-life in the body is, on average, seven years. In the environment, dioxins tend to **bio-accumulate** in the food chain. Dioxins are found throughout the world in practically all media, including **air, soil, water, sediment,** and **food**, especially dairy products, meat, fish, and shellfish.

Short-term **exposure** of human to high levels of dioxins may result in **skin lesions** such as chloracne and patch darkening of the skin, and **altered liver function**. Long-term exposure is linked to **impairment of the immune** system, the developing **nervous** system, the **endocrine** system and **reproductive** functions. **Foetuses** are most sensitive to dioxin exposure. **Newborns** may also be more vulnerable to certain effects. The **safety assurance** of food is a continuous process that begins with production and ends in consumption. Also, a balanced diet (including adequate amounts of fruits, vegetables and cereals) will help to avoid excessive exposure from a single source.

Polycyclic aromatic hydrocarbons (PAH)

Polycyclic aromatic hydrocarbons are a group of chemicals that are formed during the **incomplete burning** of **coal, oil and gas, garbage,** or other organic substances like **tobacco** or **charbroiled meat**. PAHs are found in **coal tar, crude oil, creosote, and roofing tar**, but a few are used in **medicines** or to make **dyes, plastics**, and **pesticides**. PAHs enter the air mostly as releases from **volcanoes, forest fires**, burning coal, and **automobile exhaust**.

PAHs can occur in air **attached to dust particles**. PAHs enter **water** through discharges from industrial and waste-water treatment plants. PAHs contents of **plants and animals** may be much higher than PAH contents of soil or water in which they live. Some people who have breathed or touched mixtures of PAHs and other chemicals for long periods of time have developed **cancer**.

Acrylamide

Acrylamide is a chemical which has been shown to be present in food as a result of **cooking practices**, some of which have been used for many years, even centuries. In particular, **starchy foods** have been shown to be affected, such as **potato and cereal** products, which have been **deep-fried, roasted or baked at high temperature**. The possible risk to public health is unclear.

Exercise 1b
Match the column A with the column B. Try to learn the expressions and/or sentences by heart.

A

1. Chemicals are divided into two primary categories: prohibited substances and unavoidable poisonous or deleterious substances:
2. Naturally occurring chemicals – contaminants
3. Poly-chlorinated biphenyls
4. PCBs do not readily break down in the environment
5. PCBs also bind strongly to soil
6. Processes which were considered to be possible factors in 3-MCPD formation include:
7. Domestic preparation including baking, boiling, frying, grilling, and toasting as well as commercial processing treatments like
8. Once dioxins have entered the environment or body,
9. In the environment,
10. Short-term exposure of human to high levels of dioxins
11. Long-term exposure is linked
12. Polycyclic aromatic hydrocarbons are a group of chemicals
13. PAHs occur in air attached to dust particles, they enter the air mostly as releases from
14. Acrylamide is a chemical which has been shown
15. In particular, starchy foods have been shown to be affected,

B

a) *and are taken up by small organisms and fish and also by other animals.*

b) *and thus may remain there for very long periods of time.*

c) *are mixtures of individual chlorinated compounds.*

d) *baking, evaporation, fermentation, malting, pasteurisation, roasting, smoking, spray drying, sterilization, and Ultra-High Temperature treatment were also considered to be possible factors in 3-MCPD formation*

e) *dioxins tend to bio-accumulate in the food chain.*

f) *may be present in food as a result of its production, packaging, transport or holding.*

g) *may result in skin lesions such as chloracne and patch darkening of the skin, and altered liver function.*

h) *naturally occurring levels in the raw materials, storage of raw materials or prepared products, and use of chlorinated water for washing purposes.*

i) *pesticides, herbicides, growth hormones and antibiotics, additives and processing aids, lubricants, paints, cleaners and sanitizers.*

j) *such as potato and cereal products, which have been deep-fried, roasted or baked at high temperature.*

k) *that are formed during the incomplete burning of coal, oil and gas, garbage, or other organic substances like tobacco or charbroiled meat.*

l) *they are there to stay due to their ability to dissolve in fats and to their chemical stability.*

m) *to be present in food as a result of cooking practices, some of which have been used for many years, even centuries.*

n) *to impairment of the immune system, the developing nervous system, the endocrine system and reproductive functions.*

o) *volcanoes, forest fires, burning coal, and automobile exhaust.*

Exercise 2

Translate the expressions. Try to explain their meanings in English.

Stable, spirits, grain or grapes, food chain, deemed, impair, compromise, interfere with, inhibit, groundnuts, haemorrhaging, ovulation, conception, poor thrive, abortion, mouldy or rotten, necrosis, carcinoma, medical purposes, agricultural crops, pulmonary oedema, pleural effusion, prominent, proceeds, agglutinate, permeability, trigger symptoms, soak, pour away, perspiration, bradyarrhythmia, bradycardia, nodal rhythm, atrioventricular block, circumoral, dilutes, abnormally shaped, irreversible, neurodegeneration, sensations, processing information, trigeminal ganglia, tonsils, spinal cord, dorsal, root ganglia, ileum, small intestine, prohibited substances, unavoidable, food additives, flavour enhancers, peeling aids, defoaming agents, maintenance, coatings, storage, sanitizers, intentionally added, packaging, holding, bind to soil, biliary tract, food processing, naturally occurring, evaporation, fermentation, malting, roasting, smoking, spray drying, Ultra-High Temperature treatment, baking, boiling, frying, grilling, toasting, dissolve in fats, skin lesions, altered liver function, impairment, vulnerable, safety assurance, incomplete burning, coal tar, crude oil, automobile exhaust, discharges from industrial plants.

Exercise 3
Answer the following questions. Prepare short talks and/or dialogues on these topics.

1. What are mycotoxins?
2. Characterise alfatoxins.
3. What do you know about pyrrolizidine alkaloids poisoning?
4. How to prepare beans to avoid phytohaemogglutinin (kidney bean lectin) poisoning?
5. Talk about grayanotoxin poisoning.
6. What are prions and which disease can they cause?
7. What do you understand by chemical hazards?
8. Which contaminants can we find in raw materials, in building and equipment and during processing of food?
9. Describe polychlorinated biphenyls and 3-monochloropropane diol (3-MCPD).
10. Describe dioxins and polycyclic aromatic hydrocarbons (PAH).

Vocabulary 17

Fill in the meanings in your mother language:

3-monochloropropane / 'mɒn.əʊ klɔr'prəʊ.peɪn/ **diol** / 'daɪ ɔl/ **(3-MCPD)**
abortion /ə'bɔː.ʃən/
acrylamide /ə'krɪl əˌmaɪd/
additive /'æd.ɪ.tɪv/
agglutinate /ə'glut nˌeɪt/
aid /eɪd/
alfatoxin /ˌæflə'tɒksɪn/
aquatic /ə'kwæt.ɪk/
Aspergillus /ˌæs pər'dʒɪl əs/
assurance /ə'ʃɔː.rəns/
atrioventricular / ˌaːtrɪ.ə.ven'trɪk.jə.lər/
block /blɒk/
boiler /'bɔɪ.lər/
bradyarrhythmia /'breɪ di ə'rɪð mi ə/
briskly /brɪsk li/
bovine /'bəʊvaɪn/ **spongiform** / 'spʌn dʒəˌfɔrm/ **encephalopathy** /enˌsef.ə'lɒp.ə.θi/ **BSE**
carcinoma /kɑː.sɪ'nəʊ.mə/
chlorinate /'klɔː.rɪ.neɪt/
circumoral /'sɜːkəm'ɔːrəl/
coal /kəʊl/ **tar** /tɑːr/

coating /ˈkəʊtɪŋ/
compromise /ˈkɒmprəˌmaɪz/
conception /kənˈsep.ʃən/
cooker /ˈkʊkər/
creosote /ˈkriː.ə.səʊt/
Creutzfeldt-Jacob disease /ˌkrɔɪts.feltˈjæk.ɒb.dɪˌziːz/
crock /krɒk/
crop /krɒp/
crude /kruːd/ **oil** /ɔɪl/
deem /diːm/
deep-fried /ˌdiːpˈfraɪd/
defoam /dɪˈfoʊm/
deleterious /ˌdel.ɪˈtɪə.ri.əs/
dilated /daɪˈleɪt.ɪd/
dioxin /daɪˈɒk.sɪn/
dissolve /dɪˈzɒlv/
distal /ˈdɪs.təl/
domestic /dəˈmes.tɪk/
dorsal /ˈdɔː.səl/
dust /dʌst/
dye /daɪ/
effusion /ɪˈfjuː.ʒən/
encephalopathy /enˌsef.əˈlɒp.ə.θi/
evaporation /ɪˌvæp.əˈreɪ.ʃən/
exhaust /ɪɡˈzɔːst/
fibrosis /faɪˈbrəʊ.sɪs/
forage /ˈfɒrɪdʒ/
forgetful /fəˈgetfəl/
fungicide /ˈfʌn.dʒɪ.saɪd/
ganglion /ˈɡæŋ.ɡli.ən/ pl **ganglia**
garbage /ˈɡɑːbɪdʒ/
glycoprotein /ˈɡlaɪ.kəʊˈprəʊtiːn/
grayanotoxin /greɪˈæn əˌtɒk sɪn/
groundnut /ˈɡraʊnd.nʌt/
half-life /ˈhɑːf.laɪf/
herbicide /ˈhɜː.bɪ.saɪd/
hives /haɪvz/
holding /ˈhoʊl.dɪŋ/
indirect /ˌɪn.da ɪˈrekt/
infectivity /ɪnˈfek.tɪv.ɪ.ty/
intentionally /ɪnˈten.ʃən.əl.i/
kidney /ˈkɪdni/ **bean** /biːn/
lectin /ˈlɛktɪn/
limb /lɪm/
mad /mæd/
malt /mɔːlt/
misfold /mɪˈs foʊld/
mouldy /ˈməʊldi/
nitrite /ˈnaɪ.traɪt/
nodal /ˈnəʊ.dəl/
occasional / əˈkeɪ.ʒə.nəl/
oilseed /ˈɔɪl.siːd/
ovulation /ˌɒv.jʊˈleɪ.ʃən/
particle /ˈpɑː.tɪ.kl̩/
pasteurisation /ˈpæstəˌraɪ zeɪ ʃən/
patch /pætʃ/
patulin /ˈpætʃ ʊlɪn/
phytohaemogglutinin /ˌfaɪtəʊˈˌhi məˌglut n ɪn/
pleural /ˈplʊə.rəl/
polychlorinated /ˈpɒl iˌ klɔr əˌneɪ tɪd/ **biphenyls** /baɪˈfɛn ls/ **(PCBs)**
polycyclic /ˌpɒl iˈsaɪ klɪk/ **aromatic** /əˈrəʊmə tik/ **hydrocarbons** /ˌhaɪ.drəʊˈkɑː.bəns/ **(PAHs)**
pot /pɒt/
pour /pɔːr/ **away** /əˈweɪ/
preservative /prɪˈzɜːvətɪv/
presume /prɪˈzjuːm/
raw /rɔː/ **material** /məˈtɪəriəl/
rhododendron /ˌrəʊ.dəˈden.drən/
roast /rəʊst/
rock-solid /ˌrɒkˈsɒlɪd/
roofing /ˈruːfɪŋ/ **tar** /tɑːr/
rotten /ˈrɒtən/
shaped /ʃeɪpt/
shipping /ˈʃɪp.ɪŋ/
sinus /ˈsaɪ.nəs/ **bradycardia** /ˌbræd.ɪˈkɑː.di.ə/
soaked /səʊkt/
spinal /ˈspaɪ.nəl/ **cord** /kɔːd/
spirit /ˈspɪr.ɪt/
spray /spreɪ/ **drying** /draɪŋ/
stir /stɜː/
toast /təʊst/
trigeminal /traɪˈdʒem.ɪ.nəl/
transmissible /trænzˈmɪs.ə.bəl/
spongiform /ˈspʌn dʒəˌfɔrm/

encephalopathy /enˌsef.əˈlɒp.ə.θi/ **TSEs**
ultra /ʌltrə/ **-high** /haɪ/
temperature /ˈtemprətʃər/
unavoidable /ˌʌn.əˈvɔɪ.də.bl̩/
uncanny /ʌnˈkæni/
wastewater /ˈweɪstˌwɔt̬.ər/
Wolf-Parkinson-White syndrome /ˈsɪn.drəʊm/

Solution to Exercise 1a
1x, 2i, 3h, 4s, 5r, 6k, 7b, 8f, 9a, 10j, 11m, 12l, 13q, 14d, 15o, 16t, 17n, 18e, 19g, 20u, 21w, 22p, 23c, 24v

Solution to Exercise 1b
1i, 2f, 3c, 4b, 5a, 6h, 7d, 8l, 9e, 10g, 11n, 12k, 13o, 14m, 15j

Unit 18 - Heavy metals. Added chemicals.

The term heavy metal refers to **any metallic chemical element** that has a relatively **high density** and is **toxic or poisonous at low concentrations**. The **interactions** of heavy metals with usual **elements from diet (Cu, Zn, Fe. Ca, Se)** have an important role in **acute and chronic toxicity**. Population can be contaminated with heavy metals by ingestion of contaminated or polluted food or water. According to their nutritional role the metals from food products can be divided in two categories:

1. **essential metals** (their absence or even their insufficiency in human diet induce after a period of time some modifications of **metabolic process** and will appear some **diseases**, (e.g. **Na, K, Ca, Cu, Zn, Mn**)
2. **unessential** metals (like **Pb, Hg, Al, Sn, Ag**)

For both categories, **increasing** of metal **concentration** in food over the limits can cause **toxic effects** for consumers of these products. Heavy metals are dangerous because they tend to **bioaccumulation**. Compounds accumulate **in living things** any time they are taken up and stored faster than they are broken down (metabolised) or excreted.

Cadmium

Cadmium derives its **toxicological properties** from its **chemical similarity to zinc,** an essential micronutrient for plants, animals and humans. The most significant use of cadmium is in nickel/cadmium **batteries, pigments, stabilisers for PVC, in alloys and electronic compounds**. Cadmium is **bio-persistent** and, once absorbed by an organism, remains resident for many years. In humans, long-termed exposure is associated with **renal dysfunction**. High exposure can lead to obstructive lung disease and has been linked to lung **cancer**. Cadmium may also produce bone defects (**osteomalacia, osteoporosis**) in humans and animals. Among the most important food possible **contaminated** with cadmium are **pork meat, fish, milk and beer**.

Lead

In humans exposure to lead can result in a wide range of biological effects depending on the level and duration of exposure. **High levels of exposure** may result in toxic biochemical effects in humans which in turn cause problems in the **synthesis of haemoglobin**, effects on the **kidneys, gastrointestinal tract, joints** and **reproductive** system, and acute or chronic damage to the **nervous** system. The sources of contamination with lead are: lead **piping** and **lead-lined tanks** in domestic water supplies; **canning** and using the **pottery glaze** for storage of the beverages.

Mercury

Mercury does not occur naturally in living organisms. Inorganic mercury **poisoning** is associated with **tremors, gingivitis** and/or **minor psychological changes** together with **spontaneous abortion and congenital malformation**. The usage of mercury is widespread in industrial processes and in various products. It is also widely used in **dentistry as an amalgam for fillings** and by the **pharmaceutical** industry. The main pathway for mercury to humans is through the food chain. **Monomethylmercury** and **dimethylmercury** are **highly toxic**, causing damage to the brain and the central nervous system, while foetal and postnatal exposure have given rise to abortion, congenital malformation and development changes in young children.

Copper

Copper is an **essential substance** to human life, but in **high doses** it can cause **anaemia, liver and kidney damage**, and **stomach and intestinal irritation**. The conditions for this metal to become toxic are high acidity of food and long contact time. Copper normally occurs in **drinking water** from copper pipes, as well as from additives designed to control algal growth.

Chromium

Chromium is used in **metal alloys** and pigments for **paints, cement, paper, rubber,** and other materials. Low-level exposure can irritate the skin and cause ulceration. Long-term exposure can cause kidney and liver damage, and damage to circulatory and nerve tissue.

Zinc

The distribution of zinc in our foodstuffs has much in common with copper.

Nickel

Small amounts of nickel are **needed** by the human body to produce red blood cells, however, in excessive amounts, can become mildly toxic. **Long-term exposure** can cause **decreased body weight, heart and liver damage, and skin irritation.**

Selenium

Selenium is **needed** by humans in **small amounts**, but in **larger amounts** can cause damage to the **nervous** system, **fatigue**, and

irritability. Selenium **accumulates in living tissue**, causing high selenium content in fish and other organisms, and causing greater health problems in human over a lifetime of overexposure. These health problems include **hair and fingernail loss**, damage to **kidney and liver tissue,** damage to **circulatory tissue,** and more severe damage to the **nervous** system.

Antimony

Antimony can be found in **batteries, pigments, and ceramics and glass.** Exposure to high levels of antimony for short periods of time causes nausea, vomiting and diarrhoea. It is a suspected human **carcinogen**.

Exercise 1a
Match the column A with the column B. Try to learn the expressions and/ or sentences by heart.

A

1. The term heavy metal refers to any metallic chemical element
2. The interactions of heavy metals with usual elements from diet (Cu, Zn, Fe, Ca, Se)
3. The absence of essential metals (Na, K, Ca, Cu, Zn, Mn) in human diet
4. Heavy metals are dangerous
5. The most significant use of cadmium
6. Cadmium is bio-persistent and, once absorbed by an organism,
7. Cadmium may also
8. Exposure to lead can result in toxic biochemical effects
9. The sources of contamination with lead are:
10. Mercury poisoning is associated with
11. Mercury is used in dentistry
12. Copper is an essential substance to human life,
13. Copper normally occurs in drinking water
14. Chromium is used in metal alloys
15. Small amounts of nickel are needed by the human body to produce red blood cells,
16. Selenium is needed by humans in small amounts,
17. Antimony can be found

B

a) *and pigments for paints, cement, paper, rubber, and other materials.*
b) *as an amalgam for fillings and by the pharmaceutical industry.*
c) *because they tend to bioaccumulation.*
d) *but in high doses it can cause anaemia, liver and kidney damage, and stomach and intestinal irritation.*
e) *but in larger amounts it can cause damage to the nervous system, fatigue, and irritability.*

f) *from copper pipes, as well as from additives designed to control algal growth.*
g) *have an important role in acute and chronic toxicity.*
h) *however, in excessive amounts, it can become mildly toxic.*
i) *in batteries, pigments, and ceramics and glass.*
j) *induce modifications of metabolic process and some diseases will appear.*
k) *is in nickel/cadmium batteries, pigments, stabilisers for PVC, in alloys and electronic compounds.*
l) *it remains resident for many years.*
m) *lead piping and lead-lined tanks in domestic water supplies; canning and using the pottery glaze for storage of the beverages.*
n) *on the kidneys, gastrointestinal tract, joints, nervous system and reproductive system.*
o) *produce bone defects (osteomalacia, osteoporosis).*
p) *that has a relatively high density and is toxic or poisonous at low concentrations.*
q) *tremors, gingivitis and/ or minor psychological changes together with spontaneous abortion and congenital malformation.*

Added chemicals
Food additives

Food additives comprise a large and varied groups of chemicals that are added to food to **ensure keeping quality** (thus preventing losses) and safety, nutritional quality, other qualities (taste, appearance etc.), and certain properties required for processing and/or storage.

Some **traditional measures** such as **curing and smoking** are considered to be risk factors for certain diseases (**hypertension**, some **cancers**). If possible other method of preservation should be used.

The direct food additives used at present include:

- **Processing aids** – e.g. **anticaking agents**, which are intended to aid in the processing of foods during production and after purchase.
- **Texturing agents** – e.g. **thickeners**, which provide specific food items with a desirable **consistency and texture**.
- **Preservatives** – e.g. **antioxidants**, and **antibacterials**, which prevent degradation of foods during processing and storage.
- **Flavouring and appearance agents** – e.g. **flavour enhancers**, flavouring agents, and **surface-finishing** agents, which

are used to give taste and/or smell to food.

- **Artificial sweeteners**
- **Nutritional supplements** – e.g. **vitamins and trace minerals**, which are added to replace essential nutrients lost during processing or to supplement existing levels.
- **Food colours** – of both natural and synthetic nature

Veterinary drugs and feed additives

Veterinary drugs are intended to **maintain or improve the health of animal** species. In food producing animals such as cattle, pigs, poultry and fish this may lead to **residues of the substances in the food** products (e.g. meat, milk, eggs). The residues should however not be harmful to the consumer.

Pesticides

A pesticide is any product that **kills** or controls various types of **pests**. A pest **(insect, weeds, rodents, birds, snails, fungi, algae, and bacteria)** is defined as a plant or animal that is harmful to man or the environment.

Pesticides are used primarily on crop-land to **control weeds (herbicides)**, **insects (insecticides)**, and **diseases (fungicides)** – and secondarily in storage areas to **protect the harvest**. Pesticides may cause serious health effects following excessive exposure, which range from acute fatal **poisoning** to **sensitization**, impaired immune function, **neurobehavioural** disorders, and **cancer**. Consumers can take the following steps to **reduce** their potential **exposure** to pesticide residues in food:

- **Choose a variety of foods** rather than a diet centred on only a small number of foods.
- **Rinse** all fruits and vegetables thoroughly in water. This surface cleaning will not remove pesticide residues taken up by the growing plant, but will remove residues on the **surface** as well as any dirt on the product.
- **Trim the fat** from meat and poultry and **discard the fat** in broths and pan drippings. This eliminates most residues that might concentrate in the fat.
- **Avoid** fish and game from areas where pesticides have been misused or **areas** that are known to be **contaminated**.

Physical hazards

A physical hazard is any extraneous object or foreign matter in a food item, which may cause illness or injury to a person consuming the product. These **foreign objects** include bone chips, metal flakes or fragments, injection needles, Bbs or shotgun pellet, pieces of product packaging, stones, glass or wood fragments, insects or other filth or personal items.

The following tables indicate some possible physical that may be found in meat processing operations.

Material	Injury potential	Sources
Glass	Cuts, bleeding; may require surgery to find or remove	Bottles, jars, light fixtures, gauge covers
Wood	Cuts, infection, choking; may require surgery to remove	Fields, pallets, boxes, buildings
Stones	Choking, broken teeth	Fields, buildings
Bullet/ BB shot/ needles	Cuts, infection; may require surgery to remove	Animals shot in field, hypodermic needles used for injections
Jewellery	Cuts, infection; may require surgery to remove	Pens/pencils, buttons, careless employee practices.
Metal	Cuts, infection; may require surgery to remove	Machinery, fields, wire, employees
Insects and other filth	Illness, trauma, choking	Fields, plant post-process entry
Insulation	Choking; long-term if asbestos were used	Building materials
Bone	Choking, trauma	Fields, improper plant processing
Plastic	Choking, cuts, infection; may require surgery to remove	Fields, plant packaging materials, pallets, employees.
Personal effects	Choking, cuts, broken teeth; may require surgery to remove	Employees

Exercise 1b
Match the column A with the column B. Try to learn the expressions and/or sentences by heart.

A

1. Food additives comprise a large and varied groups of chemicals
2. Some traditional measures such as curing and smoking
3. Anticaking agents are intended
4. Texturing agents – e.g. thickeners
5. Preservatives – e.g. antioxidants, and antibacterials
6. Flavouring and appearance agents – e.g. flavour enhancers, flavouring agents, and surface-finishing agents
7. Nutritional supplements – e.g. vitamins and trace minerals
8. Veterinary drugs are intended to
9. Residues of the substances in the food products
10. A pesticide is any product that
11. Pesticides are used primarily on cropland
12. Pesticides may cause serious health effects
13. Surface cleaning will remove residues of
14. Trim the fat from meat and poultry
15. A physical hazard is any extraneous object or foreign matter in a food item,

16. These foreign objects include bone chips, metal flakes or fragments,

B

a) and discard the fat in broths and pan drippings.
b) are added to replace essential nutrients lost during processing or to supplement existing levels.
c) are considered to be risk factors for certain diseases (hypertension, some cancers).
d) are used to give taste and/or smell to food.
e) injection needles, Bbs or shotgun pellet, pieces of product packaging, stones, glass or wood fragments or insects.
f) kills or controls various types of pests.
g) maintain or improve the health of cattle, pigs, poultry and fish.
h) pesticides on the surface as well as any dirt on the product.
i) prevent degradation of foods during processing and storage.
j) provide specific food items with a desirable consistency and texture.
k) should not be harmful to the consumer.
l) that are added to food to ensure keeping quality.
m) to aid in the processing of foods during production and after purchase.
n) to control weeds (herbicides), insects (insecticides), and diseases (fungicides)
o) which may cause illness or injury to a person consuming the product.
p) which range from acute fatal poisoning to sensitization, impaired immune function, neurobehavioural disorders, and cancer.

Exercise 2
Translate the expressions. Try to explain their meanings in English.

Interactions, usual elements, polluted, insufficiency, tend to, bioaccumulation, taken up and stored faster, toxicological properties, remains resident, obstructive lung disease, linked to, osteomalacia, osteoporosis, domestic water supplies, canning, pottery glaze, tremors, gingivitis, congenital malformation, amalgam for fillings, essential substance, irritation, metal alloys, excessive amounts, mildly toxic, fatigue, irritability, accumulates in living tissue, over a lifetime, comprise, taste, appearance, storage, curing and smoking, anticaking agents, intended, thickeners, consistency and texture, prevent degradation, flavouring agents, trace minerals, maintain or improve, residues, harmful, insect, weeds, rodents, birds, snails, fungi, algae, harvest, neurobehavioural disorders, rinse, trim, discard the fat, pesticides, misused, extraneous, bone chips, metal flakes, fragments, needles, shotgun pellet, jars, pallets, wire, require surgery, remove, cuts, bleeding, broken teeth, choking.

Exercise 3
Answer the following questions. Prepare short talks and/or dialogues on these topics.

1. What do you know about heavy metals?
2. Describe the effects of cadmium, lead and mercury.
3. Describe the effects of copper, chromium, nickel, selenium and antimony.
4. What do you know about food additives?
5. Talk about veterinary drugs and feed additives.
6. What do you understand by pesticides and how to reduce potential exposure?
7. Give examples of physical hazards, their sources and injury potential.

Vocabulary 18

Fill in the meanings in your mother language:

alloy /ˈæl.ɔɪ/
amalgam /əˈmæl.gəm/
anticaking /ˈæn taɪ keɪk ɪŋ/ **agent** /ˈeɪ.dʒənt/
antimony /ˈæn.tɪ.mə.ni/
artificial /ˌɑː.tɪˈfɪʃ.əl/
BB /ˈbiˌbi/ **shot** /ʃɒt/
BB /ˈbiˌbi/
bioaccumulation /baɪəʊ əˌkjuːmjəˈleɪʃən/
broth /brɒθ/
bullet /ˈbʊl.ɪt/
cadmium /ˈkæd.mi.əm/
cake /keɪk/
centred /sen.təd/
chip /tʃɪp/
comprise /kəmˈpraɪz/
consistency /kənˈsɪs.tənt .si/
cover /ˈkʌv.ə/
cropland /ˈkrɒpˌlænd/
cure /kjʊər/
degradation /ˌdeg.rəˈdeɪ.ʃən/
density /dent .sɪ.ti/
dentistry /ˈdɛntɪstrɪ/
dimethylmercury / diˌmɛθ əlˈmɜr kjə ri/
discard /dɪˈskɑːd/
disease /dɪˈziːz/
dripping /ˈdrɪp.ɪŋ/
essential /ɪˈsen.tʃəl/
extraneous /ɪkˈstreɪ.ni.əs/
feed /fiːd/
filling /ˈfɪl.ɪŋ/
filth /fɪlθ/
fingernail /ˈfɪŋ.gə.neɪl/
flavouring /ˈfleɪ.vər.ɪŋ/
fragment /ˈfræg.mənt/
gauge /geɪdʒ/
gingivitis /ˌdʒɪn.dʒɪˈvaɪ.tɪs/
glaze /gleɪz/
growth /grəʊθ/
harvest /ˈhɑː.vɪst/
have st in common /ˈkɒmən/ **with sb**
hypodermic /ˌhaɪ.pəˈdɜː.mɪk/
illness /ˈɪl.nəs/
insecticide /ɪnˈsek.tɪ.saɪd/
insufficiency /ˌin.səˈfiʃ.ən.siː/
insulation /ˌɪnsjəˈleɪʃən/
irritation /ˌɪr.ɪˈteɪ.ʃən/
jar /dʒɑːr/
lead /led/
lifetime /ˈlaɪftaɪm/
light /laɪt/ **fixtures** /ˈfɪkstʃər/

line /laɪn/
malformation /ˌmæl.fəˈmeɪ.ʃən/
mercury /ˈmɜː.kjʊ.ri/
metallic /məˈtæl.ɪk/
misuse /ˌmɪsˈjuːs/
monomethylmercury /ˈmɒn oʊˌmɛθ əlˈmɜr kjə ri/
needle /ˈniː.dl̩/
neurobehavioural /ˌnʊər oʊ bɪˈheɪv jər əl/ **disorder** /dɪsˈɔːdə/
nickel /ˈnɪkl/
obstructive /əbˈstrʌk.tɪv/
overexposure /ˈəʊvər ɪkˈspəʊʒər/
pallet /ˈpæl.ɪt/
pellet /ˈpelɪt/
pest /pest/
piping /ˈpaɪpɪŋ/
pollute /pəˈluːt/
postnatal /ˌpəʊstˈneɪ.təl/
pottery /ˈpɒt.ər.i/
property /ˈprɒp.ə.ti/
resident /ˈrez.ɪ.dənt/
rubber /ˈrʌbər/
sensitization /ˌsɛn sɪ təˈzeɪ ʃən/
shotgun /ˈʃɒt.gʌn/
similarity /ˌsɪm.ɪˈlær.ɪ.ti/
snail /sneɪl/
surface /ˈsɜː.fɪs/
sweetener /ˈswiːtənər/
tank /tæŋk/
texture /ˈteks.tʃər/
thickener /ˈθɪk.ən.ər/
tremor /ˈtrem.ər/
trim /trɪm/
weed /wiːd/
wire /waɪər/

Solution to Exercise 1a
1p, 2g, 3j, 4c, 5k, 6l, 7o, 8n, 9m, 10q, 11b, 12d, 13f, 14a, 15h, 16e, 17i

Solution to Exercise 1b
1l, 2c, 3m, 4j, 5i, 6d, 7b, 8g, 9k, 10f, 11n, 12p, 13h, 14a, 15o, 16e

Unit 19 - Food allergy and intolerances. Differential diagnosis.

Food allergies or food intolerances affect nearly everyone at some point. People often have an unpleasant reaction to something they ate and wonder if they have a food allergy. But only about three percent of children have **clinically proven allergic reactions** to foods. In adults, the prevalence of food allergy drops to about one percent of the total population. A food allergy, or **hypersensitivity**, is an **abnormal response** to a food that is triggered by the immune system. The **immune system is not responsible** for the symptoms of **food intolerance**, even though these **symptoms can resemble** those of a food allergy. It is extremely important for people who have **true food allergies** to identify them and prevent allergic reactions to food because these reactions can cause **devastating illness** and, in some cases, be fatal. Generally, such people come from **families** in which allergies are common – not necessarily food allergies but perhaps **hay fever, asthma, or hives**.

Before an allergic reaction can occur, a person **first has to be exposed** to the food. **The next time** the person eats that food the mast cells **release chemicals such as histamine**. If the mast cells release chemicals in the **ears, nose, and throat**, a person may feel itching in the mouth and may have trouble **breathing or swallowing.**

If the affected mast cells are in the **gastrointestinal tract**, the person may have **abdominal pain or diarrhoea**. The chemicals released by **skin** mast cells can prompt **hives**. Food **allergens** (the food **fragments responsible** for an allergic reaction) **are proteins within the food** that usually are not broken down by the heat of cooking or by stomach acids or enzymes that digest food. As a result, they **survive** to cross the gastrointestinal lining, **enter the bloodstream**, and **go to target organs**, causing allergic reaction throughout the body.

Common food allergies

In adults, the most common foods to cause allergic reactions include: **shellfish** such as shrimp, crayfish, lobster, and crab; **peanuts**, a legume that is one of the chief foods to cause **severe anaphylaxis**, a sudden drop in blood pressure that can be fatal if not treated quickly; tree nuts such as **walnuts**; **fish; and eggs**. The most common allergens that cause problems in children are eggs, milk, and peanuts. The foods that adults or children **react** to are those **foods they eat often**.

Cross reactivity

If someone has a **life-threatening reaction** to a certain food, the doctor will counsel the patient to **avoid similar foods** that might trigger this reaction. This is called cross-reactivity.

Exercise 1a
Match the column A with the column B. Try to learn the expressions and/ or sentences by heart.

A

1. Only about three percent of children
2. A food allergy, or hypersensitivity, is an abnormal response to a food
3. The immune system is not responsible
4. True food allergies
5. Before an allergic reaction can occur,
6. The next time the person eats that food
7. If the mast cells release chemicals in the ears, nose, and throat,
8. If the affected mast cells are in the gastrointestinal tract,
9. The chemicals released by skin mast cells
10. Food allergens (the food fragments responsible for an allergic reaction)
11. They survive to cross the gastrointestinal lining,
12. The most common allergens that cause problems in children
13. If someone has a life-threatening reaction to a certain food,

B

a) a person first has to be exposed to the food.

b) a person may feel itching in the mouth and may have trouble breathing or swallowing.
c) are eggs, milk, and peanuts.
d) are proteins within the food that usually are not broken down.
e) can cause devastating illness.
f) can prompt hives.
g) enter the bloodstream, and go to target organs.
h) for the symptoms of food intolerance, even though these symptoms can resemble those of a food allergy.
i) have clinically proven allergic reactions to foods.
j) that is triggered by the immune system.
k) the doctor will counsel the patient to avoid similar foods.
l) the mast cells release chemicals such as histamine.
m) the person may have abdominal pain or diarrhoea.

Differential diagnosis

A differential diagnosis means **distinguishing food allergy from food intolerance** or other illnesses. One possibility is the **contamination** of foods with microorganisms, such as **bacteria**, and their products, such as **toxins**. There are also **natural substances**, such as **histamine**, that can occur in foods (cheese, some wines, tuna and mackerel) and stimulate a reaction **similar to an allergic reaction**. This reaction is called **histamine toxicity**. Another cause of food intolerance is **lactase deficiency**. Lactase is an **enzyme** that is **in the lining of the gut**. This enzyme degrades lactose, which is in milk. If a person **does not have enough lactase, the body cannot digest the lactose** in most milk products. Another type of food intolerance is an **adverse reaction** to certain **products that are added to food** to enhance taste, provide colour, or protect against the growth of microorganisms. **Gluten intolerance** is associated with the disease called gluten-sensitive enteropathy or **celiac disease**. It is caused by an abnormal immune response to gluten, which is a **component of wheat** and some other grains. Some people may have a food intolerance that has a **psychological trigger**. People who experience exercise-food allergy eat a specific food before exercising. As they exercise and their body temperature goes up, they begin to itch, get light-headed, and soon have allergic reactions such as hives or even anaphylaxis.

Treatment

Food allergy is treated by **dietary avoidance**. People who have had **anaphylactic reactions** to a food should wear medical alert bracelets or necklaces stating that they have a food allergy. Such people should always carry a **syringe of adrenaline** (epinephrine), obtained by prescription from their doctors, and be prepared to self-administer it.

They should then immediately **seek medical help** by either calling the rescue squad or by having themselves transported to an emergency room. Anaphylactic allergic reactions **can be fatal** even when they start off with **mild symptoms** such as a **tingling in the mouth and throat** or **gastrointestinal discomfort**. Parents and caregivers must know how to protect children from foods to which the children are allergic and how to manage the children, including the administration of epinephrine. There are several **medications** that a patient can take to relieve food allergy symptoms. These include **antihistamines** to relieve gastrointestinal symptoms, hives, or sneezing and a runny nose. **Bronchodilators** can relieve asthma symptoms.

Infants and children

Milk and soy allergies are particularly common in infants and small children. Exclusive breast-feeding (excluding all other foods) of infants for the first 6 to 12 months of life is often suggested to avoid milk or soy allergies from developing. Such **breast-feeding** often allows parents to avoid infant-feeding problems, especially if the parents are allergic (and the infant is therefore likely to be allergic). The breast-feeding delays the onset of food allergies. By delaying the **introduction of solid foods** until the infant is 6 months old or older, parents can also prolong the child's allergy-free period.

Controversial issues

There are **several disorders** thought by some to be caused by food allergies, but the evidence is currently insufficient or contrary to such claims. There is virtually no evidence that most **rheumatoid arthritis or osteoarthritis** can be made worse by foods. **Cerebral allergy** is a term that has been applied to people who have trouble concentrating and have headaches as well as other complaints. It is controversial, for example, whether **migraine headaches** can be caused by food allergies. There are studies showing that people who are prone to migraines can have their headaches brought on by histamine and other substances in foods.

There is also no evidence that food allergies can cause a disorder called the **allergic tension fatigue syndrome,** in which people are tired, nervous, and may have problems concentrating, or have headaches. Another controversial topic is **environmental illness**. In a seemingly pristine environment, some people have many non-specific complaints such as problems concentrating or depression. Sometimes this is attributed to small amounts of allergens or toxins in the environment. Some people believe **hyperactivity in children** is caused by food allergies. But researchers have found that this behavioural disorder in children is only occasionally associated with food additives, and then only when such additives are consumed in large amounts.

Exercise 1b
Match the column A with the column B. Try to learn the expressions and/or sentences by heart.

A

1. A differential diagnosis means
2. One possibility is the contamination of foods
3. There are also natural substances, such as histamine,
4. Another cause of food intolerance
5. If a person does not have enough lactase,
6. Another type of food intolerance is an adverse reaction to certain products
7. Gluten intolerance is associated with the disease
8. It is caused by an abnormal immune response to gluten,
9. People who have had anaphylactic reactions to a food
10. Such people should always carry a syringe of adrenaline
11. Anaphylactic allergic reactions can be fatal even when they start off
12. Medications that a patient can take to relieve food allergy symptoms include antihistamines
13. Exclusive breast-feeding of infants for the first 6 to 12 months of life
14. By delaying the introduction of solid foods until the infant is 6 months
15. There are several disorders thought by some to be caused by food allergies,

B

a) *and be prepared to self-administer it.*
b) *called gluten-sensitive enteropathy or celiac disease.*
c) *distinguishing food allergy from food intolerance or other illnesses.*
d) *e.g. rheumatoid arthritis, osteoarthritis, migraine headaches, allergic tension fatigue syndrome or hyperactivity in children.*
e) *is lactase deficiency.*
f) *is often suggested to avoid milk or soy allergies from developing.*
g) *parents can prolong the child's allergy-free period.*
h) *should wear medical alert bracelets or necklaces stating that they have a food allergy.*
i) *that are added to food to enhance taste, provide colour, or protect against the growth of microorganisms.*
j) *that can occur in foods (cheese, some wines, tuna and mackerel) and stimulate a reaction similar to an allergic reaction.*
k) *the body cannot digest the lactose in most milk products.*

l) *to relieve gastrointestinal symptoms, hives, or sneezing and a runny nose and bronchodilators to relieve asthma symptoms.*
m) *which is a component of wheat and some other grains.*
n) *with microorganisms, such as bacteria, and their products, such as toxins.*
o) *with mild symptoms such as a tingling in the mouth and throat or gastrointestinal discomfort.*

Exercise 2
Translate the expressions. Try to explain their meanings in English.

Clinically proven, triggered, responsible, resemble, devastating illness, hives, release, mast cells, gastrointestinal lining, bloodstream, target organs, counsel, distinguishing, lactase deficiency, adverse reaction, gluten-sensitive enteropathy, dietary avoidance, medical alert bracelets or necklaces, prescription, self-administer, rescue squad, emergency room, gastrointestinal discomfort, relieve, sneezing and a runny nose, breast-feeding, onset, introduction of solid foods, insufficient, contrary, complaints, evidence, tension, attributed, behavioural disorder.

Exercise 3
Answer the following questions. Prepare short talks and/or dialogues on these topics.

1. What is the difference between food allergy and intolerances?
2. Describe true food allergies.
3. Describe some food intolerances.
4. What is the treatment of anaphylactic reaction?
5. Allergies in infants and small children.

Vocabulary 19

Fill in the meanings in your mother language:

administration /əd̩mɪn.ɪˈstreɪ.ʃən/
adrenaline /əˈdren.əl.ɪn/
allow /əˈlaʊ/
attribute /ˈæt.rɪ.bjuːt/
avoidance /əˈvɔɪ.dəns/
bracelet /ˈbreɪ.slət/
bronchodilator /ˌbrɒŋ.kə.daɪˈleɪ.tər/
claim /kleɪm/
complaint /kəmˈpleɪnt/
contrary /ˈkɒn.trə.ri/
counsel /ˈkaʊnsəl/
crayfish /ˈkreɪ.fɪʃ/
cross /ˈkrɒs/**-reactivity** /ˌri ækˈtɪv ɪ t̬ i/
cross /krɒs/
currently /ˈkʌr.ənt.li /
devastating /ˈdev.ə.steɪ.tɪŋ/
differential /ˌdɪf.əˈren.tʃəl/
distinguish /dɪˈstɪŋ.gwɪʃ/
emergency /ɪˈmɜː.dʒənt .si/
enteropathy /ˌɛn təˈrɒp ə θi/
epinephrine /ˌepɪˈnef.riːn/
gluten /ˈgluː.tən/ **-sensitive** /ˈsensɪtɪv/
hay /heɪ/ **fever** /ˈfiːvər/
intolerance /ɪnˈtɒl.ər.əns/
introduction /ˌɪn.trəˈdʌk.ʃən/
light-headed /ˌlaɪtˈhed.ɪd/
mast /mɑːst/ **cell** /sel/
mastocyte /mæst.ə.saɪt/
necklace /ˈnek.ləs/
osteoarthritis /ˌɒs.ti.əʊ.ɑːˈθraɪ.tɪs/
prescription /prɪˈskrɪp.ʃən/
pristine /ˈprɪstiːn/

prompt /prɒmpt/
proven /ˈpruː.vən/
relieve /rɪˈliːv/
rescue /ˈreskjuː/ **squad** /skwɒd/
researcher /rɪˈsɜːtʃə/
rheumatoid arthritis /ˌruː.mə.tɔɪd.ɑːˈθraɪ.tɪs/
runny /ˈrʌnɪ/
seemingly /ˈsiː.mɪŋ.li/
self /self/**-administer** /ədˈmɪn.ɪ.stər/
shrimp /ʃrɪmp/
sneezing /sniːz.ɪŋ/
syringe /sɪˈrɪndʒ/
target /ˈtɑː.gɪt/
tension /ˈten.ʃən/
virtually /ˈvɜː.tju.ə.li/

Solution to Exercise 1a
1i, 2j, 3h, 4e, 5a, 6l, 7b, 8m, 9f, 10d, 11g, 12c, 13k

Solution to Exercise 1b
1c, 2n, 3j, 4e, 5k, 6i, 7b, 8m, 9h, 10a, 11o, 12l, 13f, 14g, 15d,

Unit 20 - Food safety assurance. Food technologies for preservation.

International **food trade**, and **foreign travel,** are increasing, bringing important social and economic benefits. But this also makes the **spread of illness** around the world easier. **Eating habits**, too, have undergone major change in many countries over the last two decades and new food production, preparation and distribution techniques have developed to reflect this.

Effective **hygiene control**, therefore, is vital to avoid the adverse human health and economic consequences of **food-borne illness, food-borne injury, and food spoilage**. Everyone, including farmers and growers, manufacturers and processors, food handlers and consumers, has a responsibility to assure that food is safe and suitable for consumption.

Preventing of food-borne diseases

Preventing of food-borne illness requires a multi-sectoral effort by government, food industries, and consumers. The prevention strategy comprises **regulatory measures**, educational **activities**, and the surveillance of food-borne diseases and monitoring of contaminants.

The **food chain** may include the following stages:

- primary **production**
- **processing** and **manufacturing** by large or cottage industries
- transport, storage and distribution involving **retailers** and **supermarkets**
- preparation for consumption by **food service** and **catering** establishments, street food **vendors**, and **domestic** food handlers preparing family food.

The strategy for preventing food-borne illness can be described in terms of three lines of **defence**:

- improvement of the **hygienic quality** of raw foodstuffs in agriculture and aquaculture

- application of **food processing** technologies that control contaminants
- **education** of consumers and food handlers

Ten golden rules of the WHO

- Choose foods **processed for safety** (pasteurized milk)
- **Cook food thoroughly** (the temperature of all parts of the food must reach at least 70°C. Frozen meat, fish, and poultry must be thoroughly thawed before cooking).
- **Eat** cooked food **immediately** (when cooked foods cool to room temperature, microbes begin to proliferate)
- **Store** cooked **foods** carefully, either **hot** (near or above 60°C) or **cool** (near or bellow 10°C). Foods for infants should not be stores at all. A common error is putting too large quantity of warm food in the refrigerator.
- **Reheat** cooked foods **thoroughly** (all parts of the food must reach 70°C)
- **Avoid contact** between **raw foods and cooked** foods (safely cooked food can become contaminated through even the slightest contact with raw food)
- **Wash hands** repeatedly (wash hands thoroughly before you start preparing food and then after every interruption).
- Keep all kitchen **surfaces** meticulously **clean** (think of every food scrap, crumb or spot as a potential reservoir of germs)
- **protect foods** from insects, rodents, and other animals (storing foods in tightly sealed containers is your best protection)
- use **pure water** (pure water is just as important for food preparation as for drinking, boil water before adding it to food or making ice for drinks)

Exercise 1a
Match the column A with the column B. Try to learn the expressions and/or sentences by heart.

A

1. International food trade, and foreign travel
2. Effective hygiene control is vital to avoid the adverse human health and economic consequences
3. The food chain may include the following stages: primary production, processing and manufacturing,
4. Choose foods
5. Cook food thoroughly
6. Frozen meat, fish, and poultry must be
7. Eat cooked food immediately or store cooked foods carefully,

8. Avoid contact between
9. Wash hands repeatedly
10. Keep all kitchen surfaces meticulously clean;
11. Protect foods from insects, rodents, and other animals
12. Pure water is just as important for food preparation as for drinking

B

a) before you start preparing food and then after every interruption.
b) boil water before adding it to food or making ice for drinks.
c) either hot (near or above 60°C) or cool (near or bellow 10°C).
d) make the spread of illness around the world easier.
e) of food-borne illness, food-borne injury, and food spoilage.
f) processed for safety (pasteurized milk).
g) raw foods and cooked foods.
h) storing foods in tightly sealed containers.
i) the temperature of all parts of the food must reach at least 70°C.
j) think of every food scrap, crumb or spot as a potential reservoir of germs.
k) thoroughly thawed before cooking.
l) transport, storage and distribution, involving retailers and supermarkets, preparation for consumption by food service and catering establishments, street food vendors, and domestic food handlers.

Food technologies for preservation

Food preservation is achieved by:

- **Physical** techniques – include irradiation, cooking, pasteurisation, heat sterilization (canning), dehydration (drying), cooling, freezing and packaging (atmosphere control)
- **Chemical** techniques – include salting, pickling, smoking, fermentation, and additives with specific activities (antimicrobials, antioxidants)

Physical techniques

Irradiation

The radiation of interest in food preserving is **ionizing radiation**. The **energy waves** affect unwanted organisms but **are not retained in the food**. Irradiation is known as a **cold** process. "**Free radicals**" are **atoms or molecules** that are unstable and very **reactive**.

They can be **formed** during **irradiation**, and also **by toasting, frying, and freeze-drying.** There is **no evidence that** irradiated foods present **any increased risk** of exposure to harmful substances over conventionally processed foods.

Irradiation is most useful in four areas:

- **Preservation**. Irradiation has several advantages over traditional canning. The resulting products are **closer to the fresh state** in texture, flavour, and colour. Both large and small containers can be used and food can be **irradiated after being packaged or frozen.**
- **Sterilization**. Foods that are sterilized **by irradiation** can be **stored for years** without refrigeration just like canned (heat sterilized) foods. Sterilized food is useful **in hospitals** for patients with severely impaired immune systems, such as some patients with cancer or AIDS. These foods can be used by the **military** and for **space flights**.
- **Control sprouting, ripening, and insect damage. Irradiation** offers an alternative to chemicals for use with **potatoes, tropical and citrus fruits, grains, spices and seasonings**. Irradiation does not protect against re-infestation like insect sprays and fumigants do.
- **Control food-borne illness**. Irradiation can be used to effectively **eliminate** those **pathogens** that cause food-borne illness, such as Salmonella.

Cooking

Cooking is the act of preparing food for consumption. Heating can sterilize the food, in addition to **softening** the food by turning **collagen into gelatine.**
Some major hot cooking techniques.

- **Baking** (broiling)
- **Boiling** (blanching, coddling, infusion, braising, steaming, double steaming, poaching, simmering, pressure cooking, vacuum flask cooking)
- **Frying** (deep frying, hot salt frying, hot sand frying, pan frying, pressure frying, sautéing, stir frying)
- **Roasting** (grilling, searing, barbecuing)
- **Smoking**
- **Microwaving** (colloquially known as “nuking”)

Pasteurisation

The process of pasteurisation was created by Louis Pasteur. Pasteur’s aim was to **destroy bacteria, moulds, spores**, etc. He discovered that the destruction of bacteria can be performed by exposing them to certain minimum **temperature** for certain minimum **time** and the higher the temperature the shorter the exposure time required.

UHT pasteurisation, **ultra high temperature pasteurisation** is used mainly for **coffee creamers** and

boxed juices. These products are brought to over the boiling point, **120°C (under pressure**) for only a **fraction of a second.** After this is done, there is no need to refrigerate, because it sterilizes the product. The process of pasteurisation, not only **kills bacteria**, **but** it **also** kills off **nutrients**, and the essential **vitamins**. Products that can be pasteurized are: **milk, wine, beer, fruit juice, honey.**

Canning (heat sterilization)

Canning is a method of preserving food by sealing it in **air-tight jars or cans** and then **heating it** to a temperature that destroys contaminating microorganisms. Because of the danger of **botulism**, the only safe method of **canning** most foods is under condition of **both high heat and pressure**. Foods that must be pressure canned include all **vegetables, meats, seafood, poultry, and dairy products**.

The high percentage of **water** in most **fresh foods** makes them very **perishable**. They spoil or lose their quality for several reasons:

- growth of undesirable **micro-organisms** – bacteria, moulds, and yeasts
- activity of food **enzymes**
- reactions with **oxygen**
- **moisture loss**

Proper canning **practices** include:

- carefully **selecting and washing** fresh food
- **peeling** some fresh foods
- **hot packing** many foods
- adding **acids** (lemon juice or vinegar) to some foods
- using acceptable **jars and self-sealing lids**
- processing jars in a **boiling-water** or pressure canner for the correct period of time

These practices remove oxygen; destroy enzymes; prevent the growth of undesirable bacteria, yeasts, and moulds; and help form a high vacuum in jars.

Drying

Drying is a method of food preservation that works by **removing water**, which is required **for decay and** the growth of micro-organisms. Water is usually removed by **evaporation** (**air** drying, **sun** drying, **smoking** or **wind** drying) but in the case of **freeze-drying**, food is first frozen and then water is removed by **sublimation**. There are many different modes of drying and these include **drying** on a bed dryer, a fluidized bed dryers as well as an enclosed shelf-dryer. Many different foods are prepared by drying, including **Parma ham, beef jerky, and fruits such as prunes, raisins, figs, and dates.**

Water activity

The food with its specific water activity is **surrounded by a solution with lower water activity.** The driving force between the **internal** and **external water activity** produces water flow, which is known as **osmotic dehydration**.

There is also a certain amount of solute diffusion into the food resulting in a reduction of water activity to a level **sufficient to prevent microbial growth** and hence to preserve the food. When a bacterial cell is placed in a solution with low water activity, the cell dehydrates and bacterial growth is inhibited. Moisture migration in a dry food mix is a very important problem.

Exercise 1b
Match the column A with the column B. Try to learn the expressions and/or sentences by heart.

A

1. Physical techniques include
2. Chemical techniques include
3. The radiation of interest
4. The energy waves affect unwanted organisms
5. Free radicals are atoms or molecules
6. They can be formed during irradiation,
7. Irradiation has several advantages over traditional canning;
8. Foods that are sterilized by irradiation
9. Irradiation controls sprouting, ripening, and insect damage and
10. Heating can sterilize the food, in addition to softening
11. Some major hot cooking techniques are:
12. Boiling includes blanching, coddling, infusion, braising, steaming
13. Frying includes deep frying, hot salt frying, hot sand frying,
14. Roasting includes
15. Louis Pasteur discovered that the destruction of bacteria can be performed
16. In ultra high temperature pasteurisation (UHT) the products (milk, wine, beer, fruit juice, honey)
17. Canning is a method of preserving food by sealing it in air-tight jars or cans
18. Because of the danger of botulism, the only safe method of canning
19. Fresh foods spoil or lose their quality for several reasons:
20. Proper canning practices include:
21. Canning practices remove oxygen; destroy enzymes;
22. Drying is a method of food preservation that works
23. Water is usually removed by evaporation (air drying, sun drying, smoking or wind drying)
24. Many different foods are prepared by drying,
25. The driving force between the internal and external water activity

B

a) and also by toasting, frying, and freeze-drying.
b) and then heating it to a temperature that

destroys contaminating micro-organisms.

c) *are brought to over the boiling point, 120°C (under pressure) for only a fraction of a second.*

d) *baking, boiling, frying, roasting, and smoking.*

e) *but are not retained in the food.*

f) *but in the case of freeze-drying, food is first frozen and then water is removed by sublimation.*

g) *by exposing them to certain minimum temperature for certain minimum time.*

h) *by removing water, which is required for decay and the growth of micro-organisms.*

i) *can be stored for years without refrigeration just like canned (heat sterilized) foods.*

j) *carefully selecting and washing fresh food, peeling, hot packing, adding acids, using acceptable jars and self-sealing lids, and processing jars in a boiling-water or pressure canner.*

k) *double steaming, poaching, simmering, pressure cooking, or vacuum flask cooking*

l) *grilling, searing, and barbecuing.*

m) *growth of undesirable micro-organisms (bacteria, moulds, and yeasts), activity of food enzymes, reactions with oxygen, and moisture loss.*

n) *in food preserving is ionizing radiation.*

o) *including Parma ham, beef jerky, and fruits such as prunes, raisins, figs, and dates.*

p) *irradiation, cooking, pasteurisation, heat sterilization (canning), dehydration (drying), cooling, freezing and packaging (atmosphere control).*

q) *is under condition of both high heat and pressure.*

r) *offers an alternative to chemicals for use with potatoes, tropical and citrus fruits, grains, spices and seasonings.*

s) *pan frying, pressure frying, sautéing, and stir frying.*

t) *prevent the growth of undesirable bacteria, yeasts, and moulds; and help form a high vacuum in jars.*

u) *produces water flow, which is known as osmotic dehydration.*

v) *salting, pickling, smoking, fermentation, and additives with specific activities (antimicrobials, antioxidants)*

w) *that are unstable and very reactive.*

x) *the food by turning collagen into gelatine.*

y) *the resulting products are closer to the fresh state in texture, flavour, and colour.*

Exercise 2
Translate the expressions. Try to explain their meanings in English.

Trade, travel, spread of illness, eating habits, adverse consequences, food spoilage, assure, regulatory measures, retailers, catering establishments, street vendors, defence, education of consumers and food handlers, thoroughly thawed, proliferate, common error, reheat thoroughly, tightly sealed containers, pure water, irradiation, canning, drying, cooling, freezing, packaging, salting, pickling, smoking, fermentation, ionizing radiation, energy waves, retained, unstable, toasting, freeze-drying, texture, packaged, impaired, military, space flights, ripening, re-infestation, fumigants, softening, gelatine, broiling, flash-bake, blanching, coddling, infusion, braising, steaming, poaching, simmering, vacuum flask, deep frying, pan frying, stir frying, sautéing, searing, barbecuing, nuking, ultra high temperature pasteurisation, coffee creamers, boxed juices, fraction of a second, air-tight jars or cans, perishable, undesirable, moisture, jars and self-sealing lids, evaporation, bed dryer, prunes, raisins, figs, dates, solute, diffusion, moisture migration.

Exercise 3
Answer the following questions. Prepare short talks and/or dialogues on these topics.

1. Preventing of food-borne diseases.
2. List the Ten golden rules of the WHO.
3. Food technologies for preservation.
4. What do you know about physical techniques?
5. Characterize irradiation.
6. Describe major hot cooking techniques.
7. How does pasteurisation and UHT pasteurisation work?
8. What do proper canning practices include?
9. How does drying protect foods?

Vocabulary 20

Fill in the meanings in your mother language:

actinomycetes /æk͵tɪn oʊ'maɪ sits/
adverse /'æd.vɜːs/
agriculture /'æg.rɪ.kʌl.tʃər/
air-tight /'eə.taɪt/
ancient /'eɪn.tʃənt/
antimicrobial /͵æn ti maɪ'kroʊ bi əl/
antioxidant/͵æn.ti'ɒk.sɪ.dənt/
aquaculture /'æk wə͵kʌl tʃər/
arthralgia /aː'θræl.dʒɪ.ə/
ascospore /'æs kə͵spɔr/
aside /ə'saɪd/
atmosphere /'æt.mə.sfɪər/
baking /'beɪk.ɪŋ/
barbecue /'bɑː.bɪ.kjuː/
basidiospore /bə'sɪd i oʊ͵spɔr/
bed dryer /'draɪər/
bewildering /bɪ'wɪldərɪŋ/
botulism /'bɒt.jʊ.lɪ.zəm/
braise /breɪz/
broil /brɔɪl/
bud /bʌd/
can /kæn/
carbonation /'kɑːbəneɪʃən

case /keɪs/
coddle /ˈkɒd.l̩/
coffee /ˈkɒfi/ **creamer** /ˈkriː.mər/
concern /kənˈsɜːn/
confused /kənˈfjuːzd/
conventionally /kənˈvenʃənəli/
cool /kuːl/
cottage /ˈkɒt.ɪdʒ/ **industry** /ˈɪn.də.stri/
cottony /ˈkɒtən i/
creep /kriːp/
cruise /kruːz/ **ship** /ʃɪp/
crumb /krʌm/
Danish /ˈdeɪnɪʃ/ **blue** /bluː/
date /deɪt/
deep fry /ˌdiːpˈfraɪ/
defence /dɪˈfens/
dehydration /ˌdiː.haɪˈdreɪ.ʃən/
diffusion /dɪˈfjuː.ʒən/
diversity /daɪˈvɜː.sɪ.ti/
dry /draɪ/
enclose /ɪnˈkləʊz/
exceptionally /ɪkˈsep.ʃən.əl.i/
feeder /ˈfiː.dər/
fig /fɪg/
filament /ˈfɪl.ə.mənt/
filter /ˈfɪltər/
flask /flɑːsk/
fluidize /ˈflu ɪˌdaɪz/
force /fɔːs/
fraction /ˈfræk.ʃən/
freeze /friːz/ **(froze, frozen)**
freeze-dry /ˌfriːzˈdraɪ/
fry /fraɪ/
fumigant /ˈfju mɪ gənt/
gelatine /ˈdʒɛl ə tn/
geriatric /ˌdʒeriˈætrɪk/
germinate /ˈdʒɜːmɪneɪt/
grill /grɪl/
grower /ˈgrəʊər/
hepatitis /ˌhep.əˈtaɪ.tɪs/
hors d'oeuvre /ˌɔːrˈdɝːv/
hypha /ˈhaɪfə/ (plural hyphas or **hyphae** /ˈhaɪfiː/
in spite of /spaɪt/
ineffective /ˌɪn.ɪˈfek.tɪv/
inhibited /ɪnˈhɪbɪtɪd/
initiation /ɪˌnɪʃ.iˈeɪ.ʃən/
insect /ˈɪn.sekt/
interruption /ˌɪn.təˈrʌp.ʃən/
invade /ɪnˈveɪd/
ionize /ˈaɪ əˌnaɪz/
irradiation /ɪˌreɪ diˈeɪ ʃən/
log /lɒg/
mat /ˈmæt/
microwave /ˈmaɪ kroʊˌweɪv/
modification /ˌmɒd.ɪ.fɪˈkeɪ.ʃən/
moisture /ˈmɔɪs.tʃər/
mollusc /ˈmɒl əsk /
motile /ˈməʊ.taɪl/
mycelium /maɪˈsiːlɪəm/
mycotoxin /ˌmaɪkəˈtɒksɪn/
Norwalk /ˈnɔr wɔk/ **virus** /ˈvaɪ rəs/
noticeable /ˈnəʊ.tɪ.sə.bl̩/
nuke /nuːk/
offspring /ˈɒf.sprɪŋ/
oospore /ˈəʊəˌspɔː/
osmotic /ɒzˈmɒt.ɪk/
paediatric /ˌpiː.diˈæt.rɪk/
Parma ham /ˌpɑː.məˈhæm/
pasty /ˈpæs.ti/
Penicillium /ˌpɛnɪˈsɪlɪəm/
chrysogenum /krɪs əʊ dʒ.ɪ.nəm/
poisonous /ˈpɔɪ.zən.əs/
pickle /ˈpɪk.l̩/
plant /plɑːnt/
poach /pəʊtʃ/
prison /ˈprɪz.ən/
processor /ˈprəʊsesər/
proliferate /prəʊˈlɪfəreɪt/
prune /pruːn/
radiation /ˌreɪdiˈeɪʃən/
raisin /ˈreɪzən/
reactive /riˈæk.tɪv/
refrigerate /rɪˈfrɪdʒ.ər.eɪt/
reinfestation /rɪˌɪnfesˈteɪʃən/
render /ˈren.dər/
repeatedly /rɪˈpiː.tɪd.li/
ripen /ˈraɪpən/
rising /ˈraɪ zɪŋ/ **process** /ˈprəʊses/
Roquefort /ˈroʊk fərt/

rotavirus /ˈrəʊ.tə.ˈvaɪ.rəs/
safety /ˈseɪftɪ/
sauté /ˈsəʊteɪ/
scrap /skræp/
sealed /siːld/
sear /sɪər/
seasoning /ˈsiːzənɪŋ/
server /ˈsɜːvər/
simmer /ˈsɪmər/
slime /slaɪm/
slimy /ˈslaɪmi/
solute /ˈsɒl.juːt/
sporangium /spəˈræn dʒi əm/
pl **sporangia** /spəˈræn dʒi ə/
sprout /spraʊt/
stained /steɪnd/
sterilization /ˌsterəlaɪˈzeɪʃən/
stir fry /ˈstɜː.fraɪ/
surveillance /səˈveɪ.ləns/
survive /səˈvaɪv/
thoroughly /ˈθʌr.ə.li/
threadlike /θred.laɪk/
tightly /ˈtaɪt.li/
undesirable /ˌʌndɪˈzaɪərəbl/
unexploited /ʌn ɪkˈsplɔɪ təd/
unstable /ʌnˈsteɪ.bl̩/
unwanted /ʌnˈwɒntɪd/
vacuum /ˈvækjuːm/
vendor /ˈven.dər/
vigorously /ˈvɪg.ər.əs.li/
vinegar /ˈvɪn.ɪ.gər/
ward /wɔːd/
wave /weɪv/

Solution to Exercise 1a
1d, 2e, 3l, 4f, 5i, 6k, 7c,
8g, 9a, 10j, 11h, 12b

Solution to Exercise 1b
1p, 2v, 3n, 4e, 5w, 6a, 7y, 8i, 9r, 10x, 11d, 12k, 13s, 14l, 15g, 16c, 17b, 18q, 19m, 20j, 21t, 22h, 23f, 24o, 25u

Unit 21 - Cooling (refrigeration). Chemical techniques.

Refrigeration slows bacterial growth. A refrigerator set at 4°C (or below will protect most foods). There are two completely different families of bacteria:

- **pathogenic bacteria**, the kind that causes **food-borne illness**. Pathogenic bacteria can **grow rapidly** in the temperature range between 4°C and 60°C, but they **do not** generally **affect the taste, smell, or appearance** of a food.
- **spoilage bacteria**, the kind of bacteria that cause foods to deteriorate and develop **unpleasant odours, tastes, and textures**. Spoilage bacteria can grow at low temperatures, such as in the refrigerator.

Food that has been left too long on the counter may be dangerous to eat, but could seem fine. Food that has been stored too long in the refrigerator or freezer may be of lessened quality, but most likely would not make anyone sick.

Hot food cannot be placed directly in the refrigerator. It can be **rapidly chilled** in an ice or cold-water bath **before refrigerating. Cover foods** to retain moisture and prevent them from picking up odours from other foods. Raw meat, poultry, and seafood should be in a **sealed container or wrapped securely** to prevent **raw juices** from contaminating other foods. Some refrigerators have **adjustable shelves, door bins, crispers, and meat/cheese drawers**.

Freezing

Freezing is a common method of food preservation which **slows** both **food decay, and the growth of micro-organisms** and, by turning water to ice, makes it unavailable for bacterial growth and chemical reactions.

Long-term freezing requires a constant temperature of **-18°C, or less.** Freezer **doors** should be kept closed as much as possible, and only a **small amount** of unfrozen food should be **added** at one time. Unfrozen food should be placed in the coldest areas, which are near the **bottom** of the freezer. Freezing adversely affects the texture of many foods, and the **texture** of nearly all foods is damaged by **thawing and re-freezing**. Defects in the texture of thawed food can sometimes be obscured by cooking.

Packaging

Vacuum packaging

Vacuum packaging refers to packaging in containers (rigid or flexible), from which substantially all **air has been removed prior to final sealing** of the container. Normal room air is removed from the package.

Advantages of vacuum packaging:

- extends **shelf life**
- **reduces moisture loss** and freezer burn
- requires **minimal storage space**
- **leakers** are easily **detected**

Gas packaging

Gas packaging can be defined as the **alteration of the proportional volumes** of the gases, which comprise a normal atmosphere.

Controlled atmosphere (CAP)

Refers to a controlled system whereby **gases are added or removed to** maintain a **desired balance.**

Modified atmosphere (MAP)

In this process, products are packaged in **modified atmosphere** and the **oxygen removed.** The product is enclosed in a **blister package**, placed in the **vacuum chamber** and **evacuated**. The modified **atmosphere is then injected** and the blister package and food are sealed with a **protective film**. Using this method, the food retains its **original shape** and meats present a suitably red appearance to customers, even after extended storage.

Advantages of gas packaging

- allows **meat** to bloom
- extended **shelf life**
- **prevents crushing** of soft products
- retains **moisture**

Film properties

- **Nylon (PA)** – used for processed meat, cheese

packaging and boil-in-bag application

- **Polypropylene (P)** – used for fresh red meats packaging
- **Polyethylene (E)** – used for processed and fresh meats and cheese packaging
- **Surlyn (SU)** – used for processed and fresh meats packaging
- **Metallized Polyester (MES)** – used for processed meat, fish, snacks, candy and nuts packaging
- **Polyester (ES)** – used for processed meat, cheese, snacks, candy and coffee packaging
- **Poly Vinyl Chloride (PVC)** – used for processed meat, pasta.

Exercise 1a

Match the column A with the column B. Try to learn the expressions and/or sentences by heart.

A

1. Pathogenic bacteria can grow rapidly
2. Spoilage bacteria, is the kind of bacteria that cause foods
3. Food that has been left too long on the counter
4. Food that has been stored too long in the refrigerator or freezer may be of lessened quality,
5. Cover foods to retain moisture and prevent them
6. Some refrigerators have
7. Freezing is a common method of food preservation
8. Long-term freezing requires
9. Only a small amount of unfrozen food
10. Unfrozen food should be placed in the coldest areas,
11. The texture of nearly all foods
12. Vacuum packaging refers to packaging in containers (rigid or flexible),
13. Vacuum packaging
14. Gas packaging can be defined
15. Controlled atmosphere (CAP) refers to
16. Using modified atmosphere (MAP),
17. Product is enclosed in a blister package, placed in the vacuum chamber and evacuated,

B

a) *a constant temperature of -18°C, or less.*
b) *a controlled system whereby gases are added or removed to maintain a desired balance.*
c) *adjustable shelves, door bins, crispers, and meat/ cheese drawers.*
d) *as the alteration of the proportional volumes of the gases, which comprise a normal atmosphere.*
e) *but most likely would not make anyone sick.*

f) but they do not generally affect the taste, smell, or appearance of a food.

g) extends shelf life, reduces moisture loss, requires minimal storage space, and leakers are easily detected.

h) from picking up odours from other foods.

i) from which substantially all air has been removed prior to final sealing of the container.

j) is damaged by thawing and re-freezing.

k) may be dangerous to eat, but could seem fine.

l) should be added at one time.

m) the food retains its original shape and prevents crushing of soft products.

n) then the modified atmosphere is injected and the blister package and food are sealed with a protective film.

o) to deteriorate and develop unpleasant odours, tastes, and textures.

p) which are near the bottom of the freezer.

q) which slows both food decay, and the growth of micro-organisms.

Chemical techniques
Salting

Salting is the preparation of food with salt. Most **bacteria, fungi** and other potentially **toxic organisms cannot survive** in a highly salty environment. The use of "salt" to preserve meat and fish is a practice with a long history. **Salting** is often used in combination **with drying or smoking**. High intake of salt is associated with **high blood pressure** and that is why most guidelines call for a reduction in salt intake.

Pickling

Pickling is the process of preparing a food by **soaking and storing** it in a **brine (salt) or vinegar solution**, a process which can preserve otherwise perishable foods for months. Unlike the canning process, pickling **does not require the food** to be made **completely sterile** before it is sealed. The **acidity or salinity** of the solution makes it an environment in which **bacteria or fungi do not** easily **grow**.

Pickle products are subject to **spoilage from micro-organisms**, particularly **yeasts and moulds**, as well as **enzymes** that may affect flavour, colour, and texture. **Processing the pickles in a boiling-water canner** will prevent both of these problems. Standard canning jars and self-sealing lids are recommended.

Foods that are pickled include:

- **Vegetables**: onions, cabbage, cauliflower, ginger, peppers, mushrooms, lotus root, garlic, beets.
- **Fruit**: mango, plum, kumquat, lemon, watermelon, rind.
- **Meats**: beef, pork, ham
- **Fish**: herring

Smoking

Smoke treatment rivals salting, and is one of the oldest methods for preserving meat and other foodstuffs. In addition to preservation, **smoke treatment** also gives the food **flavour and colour**.

Traditional smoking is carried out by **suspending** the foodstuffs **in a kiln** where it is subjected to a **stream of smoke** generated by the controlled **combustion** of certain hard woods. "**Hot smoking**" is typically a several-hours-long process that can be used to fully cook raw meats or fish, while "**cold-smoking**" is an hours-or days-long process that is generally used to preserve or flavour foods (usually meats or fish, but sometimes cheese, vegetables, fruits, and even beer).

Because of the improvements in other preservation methods, many foods are now only **smoked commercially** for flavour and colour. This has lead to an increasing use of **liquid smoke** products as an alternative to traditional smoking. Liquid smokes are prepared by the **selective condensation of smoke constituents**. As a consequence, foods have a **much lower content of PAHs**, if any, and possible carcinogenic nitrosamine formation is eliminated.

Curing in food preparation

Curing in food preparation refers to various preservation and flavouring processes, especially of meat or fish, by the **combination of salt, sugar and either nitrate or nitrite.** Many curing processes also involve smoking. The application of pellets of salt called "corns", is often called corning. Curing in a **water solution** or brine is called **wet-curing or pickling**. The curing of **fish** is sometimes called **kippering**.

Seasoning

Seasoning is the process of **adding flavours**, or enhancing natural flavour of any type of food. Common seasonings include **black pepper, salt, and herbs**. A well designed dish will combine seasonings that complement each other. Seasoning may cause secondary contamination of food. The timing of when flavours are added will affect the food that is being cooked.

Fermentation

Many animal and vegetable foodstuffs are **fermented with bacteria, fungi, or yeasts to preserve them** as well as to produce flavour and texture. **Lactic acid** and **ethanol** are produced during fermentation and preserve by **preventing the growth of food spoilage micro-organisms.** Some bacteria used in fermentation systems also produce natural antimicrobial substance, for example nisin, which is a widely accepted food additive. Examples of fermented foodstuffs:

- **milk** products (cheese, yoghurt)
- **meat** products (fermented sausages)
- **cereal and legume** products (bread, oriental foods, soya sauce)

- **alcohol-containing** beverage (beer, wine)

Preservative additives

A preservative is a natural or synthetic chemical that is added to products such as foods, pharmaceuticals, paints, biological samples, etc. to **retard spoilage**, whether from **microbial growth**, or undesirable **chemical changes**. Food additives can be divided in two groups:

- **Anti-microbial** preservatives which function by inhibiting the growth of insects, bacteria and fungi.
- **Antioxidants** are chemicals that **prevent the oxidation** of other chemicals. In **biological systems**, the normal processes of **oxidation** (plus a minor contribution from ionizing radiation) **produce highly reactive free radicals**. These can easily react with and **damage other molecules**.

The **following vitamins and mineral** have shown **positive antioxidant effects:**

- **retinol, vitamin A or beta-carotene**. It has been discovered that beta-carotene protects **dark green, yellow and orange vegetables and fruits** from solar radiation damage and it is thought that it plays a similar role in human body. **Carrots, squash, broccoli, sweet potatoes, tomatoes, kale, collards, cantaloupe, peaches and apricots** are particularly rich sources of beta-carotene.
- **Ascorbic acid (vitamin C)** is a water soluble compound that fulfils this role, among others, in living systems. Important source includes **citrus fruits, green peppers, broccoli, green leafy vegetables, strawberries, raw cabbage, and tomatoes.**
- **Vitamin E (tocopherol)** is **fat soluble** and similarly protects lipids. Sources include **wheat germ, nuts, seeds, whole grains, green leafy vegetables, vegetable oil and fish liver oil**.
- **Selenium**. It is best to get selenium through foods, as large sources of the supplement form can be toxic. Good food sources include **fish, shellfish, red meat, grains, eggs, chicken and garlic.** Vegetables can also be a good source if grown in selenium-rich soils.

Several **food additives** (including ascorbic acid and tocopherol-derived compounds) are used as antioxidants to help guard against deterioration of food:

- **BHA** is the common abbreviation for **butylated**

hydroxyanisole, a fat-soluble antioxidant food additive. BHA is used to **preserve fats and oils** in food, cosmetics, and pharmaceuticals. Some foods in which BHA is used include: **butter, meats, cereals, chewing gum, baked goods, snack foods, dehydrated potatoes, and beer.**

- **BHT** is the common abbreviation for **butylated hydroxytoluene**, a fat soluble compound used as an antioxidant food additive. BHT **reacts with free radicals**, slowing the rate of autoxidation in food, preventing changes in the food's colour, odour, and taste.

Exercise 1a
Match the column A with the column B. Try to learn the expressions and/ or sentences by heart.

A

1. Most bacteria, fungi and other potentially toxic organisms cannot survive
2. Pickling is the process of preparing a food by soaking and storing it in a brine (salt) or vinegar solution,
3. The acidity or salinity of the solution
4. Pickle products are subject to spoilage from micro-organisms,
5. Foods that are pickled include:
6. Traditional smoking is carried out by suspending the foodstuffs in a kiln
7. Because of the improvements in other preservation methods, many foods are now only smoked commercially
8. As a consequence, foods have a much lower content
9. Curing in food preparation refers to various preservation and flavouring
10. Common seasonings include black pepper, salt, and herbs and
11. Many animal and vegetable foodstuffs are
12. Lactic acid and ethanol are produced during fermentation
13. A preservative is a natural or synthetic chemical that is added to products
14. Anti-microbial preservatives
15. In biological systems, the normal processes of oxidation
16. The following vitamins and minerals have shown positive antioxidant effects:
17. Beta-carotene protects dark green, yellow and orange vegetables and fruits
18. Carrots, squash, broccoli, sweet potatoes, tomatoes, kale, collards, cantaloupe, peaches and apricots
19. Important source of ascorbic acid (vitamin C) includes

20. Sources of vitamin E (tocopherol) include
21. Good food sources of selenium include
22. Several food additives are used as antioxidants to help guard against deterioration of food, e.g.
23. BHA is used to
24. Some foods in which BHA is used include:
25. BHT reacts with free radicals,

B

a) *a process which can preserve otherwise perishable foods for months.*

b) *and preserve by preventing the growth of food spoilage micro-organisms.*

c) *are particularly rich sources of beta-carotene.*

d) *butter, meats, cereals, chewing gum, baked goods, snack foods, dehydrated potatoes, and beer.*

e) *butylated hydroxyanisole and butylated hydroxytoluene.*

f) *citrus fruits, green peppers, broccoli, green leafy vegetables, strawberries, raw cabbage, and tomatoes.*

g) *fermented with bacteria, fungi, or yeasts to preserve them as well as to produce flavour and texture.*

h) *fish, shellfish, red meat, grains, eggs, chicken and garlic.*

i) *from solar radiation damage and it is thought that it plays a similar role in human body.*

j) *function by inhibiting the growth of insects, bacteria and fungi.*

k) *in a highly salty environment; salting is often used in combination with drying or smoking.*

l) *slowing the rate of autoxidation in food, preventing changes in the food's colour, odour, and taste.*

m) *makes it an environment in which bacteria or fungi do not easily grow.*

n) *of PAHs, and possible carcinogenic nitrosamine formation is eliminated.*

o) *particularly yeasts and moulds, as well as enzymes that may affect flavour, colour, and texture.*

p) *preserve fats and oils in food, cosmetics, and pharmaceuticals.*

q) *processes with the combination of salt, sugar and either nitrate or nitrite.*

r) *produce highly reactive free radicals which can easily react with and damage other molecules.*

s) *such as foods, pharmaceuticals, paints, biological samples, etc. to retard spoilage, whether from microbial growth, or undesirable chemical changes.*

t) *the timing of when flavours are added will affect the food that is being cooked.*

u) *vegetables, (onions, cabbage, cauliflower, ginger, peppers, mushrooms, lotus root, garlic, beets) and fruit (mango, plum, kumquat, lemon, watermelon, rind).*

v) *vitamin A, vitamin C, vitamin E and selenium.*

w) *wheat germ, nuts, seeds, whole grains, green leafy vegetables, vegetable oil and fish liver oil.*

x) *where it is subjected to a stream of smoke generated by the controlled combustion of certain hard-woods.*

y) *which has lead to an increasing use of liquid smoke products as an alternative to traditional smoking.*

Exercise 2

Translate the expressions. Try to explain their meanings in English.

Food-borne illness, affect the taste, smell, appearance, spoilage, deteriorate, odours, textures, counter, seem fine, retain moisture, picking up, odours, wrapped securely, adjustable shelves, door bins, crispers, drawers, decay, unavailable, unfrozen food, the bottom of the freezer, adversely affects the texture, thawing, re-freezing, containers (rigid or flexible), prior to final sealing, extends shelf life, minimal storage space, alteration of the proportional volumes, comprise, added or removed, desired balance, modified atmosphere, blister package, vacuum chamber, evacuated, injected, protective film, prevents crushing, boil-in-bag, snacks, candy, processed meat, pasta, guidelines, intake, soaking, brine, vinegar, acidity or salinity, cabbage, cauliflower, ginger, peppers, suspending in a kiln, combustion, liquid smoke, condensation, constituents, consequence, curing processes, seasonings, black pepper, herbs, complement, timing, lactic acid, ethanol, retard spoilage, undesirable, inhibiting, highly reactive, discovered, solar radiation, carrots, squash, sweet potatoes, tomatoes, kale, collards, cantaloupe, peaches, apricots, citrus fruits, green peppers, broccoli, green leafy vegetables, strawberries, raw cabbage, tomatoes, guard against, deterioration, abbreviation.

Exercise 3

Answer the following questions. Prepare short talks and/or dialogues on these topics.

1. What is the difference between pathogenic bacteria and spoilage bacteria?
2. How to treat the food before refrigerating?
3. Talk about freezing.
4. Describe vacuum packaging, gas packaging, controlled atmosphere packaging and modified atmosphere packaging.

5. What is the use of Nylon Polypropylene, Polyethylene, Surlyn, Metallized Polyester, Polyester, and Poly Vinyl Chloride?
6. Characterise chemical techniques salting, pickling and fermentation.
7. Describe smoking and curing.
8. What do you know about preservative additives?

Vocabulary 21

Fill in the meanings in your mother language:

abuse /ə'bjuːz/
achievement /ə'tʃiːv.mənt/
adjustable /ə'dʒʌstəbl/
adulthood /'æd.ʌlt.hʊd/
amenorrhoea /eɪˌmɛn ə'ri ə/
anorexia nervosa /
æn.əˌrek.si.ə.nə'vəʊ.sə/
anxiety /æŋ'zaɪ.ə.ti/
disorder /dɪ'sɔː.dər/
autoxidation /ɔˌtɒk sɪ'deɪ ʃən/
avoid /ə'vɔɪd/
bear /beə/ **weight** /weɪt/
beet /biːt/
behavioural /bɪ'heɪ.vjə.rəl/
beta-carotene /ˌbiː.tə'kær.ə.tiːn/
bin /bɪn/
binge /bɪndʒ/
black /blæk/ **pepper** /'pep.ər/
blister /'blɪs.tər/ **package** /'pækɪdʒ/
bloom /bluːm/
bowel /'baʊ.əl/ **movement** /
'muːv.mənt/
brine /braɪn/
bulimia /bjuː'lɪmɪə/
nervosa /nɜː'vəʊsə/
butylated /'bjut lˌeɪt ɪd/
hydroxyanisole, BHA /
haɪˌdrɒk si'æn əˌsoʊl/
butylated /'bjut lˌeɪt ɪd/
hydroxytoluene, BHT /
haɪ'drɒk sə 'tɒljʊˌiːn/
cachectic /kə'kɛk.tik/
cachexia /kə'kɛk si ə/
canner /'kænə/
cantaloupe /'kæntəˌluːp/
cauliflower /'kɒl.ɪˌflaʊ.ər/
cease /siːs/
cloning /'kloʊ.nɪŋ/
code /kəʊd/
collard /'kɒl ərd/
combustion /kəm'bʌs.tʃən/
commercially /kə'mɜː.ʃəl.i/
compensatory /ˌkɒm.pən'seɪt.ə ri/
complement /'kɒm.plɪ.ment/
compulsive /kəm'pʌl.sɪv/
conceal /kən'siːl/
condensation /ˌkɒn dɛn'seɪ ʃən/
conducive /kən'djuːsɪv/
consequence /'kɒn.sɪ.kwəns/
contempt /kən'tempt/
cor pulmonale /'kɔr ˌpʊl mə'næl i/
corn /kɔrn/
correlation /ˌkɒrə'leɪʃən/
crisper /krɪspə/
crushing /'krʌʃ.ɪŋ/
current /'kʌr.ənt/
Cushing's /'kʌʃ.ɪŋz/
syndrome /'sɪndrəʊm/
deplete /dɪ'pliːt/
deteriorate /dɪ'tɪə.ri.ə.reɪt/
determinant /dɪ'tɜː.mɪ.nənt/
deviant /'diːviənt/
dilemma /daɪ'lem.ə/
discovery /dɪ'skʌvəri/
discrimination /dɪˌskrɪm.ɪ'neɪ.ʃən/
disparagement /dɪ'spær ɪdʒ mənt/
distress /dɪ'stres/
diuretic /ˌdaɪ.jʊə 'ret.ɪk/
divide /dɪ'vaɪd/
drawer /drɔːr/

dysfunction /dɪsˈfʌŋk.ʃən/
elevation /ˌel.ɪˈveɪ.ʃən/
emphasis /ˈem.fə.sɪs/
engage /ɪnˈgeɪdʒ/
enlarge /ɪnˈlɑːdʒ/
enormous /ɪˈnɔːməs/
environment /ɪnˈvaɪə .rən .mənt/
evacuate /ɪˈvæk.ju.eɪt/
exclusive /ɪkˈskluː.sɪv/
exert /ɪgˈzɜːt/
expenditure /ɪkˈspendɪtʃər/
extend /ɪkˈstend/
film /ˌfɪlm/
flexible /ˈflek.sɪ.bl̩/
fungal /ˈfʌŋ.gəl/
genuine /ˈdʒɛn jʊ ɪn/
get /get/ **rid** /rɪd/ **of** /əv/
ginger /ˈdʒɪndʒə/
gland /glænd/
goal /gəʊl/
guideline /ˈgaɪd.laɪn/
guilt /gɪlt/
hardwood /ˈhɑrdˌwʊd/
herb /hɜːb/
hypercapnia /ˌhaɪ.pə.kæp.niə/
hypercellular /ˌhaɪ pərˈseljələr/
hypercortisolism /ˌhaɪ pərˈkɔr təˌsɔˌlɪz əm/
hyperinsulinism /ˌhaɪ pərˈɪn sə lɪˌnɪz əm/
hyperphagia /ˌhaɪ pərˈfeɪ dʒi ə/
hypothyroidism /ˌhaɪ pəˈθaɪ rɔɪˌdɪz əm
hypoventilation /ˌhaɪ.pəʊˌven.tɪˈleɪ.ʃən/
hypoxia /haɪˈpɒk.sɪə/
image /ˈɪm.ɪdʒ/
impending /ɪmˈpen.dɪŋ/
induce /ɪnˈdjuːs/
inflame /ɪnˈfleɪm/
influence /ˈɪn.flʊ.əns/
inject /ɪnˈdʒekt/
intervention /ˌɪn.təˈven.ʃən/
kale /keɪl/
kiln /kɪln/
Kumquat /ˈkʌm k̦wɒt/
lactic /ˈlæk.tɪk/ **acid** /ˈæs.ɪd/
laxative /ˈlæk.sə.tɪv/
leaker /liːkər/
leptin /ˈlɛp tɪn/
lie /laɪ/
lightheadedness /ˌlaɪtˈhed.ɪd.nəs/
lipid /ˈlɪp.ɪd/
loathsome /ˈləʊð.səm/
longitudinal /ˌlɒn.dʒɪˈtjuː.dɪ.nəl/
lotus /ˈloʊ təs/
mango /ˈmæŋ.gəʊ/
manipulative /məˈnɪp jəˌleɪ tɪv/
markedly /ˈmɑː.kɪd.li/
mature /məˈtjʊər/
Metalyzed /ˈmetəlaɪzd/ **Polyester (MES)** /ˈpɒl iˌɛs tər/
meticulous /məˈtɪk.jʊ.ləs/
mice /maɪs/
morbid /ˈmɔː.bɪd/
mutation /mjuːˈteɪ.ʃən/
neoplasm /ˈniː.ə.plæz.əm/
Nylon (PA) /ˈnaɪlɒn/
ob gene /dʒiːn/
obscure /əbˈskjʊə/
onion /ˈʌn.jən/
ought /ɔːt/
ovarian /əʊˈveə.ri.ən/
ovary /ˈəʊ.vər.i/
overeat /ˌoʊ vərˈit/
pancreatitis /ˌpæŋ.krɪ.əˈtaɪ.tɪs/
partially /ˈpɑː.ʃəl.i/
peach /piːtʃ/
peptic /ˈpep.tɪk/ **ulcer** /ˈʌl.sər/
pervade /pərˈveɪd/
pharmacotherapy /ˌfɑr mə koʊˈθɛr ə pi/
pick /ˈpɪk/ **up** /ʌp/
pick /pɪk/ **out** /aʊt/
pickwickian /pɪkˈwɪk i ən/ **syndrome** /ˈsɪn droʊm/
plum /plʌm/
Poly Vinyl Chloride (PVC) /ˌpɒlɪvaɪnəl ˈklɔːraɪd/

polycystic /ˌpɒlɪˈsɪstɪk/ **ovary** /ˈəʊvərɪ/ **syndrome** /ˈsɪndrəʊm/
Polyester (ES) /ˈpɒl iˌɛs tər/
Polyethylene (E) /ˌpɒl iˈɛθ əˌlin/
Polypropylene (P) /ˌpɒl iˈproʊ pəˌlin/
powerful /ˈpaʊə.fəl/
precision /prɪˈsɪʒən/
predispose /ˌpriː.dɪˈspəʊz/
prejudice /ˈpredʒ.ʊ.dɪs/
primarily /praɪˈmer.ɪ.li/
prior /praɪər/
prominent /ˈprɒm.ɪ.nənt/
proportional /prəˈpɔː.ʃən.əl/
psychopathology /ˌsaɪ.kəʊ.pəˈθɒl.ə.dʒi/
purge /pɜːdʒ/
pursue /pəˈsjuː/
race /reɪs/
reflect /rɪˈflekt/
refusal /rɪˈfjuː.zəl/
regulator /ˈreg.jʊ.leɪ.tər/
restriction /rɪˈstrɪk.ʃən/
rigid /ˈrɪdʒ.ɪd/
rind /raɪnd/
salinity /səˈlɪn.ɪ.t̬i/
securely /sɪˈkjʊə.lɪ/
sedentary /ˈsed.ən.tər.i/
seem /siːm/
selective /sɪˈlek.tɪv/
self-conscious /self.kɒn.ʃəs/
shame /ʃeɪm/
sheet /ʃiːt/
sleep /sliːp/ **apnoea** /ˈæp.ni.ə/
square /skweər/
squash /skwɒʃ/
substantially /səbˈstænʃəlɪ/
Surlyn (SU) /ˈsɜr lin/
suspend /səˈspend/
sweat /swet/
syndrome /ˈsɪn.drəʊm/
thaw /θɔː/
trapped /træpd/
undefined /ˌʌn dɪˈfaɪnd/
underdiagnose /ˈʌndəˈdaɪəgnəʊz/
vacuum /vækjʊəm/
chamber /tʃeɪmbə/
vigorous /ˈvɪg.ər.əs/
watermelon /ˈwɔː.təˌmel.ən/
wear /weə/ **down** /daʊn/
weigh /weɪ/
wheat /wiːt/ **germs** /dʒɜːmz/
wrap /ræp/

Solution to Exercise 1a
1f, 2o, 3k, 4e, 5h, 6c, 7q, 8a, 9l, 10p, 11j, 12i, 13g, 14d, 15b, 16m, 17n

Solution to Exercise 1b
1k, 2a, 3m, 4o, 5u, 6x, 7y, 8n, 9q, 10t, 11g, 12b, 13s, 14j, 15r, 16v, 17i, 18c, 19f, 20w, 21h, 22e, 23p, 24d, 25l

Chapter III
Basics in clinical nutrition

Unit 1 - Ethical and legal aspects. Basic concepts in nutrition

Ethical and legal aspects

Ethical codex of caring professions include not only minimal standards of behaviour but also ideals, and have been described as the 'collective conscience of our profession'. **The law,** on the other hand, **defends individual rights** and liberties and sets minimum standards below which **conduct** can be regarded as **lacking in care**, **negligent**, or downright **criminal**. It also **protects**

those who are **unable or incompetent** to make decisions for themselves.

Medical ethics are based on the four principles:

1. **Beneficence** – do good
2. **Non maleficence** – do no harm
3. **Autonomy** – the patient's right to self-determination
4. **Justice** – equal access to all

Ethical and legal considerations increasingly influence clinical decisions.

- Increased **complexity of decisions** in our technical and medico-legal climate in which the patient is better informed.
- The physician's **first duty** is to the patient (beneficence, non maleficence) but he or she also has a duty to society (justice),
- It is the **responsibility of society** as a whole to decide what resources are to be devoted to health care after full and public discussion and consultation.
- The **patient's autonomy** must be respected but no physician can be forced to undertake treatment that is futile or that he or she considers against the patient's interest.
- The **interest of the individual** must however be protected against arbitrary action or decisions by government, purchasing bodies, insurance companies or individuals by a **Bill of Rights** which is safeguarded by the courts acting independently of government.
- Care of the sick entails the basic duty of providing adequate and appropriate **fluid and nutrients by mouth**.
- As long as a patient can swallow and expresses a **desire or willingness to drink or eat**, fluid and nutrients should be given provided that there is no medical contraindication. This is **basic care**. **Artificial feeding** by tube or by vein is a **medical treatment**.
- A treatment for any patient should include provision for fluid and nutrition. Health carers should work as a team.
- If the plan is to maintain an **adequate intake** the ethical duty is to provide this, with the patient's consent, orally or by artificial means.
- Although **nutritional support** may be of value in the early stages of **terminal illness** there comes a point where intervention becomes more burden than benefit. Under these circumstances religious, ethical and legal authorities

consider that compassionate care should include only measures to **ensure comfort.** Prolongation of misery or dying by burdensome technology is unethical.

- Fluid or food given by tube **enterally or parenterally** is legally **medical treatmen**t and not basic care.
- For an incompetent **adult**, the doctor is responsible in law for doing of what is in the patient's best interest. He should seek to ascertain the previously expressed views of the patient, consulting the other members of the team and family. The legal position of **living wills** and the family varies between countries.
- Special considerations apply regarding the **responsibility of parents** to make a decision on behalf of their child and consent for the treatment by adolescents.
- Application to the court should be made regarding the **legality of withdrawing** artificial hydration and nutrition from a patient in vegetative state.
- Under carefully specified circumstances, it can be legal to **enforce nutritional treatment** on an unwilling patient, e.g. anorexia nervosa or hunger strikers.
- It could be construed as unethical not to be able to conduct a time-limited **trial of treatment** for fear of being unable to withdraw it if it proves of no benefit.
- When **tube feeding** is continued **outside hospital**, there is an ethical duty to ensure that the patient, daily carers and the community health team are adequately instructed in the technique and possible complications.

Organisation of nutritional care

Studies have shown that between 15 and 60% of **hospital admissions** are **undernourished**, half severely so. Furthermore such malnutrition is associated with increased complications and costs of illness, longer hospital stay and slower convalescence.

In many cases appropriate **nutritional support** can improve all these parameters. Unfortunately the condition goes largely unrecognised since few hospitals have a nutritional care policy or system of nutritional screening and assessment of patients at admission.

Although the prevalence of **undernutrition** in the community in European countries is less than 5%, it is higher than this in particular groups, e.g. in those suffering from disease or old age. In view of the serious clinical and economic consequences of undernutrition, health services and hospital authorities should be urged to develop proper strategies for managing nutrition in hospital and the community.

Improved organisation of nutritional care will have both clinical and economic benefits in the hospital service. Certain groups e.g. **the elderly** and those with **chronic disease** are at risk of malnutrition in the community and should also be identified and treated.

Exercise 1a
Match the column A with the column B. Try to learn the expressions and/or sentences by heart.

A

1. Ethical codex of caring professions
2. The law, on the other hand, defends individual rights and liberties and sets minimum standards below which conduct
3. Medical ethics are based on the four principles:
4. The physician's first duty is to the patient
5. The patient's autonomy must be respected
6. Bill of Rights is safeguarded
7. As long as a patient can swallow and expresses a desire or willingness to drink or eat,
8. Although nutritional support may be of value in the early stages of terminal illness
9. Fluid or food given by tube enterally or parenterally
10. The doctor should seek to ascertain the previously expressed views of the patient,
11. Special considerations apply regarding the responsibility of parents
12. Application to the court should be made regarding the
13. It can be legal to enforce nutritional treatment
14. When tube feeding is continued outside hospital, there is an ethical duty to ensure that the patient and daily carers
15. Between 15 and 60% of hospital admissions are undernourished;
16. Health services and hospital authorities should be urged
17. The elderly and those with chronic disease
18. Homoeostasis refers to the metabolic regulatory mechanisms
19. Homoeorhesis refers to regulatory mechanisms that allow the body to change from one homoeostatic, stable condition to another
20. Mild disturbances of homoeostasis or homoeorhesis lead to adaptation, without loss of function,
21. Attempts to establish recommended intakes for protein and energy intakes in various disease states
22. In disease states there is also a need

23. Body composition measurements are always indirect and are based on one or more assumptions
24. The starting point is the measurement
25. During the last twenty years a lot of research has been done
26. Basic rules should include the use of an equation

B

a) *are adequately instructed in the technique and possible complications.*
b) *are at risk of malnutrition in the community and should also be identified and treated.*
c) *beneficence – do good; non maleficence – do no harm; autonomy – the patient's right to self-determination and justice – equal access to all.*
d) *but he or she also has a duty to society.*
e) *but no physician can be forced to undertake treatment that is futile or that he or she considers against the patient's interest.*
f) *by the courts acting independently of government.*
g) *can be regarded as lacking in care, negligent, or downright criminal.*
h) *consulting the other members of the team and family; the legal position of living wills and the family varies between countries.*
i) *fluid and nutrients should be given provided that there is no medical contraindication (this is basic care).*
j) *include not only minimal standards of behaviour but also ideals.*
k) *is legally medical treatment and not basic care.*
l) *legality of withdrawing artificial hydration and nutrition from a patient in vegetative state.*
m) *on an unwilling patient, e.g. anorexia nervosa or hunger strikers.*
n) *such malnutrition is associated with increased complications and costs of illness, longer hospital stay and slower convalescence.*
o) *there comes a point where intervention becomes more burden than benefit.*
p) *to develop proper strategies for managing nutrition in hospital and the community.*
q) *to make a decision on behalf of their child and consent for the treatment by adolescents.*

Basic concepts in nutrition.
Energy and protein balance.
Basic concepts

Homoeostasis refers to the metabolic regulatory mechanisms that act to keep the body in constant condition with respect to **physiological function and reserves** of energy and other nutrients.

Homoeorhesis refers to **regulatory mechanisms** that allow the body to change from one homoeostatic, stable condition to another in an **organised fashion**, e.g. **growth during childhood**, or the onset of lactation.

The concept can be extended to weight gain after a period of weight loss, and perhaps also to weight loss itself, as far as it follows an organised pattern. **Mild disturbances** of homoeostasis or homoeorhesis **lead to adaptation**, without loss of function, e.g. the decrease in resting energy expenditure during starvation, while **more severe disturbances** lead to **accommodation**, or **changes in function**, (e.g. reduction in physical activity during prolonged semi-starvation), with the aim of maintaining other more vital functions.

Attempts to establish **recommended intakes** for protein and energy intakes in various disease states originated from attempts to establish requirements in **healthy subjects** where the aim was to preserve a **healthy weight by maintaining nutrients and energy balances.** However, in **disease states** there is also a need to consider **desirable changes** in body composition.

Body composition

In vivo body composition measurements are always **indirect** and are based on one or more assumptions concerning the **nature of the body components,** i.e. **fat mass** and fat-free mass including **water, protein and bone**. Examples of indirect methods based on assumption derived from carcass analysis, are **densitometry** and the measurement of **total body water**. The other methods are all double-indirect, validated against indirect methods, and therefore based on more assumptions. Whatever method is used, **the starting point** is the measurement of body mass with a **calibrated scale**. Subsequent subdivision of body mass into components like fat mass and fat-free mass has an **accuracy of 1 kg** or less, especially in patients in whom these assumptions are violated by the effects of disease.

Bioelectrical impedance analysis

Several methods have been developed for measurement of body composition. However, many of them are used almost exclusively for **research purposes** because they are time consuming and often expensive. During the last twenty years a lot of research has been done on bioelectrical impedance analysis (BIA) of body compartments. This is a **relatively accessible** method of measurement of body composition, which is increasingly frequently used in clinical practice. BIA can be considered a suitable option for body composition assessment so long as some **basic rules** are respected. These should include the use of an **equation** developed for the specific **population concerned,** preferably without fluid imbalance or abnormalities in body shape and with a BMI in the range 18 to 34kg·m^{-2}.

Exercise 1b
Match the column A with the column B. Try to learn the expressions and/or sentences by heart.

A

1. Homoeostasis refers to the metabolic regulatory mechanisms
2. Homoeorhesis refers to regulatory mechanisms that allow the body to change from one homoeostatic, stable condition to another
3. Mild disturbances of homoeostasis or homoeorhesis lead to adaptation, without loss of function,
4. Attempts to establish recommended intakes for protein and energy intakes in various disease states
5. In disease states there is also a need
6. Body composition measurements are always indirect and are based on one or more assumptions
7. The starting point is the measurement
8. During the last twenty years a lot of research has been done
9. Basic rules should include the use of an equation

B

a) *concerning the nature of the body components, i.e. fat mass and fat-free mass including water, protein and bone.*
b) *developed for the specific population concerned, preferably without fluid imbalance or abnormalities in body shape and with a BMI in the range 18 to 34kg·m^{-2}.*
c) *in an organised fashion, e.g. growth during childhood, or the onset of lactation.*
d) *of body mass with a calibrated scale.*
e) *on bioelectrical impedance analysis (BIA) of body compartments.*
f) *originated from attempts to establish requirements in healthy subjects.*
g) *that act to keep the body in constant condition with respect to physiological function and reserves of energy and other nutrients.*
h) *to consider desirable changes in body composition.*
i) *while more severe disturbances lead to accommodation, or changes in function.*

Exercise 2
Translate the expressions. Try to explain their meanings in English.

Caring professions, conscience, defends individual rights, liberties, conduct, be regarded as, lacking in care, negligent, criminal, unable or incompetent, beneficence, non maleficence, autonomy, self-determination, justice, complexity, duty to society, responsibility, resources, devoted, undertake treatment, futile, arbitrary action, government, purchasing bodies, insurance companies, safeguarded, by the courts, independently, entails, swallow, desire or willingness, medical contraindication, artificial feeding, by tube or vein, medical treatment, provision, health carers, adequate intake, consent, orally or by artificial means, support, intervention, burden, compassionate, care measures, to ensure comfort, misery, dying, medical treatment, incompetent adult, ascertain, expressed views, living wills, responsibility of parents, decision on behalf of, consent for, application to the court, legality of withdrawing, artificial hydration and nutrition, enforce nutritional treatment, anorexia nervosa, hunger strikers, construed as unethical, conduct a trial of treatment, unable to withdraw it, proves of no benefit, tube feeding, outside hospital, daily carers, adequately instructed, hospital admissions, undernourished, costs, slower convalescence, goes unrecognised, nutritional screening, prevalence, consequences, be urged to, constant condition, with respect to, homoeorhesis, stable condition, organised fashion, growth, onset of lactation, concept, pattern, disturbances, adaptation, resting energy, expenditure, starvation, accommodation, maintaining vital functions, recommended, attempts to establish, requirements, desirable, assumptions, nature of components, derived from carcass analysis, validated against, calibrated scale, subsequent, subdivision, accuracy, violated, impedance, research purposes, time consuming, expensive, body compartments, considered a suitable option, basic rules, equation.

Exercise 3
Prepare short talks and/or dialogues on these topics:

1. Energy and protein balance
2. Homoeostasis, homoeorhesis, adaptation and accommodation
3. Body composition and its measurement
4. Bioelectrical impedance analysis
5. Medical ethics
6. Practice of nutritional care
7. Legal aspects
8. Disease related malnutrition
9. Organisation of nutritional care

Vocabulary 1

Fill in the meanings in your mother language:

accommodation /əˌkɒm.əˈdeɪ.ʃən/
accuracy /ˈæk.jʊ.rə.si/
act /ækt/
adaptation /ˌæd.əpˈteɪ.ʃən/
admission /ədˈmɪʃ.ən/
adolescent /ˌæd.əˈles.ənt/
affect /əˈfekt/
aim /eɪm/ **at** /ət/
analysis /əˈnæl.ə.sɪs/
appreciate /əˈpriː.ʃi.eɪt/
approach /əˈprəʊtʃ/
arbitrary /ˈɑː.bɪ.trər.i/
artificial /ˌɑː.tɪˈfɪʃ.əl/

ascertain /ˌæs.əˈteɪn/
aspect /ˈæs.pekt/
assessment /əˈses.mənt/
assumption /əˈsʌmp.ʃən/
attempt /əˈtempt/
authority /ɔːˈθɒr.ɪ.ti/
autonomy /ɔːˈtɒn.ə.mi/
balance /ˈbæl.əns/
barrier /ˈbær.i.ər/
beneficence /bɪˈnef.ɪ.sən.ts/
Bill /bɪl/ **of Rights** /raɪts/
body /ˈbɒdɪ/
burdensome /ˈbɜː.dən.səm/
calibrate /ˈkæl.əˌbreɪt/
carcass /ˈkɑː.kəs/
comfort /ˈkʌm.fət/
compartment /kəmˈpɑːt.mənt/
compassionate /kəmˈpæʃ.ən.ət/
complexity /kəmˈplek.sɪ.ti/
component /kəmˈpəʊ.nənt/
composition /ˌkɒm.pəˈzɪʃ.ən/
concept /ˈkɒn.sept/
conduct /kənˈdʌkt/
conscience /ˈkɒn.tʃənt s/
consent /kənˈsent/
construe /kənˈstruː/
convalescence /ˌkɒn.vəˈles.əns/
coordinate /kəʊˈɔː.dɪ.neɪt/
court /kɔːt/
criminal /ˈkrɪm.ɪ.nəl/
densitometry /den.siˈtom.i.tri/
desire /dɪˈzaɪər/
devoted /dɪˈvəʊ.tɪd/
disturbance /dɪˈstɜː.bəns/
double /ˈdʌb.lˌ/
downright /ˈdaʊn.raɪt/
enforce /ɪnˈfɔːs/
entail /ɪnˈteɪl/
equal /ˈiːkwəl/
equation /ɪˈkweɪ.ʒən/
ethical /ˈeθ.ɪ.kəl/
exclusively /ɪkˈskluː.sɪv.li/
expenditure /ɪkˈspen.dɪ.tʃər/
failure /ˈfeɪ.ljər/
feeding /ˌfiː.dɪŋ/
futile /ˈfjuːtaɪl/
homeorhesis /ˌhəʊ.mi.əʊ.riː.sis/
homeostasis /ˌhəʊ.mi.əʊˈsteɪ.sɪs/
hunger /ˈhʌŋ.gər/ **striker** /ˈstraɪ.kər/
ideal /aɪˈdɪəl/
identify /aɪˈden.tɪ.faɪ/
impedance /ɪɪmˈpiː.dənts/
implementation /ˌɪm.plɪ.menˈteɪ.ʃən/
improve /ɪmˈpruːv/
in vivo /ˈviː.vəʊ/
incompetent /ɪnˈkɒm.pɪ.tənt/
independently /ˌɪn.dɪˈpen.dənt.li/
indirect /ˌɪn.da ɪˈrekt/
instruct /ɪnˈstrʌkt/
insurance /ɪnˈʃɔː.rəns/
company /ˈkʌm.pə.ni/
justice /ˈdʒʌs.tɪs/
lactation /lækˈteɪ.ʃən/
legal /ˈliː.gəl/
legality /liːˈgæl.ə.ti/
liberty /ˈlɪb.ə.ti/
living /ˈlɪv.ɪŋ/ **will** /wɪl/
maintain /meɪnˈteɪn/
malnutrition /ˌmæl.njuːˈtrɪ.ʃən/
manage /ˈmæn.ɪdʒ/
measurement /ˈmeʒ.ə.mənt/
misery /ˈmɪz.ər.i/
model /ˈmɒdəl/
multidisciplinary /ˌmʌl.ti.dɪs.əˈplɪn.ər.i/
nature /ˈneɪ.tʃə/
negligent /ˈneg.lɪ.dʒənt/
nitrogen /ˈnaɪ.trə.dʒən/
non-maleficence /nɒn-məˈlef.ɪ.sən.ts/
objective /əbˈdʒek.tɪv/
on behalf of sb /bɪˈhɑːf/
option /ˈɒp.ʃən/
organisational /ˌɔːgənaɪˈzeɪʃənəl/
originate /əˈrɪdʒ.ɪ.neɪt/
particular /pəˈtɪk.jʊ.lər/
phase /feɪz/
policy /ˈpɒl.ə.si/
practice /ˈpræk.tɪs/
precision /prɪˈsɪʒ.ən/
prevalence /ˈprevələns/

principle /ˈprɪn.sɪ.pl̩/
prognostic /prɒgˈnɒs.tɪk/
prolongation /ˈpɜː.tʃəs/
regard /rɪˈgɑːd/ **for** /fɔː/
regarding /rɪˈgɑː.dɪŋ/
related /rɪˈleɪ.tɪd/
religious /rɪˈlɪdʒəs/
resource /rɪˈzɔːs/
responsibility /rɪˌspɒn.sɪˈbɪl.ɪ.ti/
safeguard /ˈseɪfˌgɑːd/
scale /skeɪl/
screening /ˈskriː.nɪŋ/
semi- /ˈsem.i/
severely /sɪˈvɪə.li/
stable /ˈsteɪ.bl̩/
standard /ˈstæn.dəd/
starvation /stɑːˈveɪ.ʃən/
state /steɪt/
subdivision /ˈsʌb.dɪˌvɪʒ.ən/
subsequent /ˈsʌb.sɪ.kwənt/
suitable /ˈsj uː.tə.bl̩/
terminal /ˈtɜː.mɪ.nəl/ **illness** /ˈɪlnɪs/
time-consuming /ˈtaɪm.kənˌsjuː.mɪŋ/
tool /tuːl/
treated /ˈtriː.tɪd/
trial /traɪl/
tube /tjuːb/
undernourished /ˈʌndəˈnɜːrɪʃt/
undertake /ˌʌndəˈteɪk/
unrecognised /ʌnˈrekəgˌnaɪzd/
unwilling /ʌnˈwɪl.ɪŋ/
urge /ɜːdʒ/
validate /ˈvæl.ɪ.deɪt/
value /ˈvæl.juː/
vegetative /ˈvedʒ.ɪ.tə.tɪv/
violate /ˈvaɪə.leɪt/
weight /weɪt/ **gain** /geɪn/
willingness /ˈwɪl.ɪŋ.nəs/
withdraw /wɪðˈdrɔː/

Solution to Exercise 1a
1j, 2g, 3c, 4d, 5e, 6f, 7i, 8o, 9k, 10h, 11q, 12l, 13m, 14a, 15n, 16p, 17b

Solution to Exercise 1b
1g, 2c, 3i, 4f, 5h, 6a, 7d, 8e, 9b

Unit 2 - Diagnosis of malnutrition - screening and assessment

Nutritional screening is increasingly practised in hospitals, but a large number of cases of malnutrition still remain **undiagnosed and untreated**. This is mainly due to lack of training and awareness among staff, but also due to the former **lack of validated protocols** for screening, assessment and treatment. Another problem has also been lack of **consensus** concerning the definition of malnutrition. **Undernutrition** not only causes weight loss and changes in body composition but also impairs **physiological function** and a higher risk of complications and poor outcome from illness. **Disease** predisposes to malnutrition not only by its effects on **food intake**, but in the case of trauma and inflammatory disease, by **increased metabolic rate** and **protein catabolism.**

All patients should undergo nutritional screening **on admission** using a validated screening tool. Those found to be nutritionally at risk should have a more detailed assessment, combining **history, examination, bedside tests** of physical and mental function, and relevant **laboratory tests**. **All data** should be **recorded** digitally or on serial data charts in an easily accessible way, so that **trends** in the different parameters can be **readily observed**. Screening and assessment should lead to the development of a **nutritional management plan**, including continued monitoring.

Influence of malnutrition on function

The effects of **starvation** on the **structure and function of organs** is considerable. The degree of wasting of various organs has been determined in Krieger's **autopsy study** of patients **dying from malnutrition**. The **heart and liver** lost approximately 30% of their usual weight, but **spleen, kidney and pancreas** were also affected. In the Keys study, in which 32 healthy men underwent partial starvation for 24 weeks, each volunteer lost approximately 25% of his initial body weight, fat mass declined to about 30% of baseline value and fat-free mass to about 82% of baseline. Clinical observation shows that the **largest component** in the loss of FFM is **skeletal muscle**. In the response to stress muscle protein supplies not only the precursors for glucogenesis but also the amino acids for the synthesis of proteins for repair and for the immune response. This **loss of muscle mass** may be one reason why depleted persons have a higher **risk of developing complications following surgery or in acute illness.** Loss of both structure and **mental and physical function** occurs in proportion to the **degree and severity of undernutrition**. Cognition and mood are impaired. Changes are also seen in skeletal and cardiac muscle and in respiratory, thermoregulatory, gastrointestinal, immune, and other organ functions.

Overnutrition – functional and clinical consequences

Overfeeding can be defined as supplying **nutrients in excess of requirements** leading to increased storage of fat as well as other **undesirable effects**. Practically **every component** of nutrition, entering the body enterally or parenterally, **has to be processed metabolically**, unless it exceeds the renal clearance threshold and is excreted in urine. **Surplus energy** given acutely or chronically has numerous **detrimental effects** on the body. In chronic overnutrition, the body accumulates **excessive fat** leading to obesity. Nowadays the vast majority of the population in the developed world consumes more food than it needs and only a **minority** take enough **exercise to burn off** this excess. **Adipose tissue** stores **energy** in the form of **triglycerides** synthesised from the excess of ingested fats and carbohydrates.

The main complication of chronic overnutrition is **obesity**, which is associated with serious complications, e.g. **diabetes, cardiovascular disease** and **cancer**. These can be decreased **by losing 5-10% of weight**, thereby reducing insulin resistance, and the production of many atherogenic, pro-coagulatory, diabetogenic, hormonal and metabolically active substances. Even with such a small reduction in weight, **adipose tissue**

regains its capacity to **protect organs** such as liver, pancreas and muscles **from fat accumulation.**

In catabolic illness, obese patients are just as vulnerable to malnutrition as lean individuals and should be screened and given appropriate nutritional support. The incidence of **peri-operative complications** is higher in the obese, but has been significantly reduced by development of laparoscopic surgery. The risks of **morbid obesity** are high and can be significantly reduced by **bariatric surgery.** To be fully successful **gastric banding** requires appropriate perioperative nutritional support and dietary education.

Prevalence of malnutrition

Malnutrition can be defined as a state of nutrition in which a **deficiency or excess (or imbalance) of energy, protein and other nutrients** causes measurable **adverse effects** on tissue/body form (**body shape, size, composition**), body **function** and clinical outcome. Malnutrition is a broad term and can include not only **protein-energy** malnutrition (both over- and under-nutrition) but also malnutrition due to **specific nutrients**, such as **micronutrients**. The prevalence of malnutrition will also depend on which cut-off values are used to identify risk of malnutrition (to identify normal versus abnormal status or low versus high risk). Therefore, it is **essential that the criteria** used to define malnutrition are **documented** in epidemiological studies. It is well recognized that malnutrition of micronutrients is widespread in the elderly and in those with acute and chronic disease. Furthermore, individuals who have an acceptable protein-energy status or who are obese (overnutrition) may also have deficiencies in one or more micronutrients.

Protein-energy malnutrition is a major global public health problem in the 21st century. In most Western populations (including Europe, America, Australia, New Zealand), it is likely that the majority of individuals have some form of protein-energy malnutrition (undernutrition or overnutrition). Malnutrition (both undernutrition and overnutrition) is a **public health problem** and major national and international initiatives are needed to improve both the **prevention and the treatment** of this condition. **Overnutrition** (both overweight and obesity) is **widespread** and continues to increase in Europe and beyond and is costly to society. **Undernutrition**, most commonly **caused by disease** (disease-related malnutrition) is also a significant and more costly problem than obesity. Undernutrition occurs in individuals with a wide variety of acute and chronic illness, across all ages and settings.

Routine and regular screening for risk of malnutrition (both over- and undernutrition) in individuals **in hospitals, care homes and in out patient clinics and general practice is essential.** A universal, simple, evidence based and validated screening tool to detect malnutrition is recommended for use across all settings. The screening programme needs to be multidisciplinary and the results of the screening test must be linked to appropriate action including a **nutritional care plan.** An effective treatment for obesity that helps people lose weight can lead to **significant health benefits**. Similarly, the **use of nutritional support** to treat undernutrition can improve body structure and function and **improve clinical outcome,** decreasing complication rates and mortality. Successful treatment of undernutrition and overnutrition results in substantial clinical improvements for individuals and substantial cost savings to healthcare systems and society.

Exercise 1
Match the column A with the column B. Try to learn the expressions and/or sentences by heart.

A

1. Nutritional screening is increasingly practised in hospitals,
2. Undernutrition not only causes weight loss and changes in body composition
3. Disease predisposes to malnutrition not only by its effects on food intake,
4. Those found to be nutritionally at risk should have a more detailed assessment,
5. The loss of muscle mass may be one reason why depleted persons
6. Loss of both structure and mental and physical function
7. Overfeeding can be defined as supplying nutrients in excess of requirements
8. Surplus energy given acutely or chronically
9. The vast majority of the population in the developed world consumes more food than it needs
10. The main complication of chronic overnutrition
11. In catabolic illness, obese patients are just as vulnerable to malnutrition
12. The incidence of peri-operative complications is higher in the obese,
13. The risks of morbid obesity are high
14. Malnutrition can be defined as a state of nutrition in which a deficiency or excess (or imbalance) of energy, protein and other nutrients
15. Malnutrition of micronutrients is widespread
16. Undernutrition, most commonly caused by disease (disease-related malnutrition)
17. Routine and regular screening for risk of malnutrition
18. The screening programme needs to be multidisciplinary and the results of the screening test

19. The use of nutritional support to treat undernutrition can improve body structure and function
20. Successful treatment of undernutrition and overnutrition results in

B

a) *and can be significantly reduced by bariatric surgery.*
b) *and improve clinical outcome, decreasing complication rates and mortality.*
c) *and only a minority take enough exercise to burn off this excess.*
d) *as lean individuals and should be screened and given appropriate nutritional support.*
e) *but a large number of cases of malnutrition still remain undiagnosed and untreated.*
f) *but also impairs physiological function and a higher risk of complications and poor outcome from illness.*
g) *but has been significantly reduced by development of laparoscopic surgery.*
h) *but in the case of trauma and inflammatory disease, by increased metabolic rate and protein catabolism.*
i) *causes measurable adverse effects on tissue/body form (body shape, size, composition), body function and clinical outcome*
j) *combining history, examination, bedside tests of physical and mental function, and relevant laboratory tests.*
k) *has numerous detrimental effects on the body.*
l) *have a higher risk of developing complications following surgery or in acute illness.*
m) *in individuals in hospitals, care homes and in out patient clinics and general practice is essential.*
n) *in the elderly and in those with acute and chronic disease.*
o) *is also a significant and more costly problem than obesity.*
p) *is obesity, which is associated with serious complications, e.g. diabetes, cardiovascular disease and cancer.*
q) *leading to increased storage of fat as well as other undesirable effects.*
r) *must be linked to appropriate action including a nutritional care plan.*
s) *occurs in proportion to the degree and severity of undernutrition.*
t) *substantial clinical improvements for individuals and substantial cost savings to healthcare systems and society.*

Exercise 2
Translate the expressions. Try to explain their meanings in English.

Training, awareness, former, validated protocols, assessment, consensus, impairs physiological function, poor outcome, predisposes, trauma, inflammatory disease, metabolic rate, protein catabolism, data charts, accessible way, readily observed, continued monitoring, starvation, degree of wasting, approximately, spleen, kidney, pancreas, baseline value, precursors, depleted persons, following surgery, in proportion to, degree and severity, cognition, consequences, excess of requirements, storage of fat, undesirable, component, enterally or parenterally, processed metabolically, exceeds, renal clearance, surplus, detrimental, vast majority, burn off, adipose tissue, insulin resistance, regains its capacity, accumulation, vulnerable, peri-operative, gastric banding, prevalence, deficiency, excess, imbalance, measurable, adverse effects, clinical outcome, cut-off values, recognized, international initiatives, validated, screening tool, detect, linked to, substantial clinical improvements, cost savings.

Exercise 3
Prepare short talks and/or dialogues on these topics.

1. Principles and practice of nutritional screening
2. Effect of malnutrition on function of different organs
3. Risk of chronic overfeeding
4. Prevalence of undernutrition and overnutrition
5. The main causes of malnutrition

Vocabulary 2

Fill in the meanings in your mother language:

adipose /'æd.ɪ.pəʊz/
adverse /'æd.vɜːs/
approximately /ə'prɒk.sɪ.mət.lɪ/
atherogenic /ˌæθərəʊ'dʒɛnɪk/
autopsy /'ɔː.tɒp.si/
aware /ə'weər/
awareness /ə'weə.nəs/
bariatric /bær.i'æt.rɪk/
bonding /'bɒn.dɪŋ/
baseline /'beɪsˌlaɪn/
bedside /'bedˌsaɪd/
beyond /bi'jɒnd/
broad /brɔːd/
catabolic ˌ/kætə'bɒlɪc/
catabolism /kə'tæbəˌlɪzəm/
chart /tʃɑːt/
cognition /kɒg'nɪʃ.ən/
consensus /kən'sen.səs/
consequence /'kɒn.sɪ.kwəns/
considerable /kən'sɪd.ər.ə.bḷ/
costly /'kɒst.li/
cut-off /kʌtˌɒf/ **value** /'væljuː/
decline /dɪ'klaɪn/
deficiency /dɪ'fɪʃ.ənt .si/
define /dɪ'faɪn/
depleted /dɪ'pliː.tɪd/
detrimental /ˌdet.rɪ'men.təl/
diabetogenic /ˌdaɪə'bet.ə'dʒen.ɪk/
educated /'ed.jʊ.keɪ.tɪd/
effect /ɪ'fekt/
elderly /'el.dəl.i/
epidemiological /ˌep.ɪ.diː.mi.ə'lɒdʒ.ɪ.kəl/
essential /ɪ'sen.tʃəl/
exceed /ɪk'siːd/

excess /ek'ses/
excrete /ɪk'skriːt/
furthermore /'fɝː.ðɚ.mɔːr/
gastric /'gæs.trɪk/ **banding** /'bændɪŋ/
glucogenesis /ˌgluːkə'dʒe.nɪ.sɪs/
history /'hɪs.tər.i/
imbalance /ˌɪm'bæl.ənt s/
impaired /ɪm'peəd/
incidence /'ɪnt .sɪ.dənts/
individual /ˌɪn.dɪ'vɪd.ju.əl/
initial /ɪ'nɪʃ.əl/
laparoscopic /ˌlæp.ər.əs'kɒp.ɪk/
lean /liːn/
limitation /ˌlɪm.ɪ'teɪ.ʃən/
link /lɪŋk/
majority /mə'dʒɒrɪtɪ/
metabolic /ˌmet.ə'bɒl.ɪk/
syndrome /'sɪndrəʊm/
micronutrient /ˌmaɪ.krəʊ'njuː.tri.ənt/
mood /muːd/
muscle /mʌsəl/
outcome /'aʊt.kʌm/
overfeeding /'əʊ.vərfiːdɪŋ/
overnutrition /'əʊ.vər.njuː'trɪʃ.ən/
partial /'pɑː.ʃəl/
perioperative /ˌper.ɪ'ɒp.ər.ə.tɪv/
precursor /ˌpriː'kɜː.sər/
predispose /ˌpriː.dɪ'spəʊz/
pro /prəʊ/ **-coagulatory** /
koʊ'æg jə ləˌtɔr i/
readily /'red.ɪ.li/
record /'rekɔːd/
renal /'riː.nəl/ **clearance** /kliər.əns/
repair /rɪ'peə/
resistance /rɪ'zɪs.tənts/
setting /'setɪŋ/
shape /ʃeɪp/
skeletal /'skel.ɪ.təl/
spleen /spliːn/
storage /'stɔː.rɪdʒ/
store /stɔːr/
summarize /'sʌm.ər.aɪz/
surplus /'sɜː.pləs/
threshold /'θreʃ.h əʊld/
tissue /'tɪʃ.uː/
training /'treɪ.nɪŋ/
trend /trend/
triglyceride /traɪ.glɪs.ə.raɪd/
undergo /ˌʌn.də'gəʊ/
(underwent, undergone)
undesirable /ˌʌn.dɪ'zaɪə.rə.bl̩/
undiagnosed /ʌn'daɪ.əg.nəʊzd/
untreated /ʌn'triː.tɪd/
vast /vɑːst/
volunteer /ˌvɒl.ən'tɪər/
vulnerable /'vʌl.nər.ə.bl̩/
wasting /weɪst.ɪŋ/
widespread /ˌwaɪd'spred/

Solution to Exercise 1
1e, 2f, 3h, 4j, 5l, 6s, 7q, 8k, 9c, 10p, 11d, 12g, 13a, 14i, 15n, 16o, 17m, 18r, 19b, 20t

Unit 3 - Nutritional requirements for health at rest and upon exercise

Adult subjects
Macronutrients

Total **energy requirements** vary between individuals. Requirements of **CHO and fat** are set at 50-55% and 30-35%, respectively, of total energy intake for healthy subjects at rest. **Protein** allowances should be 0.8g·kg^{-1}body weight. Further research is needed to determine the precise needs for different types of CHOs, fats, and proteins as well as their consequences for health. **Physical exercise** increases energy requirements. The **ratio of macronutrients** required by physically active subjects is similar as in resting subjects, although an increased intake of CHOs may be recommended. During exercise lasting less than

1h, **carbohydrate supplementation** may help to delay fatigue.

Micronutrients

Trace elements (essential **inorganic** micronutrients) and **vitamins** (essential **organic** micronutrients) are required in the diet in very **small amounts**. The fact that only a small intake is necessary is in contrast to their critical importance in both health and disease. **The role** of these micronutrients can be classified as follows:

- As **cofactors** in **metabolism** – many trace elements are required to **modulate enzyme** activity as an integral part of enzyme prosthetic groups - e.g. **zinc** is a cofactor for many enzymes whereas **selenium** is required in the form of selenocysteine within the enzyme glutathione peroxidase.
- As **coenzymes** in **metabolism** – many **vitamins** or **metabolites** of vitamins are required to play an active part within complex **biochemical reactions** e.g. **riboflavin** and **niacin** within the electron transport chain, or **folic acid** as a part of the reactions, which transfer methyl groups. These reactions are critical to intermediary metabolism and ensure **utilisation** of the major **nutrients** to provide energy, **proteins, nucleic acids and other** compounds.
- Control functions – zinc plays an essential role as part of the zinc fingers, transcription control factors which **control gene expression.**
- **Structural** components – certain elements are required to provide a structural role within proteins to obtain the necessary **folding of the protein** molecule.
- **Antioxidants** (a by-product of **oxidative metabolism**); their role is the **generation of species**, which have the potential to **cause further oxidative reactions**, especially to **organic parts of the cell** (cell membranes and nucleic acids) in a relatively **reduced state.** The body has a sophisticated **system to limit the potential damage** caused by this: mechanisms include **quenching of oxidant activity via** complex molecules such as **vitamin E and vitamin A**, or **enzyme systems** to **dispose of the products of oxidation** – superoxide dismutase (either **zinc/copper or manganese dependent**) and glutathione peroxidase **(selenium dependent)**.

Nutritional needs of infants, children and adolescents

Substrate supply and **utilisation** are of greater biological relevance during early childhood than during any other period of life. Nutrient supply to adults only needs to cover maintenance requirements and the needs of physical activity.

In contrast, **infants, children and adolescents** require **additional** large energy and substrate supplies for **body growth** and **deposition** of newly **forming tissues.** These requirements are very high in **healthy newborn** infants who **double** their **body weight** extremely rapidly in only **4-5 months**. Even greater are the needs of **preterm infants** who grow even faster and, if born at 30 weeks of gestation, need only 6 weeks to double their birth weight if their extrauterine growth rate is to match foetal growth in utero. Such rapid growth rates require a very high substrate supply per kg body weight. In addition to supporting **weight gain**, the **quantity and quality of nutrient** supply during early life also **modulates** the **development and differentiation of tissues** and has short- and long-term consequences for health. **Nutrient intake values** (NIVs) for populations of healthy children may provide some **preliminary guidance** for designing **enteral or parenteral feeds** for paediatric patients, even with all the reservations concerning the derivation of NIVs for children because of a lack of systematic studies. The needs of individual patients may differ markedly from NIV for the group.

Exercise 1a
Match the column A with the column B. Try to learn the expressions and/ or sentences by heart.

A

1. The ratio of macronutrients required by physically active subjects is similar
2. During exercise lasting less than 1h,
3. Trace elements (essential inorganic micronutrients) and vitamins (essential organic micronutrients)
4. The role of micronutrients can be classified as:
5. Many trace elements are required
6. Many vitamins or metabolites of vitamins are required to play an active part within complex biochemical reactions
7. Biochemical reactions are critical to intermediary metabolism and ensure
8. Zinc plays an essential role as part of the zinc fingers,
9. Certain elements are required to provide a structural role
10. The role of antioxidants is the generation of species
11. The mechanisms to limit the potential damage include quenching of oxidant activity via complex molecules such as vitamin E and vitamin A,

12. Nutrient supply to adults only needs to cover
13. Infants, children and adolescents require additional large energy and substrate supplies
14. Healthy newborn infants double their body weight extremely rapidly in only 4-5 months;
15. The quantity and quality of nutrient supply during early life
16. Nutrient intake values (NIVs) for populations of healthy children may provide

B

a) *are required in the diet in very small amounts.*

b) *as in resting subjects, although an increased intake of CHOs may be recommended.*

c) *carbohydrate supplementation may help to delay fatigue.*

d) *cofactors in metabolism, coenzymes in metabolism, structural components, and antioxidants, and they have control functions*

e) *e.g. riboflavin and niacin or folic acid.*

f) *for body growth and deposition of newly forming tissues.*

g) *is in contrast to their critical importance in both health and disease.*

h) *maintenance requirements and the needs of physical activity.*

i) *modulates the development and differentiation of tissues and has short- and long-term consequences for health.*

j) *or enzyme systems to dispose of the products of oxidation – superoxide dismutase (either zinc/copper or manganese dependent) and glutathione peroxidase (selenium dependent).*

k) *some preliminary guidance for designing enteral or parenteral feeds for paediatric patients.*

l) *such rapid growth rates require a very high substrate supply per kg body weight.*

m) *to modulate enzyme activity e.g. zinc or selenium.*

n) *transcription control factors which control gene expression.*

o) *utilisation of the major nutrients to provide energy, proteins, nucleic acids and other compounds.*

p) *which have the potential to cause further oxidative reactions, especially to organic parts of the cell in a relatively reduced state.*

q) *within proteins to obtain the necessary folding of the protein molecule.*

Nutritional physiology and biochemistry

Appetite and its control

Survival for organisms is dependent upon the preservation of energy homoeostasis. Consequently, **food intake and energy expenditure** are tightly controlled and modulated by several **peripheral and central factors**. The **integrating centre** is located in the **hypothalamus**, where peripheral signals are conveyed and transduced into **neuronal activity** and **behavioural responses. Appetite and satiety**, the 'ying and yang' of the control of food intake are, in general, considered to be opposing symptoms, and may appear to be mediated by separate neuronal pathways. In contrast with this hypothesis, data consistently show that they should be considered to be **different sides of the same coin**. Indeed, it appears more consistent with the available evidence to state that food intake is controlled by the balance between more appetite/less appetite (or more satiety/less satiety) rather than by the balance between appetite and satiety.

Digestion and absorption of nutrients

In order for food to yield its nutrients there must be a **functional gastrointestinal (GI) tract**. Most nutrients require digestion by the GI tract, and all nutritional **substances** must be **absorbed** for their subsequent **utilisation**. **Digestion** occurs intraluminally and the mucosal surface of the enterocytes, and is **initiated by gastric acid** as well as by a series of nutrient specific **enzymes (disaccharidases, proteases, lipases,** etc.). Absorption is the process by which the products of digestion and other **small molecules** are transported into the **epithelial cells that line the GI tract,** and from there ultimately **into the blood and lymphatic vessels** which drain the tract and serve **the rest of the body**.

These processes depend also on normal gastrointestinal **motility**, both physically to **mix the contents** of the GI tract, and to **move these contents along** its length. Digestion and absorption of **macronutrients** take place mainly in the **small intestine**, with the stomach and the colon involved much less in this procedure. The **colon (large intestine)** plays a significant role however in **electrolyte and water absorption.**

The digestion and absorption of **macronutrients (carbohydrates, lipids, proteins)** and **micronutrients (vitamins and minerals)**, essential for the requirements of the human body, **take place** mostly **in the small intestine.** In most cases digestion occurs both in the gastrointestinal lumen and at the mucosal surface, continuing in some cases within the enterocytes themselves. Substrate-**specific enzyme processes** exist for **polysaccharide carbohydrates** and **polypeptides,** linked with digest-specific active co-transporters to aid absorption at the cellular level. The hydrophobicity of fats makes **lipid handling** more complex, requiring the **creation of intraluminal emulsions and micelles** which present lipid **degradation** products to the electrolytes. The **intestine (small bowel and colon)** has additional mechanisms for absorption and re-absorption **of water and key electrolytes**. In most cases **micro-nutrients** are liberated from dietary macromolecules by non-specific digestion and then **absorbed passively** (or as other **lipid-soluble moieties** in the case of the fat-soluble vitamins) but some specific **transporters** are also involved as in the case of vitamin B_{12}. Quantitatively minor but important digestion and nutrient absorption also occur in the colon.

Exercise 1b
Match the column A with the column B. Try to learn the expressions and/or sentences by heart.

A

1. Food intake and energy expenditure are tightly controlled
2. The integrating centre is located in the hypothalamus,
3. Food intake is controlled by the balance between
4. Most nutrients require digestion by the GI tract, and all nutritional substances
5. Digestion is initiated by gastric acid
6. The products of digestion and other small molecules are transported into the epithelial cells that line the GI tract,
7. These processes depend also on normal gastrointestinal motility both
8. Digestion and absorption of macronutrients
9. The colon (large intestine) plays a significant role
10. The digestion and absorption of macronutrients (carbohydrates, lipids, proteins) and micronutrients (vitamins and minerals),
11. Substrate-specific enzyme processes
12. The hydrophobicity of fats makes lipid handling more complex,
13. Micro-nutrients are liberated from dietary macromolecules

B

a) *and from there ultimately into the blood and lymphatic vessels which drain the tract and serve the rest of the body.*
b) *and modulated by several peripheral and central factors.*
c) *and then absorbed passively (or as other lipid-soluble moieties in the case of the fat-soluble vitamins).*
d) *as well as by a series of nutrient specific enzymes (disaccharidases, proteases, lipases, etc.).*
e) *exist for polysaccharide carbohydrates and polypeptides.*

f) in electrolyte and water absorption.

g) more appetite/less appetite (or more satiety/less satiety) rather than by the balance between appetite and satiety.

h) must be absorbed for their subsequent utilisation.

i) requiring the creation of intraluminal emulsions and micelles which present lipid degradation products to the electrolytes.

j) take place mostly in the small intestine.

k) to mix the contents of the GI tract, and to move these contents along its length.

l) where peripheral signals are conveyed and transduced into neuronal activity and behavioural responses.

Exercise 2

Translate the expressions. Try to explain their meanings in English.

Protein allowances, precise needs, ratio of macronutrients, resting subjects, lasting less than 1h, supplementation, delay fatigue, trace elements, critical importance, cofactors, modulate, integral part, electron transport chain, transfer, intermediary utilisation, gene expression, folding of the protein molecule, generation of species, cell membranes and nucleic acids, limit the potential damage, quenching of oxidant activity, dispose of, substrate supply, relevance, cover maintenance requirements, double, preterm infants, gestation, extrauterine growth rate, foetal growth, in utero, modulates differentiation of tissues, large additional energy, long-term consequences, nutrient intake values, preliminary guidance for designing, reservations concerning, derivation, survival, preservation, food intake, energy expenditure, integrating centre, conveyed, transduced, neuronal activity and behavioural responses, satiety, mediated by, separate neuronal pathways, consistently, available evidence, to state that, utilisation, mucosal surface, enterocytes, disaccharidases, proteases, lipases, epithelial cells, line, ultimately, lymphatic vessels, motility, small intestine, stomach, colon, large intestine, take place, linked with, emulsions and micelles, lipid degradation, liberated from, lipid-soluble moieties, transporters.

Exercise 3

Prepare short talks and/or dialogues on these topics.

1. The energy requirements of healthy adults
2. Macronutrient requirements at rest and during physical activity
3. Macronutrients beneficial for health
4. The classification of micronutrients
5. Micronutrient requirements in adult healthy subjects
6. Nutritional needs of infants, children and adolescents

7. Adequate nutrient supply for growth, development and long term health
8. Appetite and satiety as determinants of food intake
9. Neurochemical mediators of appetite and satiety
10. The role of the hypothalamus in the regulation of food intake
11. Normal topography of the gastrointestinal tract
12. Digestion and absorption of nutrients
13. The digestive metabolism of the principal macronutrients and micronutrients
14. The relevance and importance of the colon as a nutritional organ

Vocabulary 3

Fill in the meanings in your mother language:

additional /ə'dɪʃ.ən.əl/
allowance /ə'laʊ.əns/
appreciation /əˌpriː.ʃi'eɪ.ʃən/
behavioural /bɪ'heɪ.vjə.rəl/
beneficial /ˌben.ɪ'fɪʃ.əl/
by-product /'baɪˌprɒd.ʌkt/
cell /sel/ **membrane** /'mem.breɪn/
chain /tʃeɪn/
challenge /'tʃæl.ɪndʒ/
classification /ˌklæs.ɪ.fɪ'keɪ.ʃən/
co /'kəʊ/ **-transporter** /træn'spɔː.tər/
cofactor /kəʊ 'fæk.tər/
coin /kɔɪn/
colon /'kəʊ.lɒn/
consistently /kən'sɪs.tənt.li/
content /kən'tent/
cover /'kʌv.ə/
degradation /ˌdeg.rə'deɪ.ʃən/
delay /dɪ'leɪ/
deposition /ˌdep.ə'zɪʃ.ən/
derivation /ˌder.ɪ'veɪ.ʃən/
determinant /dɪ'tɜː.mɪ.nənt/
determine /dɪ'tɜː.mɪn/
dietary /'daɪ.ə.tər.i/
differ /'dɪf.ər/
differentiation /ˌdɪf.ər.en.ʃi'eɪ.ʃən/
digestion /da ɪ'dʒes.tʃən/
disaccharidase /daɪ'sækəˌraɪd.eiz/
dispose of /dɪ'spəʊz/
drain /dreɪn/
electrolyte /ɪ'lek.trə.laɪt/
electron /ɪ'lek.trɒn/
emulsion /ɪ'mʌl.ʃən/
epithelial /ˌep.ɪ'θiː.li.əl/
establish /ɪ'stæb.lɪʃ/
estimate /'es.tɪ.meɪt/
expression /ɪk'spreʃ.ən/
extrauterine /'ek.strə/'juː.t̬ər.ɪn/
fatigue /fə'tiːg/
folding /'fəʊl.dɪŋ/
folic acid /ˌfəʊ.lɪk'æs.ɪd/
gene /dʒiːn/
glutathione /ˌgluːtə'θaɪəʊn/
peroxidase /pə'rɒksɪˌdeɪs/
growth /grəʊθ/ **rate** /reɪt/
guidance /'gaɪ.dəns/
hydrophobicity /ˌhaɪ.drə.foʊ'bɪs.ɪ.ti/
hypothalamus /ˌhaɪ.pəʊ'θæl.ə.məs/
indeed /ɪn'diːd/
initiate /ɪ'nɪʃ.i.eɪt/
integral /'ɪn.tɪ.grəl/
intermediary /ˌɪn.tə'miː.di.ə.ri/
intraluminal /'ɪn trə'lu mə nl/
involved /ɪn'vɒlvd/
knowledge /'nɒl.ɪdʒ/
liberated /'lɪb.ər.eɪ.tɪd/
line /laɪn/
maintenance /'meɪn.tɪ.nəns/
markedly /'mɑː.kɪd.li/
methyl /ˌmeθəl/
micelle /mɪ'sɛl/
modulate /'mɒd.jʊ.leɪt/

mucosal /mjuːˈkəʊ.səl/
neurochemical /nʊr.oʊˈkem.ɪ.kəl/
neuronal /nʊˈroʊ.nəl/
nucleic acid /njuːˌkleɪ.ɪkˈæs.ɪd/
obtain /əbˈteɪn/
oxidant /ˈɒk.sɪ.dənt/
oxidative /ɒkˈsɪd.ə.tɪv/
pathway /ˈpɑː.θ.weɪ/
polypeptide /ˌpɒl.ɪˈpep.taɪd/
polysaccharide /ˌpɒl.ɪˈsæk.ər.aɪd/
potential /pəˈten.ʃəl/
precise /prɪˈsaɪs/
preliminary /prɪˈlɪm.ɪ.nər.i/
preterm /ˌpriːˈtɜːm/
principal /ˈprɪnt.sɪ.pəl/
prosthetic /ˈprɒs.θə.tɪk/
quench /kwentʃ/
ratio /ˈreɪ.ʃi.əʊ/
regulation /ˌreg.jʊˈleɪ.ʃən/
relevance /ˈrel.ə.vəns/
requirement /rɪˈkwaɪə.mənt/
research /rɪˈsɜːtʃ/
respectively /rɪˈspek.tɪv.li/
resting /ˈrest.ɪŋ/
selenocysteine /ˌsiːlɪˈnɒˈsɪstɪˌiːn/
sophisticated /səˈfɪs.tɪ.keɪ.tɪd/
species /ˈspiː.ʃiːz/
stage /steɪdʒ/
structural /ˈstrʌk.tʃər.əl/
subject /ˈsʌb.dʒekt/
substrate /ˈsʌb.streɪt/
superoxide /ˌsuːpərˈɒksaɪd/
dismutase /dɪs.mjʊ.təɪz/
supplementation /sʌp.lɪ.menˈteɪ.ʃən/
surface /ˈsɜː.fɪs/
topography /təˈpɒg.rə.fi/
trace /treɪs/ **element** /ˈel.ɪ.mənt/
transcription /trænˈskrɪp.ʃən/
transfer /trænsˈfɜːr/
transform /trænsˈfɔːm/
transport /ˈtræn.spɔːt/
utilisation /ˌjuː.tɪ.laɪˈzeɪ.ʃən/
vary /ˈveə.ri/
via /ˈvaɪə/
whereas /weərˈæz/
yield /jiːld/
ying /jɪn/ **and yang** /yɑŋ/
zinc /zɪŋk/ **finger** /ˈfɪŋ.gər/

Solution to Exercise 1a
1b, 2c, 3a, 4g, 5d, 6m, 7e, 8o, 9n, 10q, 11p, 12j, 13h, 14f, 15l, 16i, 17k

Solution to Exercise 1b
1b, 2m, 3g, 4h, 5d, 6a, 7k, 8f, 9j, 10e, 11i, 12c

Unit 4 - Metabolism

Carbohydrate metabolism

Glucose metabolism is primarily regulated by the **balance** between **anabolic** (insulin) and **catabolic** (adrenalin, glucagon, cortisol, growth hormone) **hormones**, and by the **cell energy status**. In **fasting** conditions, catabolic hormones **enhance hepatic glucose production** and **decrease glucose utilisation** in skeletal muscle and adipose tissue. In **postprandial** conditions, **insulin** stimulates glucose oxidation in skeletal muscle and glucose storage in liver, skeletal muscle and adipose tissue, and **inhibits hepatic glucose production**. **Stress**, by increasing catabolic hormones, causes **insulin resistance** and **hyperglycaemia**. In addition, inflammatory mediators are generally activated during **critical illness** and antagonize insulin's actions. The results are marked insulin resistance and hyperglycaemia, which may have **deleterious** effects in the **long term.**

Lipid metabolism

Lipids represent the major form of **energy storage** in the body. This is due to their **high content of energy** and **low hydration**; thus, fat is an ideal form of energy storage both in animals and in plants (seeds and nuts).

Adipose tissue can accumulate **large amounts of energy.** The average amount of energy stored in adipose tissue in a healthy adult is 150,000 kcal; however, this amount depends on the total quantity of accumulated fat. **Fatty acids** released from adipose tissue are **insoluble in water** and **circulate bound to plasma albumin;** moreover, they can **destabilize plasma membranes.** While **fatty acids** can be **oxidised** by many, but not all tissues, **ketone bodies** produced in the **liver** from fatty acids are a **suitable substrate** for almost all cells.

Lipids constitute an important part of **cell structure**. The phospholipid bilayers are a fundamental part of all membrane structures in all cells. In addition to their structural role, **membrane phospholipids** are metabolically important molecules, which are **split by various enzymes** connected with cell receptors to yield **bioactive molecules** such as prostaglandins, leukotrienes, inositol phosphate, etc. Via such mechanisms, lipids can serve as second messengers of many **hormones** and bioactive molecules. Lipids are not only very important **energy substrates**, but some **fatty acids and lipid-soluble vitamins** act also as **metabolic regulators**. After **ingestion** of a mixed meal, **fat** is preferentially **stored** in adipose tissue whereas **carbohydrates** are **oxidised**. During **fasting**, fatty acids are **released** from adipose tissue and **utilised** as energy substrates **in liver and extra-hepatic tissue**. This process is effectively **controlled** by **catecholamines** and **insulin**, which regulate hormone sensitive lipase and lipoprotein lipase.

During critical illness, increased adipose tissue **lipolysis** together with **decreased fatty acid oxidation** leads to **increased triglyceride production** and deposition in the liver (and in other tissues), with an augmented production of **VLDL**. This may contribute to the aggravation of **organ dysfunction**. In addition, several major changes are observed with respect to the concentration and composition of plasma cholesterol-rich lipoproteins.

Protein and amino acid metabolism

Proteins are cellular and extracellular constituents and play a **crucial part in most biological processes**. Proteins have a role in: **structure** (e.g. collagen, actin, myosin); **biochemical reactions** (enzymes); **transport** (e.g. haemoglobin); **immune responses** (immuoglobulins, C-reactive protein (CRP), opsonins); the **translation process** (e.g. histones). Proteins are continuously **produced and broken down,** each at specific rates but varying depending on conditions such as **starvation, stress, and undernutrition.** The building blocks of proteins consist of 20 amino acids. **Proteins** are 'strings' of **amino acids (peptides)**

folded into **a tree-dimensional** structure. This structure is usually maintained by disulphide **bridges** between the amino acid cysteine, which is present in the peptide chain. This tree-dimensional structure is crucial for protein function.

Proteins play a crucial part in biological processes and are continuously **synthesised and broken down** by different routes. On a whole-body level, the synthesis and breakdown of proteins are measured with the use of amino-acid isotopes. Whole-body synthesis and breakdown of proteins are each the net result of the synthesis and breakdown of all the different proteins in the body.

In health, adults remain in **zero protein balance**. However, synthesis and breakdown are differentially **affected by** the stages of **disease** and prevailing **conditions** (e.g. **starvation, feeding, sepsis, growth, convalescence, and activity**) resulting in net **catabolism or anabolism**.

In stress situations, **peripheral organs (muscle, skin, bone)** are **catabolic**, whereas **central** organs (e.g. **liver, spleen, immune cells, wounds)** are **anabolic**.

Exercise 1a
Match the column A with the column B. Try to learn the expressions and/or sentences by heart.

A

1. Glucose metabolism is primarily regulated by the balance between anabolic (insulin) and
2. In fasting conditions, catabolic hormones enhance hepatic glucose production
3. In postprandial conditions, insulin stimulates glucose oxidation in skeletal muscle
4. Stress
5. During critical illness marked insulin resistance and hyperglycaemia
6. Inflammatory mediators are generally activated during critical illness and the results are
7. Lipids represent the major form of energy storage in the body;
8. Adipose tissue can
9. Fatty acids released from adipose tissue are insoluble in water
10. Lipids constitute an important part of cell structure;
11. Membrane phospholipids are metabolically important molecules, which are split by various enzymes
12. Lipids are not only very important energy substrates,
13. After ingestion of a mixed meal,
14. During fasting, fatty acids are released from adipose tissue
15. During critical illness, increased adipose tissue lipolysis together with decreased fatty acid oxidation

16. Proteins are cellular and extracellular constituents
17. Proteins have a role in: structure (e.g. collagen, actin, myosin); biochemical reactions (enzymes); transport (e.g. haemoglobin);
18. Proteins are continuously produced and broken down, each at specific rates
19. Proteins are 'strings' of amino acids (peptides)
20. Synthesis and breakdown are differentially affected by the stages of disease
21. In stress situations, peripheral organs (muscle, skin, bone) are catabolic,

B

a) *accumulate large amounts of energy.*
b) *and circulate bound to plasma albumin; moreover, they can destabilize plasma membranes.*
c) *and decrease glucose utilisation in skeletal muscle and adipose tissue.*
d) *and glucose storage in liver, skeletal muscle and adipose tissue.*
e) *and play a crucial part in most biological processes.*
f) *and prevailing conditions (e.g. starvation, feeding, sepsis, growth, convalescence, and activity) resulting in net catabolism or anabolism.*
g) *and utilised as energy substrates in liver and extra-hepatic tissue.*
h) *but some fatty acids and lipid-soluble vitamins act also as metabolic regulators.*
i) *but varying depending on conditions such as starvation, stress, and undernutrition.*
j) *catabolic (adrenalin, glucagon, cortisol, growth hormone) hormones, and by the cell energy status.*
k) *causes insulin resistance and hyperglycaemia.*
l) *connected with cell receptors to yield bioactive molecules such as prostaglandins, leukotrienes, inositol phosphate, etc.*
m) *fat is preferentially stored in adipose tissue whereas carbohydrates are oxidised.*
n) *folded into a tree-dimensional structure, this structure is crucial for protein function.*
o) *immune responses (immuoglobulins, C-reactive protein (CRP), opsonins); the translation process (e.g. histones).*
p) *leads to increased triglyceride production and deposition in the liver (and in other tissues).*
q) *marked insulin resistance and hyperglycaemia, which may have deleterious effects in the long term.*

r) *may have deleterious effects in the long term.*

s) *the phospholipid bilayers are a fundamental part of all membrane structures in all cells.*

t) *this is due to their high content of energy and low hydration.*

u) *whereas central organs (e.g. liver, spleen, immune cells, wounds) are anabolic.*

Water and electrolytes in health and disease

Water and electrolytes are essential components of the 'milieu interieur' of the body, creating an **environment which surrounds nearly all cells** through which the **metabolites and gases** pass to and from. They are also major intracellular components, being 75% of muscle cells but less than 5% of fat cells. The **electrolyte gradient** across cell membranes is a prerequisite for **cell excitability, signal conduction, transport processes and cell movement**. Electrolytes also serve as second messengers, coenzymes or have structural functions. It is important to consider **fluid and electrolyte balance** in terms not only external gain or loss, but also in relation to the shifts which occur between the internal fluid compartments as a consequence of disease. Fluid balance should be considered in terms not only of **external loss or gain** but also of the **intercompartmental shifts**, which occur with **disease. Injury and starvation** are associated with **retention of salt and water** and expension of ECF. The ability to **excrete an excess salt and water** load **returns** during **convalescence. Potassium, phosphate and Mg are lost** during catabolic illness and **require replacement** during the anabolic convalescent phase. A proper understanding of normal and abnormal fluid and electrolyte physiology is necessary in the proper management of patients **receiving nutritional support** as both fluid (and sodium) **deficit and overload** can be detrimental to clinical outcome.

Trace elements are essential **inorganic micronutrients**, which are required in the diet in very small amounts. Although only small amounts are necessary they are critical in both health and disease.

Vitamins are essential **organic micronutrients**, which are required in the diet in relatively small amounts. However, they are necessary for both healthy and diseased organism.

Antioxidants in health and disease

In parallel with recent technological developments, the role of 'oxidative stress', the **imbalance** between **pro-oxidant** species and **anti-oxidant defence mechanisms**, has progressively emerged as a central pathogenic event for several acute and chronic conditions and diseases. Known conditions presenting higher **risk of oxidative stress include**: old age, strict vegetarianism, chronic (high) alcohol intake, obesity, dietary restriction, diabetes/hyperglycaemia, chronic obstructive pulmonary disease, chronic and acute inflammation, cancer, malabsorption, ischaemia/reperfusion, trauma, chronic exposure to air pollutants.

However, primary and secondary **prevention** with dietary **supplementations** of anti-oxidant vitamins and trace elements in the general population is **mostly inefficient**. Contrasted findings are reported from large-scale studies of supplementation, stressing the complexities of the roles and the regulation of the components of oxidative stress in vivo. Recent findings allow a better understanding of the **roles of oxidative stress in physiological and pathological conditions.** The release of RNOS is tightly regulated and required for several cell functions, including the **anti-infectious defence mechanisms**. When the anti-oxidant defence mechanisms are overwhelmed by a massive or sustained release of RNOS and/or by defective or insufficient stores of anti-oxidants, **oxidative damage can occur at the cell and tissue level.** Avoiding excessive exposure to oxidative conditions and ensuring adequate provision of **dietary anti-oxidants** limits the risk of oxidative stress.

Exercise 1b
Match the expressions in column A with the expressions in column B to create full sentences. Try to learn them by heart.

A

1. Water and electrolytes are essential components creating an environment which surrounds nearly all cells
2. The electrolyte gradient across cell membranes is a prerequisite
3. Fluid balance should be considered in terms not only of external loss or gain
4. Injury and starvation are associated with retention of salt and water;
5. Potassium, phosphate and Mg are lost during catabolic illness
6. Both fluid (and sodium) deficit and overload
7. Trace elements are essential inorganic micronutrients;
8. Vitamins are essential organic micronutrients, which are
9. The imbalance between pro-oxidant species and anti-oxidant defence mechanisms, has progressively emerged
10. Higher risk of oxidative stress include: old age, strict vegetarianism, chronic (high) alcohol intake, obesity, dietary restriction, diabetes/hyperglycaemia,
11. When the anti-oxidant defence mechanisms are overwhelmed by a massive or sustained release of RNOS

B

a) although only small amounts are necessary they are critical in both health and disease.

b) and require replacement during the anabolic convalescent phase.

c) and/or by defective or insufficient stores of anti-oxidants, oxidative damage can occur at the cell and tissue level.

d) as a central pathogenic event for several acute and chronic conditions and diseases.

e) but also of the intercompartmental shifts, which occur with disease.

f) can be detrimental to clinical outcome.

g) chronic obstructive pulmonary disease, chronic and acute inflammation, cancer, malabsorption, ischaemia/reperfusion, trauma, and chronic exposure to air pollutants.

h) for cell excitability, signal conduction, transport processes and cell movement.

i) necessary for both healthy and diseased organism.

j) the ability to excrete an excess salt and water load returns during convalescence.

k) through which the metabolites and gases pass to and from.

Exercise 2

Translate the expressions. Try to explain their meanings in English.

Status, in fasting, enhance, hepatic glucose production, utilisation in skeletal muscle, adipose tissue, in postprandial conditions, storage, inhibits insulin resistance, inflammatory mediators, antagonize, marked, deleterious, content, hydration, accumulate large amounts, average amount, insoluble, circulate, bound to plasma albumin, destabilize, suitable substrate, constitute, fundamental part, split, preferentially, extra-hepatic tissue, sensitive, lipolysis, deposition, augmented production, aggravation, extracellular constituents, play a crucial part in, produced and broken down, strings, folded, tree-dimensional, different routes, net result, affected by, environment, surrounds, pass to and from, intracellular components, electrolyte gradient, prerequisite, excitability, signal conduction, shifts internal fluid compartments, consequence, retention of salt and water, expension, convalescence, replacement, deficit and overload, detrimental, outcome, trace elements, in parallel with, recent, defence mechanisms, emerged, dietary restriction, large-scale studies, in vivo, recent findings, overwhelmed, sustained, release of, defective or insufficient, exposure, ensuring provision.

Exercise 3
Prepare short talks and/or dialogues on these topics.

1. Basic concepts in water and electrolyte metabolism.
2. Influence of starvation, trauma and sepsis on fluid and electrolyte physiology.
3. Normal roles of minerals and trace elements.
4. Physiological roles of vitamins and the effects of deficiency of vitamins.
5. Oxidative stress and antioxidant defence mechanisms.
6. Glucose metabolism in humans and alterations of glucose metabolism
7. Pathways of lipid metabolism
8. Basic routes of protein synthesis and degradation in cells

Vocabulary 4

Fill in the meanings in your mother language:

actin /'æk tən/
adrenaline /ə'dren.əl.ɪn/
aggravation /ˌægrə'veɪʃən/
aggression /ə'greʃ.ən/
albumin /'æl.bjʊ.mɪn/
alteration /ˌɒl.tə'reɪ.ʃən/
anabolic /ˌæn.ə.bɒl.ɪk/
assess /ə'ses/
augment /ɔ:g'ment/
average /'æv.ər.ɪdʒ/
bind /baɪnd/ **(bound, bound)**
bridge /brɪdʒ/
calorimetry /ˌkæl.ə'rɪm.ə.tri/
characterize /'kær.ɪk.tə.raɪz/
collagen /'kɒl.ə.dʒən/
constituent /kən'stɪt.ju.ənt/
convalescent /ˌkɒn.və'les.ənt/
cortisol /'kɔ:.tɪ.sɒl/
critical /'krɪt.ɪ.kəl/
cysteine /'sɪstɪˌi:n/
decrease /dɪ'kri:s/
defective /dɪ'fek.tɪv/
defence /dɪ'fens/
deleterious /ˌdel.ɪ'tɪə.ri.əs/
destabilize /ˌdi:'steɪ.bəl.aɪz/
dilution /daɪ'lu:ʃən/
dimensional /-daɪ.men.ʃən.əl/
disulfide /daɪ'sʌl faɪd/
environment /ɪn'vaɪə .rən .mənt/
excessive /ek'ses.ɪv/
excitability /ɪkˌsaɪ.tə'bɪl.ə.tɪ/
exposure /ɪk'spəʊ.ʒər/
extrarenal /ˌek.strə'ri:.nəl/
familiar /fə'mɪl.i.ər/ **with** /wɪð/
fatty /'fæt.i/ **acids** /'æs.ɪds/
finding /'faɪn.dɪŋ/
fold /fəʊld/
fundamental /ˌfʌn.də'men.təl/
glucagon /glu:kə.gən/
gradient /'greɪ.di.ənt/
growth /grəʊθ/ **hormone** /'hɔ:.məʊn/
histone /'hɪstəʊn/
human /hju:mən/
hyperglycaemia /ˌhaɪ.pə.glaɪ'si:mi.ə/
illness /'ɪl.nəs/
inflammation /ˌɪn.flə'meɪ.ʃən/
influence /'ɪn.flʊ.əns/
injury /'ɪn.dʒər.i/
inositol /ɪ'nəʊsɪˌtɒl/
phosphate /'fɒs.feɪt/
insoluble /ɪn'sɒl.jʊ.blˌ/
insufficient /ˌɪn.sə'fɪʃ.ənt/
intercompartmental / ɪn'tɜ:r.kəm'pɑ:t.mənt.əl/
intracellular /ˌɪn.trə'sel.jə.lər/
isotope /'aɪ.sə.təʊp/
leukotriene /ˌlu:kəʊ'traɪi:n/
lipase /'laɪ.peɪz/
lipolysis /lɪ'pɒlɪsɪs/
lipoprotein /ˌlɪp.ə .'prəʊ.ti:n/

load /ləʊd/
messenger /ˈmes.ɪn.dʒər/
milieu /mɪlˈjʊ/ **interieur** /ɪnˈtɪə.ri.ər/
mineral /ˈmɪn.ər.əl/
myosin /ˈmaɪəsɪn/
net /net/ **effect** /ɪˈfekt/
nitrogenous /nɑɪˈtrɑdʒ.ə.nəs/
opsonin /ˈɒpsənɪn/
overwhelm /ˌəʊ.vəˈwelm/
oxidative /ɒkˈsɪd.ə.tɪv/
peptide /ˈpep.taɪd/
peripheral /pəˈrɪf.ər.əl/
phospholipid /ˌfɒsfəˈlɪpɪd/
postprandial /ˌpəʊstˈpræn.di.əl/
preferentially /ˌpref.ərˈen.ʃəl.i/
prerequisite /ˌpriːˈrek.wɪ.zɪt/
prevailing /prɪˈveɪ.lɪŋ/
prostaglandins /ˌprɒstəˈglændɪn/
relation /rɪˈleɪ.ʃən/
reperfusion /ˌriː.pəˈfjuː.ʒən/
replacement /rɪˈpleɪs.mənt/
retention /rɪˈten.ʃən/
route /ruːt/
sepsis /ˈsep.sɪs/
shift /ʃɪft/
status /ˈsteɪ.təs/
vegetarianism /ˌvedʒ.ɪˈteə.ri.ə.nɪ.zəm/

Solution to Exercise 1a
1j, 2c, 3d, 4k, 5r, 6q, 7t, 8a, 9b, 10s, 11l, 12h, 13m, 14g, 15p, 16e, 17o, 18i, 19n, 20f, 21u

Solution to Exercise 1b
1k, 2h, 3e, 4j, 5b, 6f, 7a, 8i, 9d, 10g, 11c

Unit 5 - Simple and stress starvation. Injury and sepsis.

Dietary fibre: metabolism and physiological effects

Dietary fibre, resistant carbohydrates (saccharides) is a term used to describe substrates which are **not digested by enzymes** produced in the human **small intestine** or which are **poorly absorbed or metabolised**. They are needed to **maintain normal functioning** of the gastrointestinal (GI) tract. Sources of fibre **vary** considerably in **chemical structure**, as does the **composition** of the fibre-containing matrix in foods. The **response** within the GI tract is defined by the **physiochemical properties** of the fibre and on the **location within the gut.** These factors are important for the physiological responses in the gut because **fibre can affect** various physiological functions such as **appetite and satiety**, the **metabolism of lipids and carbohydrates, bowel function** as well as **inflammatory**, and **proliferation processes**.

Dietary fibre is essential for the **general health** and normal function of the gut. Several beneficial effects are known. The intake of different fibres can modulate **blood glucose and lipid metabolism.** The main activity of fibre can be found in the **large bowel.** Due to their distinct **chemical structure,** the various fibres show **different effects**. The **non-fermentable fibres** regulate bowel function mainly by **increasing colonic bulk**. **Fermentable** fibres are, however, also important **metabolic substrates**. The production of SCFAs is crucial: these agents are necessary for the maintenance of a healthy gut. In general, the **beneficial attributes** of dietary fibre include **weight control**, as well as the **prevention of**

constipation, diabetes, CVD, colonic adenomas and colorectal cancer.

Simple and stress starvation

Food intake in humans is an **intermittent process**, but **energy is expended continually**. Therefore, humans **adapt well** to short or long-term **starvation, using their stores** of carbohydrates, fat (mainly) and protein, by mechanisms, which **reduce energy expenditure** as well as **conserving protein.** The adaptation to fasting is dependent on energy reserves, duration of starvation and additional stressful influences. **Long-term** partial or total **cessation of energy intake** without additional stress leads to **marasmic wasting**. Although confirmed report has described very obese individual surviving fasting for 249 and 382 days, individuals with normal initial body weight and composition rarely survive for more than three months' starvation (40% body weight loss or a BMI less than 10 in women and 11 in men).

With the addition of the **stress response, catabolism and wasting** are **accelerated. Protein losses rise** due to the **increased requirements for glucose** (via gluconeogenesis), **glutamine**, and for **aminoacids** for **synthesis of visceral proteins** and for **repair of injured tissue. Weight loss** in either situation results in **impaired** mental and physical **function**, as well as in poorer clinical outcome with increased **complications. Previously malnourished** subjects have **less reserves** with which to face an acute illness or trauma and consequently have poorer outcome. If **surgery** is planned in these patients, **pre-operative nutritional support for 10 days** improves physiological functions and lessens surgical risk.

Exercise 1a
Match the column A with the column B. Try to learn the expressions and/ or sentences by heart.

A

1. Dietary fibre is a term used to describe substrates
2. The response within the GI tract is defined by the physiochemical properties
3. Fibre can affect various physiological functions such as
4. The intake of different fibres
5. The main activity of fibre can be found in the large bowel;
6. The non-fermentable fibres regulate bowel function mainly by increasing colonic bulk;
7. The beneficial attributes of dietary fibre include
8. Food intake in humans is an intermittent process, but energy is expended continually;
9. The adaptation to fasting is dependent on
10. Long-term partial or total cessation of energy intake
11. With the addition of the stress response,

12. Weight loss in either situation results in impaired mental and physical function,
13. If surgery is planned, pre-operative nutritional support

B

a) *appetite and satiety, the metabolism of lipids and carbohydrates, bowel function as well as inflammatory, and proliferation processes.*
b) *as well as in poorer clinical outcome with increased complications.*
c) *can modulate blood glucose and lipid metabolism.*
d) *catabolism and wasting are accelerated:*
e) *due to their distinct chemical structure, the various fibres show different effects.*
f) *energy reserves, duration of starvation and additional stressful influences.*
g) *fermentable fibres are also important metabolic substrates.*
h) *for 10 days improves physiological functions and lessens surgical risk.*
i) *of the fibre and on the location within the gut.*
j) *therefore, humans adapt well to short or long-term starvation, using their stores of carbohydrates, fat (mainly) and protein.*
k) *weight control, the prevention of constipation, diabetes, CVD, colonic adenomas and colorectal cancer.*
l) *which are not digested by enzymes produced in the human small intestine or which are poorly absorbed or metabolised.*
m) *without additional stress leads to marasmic wasting.*

Influence of genotype on inflammation and metabolism

It has been noted that some families were **more prone** to appearance of **inflammatory disease** than others. The characteristics of an individual's major **histocompatibility complex** alter the risk of acquiring inflammatory diseases and are associated with **raised or lowered capacities for cytokine production.** The **genomic differences** modulate the ability of **nutrients** to **interact beneficially** in health and disease.

Injury and sepsis

Many types of **micro-organisms** exert **pathological effects** if they succeed in **penetrating** the surface defences of the body. Once entry is gained, rapid **multiplication** occurs, which, if unchecked, can end in death. However we possess an **immune system** that has great capacity for **immobilising invading microbes**, creating a hostile environment for them and bringing about **their destruction.** Humans and warm-blooded animals have the ability to **focus** a **range of lethal activities** upon the invader. This **biological property** is important since many microbes can multiply at least 50 times faster than the cells of the system.

The immune system can also become **activated**, in a similar way to the response to microbial invasion, by a wide range of **stimuli** and **conditions**; these **include burns, penetrating and blunt injury**, the presence of **tumour** cells, environmental **pollutants, radiation**, exposure to **allergens** and the presence of **chronic inflammatory diseases**. In the normal response the immune system goes from a state of **activation to deactivation** as the body becomes repaired from the effects of the invasion. However in **chronic inflammatory disease** the initial activation continues unchecked. This can be seen in the **end stages** of many chronic conditions which have, as a root cause, **an on-going systemic inflammatory response.**

The **pro-inflammatory cytokines** are produced in response to a wide range of **stimuli (injury, infection, extreme exercise** etc.) They bring about a **powerful, purposeful and focussed response** aimed at **defeating invading organisms** and restoring body function to normal. Profound **metabolic changes** occur due to their actions. The changes influence **protein, fat, carbohydrate, energy and micronutrient metabolism**. While **pro-inflammatory cytokine** production is an **essential part of the response** to **infection, injury and surgery** these **molecules** may have **adverse effects** upon patients. **Anti-oxidant defences become depleted** during the response to cytokines increasing the risk of **up-regulation of the inflammatory process** and tissue damage. Variations in **phenotype, age, and gender** influence the level of **cytokine production** at an **individual** level and have been linked with increased morbidity and mortality.

The neuroendocrine response

The **trauma response** has a large **impact on nutritional treatment** and on substrate metabolism. In essence, following **accidental trauma, surgical operations** and during **acute illness, substrates are diverted** from non-essential tasks, e.g. muscular activity, to the **healing of wounds**, to **support** metabolism of the **immune system** and the **splanchnic organs**, and to other metabolic tasks **involved in survival** from the disease. These **metabolic changes** are mediated both by the **neuroendocrine system** and by **cytokines released** in response to inflammation. A **multimodal approach,** reducing the catabolic stimulus by aggressive **treatment** of infection, optimizing **fluid management** to avoid deficit or excess, by **control of pain and anxiety**, by nursing in a **warm environment,** and by appropriate **surgery**, combined with optimal **nutrition** can **ameliorate** the **neuroendocrine and cytokine responses** mediating catabolism. These concepts have been incorporated in ERAS (**enhanced**

recovery after surgery) programs. **Feeding** alone cannot reverse the catabolic response, although it can **reduce net tissue loss** and **maintain function**. Additional **pharmacological measures,** particularly the use of insulin, may diminish catabolism and improve outcome. Knowledge of the **actions of the neuroendocrine system** in trauma either accidental or elective is important when designing **programmes to optimize nutrition and improve outcome** following trauma and surgery (ERAS) and during acute illness.

Exercise 1b
Match the column A with the column B. Try to learn the expressions and/ or sentences by heart.

A

1. It has been noted that some families
2. The genomic differences modulate
3. Many types of micro-organisms exert pathological effects
4. Once entry is gained, rapid multiplication occurs,
5. The immune system can also become activated by a wide range of stimuli and conditions;
6. In the normal response the immune system goes from a state of activation to deactivation
7. The pro-inflammatory cytokines are produced in response to a wide range of stimuli (injury, infection, extreme exercise etc.)
8. Profound metabolic changes occur due to their actions
9. Anti-oxidant defences become depleted during the response to cytokines,
10. Following accidental trauma, surgical operations and during acute illness, substrates are diverted from non-essential tasks, e.g. muscular activity,
11. These metabolic changes are mediated both by the neuroendocrine system
12. Feeding alone cannot reverse the catabolic response,
13. Knowledge of the actions of the neuroendocrine system in trauma either accidental or elective

B

a) although it can reduce net tissue loss and maintain function.
b) and by cytokines released in response to inflammation.
c) and they bring about a powerful, purposeful and focussed response aimed at defeating invading organisms and restoring body function to normal.
d) as the body becomes repaired from the effects of the invasion.

e) *burns, penetrating and blunt injury, the presence of tumour cells, environmental pollutants, radiation, exposure to allergens and the presence of chronic inflammatory diseases.*

f) *but we possess an immune system that has great capacity for immobilising invading microbes, creating a hostile environment for them and bringing about their destruction.*

g) *if they succeed in penetrating the surface defences of the body.*

h) *increasing the risk of up-regulation of the inflammatory process and tissue damage.*

i) *is important when designing programmes to optimize nutrition and improve outcome following trauma and surgery (ERAS) and during acute illness.*

j) *the ability of nutrients to interact beneficially in health and disease.*

k) *to the healing of wounds, to support metabolism of the immune system and the splanchnic organs, and to other metabolic tasks involved in survival from the disease.*

l) *were more prone to appearance of inflammatory disease than others.*

m) *which can influence protein, fat, carbohydrate, energy and micronutrient metabolism.*

Exercise 2

Translate the expressions. Try to explain their meanings in English.

Vary considerably, physiochemical properties, location within the gut, bowel function, inflammatory, proliferation, beneficial effects, modulate, distinct, increasing colonic bulk, fermentable fibres, beneficial attributes, prevention of constipation, colonic adenomas, colorectal cancer, intermittent process, expended continually, adapt well, using their stores, reduce energy expenditure, conserving protein, fasting, partial or total, cessation of energy intake, confirmed report, surviving fasting, catabolism and wasting, accelerated, increased requirements, visceral proteins, repair of injured tissue, face an acute illness or trauma, outcome, noted, prone to, acquiring, interact, succeed in, penetrating defences, multiplication, unchecked, possess, immobilising, invading, hostile environment, bringing about, biological property, penetrating and blunt injury, environmental pollutants, chronic inflammatory disease, end stages, on-going, systemic inflammatory response, bring about, defeating invading organisms, restoring to normal, essential part, response to infection, injury and surgery, adverse effects, anti-oxidant defences, become depleted, phenotype, age, gender, linked with, impact on, accidental trauma, diverted from, healing of wounds, mediated by, approach, treatment, fluid management, control of pain and anxiety, incorporated, enhanced recovery after surgery, reverse the catabolic response, pharmacological measures, diminish, improve outcome, accidental or elective, designing programmes, improve outcome.

Exercise 3
Prepare short talks and/or dialogues on these topics.

1. The metabolism of fibre
2. Different physiological effects of fibre
3. Short and long-term starvation during non-stress conditions
4. Difference between simple and stress starvation
5. Injury and sepsis
6. The neuroendocrine response

Vocabulary 5

Fill in the meanings in your mother language:

accidental /ˌæk.sɪˈden.təl/
acquire /əˈkwaɪər/
ameliorate /əˈmiː.l.jə.reɪt/
appearance /əˈpɪə.rənt s/
associate /əˈsəʊ.si.eɪt/
attribute /ˈæt.rɪ.bjuːt/
blunt / blʌnt/
bring /brɪŋ/ **about** /əˈbaʊt/
bulk /bʌlk/
burn /bɜːn/
carbohydrate /ˌkɑː.bəʊ ˈhaɪ.dreɪt/
catecholamine /kat.ə.kəl.am.in/
cessation /sesˈeɪ.ʃən/
confirmed /kənˈfɜːmd/
conserve /kənˈsɜːv/
cytokine /ˈsaɪtəʊˌkaɪn/
deficit /ˈdef.ɪ.sɪt/
design /dɪˈzaɪn/
destruction /dɪˈstrʌk.ʃən/
devise /dɪˈvaɪz/
diminish /dɪˈmɪn.ɪʃ/
distinct /dɪˈstɪŋkt/
diversion /da ɪˈvɜː.ʃən/
divert /daɪˈvɜːt/
elective /ɪˈlek.tɪv/
enteral /ˈen.tə.rəl/
expend /ɪkˈspend/
face /feɪs/
fermentable /fəˈment.ə.bl̩/
fibre /ˈfaɪ.bər/
fluid /ˈfluː.ɪd/
gender /ˈdʒen.dər/
genome /ˈdʒiː.nəʊm/
glutamine /ˈgluːtəˌmiːn/
heal /hiːl/
histocompatibility / ˌhɪstəʊkəmˌpætɪˈbɪlɪtɪ/
hostile /ˈhɒs.taɪl/
immobilize /ɪˈməʊ.bəl.aɪz/
impact /ˈɪm.pækt/
incorporate /ɪnˈkɔː.pər.eɪt/
inflammatory /ɪnˈflæm.ə.tər.i/
insulin /ˈɪn.sjʊ.lɪn/
intermittent /ˌɪn.təˈmɪt.ənt/
invade /ɪnˈveɪd/
invader /ɪnˈveɪ.dər/
large /lɑːdʒ/ **bowel** /ˈbaʊ.əl/
lessen /ˈles.ən/
lethal /ˈliː.θəl/
malnourished /ˌmælˈnʌr.ɪʃt/
marasmic /məˈræzmɪk/
mass /mæs/
matrix /ˈmeɪt.rɪks/
mechanism /ˈmekəˌnɪzəm/
mediate /ˈmiː.di.eɪt/
microbe /ˈmaɪ.krəʊb/
multimodal /ˌmʌl tiˈmoʊd.l/
multiplication /ˌmʌl.tiˈ p.lɪˈkeɪ.ʃən/

neural /ˈnjʊə.rəl/
neuroendocrine /ˌnjʊə.rəʊ.ˈen.də.krɪn/
nucleotide /ˈnjuːkli.ə.taɪd/
optimize /ˈɒp.tɪ.maɪz/
parenteral /pəˈren.tə.rəl/
penetrating /ˈpen.ɪ.treɪ.tɪŋ/
permit /pəˈmɪt/
physiochemical /ˌfɪz.iˈɒˈkem.ɪ.kəl/
physiological /ˌfɪz.iˈɒl.ə.dʒi.kəl/
pollutant /pəˈluːtənt/
polymorphism /ˌpɒl.ɪˈmɔː.fɪ.zəm/
presence /ˈprez.ənt s/
previous /ˈpriː.vi.əs/
profound /prəˈfaʊnd/
prolactin /proʊˈlæk tɪn/
proliferation /prəˌlɪf.ərˈeɪ.ʃən/
prolonged /prəˈlɒŋd/
property /ˈprɒp.ə.ti/
purposeful /ˈpɜː.pəs.fəl/
radiation /ˌreɪ.diˈeɪ.ʃən/
range /reɪndʒ/
re-esterification /riː.eˌster.ə.fɪˈkeɪ.ʃən/
release /rəˈliːs/
replenish /rɪˈplen.ɪʃ/
response /rɪˈspɒns/
result /rɪˈzʌlt/
reverse /rɪˈvɜːs/
root /ruːt/
satiety /səˈtaɪə.ti/
severe /sɪˈvɪər/
short /ʃɔːt/ **-chain** /tʃeɪn/
splanchnic /ˈsplæŋk.nɪk/
stimulus /ˈstɪm.jʊ.ləs/ pl **stimuli**
support /səˈpɔːt/
surgical /ˈsɜː.dʒɪ.kəl/
survival /səˈvaɪ.vəl/
threaten /ˈθret.ən/
tumour /ˈtjuː.mər/
unchecked /ʌnˈtʃekt/
visceral /ˈvɪs.ər.əl/
withstand /wɪðˈstænd/
(withstood, withstood)
wound /wuːnd/

Solution to Exercise 1a
1l, 2i, 3a, 4c, 5e, 6g, 7k, 8j,
9f, 10m, 11d, 12b, 13h

Solution to Exercise 1b
1l, 2j, 3g, 4f, 5e, 6d, 7c, 8m,
9h, 10k, 11b, 12a, 13i

Unit 6 - Metabolic response to injury and sepsis

All **processes**, in living animal cells, are dependent on a constant **supply of substrate** to generate **high-energy phosphate bonds**. Energy is then harnessed to **cellular activity** by the **hydrolysis** of ATP. It can be **estimated** that the mass of **ATP hydrolysed daily** is **equivalent to the body weight** of the individual and that **insufficient generation** of ATP leads to **irreversible destruction** of the whole organism within less than one minute. **Continuous regeneration** of ATP is therefore essential for survival under all conditions. **Carbohydrates** (CHO), **fat** and **proteins** are the substrates, which are **oxidised to generate ATP**. Under normal circumstances these substrates are supplied in **food**, which is, after **absorption**, processed by different **metabolic** pathways. As food intake is not a continuous process **between meals** the organism has to **utilise energy substrates** from its reserves. Under normal **(non-stress) situations** ingested CHO, fat and protein are partly **stored as glycogen and lipid.** Accumulation **of protein** can only occur in an quantitatively modest manner, and may happen **during growth** of the individual, **recovery** after illness, **training** or **postprandially**. In **healthy individuals** eating food of normal quantity and composition, **as much nitrogen is excreted** in urine, stools, skin, hair and sweat **as is eaten** during the day. **The non-nitrogen part** is **oxidised or stored** as fat or glycogen.

During **fasting**, the body **mobilizes these stores** for tissue energy supply. Especially during **long-term starvation fat is utilised** preferably to furnish **energy needs** and **proteins are spared. Brain** and other tissue which **normally utilise glucose increase utilisation of ketone bodies. Glucose** is formed **from glycerol,** and, to a lesser extent, from **amino acids. In this way proteins diminish slowly** during uncomplicated starvation. The **metabolic response to stress** is mediated by **catabolic hormones** (glucagon, catecholamines and corticoids), and **insulin resistance**, as well as by **cytokines, eicosanoids, oxygen radicals**, and other local mediators. The **stress response** can only be **reversed** effectively by **reducing infection, inflammation, heat loss** etc. **Nutritional support** can **compensate** by reducing negative energy and protein balance, but it **cannot reverse** a negative protein balance **until the convalescent phase** begins.

Nutritional aspects of chronic inflammatory disease

There is a growing appreciation that **chronic inflammation** is central to the pathophysiology of much of the **chronic disease** burden that afflicts human kind. If left unchecked, chronic inflammation is associated with **sustained erosion of body cell mass** that culminates in the severe loss of body cell mass and ultimately to **cachexia.** The National Cancer Institute in the USA has described **cachexia** as a '**loss of body weight and muscle mass, and weakness** that may occur in patients with advanced cancer, AIDS, or other chronic diseases'. The European Society for Parenteral and Enteral Nutrition recently highlighted the key role of inflammation by characterizing cachexia as a '**systemic pro-inflammatory process** with associated **metabolic derangements** that include insulin resistance, increased lipolysis, increased lipid oxidation, increased protein turnover, and loss of body muscle and fat tissue'.

Weight loss is relatively common **in chronic disease,** but the full-blown appearance of the **truly cachectic state** with clear manifestations of systemic inflammation and severe losses of muscle and adipose tissue is less prevalent. Nevertheless, it is strongly associated with **adverse outcomes** that include functional decline, compromised tolerance and efficacy of treatment, and increased mortality. The most unfortunate outcome is all too often **deteriorating quality-of-life** for the final years, months, or weeks of life.

Even if nutrition remains adequate, loss of body cell mass

may occur. In later stages, fat mass is also lost, leading to the characteristic cachectic appearance. Cachexia is usually associated with mono-organ **failure** syndromes (**cardiac, lung, hepatic or renal**); advanced malignancies such as **gastric or pancreatic cancer;** advanced **HIV/AIDS**; and advanced **rheumatoid arthritis.** Nutritional support alone only partly reverses or prevents cachexia. Benefit can be greatly enhanced if the **underlying condition** is amenable to successful treatment. To improve outcome, **integrated approaches** that **target the underlying condition** or associated inflammation are required.

Metabolic aspects of neurological diseases

The development and maintenance of the entire neuromuscular apparatus, of its properties and inherent characteristics, are closely related to the **mutual communication between motor neurons and muscles**. If this communication is **disrupted**, muscle undergoes several changes. These changes are referred to as **denervation**, and are a common feature of several **degenerative or post- traumatic neurological disorders**. Recently, the **activity of motor neurons and neurotrophic factors** have been recognised to influence **muscle trophism** and to **preserve neuromuscular function**, even though the underlying mechanisms are incompletely understood. The **connection** between **motor neurons and muscle** is the crucial element in the maintenance of the **normal mass and function** of muscle. If this communication is disrupted, muscles undergo several structural and histological alterations that significantly influence metabolism.

Exercise 1
Match the column A with the column B. Try to learn the expressions and/or sentences by heart.

A

1. All processes, in living animal cells, are dependent on a constant supply of substrate to generate high-energy phosphate bonds;
2. Insufficient generation of ATP leads to irreversible destruction of the whole organism within less than one minute,
3. Carbohydrates (CHO), fat and proteins are the substrates,
4. Under normal (non-stress) situations ingested CHO, fat and protein
5. In healthy individuals eating food of normal quantity and composition
6. During long-term starvation fat is utilised preferably
7. The metabolic response to stress is mediated by catabolic hormones (glucagon, catecholamines

and corticoids), and insulin resistance,
8. Nutritional support can compensate by reducing negative energy and protein balance,
9. Chronic inflammation is associated with sustained erosion of body cell mass
10. Weight loss is relatively common in chronic disease;
11. Even if nutrition remains adequate, loss of body cell mass may occur;
12. Cachexia is usually associated with mono-organ failure syndromes (cardiac, lung, hepatic or renal); advanced malignancies
13. The development and maintenance of the entire neuromuscular apparatus,
14. If this communication is disrupted, muscle undergoes several changes;
15. The connection between motor neurons and muscle is the crucial element

B

a) are closely related to the mutual communication between motor neurons and muscles.
b) are partly stored as glycogen and lipid.
c) as much nitrogen is excreted in urine, stools, skin, hair and sweat as is eaten during the day.
d) as well as by cytokines, eicosanoids, oxygen radicals, and other local mediators.
e) but it cannot reverse a negative protein balance until the convalescent phase begins.
f) energy is then harnessed to cellular activity by the hydrolysis of ATP.
g) in later stages, fat mass is also lost, leading to the characteristic cachectic appearance.
h) in the maintenance of the normal mass and function of muscle.
i) it is strongly associated with adverse outcomes that include functional decline, compromised tolerance and efficacy of treatment, and increased mortality.
j) such as gastric or pancreatic cancer; advanced HIV/AIDS; and advanced rheumatoid arthritis.
k) that culminates in the severe loss of body cell mass and ultimately to cachexia.
l) therefore continuous regeneration of ATP is essential for survival under all conditions.
m) these changes are referred to as denervation, and are a common feature of several degenerative or post- traumatic neurological disorders.
n) to furnish energy needs and proteins are spared.

o) *which are oxidised to generate ATP.*

Exercise 2
Translate the expressions. Try to explain their meanings in English.

Phosphate bonds, harnessed, hydrolysis, estimated, equivalent to, insufficient, generation, irreversible destruction, continuous regeneration, essential for survival, under all conditions, generate, processed by metabolic pathways, accumulation, modest manner, postprandially, urine, stools, sweat, oxidised or stored, mobilizes these stores, fat is utilised, furnish energy needs, proteins are spared, to a lesser extent, mediated by, destructive, prolonged or severe, reversed effectively, convalescent phase, growing appreciation, disease burden, erosion of body cell mass, cachexia, consensus is lacking, invariably comprises, altered body composition, diminished biological function, highlighted, associated metabolic efficacy of treatment, deteriorating quality-of-life, cachectic appearance, failure syndromes (cardiac, lung, hepatic or renal), advanced malignancies, target the underlying condition, resistance strength training, development and maintenance, mutual communication disrupted, degenerative neurological disorders, muscle trophism, crucial element, mass and function of muscle.

Exercise 3
Prepare short talks and/or dialogues on these topics.

1. Metabolic response to injury and sepsis
2. Chronic inflammation as a key component of the severe malnutrition syndrome cachexia
3. Disease states associated with cachexia
4. Metabolic aspects of neurological diseases
5. The mass and function of muscle

Vocabulary 6

adaptive /ə'dæp.tɪv/
adenine /'æd.əˌnin/
adenosine /ə'dɛn əˌsin/
advanced /əd'vɑːnt st/
afflict /ə'flɪkt/
amenable /ə'miː.nə.bl̩/
Amyotrophic /æ.mi.əʊˌtrɒfɪk/ **Lateral** /læt.ər.əl/ **Sclerosis** sclerosis /sklə'rəʊ.sɪs/ **ALS**
anoxia /æn'ɒk.si.ə/
apparatus /'æpəˌreɪtəs/
atrophy /'æt.rə.fi/
burden /'bɜː.dən/
cachexia /kə'kɛksɪə/
compound /'kɒm.paʊnd/
comprise /kəm'praɪz/
condition /kən'dɪʃən/
connection /kə'nek.ʃən/
consumption /kən'sʌmp .ʃən/
corticoid /'kɔr təˌkɔɪd/
culminate /'kʌl.mɪ.neɪt/
decline /dɪ'klaɪn/
delineate /dɪ'lɪn.i.eɪt/
denervation /dɪ.nɜː'veɪ.ʃən/
derangement /dɪ'reɪndʒd.mənt/

destructive /dɪˈstrʌk.tɪv/
deteriorate /dɪˈtɪə.ri.ə.reɪt/
dinucleotide /daɪˈnu kli əˌtaɪd/
disrupt /dɪsˈrʌpt/
distinguish /dɪˈstɪŋ.gwɪʃ/
drive /draɪv/
efficacy /ˈef.ɪ.kə.si/
efficiency /ɪˈfɪʃ.ən.si/
eicosanoid /aɪ.kəʊ.sə.noid/
either /ˈiːðə/
electrochemical /ɪˌlek.troʊˈkem.ɪ.kəl/
entire /ɪnˈtaɪə/
erosion /ɪˈrəʊ.ʒən/
estimated /ˈes.tɪ.meɪt.ɪd/
evidence /ˈev.ɪ.dəns/
examine /ɪgˈzæm.ɪn/
explore /ɪkˈsplɔːr/
extent /ɪkˈstent/
fast /fɑːst/
feature /ˈfiː.tʃər/
flavin /ˈfleɪvɪn/
furnish /ˈfɜː.nɪʃ/
generate /ˈdʒen.ər.eɪt/
genotype /ˈdʒen.ə.taɪp/
glycerol /ˈglɪs.ə.rɒl/
glycolysis /glaɪˈkɒlɪsɪs/
growing /ˈgrəʊ.ɪŋ/
harmful /ˈhɑːm.fəl/
harness /ˈhɑː.nəs/
highlight /ˈhaɪ.laɪt/
histological /ˌhɪs.təˈlɒdʒ.ɪ.kəl/
hydrolysis /haɪˈdrɒl.ə.sɪs/
hyperoxia /ˌhaɪ.pəˈɒk.sɪə/
hypoxia /haɪˈpɒk.sɪə/
incomplete /ˌɪn.kəmˈpliːt/
ingest /ɪnˈdʒest/
inherent /ɪnˈher.ənt/
integrated /ˈɪn.tɪ.greɪ.t̬ ɪd/
intervention /ˌɪn.təˈven.ʃən/
invariably /ɪnˈveə.ri.ə.bli/
irreversible /ˌɪr.ɪˈvɜː.sɪ.bl̩/
ketone /ˈkiː.təʊn/ **body** /ˈbɒd.i/
kind /kaɪnd/
lack /læk/
lactate /lækˈteɪt/
latter /ˈlæt.ər/
limiting /ˈlɪm.ɪ.tɪŋ/
mediator /ˈmiː.di.eɪ.tər/
mitochondrial /ˌmaɪ.təˈkɒn.dri.əl/
modest /ˈmɒd.ɪst/
modify /ˈmɒd.ɪ.faɪ/
multifaceted /ˌmʌl.tiˈfæs.ɪ.tɪd/
neurotrophic /njʊə.rəʊˈtrəʊfɪk/
nevertheless /ˌnev.ə.ðəˈles/
nicotinamide /ˌnɪkəˈtɪnəˌmaɪd/
orbital /ˈɔː.bɪˌtəl/
oxidize /ˈɒk.sɪ.daɪz/
oxygen /ˈɒk.sɪ.dʒən/
pass /pɑːs/ **through** /θruː/
pathophysiology /ˌpæθ.əˌfɪz.iˈɒl.ə.dʒi/
persistent /pəˈsɪs.tənt/
phenotype /ˈfiː.nəʊ.taɪp/
phosphorylation /fɒsˈfɒr.ɪ.leɪ.ʃən/
pool /puːl/
practitioner /prækˈtɪ.ʃən.ər/
pre-cachexia /priː.kəˈkɛksɪə/
prebiotic /priː.baɪˈɒt.ɪk/
prevalent /ˈprev.əl.ənt/
priority /praɪˈɒr.ɪ.ti/
probiotic /ˌprəʊ.baɪˈɒt.ɪk/
promising /ˈprɒm.ɪ.sɪŋ/
proton /ˈprəʊ.tɒn/
quantitatively /ˈkwɒn.tɪ.tə.tɪv.li/
radical /ˈræd.ɪ.kəl/
recognize /ˈrek.əg.naɪz/
recycled /ˌriːˈsaɪ.kl̩d/
role /rəʊl/
selection /sɪˈlek.ʃən/
spare /speər/
sustain /səˈsteɪn/
sweat /swet/
synthesis /ˈsɪn.θə.sɪs/
synthesize /ˈsɪn.θə.saɪz/
target /ˈtɑː.gɪt/
tightly /ˈtaɪt.li/
transduced /trænzˈdjuː.səd/
transmembrane /trænsˈmem.breɪn/
treatment /ˈtriːt.mənt/
triphosphate /ˈtrɪ ˈfɒs.feɪt/
trophism /ˈtrəʊpɪzəm/

truly /ˈtruː.li/
turnover /ˈtɜːnˌəʊ.vər/
ultimately /ˈʌl.tɪ.mət.li/
underlying /ˌʌn.dəˈlaɪ.ɪŋ/
unfortunate /ʌnˈfɔː.tʃən.ət/
utilize /ˈjuː.tɪ.laɪz/
vigorous /ˈvɪg.ər.əs/

Unit 7 - Substrates used in parenteral and enteral nutrition

Energy

- Energy **needs** should be determined in relation to **expenditure**, but also to the ability of a patient to **metabolize** substrates.
- Most **hospitalised patients** present a combination of **stress and malnutrition**.
- Aiming at achieving **positive or zero nitrogen balance** via hypercaloric support **should be discouraged** during the acute catabolic phase of sepsis or trauma.
- **Overfeeding** during acute illness may be associated with major **complications and side effects** including respiratory, cardiovascular and hepatic problems.
- The main goal of feeding, **in the acute phase** of illness, should be to **preserve function** and to **reduce**, but not abolish **the loss of lean body mass**. Feeding should be **started early** (first 48 hours) and introduced cautiously, increasing slowly over a few days. During the **convalescent phase, anabolism returns**, and both energy and protein intakes can be increased with advantage.

Negative energy balance and severe body depletion is a matter of serious concern since **losses of 30-40% of proteins** are **life-threatening**. Such losses occur **after 50-70 days** of uncomplicated fasting; however during period of **critical illness** the **interval** is significantly **shorter** due to reduced adaptation to negative energy balance and increased protein catabolism. During negative energy balance the organism always **loses fat tissue together with body protein** – with consequent loss of organ and muscle functions.

Nutritional support is indicated to preserve or improve body functions, to **avoid** undue **losses of body weight** (especially body cell mass) and to **restore** normal **body composition and function** in depleted subjects. Moreover, in **growing children** energy intake is required for normal growth. In critical illness energy intake should minimize negative energy balance and losses of lean body mass. While it is difficult to overfeed patients enterally because of the limits of gastro-intestinal tolerance, it is only too **easy to overfeed by the parenteral route**. In the early days of parenteral nutrition, following the concept of so-called **hyperalimentation** (i.e. hypercaloric nutrition), large energy loads were administered, particularly in the form of carbohydrate. This **concept** was essentially based on three factors:

- the assumption that obtaining a positive nitrogen balance is an important goal to achieve in severely ill patients and that large **energy loads** could **reverse the catabolism of injury**.
- the idea that 'if some is good, **more is better**'
- the notion that conditions such as **injury and sepsis** are associated with marked **increases in energy expenditure** and that it was possible to reverse this by metabolic manipulation, thus preserving lean mass.

Carbohydrates

The **classical view** considers two major **energy substrates**: **carbohydrates** (CHO) and fat (especially **fatty acids**). However, this does not take into account that **other nutrients** (e.g. some aminoacids and ketone bodies) may be used as fuel and that **requirements** of various energy substrates may **vary considerably** between different tissues as well as in differing conditions. While **non-glucose carbohydrates and glucose derivatives** play an important role as structural **components of cells** and **extracellular matrix** (proteoglycans and glucosamines), **glucose** represents the **major circulating carbohydrate fuel.** Carbohydrates should **cover 50-60%** of total energy requirements during nutritional support. **Maltodextrins** are the major sources of CHO energy in **enteral** nutrition whereas, at present, **glucose** is the only carbohydrate used **in parenteral nutrition mixtures.**

Glucose is the major **circulating** carbohydrate fuel, and is used by most cells in the body. In spite of markedly elevated glucose turnover in conditions of stress, oxidative metabolism is not increased in the same proportion. Hence, **large loads of glucose may represent an additional stress**, increasing the demands for gas exchange.

Lipids

Lipids are important **energy substrates** and are the main **energy store** in our body. Moreover, **phospholipids** are essential **structural components** of cell membranes including plasma membrane and the vacuoles and other organelles; this is particularly relevant to the central and peripheral **nervous system.**

Fatty acids may markedly **affect cell function**, and some also are **precursors** of **eicosanoid** (prostaglandins, leukotrienes, tromboxanes) **synthesis**; **cholesterol** is a **precursor** for **steroid hormone synthesis.** Thus, lipids may **modulate metabolic processes** at local, regional, and distant sites. The **rate of lipid oxidation** is

dependent not only **on energy expenditure** but also on **hormonal status**, the **clinical situation** and the presence of other energy substrates (especially) glucose. Lipid intake should cover **20 to 40% of energy needs**, depending on individual tolerance and the clinical situation. In artificial nutrition lipids can be administered either enterally and/or parenterally. During the first few days of **lipid infusion**, particularly in stressed patients, the prescribed lipid load should be **infused as slowly as possible. Plasma triglyceride levels** should be **monitored** during this initial period and **infusion rate adjusted** to measured values. In the future, lipid preparations may be provided to modify the fatty acid pattern of cell membranes and to supply important lipid-soluble vitamins.

Exercise 1a
Match the column A with the column B. Try to learn the expressions and/or sentences by heart.

A

1. Energy needs should be determined in relation to expenditure, but also to the
2. Overfeeding during acute illness may be associated with
3. The main goal of feeding, in the acute phase of illness,
4. During the convalescent phase, anabolism returns,
5. Losses of 30-40% of proteins are life-threatening; such losses occur after 50-70 days of uncomplicated fasting;
6. Nutritional support is indicated to preserve or improve body functions, to avoid undue losses of body weight
7. In critical illness energy intake should minimize
8. While it is difficult to overfeed patients enterally because the limits of gastrointestinal tolerance,
9. In the early days of parenteral nutrition, following the concept
10. The classical view considers two major energy substrates:
11. Other nutrients (e.g. some aminoacids and ketone bodies) may be used as fuel and
12. Non-glucose carbohydrates and glucose derivatives play an important role as structural components of cells and extracellular matrix,
13. Glucose is the only carbohydrate used
14. Large loads of glucose may represent an additional stress,
15. Lipids are important energy substrates
16. Phospholipids are essential structural components of cell membranes including plasma membrane
17. Fatty acids may markedly affect cell function,

18. The rate of lipid oxidation is dependent not only on energy expenditure
19. Lipid intake should cover 20 to 40% of energy needs,
20. During the first few days of lipid infusion, particularly in stressed patients,

B

a) *ability of a patient to metabolize substrates; most hospitalised patients present a combination of stress and malnutrition.*

b) *and are the main energy store in our body.*

c) *and both energy and protein intakes can be increased with advantage.*

d) *and some also are precursors of eicosanoid synthesis; cholesterol is a precursor for steroid hormone synthesis.*

e) *but also on hormonal status, the clinical situation and the presence of other energy substrates (especially) glucose.*

f) *and the vacuoles and other organelles; this is particularly relevant to the central and peripheral nervous system.*

g) *and to restore normal body composition and function in depleted subjects.*

h) *carbohydrates (CHO) and fat (especially fatty acids).*

i) *depending on individual tolerance and the clinical situation.*

j) *during period of critical illness the interval is significantly shorter due to reduced adaptation to negative energy balance and increased protein catabolism.*

k) *glucose represents the major circulating carbohydrate fuel.*

l) *in parenteral nutrition mixtures.*

m) *increasing the demands for gas exchange.*

n) *it is easy to overfeed by the parenteral route.*

o) *major complications and side effects including respiratory, cardiovascular and hepatic problems.*

p) *negative energy balance and losses of lean body mass.*

q) *of so-called hyperalimentation, large energy loads were administered, particularly in the form of carbohydrate.*

r) *requirements of various energy substrates may vary considerably between different tissues as well as in differing conditions.*

s) *should be to preserve function and to reduce the loss of lean body mass.*

t) *the prescribed lipid load should be infused as slowly as possible.*

Proteins and aminoacids

The name protein is derived from the Greek word 'proteinon' meaning the best, the first price. Proteins are associated with **all forms of life**, an observation that dates back to the original identification of proteins as a class by Mulder in 1838. Indeed, the philosopher Engels defined life as the living form of protein. The importance of proteins lies in the fact that they are the **most abundant solid in every cell** in the body. They are subject to continuous wear-and-tear, and are therefore continuously broken down and **simultaneously replaced.** Proteins are indispensable for life and growth. **Amino acids** are not only the **building blocks** of protein, but also serve as **precursors** for the **biosynthesis** of numerous important biological compounds.

Water and electrolytes during nutritional support

The intake of **fluid and electrolytes** is **inseparable from** the administration of **nutrients** by natural or artificial means. The calculation of appropriate requirements should, therefore, be assigned the **same importance** as those of macro- and micronutrients. Despite the fact that **intravenous fluids** are the most common prescription in hospital patients, **fluid balance** is often managed badly, with adverse consequences for the patient. It is only too easy to give **excess** by the parenteral route without regard to appropriate considerations of balance and without **understanding the risks.** As little as a two litre deficit or excess saline may cause **physiological and functional problems** for the patient. Excess causes, for example, delayed return of GI function and increased complications after surgery.

Patients requiring nutritional support will often already be depleted with respect to **trace elements and vitamins,** and moreover may have increased requirements as a result of illness. **Inadequate micronutrient status** can have a wide range of clinical and subclinical effects. All patients requiring nutritional support should therefore receive a **complete intake** of essential micronutrients from the beginning of their episode of feeding. This will usually be present within the composition of complete enteral feeds, but specific complete **additives** of trace elements and vitamins should be included in PN regimens.

Dietary fibre: definition and classification

The definition and classification of dietary fibre has been changed several times. Dietary carbohydrates should probably best be classified according to their chemical structure. However, the **physiological and health effects** of dietary, non-digestible carbohydrates are dependent upon not only their primary **chemical structure**, but also on their **physical properties**, including **water solubility, fermentation** and formation of a **viscous gel.**

Special substrates
Antioxidants and phytochemicals in nutrition

The implication of **oxidative stress**, the imbalance between **pro-oxidant species** and **anti-oxidant defence mechanisms**, has progressively emerged as a central pathogenic event for **several acute and chronic conditions**. This evidence is consistent with epidemiological findings linking a **depletion of the stores of antioxidants** with an increased **prevalence** of various disorders including **cancer, heart disease,** accelerated **ageing** and **neurodegenerative diseases**. Conversely, an increased consumption of **fruits and vegetables** exert **synergistic effects** on **antioxidant activities**, and reduce the risk of chronic disease, at least for cancer and heart disease. Antioxidants are important compounds to **protect cells** and **tissues from oxidative and nitrosative stress**. It has been becoming more and more clear that the major antioxidants, **vitamins E, C, and glutathione** may act in a synergistic or complementary fashion. The present accumulated **knowledge** about antioxidants undoubtedly represents a great challenge for **physicians, nutritional scientists, pharmacists, food technologists and food chemists.** Continued rigorous critical evaluation of assumptions and hypotheses about **relationship** between **diet, nutrition, health and disease** should provide us with reliable knowledge of what can and what cannot be achieved through clinical nutrition.

Nutrients that influence inflammation and immunity: ω-3 fatty acids

The **response** to **surgery** and to **traumatic insult** may involve excessive inflammation and an **immunosuppressed state** in some patients. **ω-6 fatty acids** provided in **artificial nutrition** may play a part in **creating this state.**

One approach to **decrease** the amount of **linoleic acid** used is to partly **replace vegetable oil with fish oil. Long chain ω-3 fatty acids** found in fish oil can **decrease the production** of inflammatory **eicosanoids and cytokines**. They act directly and indirectly. Thus, long chain ω-3 fatty acids are potentially **useful anti-inflammatory agents**, and may be of benefit in patients at risk of developing a hyper-inflammatory state and sepsis. **Fish oil containing lipid emulsions** have been used in **parenteral nutrition** provided to adult patients **after** (mainly gastrointestinal) **surgery**. **Perioperative administration** of fish oil may be superior to postoperative administration. Fish oil has been used parenterally **in critically ill** adults. Here the influence on inflammatory processes, immune function, and endpoints **is not clear** because there are too few studies and those that are available report contradictory findings. One important factor is **the dose** of fish oil required to influence outcomes. Fish oil has been included in **enteral formula** used **in post-surgery and critically ill** patients. Benefits are clear with some formulas in particular patient groups, and these benefits are consistent with ω-3 fatty acids being an active ingredient.

Nutrients that influence immunity: experimental and clinical data

Nutritional **formula enriched** with **glutamine** (Gln), **arginine** (Arg), **nucleotides, ω-3 polyunsaturated fatty acids** (ω-3 PUFAs) and **micronutrients** has been proposed to **improve the immune system** and gastrointestinal (GI) trophism of patients undergoing major surgery or who are in the **intensive care unit** (ICU). Such a **nutritional strategy** has been reported to reduce late postoperative infections, wound complications, time on mechanical ventilation, length of stay in hospital, and treatment costs. Although these **positive effects** have been observed in many clinical trials, several studies have indicated **potential harm** to patients with severe sepsis or GI intolerance. **Recent studies** in experimental animals and humans concerning **immunonutrients** have been reviewed. Many of the pre-clinical data support a strong immunomodulatory effect of **Gln, Arg, nucleotides, PUFAs and micronutrients**. Several meta-analyses have confirmed that an immune-enhancing diet enriched with such nutrients shows beneficial effects in different types of patients. However, their **individual mechanisms** of action remain **unclear** due to determine more precisely their specific effects in different diseases. Immunonutrients may also include **flavonoids, prebiotics, and probiotics,** and it is likely that future studies will uncover important roles for various nutrients in immune function.

Exercise 1b
Match the column A with the column B. Try to learn the expressions and/or sentences by heart.

A

1. Proteins are the most abundant solid in every cell in the body,
2. Amino acids are not only the building blocks of protein,
3. The intake of fluid and electrolytes is inseparable
4. The calculation of appropriate requirements should
5. Patients requiring nutritional support will often already be depleted with respect to trace elements and vitamins,
6. All patients requiring nutritional support should receive a complete intake
7. The physiological and health effects of dietary, non-digestible carbohydrates are dependent upon
8. The implication of oxidative stress, the imbalance between pro-oxidant species and anti-oxidant defence mechanisms

9. An increased consumption of fruits and vegetables exert synergistic effects on antioxidant activities,
10. The major antioxidants, vitamins E, C, and glutathione
11. The response to surgery and to traumatic insult may involve excessive inflammation and an immunosuppressed state,
12. One approach to decrease the amount of linoleic acid used
13. Long chain ω-3 fatty acids found in fish oil
14. Fish oil containing lipid emulsions
15. Fish oil has been included in enteral formula
16. Nutritional formula enriched with glutamine (Gln), arginine (Arg), nucleotides, ω-3 polyunsaturated fatty acids (ω-3 PUFAs) and micronutrients
17. Many of the pre-clinical data support
18. Immunonutrients may also include

B

a) a strong immunomodulatory effect of Gln, Arg, nucleotides, PUFAs and micronutrients.

b) and moreover may have increased requirements as a result of illness.

c) and reduce the risk of chronic disease, at least for cancer and heart disease.

d) and ω-6 fatty acids provided in artificial nutrition may play a part in creating this state.

e) be assigned the same importance as those of macro- and micronutrients.

f) but also serve as precursors for the biosynthesis of numerous important biological compounds.

g) can decrease the production of inflammatory eicosanoids and cytokines.

h) flavonoids, prebiotics, and probiotics.

i) from the administration of nutrients by natural or artificial means.

j) has been proposed to improve the immune system and gastrointestinal (GI) trophism of patients undergoing major surgery or who are in the intensive care unit (ICU).

k) has progressively emerged as a central pathogenic event for several acute and chronic conditions.

l) have been used in parenteral nutrition provided to adult patients after (mainly gastrointestinal) surgery.

m) is to partly replace vegetable oil with fish oil.

n) may act in a synergistic or complementary fashion.

o) not only their primary chemical structure, but also on their physical properties, including water solubility, fermentation and formation of a viscous gel.

p) of essential micronutrients from the beginning of their episode of feeding.

q) they are continuously broken down and simultaneously replaced.

r) used in post-surgery and critically ill patients.

Exercise 2

Translate the expressions. Try to explain their meanings in English.

Aiming at, achieving, via, hypercaloric support, discouraged, catabolic phase of sepsis or trauma, overfeeding, side effects, goal, loss of lean body mass, introduced cautiously, with advantage, body depletion, serious concern, life-threatening, consequent loss, preserve or improve body functions, body composition, in depleted subjects, critical illness, overfeed, the limits of gastrointestinal tolerance, hypercaloric nutrition, assumption that, reverse, notion, preserving lean mass, take into account, used as fuel, vary considerably, extracellular matrix, circulating carbohydrate fuel, maltodextrins, enteral nutrition, parenteral nutrition mixtures, markedly elevated, glucose turnover, oxidative metabolism, the same proportion, additional stress, demands for gas exchange, phospholipids, cell membranes, vacuoles and other organelles, affect cell function, precursors of eicosanoid synthesis, steroid hormone synthesis, modulate, local, regional, and distant sites, clinical situation, individual tolerance, artificial nutrition, administered enterally and/or parenterally, prescribed lipid load, infusion rate, adjusted to, measured values, derived, observation, abundant, simultaneously, replaced, indispensable, precursors, inseparable from, natural or artificial means, appropriate requirements, assigned, adverse consequences, without regard to, deficit or excess, depleted, with respect to, enteral feeds, non-digestible carbohydrates, viscous gel, phytochemicals, species, defence mechanisms, emerged, evidence, consistent with, findings, depletion of the stores, conversely, synergistic effects, complementary, rigorous, critical evaluation, assumptions, relationship, reliable, excessive, immunosuppressed state, replace, useful anti-inflammatory agents, perioperative administration, superior to, report contradictory findings, influence, outcomes, formula, in particular, consistent with, proposed, gastrointestinal trophism, intensive care unit, clinical trials, potential harm, meta-analyses, confirmed, precisely.

Exercise 3

Prepare short talks and/or dialogues on these topics.

1. The effects of low or very high energy intake during nutritional support
2. The difference between energy needs in stable and critically ill patient

3. Carbohydrates used in parenteral and enteral nutrition support
4. Negative effects of glucose overdose
5. Optimal lipid intake during nutritional support
6. Requirements of protein and amino acids during nutritional support
7. Important functions of proteins
8. Water and electrolyte requirements in patients receiving artificial nutrition
9. Definition and classification of fibre
10. The basics of the antioxidant defence system
11. The nature, dietary source and typical intake of ω-3 fatty acids
12. The rationale for the use of long chain ω-3 fatty acids in artificial nutrition
13. Actions of immunonutrients

Vocabulary 7

Fill in the meanings in your mother language:

abolish /ə'bɒl.ɪʃ/
abundant /ə'bʌn.dənt/
accelerated /ək'sel.ə.reɪt.ɪd/
achieve /ə'tʃiːv/
acquired /əˌkwaɪ.əd/
adjust /ə'dʒʌst/
administer /əd'mɪn.ɪ.stər/
arginine /'ɑːdʒɪˌnaɪn/
assign /ə'saɪn/
be subject to /'sʌb.dʒekt/
building /'bɪl.dɪŋ/ **blocks** /blɒks/
cautiously /'kɔː.ʃəs.li/
cohesive /kəʊ'hiː.sɪv/
complementary /ˌkɒm.plɪ'men.tər.i/
consequent /'kɒn.sɪ.kwənt/
contradictory /ˌkɒn.trə'dɪk.tər.i/
conversely /kən'vɜːs.li/
depletion /dɪ'pliː.ʃən/
derivative /dɪ'rɪv.ə.tɪv/
despite /dɪ'spaɪt/
discouraged /dɪ'skʌr.ɪdʒd/
distant /'dɪs.tənt/
elevated /'el.ɪ.veɪ.tɪd/
endpoint /'ɛndˌpɔɪnt/
enriched /ɪn'rɪtʃt/
event /ɪ'vent/
exert /ɪg'zɜːt/
fashion /'fæʃ.ən/
fermentation /ˌfɜr.men'teɪ.ʃən/
flavonoid /'fleɪ vəˌnɔɪd/
glucosamine /gluː'kəʊz'əmiːn/
hyperalimentation /ˌhaɪ pərˌæl ə mɛn'teɪ ʃən/
hypertriglyceridaemia /ˌhaɪ. pə.traɪ'glɪs əˌraɪd.i mi ə/
immunomodulatory /ˌɪm. jə'nɒ'mɑː.djə'leɪ.tər.i/
immunosuppressed / ˌɪm.jə.nəʊ.sə'presd/
implication /ˌɪm.plɪ'keɪ.ʃən/
indispensable /ˌɪn.dɪ'spen.sə.bl̩/
infuse /ɪn'fjuːz/
infusion /ɪn'fjuː.ʒən/
ingredient /ɪn'griː.di.ənt/
inseparable /ɪn'sep.rə.bl̩/
insult /'ɪn.sʌlt/
intensive /ɪn'ten.sɪv/ **care** / keər/ **unit** /'juː.nɪt/
linoleic /lɪ'noʊ li ɪk/ **acid** /æs.ɪd/
maltodextrin /'mɔːl.tə'dɛkstrɪn/
marked /mɑːkt/
mixture /mɪks.tʃər/
moderately /'mɒd.ər.ət.li/
neurodegenerative /ˌnjʊə. rəʊ.dɪ'dʒen.ər.ə.tɪv/
nitrosative /'naɪ troʊ'seɪ tɪv/

non-digestible /ˌnɒnˌ daɪˈdʒes.tə.bl̩/
notion /ˈnəʊ.ʃən/
observation /ˌɒb.zəˈveɪ.ʃən/
organelle /ˌɔː.gənˈel/
overfeed /ˌəʊ.və.fiːd/
parenterally /ˈpæ.ren.tə.rəl.i/
phytochemical /ˌfaɪtəʊˈkɛmɪkəl/
pistachio /pɪˈstɑːʃɪˌəʊ/
play /pleɪ/ a **part** /pɑːt/
polyunsaturated /ˌpɒl.i.ʌnˈsætʃ.ər.eɪ.tɪd/
propose /prəˈpəʊz/
proteoglycan /ˌproʊ ti oʊˈglaɪ kæn/
rate /reɪt/
reward /rɪˈwɔːd/
rigorous /ˈrɪg.ər.əs/
side /saɪd/ **effect** /ɪˈfekt/
simultaneously /ˌsɪm.əlˈteɪ.ni.əs.li/
solid /ˈsɒl.ɪd/
solubility /ˌsɒl.jʊˈbɪl.ɪ.ti/
steroid /ˈste.rɔɪd/
subclinical /sʌbˈklɪn.ɪ.kəl/
superior /suːˈpɪə.ri.ər/
synergistic /sɪn.əˈdʒɪs.tɪk/
thromboxane /θrɒmˈbɒk seɪn/
undoubtedly /ʌnˈdaʊ.tɪd.li/
undue /ʌnˈdjuː/
vacuole /ˈvæk.ju.əʊl/
viscous /ˈvɪs.kəs/
wear /weə/ **and tear** /tɪə/

Solution to Exercise 1a
1a, 2o, 3s, 4c, 5j, 6g, 7p, 8n, 9q, 10h, 11r, 12k, 13l, 14m, 15b, 16f, 17d, 18e, 19i, 20t

Solution to Exercise 1b
1q, 2f, 3i, 4e, 5b, 6p, 7o, 8k, 9c, 10n, 11d, 12m, 13g, 14l, 15r, 16j, 17a, 18h

Unit 8 - Techniques of nutritional support

Enteral nutrition

A selection of commercially produced **enteral feeding solutions** is widely available. The most suitable solution should be **selected on an individual basis** and it should be delivered as **high up the GI tract** as possible while ensuring maximum absorption.

Oral nutritional supplements

Oral feeding is the **first-choice** intervention for nourishing patients. Use of **nutritional supplements** should be considered if the intake of oral feeding ad libitum is deficient in macronutrients or micronutrients. This is especially important **if the patient loses weight or cannot eat** a sufficient amount of normal food throughout **5-7 days.** The **oral route** is primary one due to stimulating **salivary secretions** with their formidable **antibacterial** properties. The use of **oral nutritional supplements** (ONS; sip feeds) is dependent upon the **ability to swallow** and the absence of oesophageal or gastric obstructions. **ONS** may be used to provide the entire nutritional requirements or, more commonly, to **supplement the diet** if the patient is **unwilling or unable to take** sufficient quantities of **normal food**. ONS are used to improve nutritional intake in older adults and patients with various problems related to health and eating. Consideration of patient

preferences regarding flavour, style and presentation are necessary for compliance of ONS supplementation. Particular care is required when selecting **sip-feeds** for patients with diabetes because these products are high in carbohydrates. Difficulties with **compliance** are, however, considerable **unless** administration is **carefully supervised.** Moreover, ONS should not decrease or replace a voluntary intake of normal or fortified food. **Palatability** has been a problem (although there has been some improvement recently). Oral feeding does, however, obviate the **problems** associated with **nasogastric tubes** (although it may be more demanding in staff time).

Endoscopic access: PEG, PEG-J, and D-PEJ

There are several routes and methods for the delivery of enteral nutrition. The general rule is to obtain **maximum safety and comfort** for the patient using the wide range of **equipment** available. Enteral delivery systems are **medical devices** and **tube feeding** is therefore, by law, a **medical treatment**. Directives in different countries set out the legal requirements for medical devices. There are also recommendations contained in a directive from the European Union (EU) Commission. **Percutaneous endoscopic techniques** should be considered if enteral feeding is **necessary for more than 3-4 weeks. Gastrostomy** used to be the preserve of the surgeon but is now primarily **undertaken by gastroenterological physicians**. Percutaneous endoscopic gastrostomy **(PEG)** was first introduced in 1980 and became the technique of choice to provide **long-term** enteral nutrition support. **Tube placement** is usually carried out in the **endoscopic suite** or **at the bedside** using intravenous conscious **sedation** and **local anaesthesia**. PEG, or a **PEG-jejunostomy (PEG-J)** and **direct percutaneous jejunostomy (D-PEJ)** are used today. A PEG is usually carried out. A (D-PEJ) is used in cases after gastric resections or if a (PEG-J) is dislocated. The **direct puncture procedure** is more difficult, is not always possible, and requires considerable skill.

If the endoscope cannot be inserted into the stomach, percutaneous tubes can also be **placed under radiographic or sonographic guidance.** This can sometimes be avoided if the **stenosis in the oesophagus** can be dilated or if a **metallic stent** can be inserted. PEG and PEG-J are **widely used.** PEG is particularly easy to carry out, with a low prevalence of procedure-related complications. The most widely used method is the **pull procedure**. **Impairment in swallowing** due to neurological causes, **neoplasm** in the upper GI tract, polytrauma, **long-term ventilation**; and the perioperative period in **oropharyngeal surgery** are the major **indications**. Contraindications are rare. If the tubes are carefully managed, the complications are minor. In several selected patients, a D-PEJ can be attempted. This method is less successful in terms of tube placement and has more complications.

Surgical access: gastrostomy, needle catheter jejunostomy

Surgical techniques for enteral feeding are necessary **if percutaneous endoscopic placement is not possible.** This is usually the case if endoscopy is not possible due to **tumour obstruction**. However, most surgical gastrostomies and jejunostomies are done as concomitant procedure **at the time of major surgery** for trauma or disease of the upper GI tract. The use of a **catheter jejunostom**y for **postoperative alimentation** was first described more than 100 years ago. However, use of this method has been limited by the mistaken belief in complete postoperative gastrointestinal atony. Since the end of the 1960s, the results of experimental and clinical studies have shown that **postoperative atony** primarily affects the **stomach and the colon, but the digestive function** of the **small intestine is almost physiological** 2 h after abdominal surgery. These observations gave a new viewpoint for **early postoperative enteral feeding.** Surgical techniques to allow enteral feeding vary, but can be classified as temporary or permanent. **Permanent and temporary gastrostomies** and **permanent jejunostomies** are done by classical **surgical method**. They are more technically demanding and require more extensive surgical procedures compared with temporary techniques. **Temporary jejunostomies (needle catheter jejunostomy (NCJ)** are carried out after **major surgery** before closing the abdomen **or by laparoscopic means** if other surgery is not required. Laparoscopic techniques should also be considered in patients in whom endoscopic procedures are not possible. Several **surgical technique**s for **long-term feeding** are available if endoscopic techniques are not possible. Compared with endoscopic techniques, **surgical procedures** have a **higher** prevalence of **morbidity and mortality**. NCJ is relatively easy to carry out after major surgery or via the laparoscopic approach, and is associated with fewer problems than other surgical techniques. If the tubes are handled with care, complications are rare.

Administration of enteral tube feeds

The success of enteral tube feeding is dependent upon **close co-operation** between clinical staff and the patient. Nutritional principles must be observed while providing the regimen best suited to the individual needs of each patient.

Homemade enteral (tube) nutrition

If it is not possible for a person to obtain nutrition by the oral route, enteral feeding tubes can be used to provide the nutrition the body needs. The food industry provides a **broad spectrum of ready-to-use, sterile formulas. Powdered** formulas are also available. These must be mixed with clean (cooked or sterile) **water** before use. This broad range of available products means that there will always be a formula for the need of your patient. These products **are available** in almost all countries. The price of these formulas varies based on the specific nutrients used. However, these ready-to-use liquid diets may sometimes not be available due to cost of logistics. In undeveloped countries and **if industrially produced formulas are not available** (e.g. during catastrophes and humanitarian missions), **'homemade diets'** can be an alternative. Educated specialists in nutrition support should be able to prepare such food as well to educate people on how to make it.

Commercially prepared diets for enteral nutrition

Commercially prepared formulas for enteral nutrition are those produced by industry and called **dietary foods for special medical purposes** as defined in the European legal regulation of commission directive 1999. They are delivered as liquids of various viscosities or in a powder form. Commercially prepared formulas are always **sterile**. They usually fall under one of the following categories:

- **Polymeric** formulas
- **Oligomeric and monomeric** diets
- Special formulas (**disease-specific** or **organ-specific**)
- **Modular** diets

There has been an unprecedented evolution of commercial enteral diets. These diets have become a very **strong means** of **nutritional intervention**. The large spectrum of enteral formulas has been prompted by evidence-based insights into the prevention and **treatment benefits** of enteral nutrition. The **objectives** and formulation of enteral nutrition therapy should be patient-driven, i.e. **adjusted to the specific requirements** of the **patient and the disease.** Nevertheless, as the ESPEN guidelines on enteral nutrition clearly show, **most patients** can be treated with **standard polymeric formulas.** Healthcare institutions should identify the needs of their patients, and devise an enteral product (similar to a diet manual), adapting the **number and variety of products** to the **type and frequency of the disease**.

Complications of enteral nutrition

The type and frequency of **complications** during EN may be related to the formulation and delivery of the **diet provided**, as well as to the **underlying disease**. There are three major categories of EN complications: gastrointestinal, mechanical and metabolic. **Gastrointestinal complications** are undoubtedly the most frequently described. Careful consideration should be given to the use of enteral nutrition therapy, but once implemented,

close monitoring of patients is an efficient **safeguard against** most **complications and side effects**.

Exercise 1
Match the column A with the column B. Try to learn the expressions and/or sentences by heart.

A

1. Oral feeding is the first-choice intervention for nourishing patients
2. The oral route is primary one
3. Oral nutritional supplements (ONS) may be used to provide the entire nutritional requirements or to supplement the diet
4. ONS are used to improve nutritional intake
5. ONS should not decrease or replace
6. Enteral delivery systems are medical devices
7. Percutaneous endoscopic gastrostomy (PEG) became the technique of choice
8. Tube placement is usually carried out
9. Percutaneous tubes can also be placed
10. PEG is particularly easy to carry out,
11. Impairment in swallowing due to neurological causes, neoplasm in the upper GI tract, polytrauma,
12. Surgical techniques for enteral feeding
13. Most surgical gastrostomies and jejunostomies are done as concomitant procedure
14. Postoperative atony primarily affects the stomach and the colon,
15. Permanent and temporary gastrostomies and permanent jejunostomies
16. Temporary jejunostomies (needle catheter jejunostomy (NCJ) are carried out after major surgery
17. Compared with endoscopic techniques,
18. If it is not possible for a person to obtain nutrition by the oral route,
19. The food industry provides a broad spectrum of ready-to-use, sterile formulas;
20. If industrially produced formulas are not available (e.g. during catastrophes and humanitarian missions),
21. Commercially prepared formulas for enteral nutrition
22. The objectives and formulation of enteral nutrition therapy should be
23. There are three major categories of EN complications:

B

a) a voluntary intake of normal or fortified food.

b) adjusted to the specific requirements of the patient and the disease.

c) *and tube feeding is therefore, by law, a medical treatment.*
d) *are done by classical surgical method.*
e) *are necessary if percutaneous endoscopic placement is not possible.*
f) *are those produced by industry and called dietary foods for special medical purposes.*
g) *at the time of major surgery for trauma or disease of the upper GI tract.*
h) *before closing the abdomen or by laparoscopic means if other surgery is not required.*
i) *but the digestive function of the small intestine is almost physiological 2 h after abdominal surgery.*
j) *due to stimulating salivary secretions with their formidable antibacterial properties.*
k) *enteral feeding tubes can be used to provide the nutrition the body needs.*
l) *gastrointestinal, mechanical and metabolic.*
m) *homemade diets can be an alternative.*
n) *if the patient is unwilling or unable to take sufficient quantities of normal food.*
o) *in older adults and patients with various problems related to health and eating.*
p) *long-term ventilation; and the perioperative period in oropharyngeal surgery are the major indications.*
q) *powdered formulas must be mixed with clean (cooked or sterile) water before use.*
r) *surgical procedures have a higher prevalence of morbidity and mortality.*
s) *to provide long-term enteral nutrition support.*
t) *under radiographic or sonographic guidance.*
u) *use of nutritional supplements should be considered if the intake of oral feeding is deficient in macronutrients or micronutrients.*
v) *using intravenous conscious sedation and local anaesthesia.*
w) *with a low prevalence of procedure-related complications.*

Exercise 2

Translate the expressions. Try to explain their meanings in English.

Commercially produced, enteral feeding, solutions available, suitable intervention, for nourishing, sufficient amount, salivary secretions, formidable antibacterial properties, ability to swallow, oesophageal or gastric obstructions, unwilling or unable to, preferences regarding flavour, sip-feeds, difficulties with compliance, administration is carefully supervised, voluntary intake, palatability, obviate the problems, safety and comfort, equipment, medical devices, tube feeding, directives, percutaneous endoscopic techniques, gastroenterological physicians, percutaneous endoscopic gastrostomy, tube placement, intravenous conscious sedation, local anaesthesia, jejunostomy, carried out, resections, is dislocated, direct puncture procedure, under radiographic or sonographic guidance, stenosis in the oesophagus, dilated, metallic stent, inserted, impairment, carefully managed, be attempted, surgical techniques, endoscopy, tumour obstruction, concomitant procedure, catheter jejunostomy, postoperative alimentation, postoperative atony, stomach, colon, small intestine, permanent, temporary, technically demanding, by laparoscopic means, handled with care, obtain nutrition by the oral route, enteral feeding tubes, ready-to-use sterile formulas, powdered formulas, catastrophes and humanitarian missions, homemade diets, commercially prepared, dietary foods, special medical purposes, various viscosities, nutritional intervention, treatment benefits, adjusted to the specific requirements, guidelines, complication gastrointestinal, mechanical and metabolic, safeguard against, side effects.

Exercise 3
Prepare short talks and/or dialogues on these topics.

1. Indications and benefits of enteral feeding
2. Contraindications to enteral nutrition
3. Delivery of enteral tube feeds
4. Indications of tube feeding
5. Tube feeding insertion techniques
6. Percutaneously inserted feeding tubes
7. Different surgical techniques
8. Needle catheter jejunostomy
9. The basic principles and regiments of tube feeding
10. Equipment for enteral nutrition delivery
11. The basics of homemade enteral nutrition
12. The different types of commercially prepared formulas
13. The main types of complications associated with tube feeding

Vocabulary 8

Fill in the meanings in your mother language:

ad libitum /ˈlɪbɪtəm/
alimentation /ælɪmenˈteɪʃən/
alternative /ɒlˈtɜː.nə.tɪv/
atony /ˈæt.ən.i/
catheter /ˈkæθ.ɪ.tər/
compliance /kəmˈplaɪ.ənt s/
concomitant /kənˈkɒm.ɪ.tənt/
conscious /ˈkɒn.t ʃəs/
cost /kɒst/
device /dɪˈvaɪs/
dilated /daɪˈleɪt.ɪd/
dislocate /ˈdɪsləʊkeɪt/
endoscope /enˈdɒs.kəʊp/
endoscopic /ˌɛndəʊˈskɒp.ɪk/
equipment /ɪˈkwɪp.mənt/
flavour /ˈfleɪ.vər/
formidable /ˈfɔːmɪdəbl/
formula /ˈfɔː.mjʊ.lə/
formulation /ˌfɔːmjʊˈleɪ.ʃən/

fortified/ˈfɔː.tɪˌfaɪd/
gastric /ˈgæs.trɪk/
gastroenterological /ˌgæs troʊˌɛn tər əˈlɒdʒ ɪk.əl/
gastrostomy /gæsˈtrə.stə.mi/
impairment /imˈpeərˌmənt/
implement /ˈɪm.plɪ.ment/
indication /ˌɪn.dɪˈkeɪ.ʃən/
insight /ˈɪn.saɪt/
jejunostomy /dʒɪdʒuːˈnɒstəmɪ/
logistics /lɒˈdʒɪ.stɪks/
long-term /ˌlɒŋˈtɜːm/
manual /ˈmæn.ju.əl/
means /miːnz/
metallic /məˈtæl.ɪk/
modular /ˈmɒdjʊlə/
monomeric /ˌmɒnəˈmɛrɪk/
needle /ˈniː.dl̩/
neoplasm /ˈniː.ə.plæz.əm/
obviate /ˈɒb.vi.eɪt/
oesophageal /iːˌsɒfəˈdʒiːəl/
oligomeric /əˌlɪg əˈmɛr ɪk/
palatability /ˈpæl ə tə.bəˈbɪlɪtɪ/
percutaneous /ˌpəːr.kjʊˈteɪ.ni.əs/
permanent /ˈpɜː.mə.nənt/
physician /fɪˈzɪʃ.ən/
polymeric /ˌpɒlɪˈmɛrɪk/
polytrauma /ˈpɒl.iˈtrɔːmə/
powdered /ˈpaʊ.dəd/
preserve /prɪˈzɜːv/
prompt /prɒmp t/
pull /pʊl/
radiographic /ˌreɪ.diˈɒg.rəf.ɪk/
resection /rɪˈsek.ʃən/
rule /ruːl/
salivary /səˈlaɪ.vər.i/
sedation /sɪˈdeɪʃən/
signify /ˈsɪg.nɪ.faɪ/
sip /sɪp/
skill /skɪl/
sonographic /səʊ.nəˈgræf.ɪk/
stenosis /steˈnəʊ.sɪs/
stent /stɛnt/
suite /swiːt/
supervise /ˈsuːpəˌvaɪz/
supplement /ˈsʌp.lɪ.mənt/
surgeon /ˈsɜː.dʒən/
swallow /ˈswɒl.əʊ/
temporary /ˈtem.pər.ər.i/
undeveloped /ʌndɪˈveləpt/
ventilation /ˌven.tɪˈleɪ.ʃən/
viewpoint /ˈvjuːˌpɔɪnt/
viscosity /vɪˈskɒs.ɪ.ti/
voluntary /ˈvɒl.ən.tər.i/

Solution to Exercise 1
1u, 2j, 3n, 4o, 5a, 6c, 7s, 8v, 9t, 10w, 11p, 12e, 13g, 14i, 15d, 16h, 17r, 18k, 19q, 20m, 21f, 22b, 23l

Unit 9 - Parenteral nutrition

Peripheral parenteral nutrition

Parenteral nutrition **(PN)** is the means by which **nutrients** are provided **intravenously**. Therefore, when PN is used, **venous access** is necessary, and an appropriate **infusion technique** is mandatory for successful feeding. **Peripheral parenteral nutrition (PPN)** has been developed for easy and safe PN and as an **alternative to central PN,** avoiding the risks of central catheterisation. In fact, less energy and protein can be infused than by a central vein, and serious complications may still occur. However, this is a **rational method** for patients requiring **short-term PN** and in those **in whom central catheterisation should be avoided** for some period of time. It is a very attractive method for small hospitals, lacking experience in parenteral nutrition. The **majority of hospital patients** can be **fed**

successfully using a **PPN formula** of low osmolarity by dilution or via a high fat content, infused via a **narrow** (18-20) **cannula** inserted into a **peripheral vein** and **re-sited every 24 hours,** or by using a **15 cm paediatric 22g polyurethane catheter** which will usually last longer. It is necessary to consider benefits and risks and to follow precisely the management recommendations aimed at avoiding complications.

Central parenteral nutrition

Central venous access is usually necessary for parenteral nutrition. The factors to consider when selecting a catheter are the **expected duration and kind of therapy, access site, safety** and **cost**. A well-trained operator, using a sterile technique under **strict aseptic conditions**, should perform insertion of the catheter for parenteral nutrition as an elective procedure **in the operating theatre** or comparable environment. The **right internal jugular vein** and **right subclavian vein** are the access points of choice. The **catheter tip** should be **located under fluoroscopic guidance** to lie in the **superior vena cava just above the right atrium.** If this has not been possible, the catheter position should be **confirmed by x-ray** after insertion. When classical access to the superior vena cava is not possible, the catheter may be introduced **via the femoral vein**; alternatively, special **small diameter catheters** my be introduced **via a peripheral vein**. Proper **selection** of the **catheter**, skilful **insertion**, and quality of **catheter aftercare** are key factors for safe, **successful** and complication-free **therapy**.

Complications associated with central catheter insertion and care

CVC related complications may cause serious **clinical problems** during insertion, maintenance or after CVC removal. A thorough **knowledge** of the **aetiology and of preventive principles** and rules is essential for proper prophylaxis, diagnosis and management of central venous catheters.

Pharmaceutical aspects of parenteral nutrition support

The aim of **parenteral nutrition (PN)** is to administer the **essential nutrients** by the **intravenous route** to treat or prevent malnutrition when oral/enteral nutrition is not possible – **total parenteral nutrition or TPN** or insufficient for complete nutrition – **partial parenteral nutrition or PPN.** The individual **substrates (carbohydrates, lipids, amino acids, water, electrolytes, vitamins and trace elements**) may be administered parenterally from:

- separate **containers - 'multi-bottle system'**
- preferably as an **admixture**, and, if possible, in a **single container unit** of PN admixture usually referred to as: **Two in One (TIO –** an **amino acid-glucose** system). TIO is an aqueous

formulation excluding lipid emulsion. **All-in-One (AIO** – an **amino acid-glucose-lipid system)**. AIO infusion contains all the required PN components, including lipids in the form of an **emulsion**.

AIO admixtures are **safe, effective and low-risk** formulations for practically all indications and applications. They are **sterile large volume parenteral infusions either** aseptically **compounded for immediate use upon** individual **prescription** from stable and **sterile nutritional components** (e.g. **amino acids, glucose, lipid, electrolytes, trace elements and vitamins**) **or** they are manufactured in a serial industrial production as standard regimens **in multi-compartment containers with extended expiry date,** but not yet individually adapted and **ready-to-use admixed.** The limiting (quality) aspects of PN (i.e., not just AIO) admixtures are their **physico-chemical compatibility and stability**, and the risk of microbial contamination. **The risk of microbial contamination** and subsequent microbial growth is **greatest in PPN** given their lower osmolarity compared to TPN admixtures, whereas **the risk of instability** is greatest **when any PN admixture contains lipids**, as the **admixture** is no longer a solution but an **emulsion** that **engenders** additional issues associated with the stability of the **final dispersion.**

PN admixture compounding and preparation should normally be performed in the **hospital pharmacy department** because:

- Well-trained staff, under the supervision of a pharmacist, will have **knowledge of the possible chemical/pharmaceutical interactions** between PN components, thereby helping to resolve potential life-threatening stability problems prior to compounding.
- Compounding **conditions that are strictly controlled and validated**, allow **aseptic handling** of the sterile components (e.g. within isolators or laminar flow cabinets) and minimize the risk of microbial contamination.
- **Documented protocols** for compounding and completion of ready-to-use preparations can easily be implemented
- Use of validated **automated filling devices** in larger hospital pharmacies allows the production of an **increased quantity** of PN admixtures at a decreased cost, so that a greater number of patients can be served and cared for. The compounding may be assisted efficiently by **computer aided instrumentation.**

Stability and compatibility of parenteral nutrition (PN) admixtures

AIO **admixtures** are parenteral nutrition formulations containing **water, glucose,** 15-20 **amino acids, lipids** of variable fatty acid composition, 10-12 **electrolytes,** 9 **trace elements** and 11-12 **vitamins** in a single container as **a daily prescription.** For practical reasons some nutraceuticals or medications or proton pump inhibitors may be added to the admixture in order to **maintain effective drug concentration** in the body, to **decrease total volume of liquids** administered to fluid-restricted patients, to **reduce the risk of contamination** from excess manipulations of the intravenous infusion **catheter** for multiple running infusions and/or the **associated costs** of additional infusion-related equipment. All these **ingredients and additives**, the **order** in which they are added, and the **means of delivery** influence the overall PN admixture **stability and quality**. Stability and compatibility of AIO involves a number of complex chemical and physical **interactions** and the net effect of adding various ingredients in wide ranges is not yet fully understood. It is not sage therefore simply to **mix all components** in the **amounts desired by clinicians,** but only within limits based on reliable **information from the manufacturers,** specific analytical tests and/or the peer-reviewed literature. The recommendation is to prepare AIO admixtures under **pharmaceutical supervision**, following **validated guidelines** for types and amounts of macro- and micronutrients under rigorously controlled order and conditions of mixing (standard operation procedures, GMP). Visual and appropriate instrumental **inspection** for signs of instability or incompatibility, such as **precipitation, discolouration, gas formation, aggregation, creaming and coalescence,** prior to and during administration is essential for PN quality and for safe and efficacious delivery of PN therapy.

Exercise 1

Match the column A with the column B. Try to learn the expressions and/or sentences by heart.

A

1. Parenteral nutrition (PN) is the means
2. Peripheral parenteral nutrition (PPN) has been developed for easy and safe PN
3. Peripheral parenteral nutrition is a rational method for patients requiring short-term PN and in those
4. It is necessary to consider benefits and risks
5. A well-trained operator should perform insertion of the catheter for parenteral nutrition
6. The right internal jugular vein and right

subclavian vein are the access points of choice;
7. The catheter may be introduced via the femoral vein;
8. CVC related complications may cause
9. The aim of parenteral nutrition (PN) is to administer the essential nutrients by the intravenous route
10. The individual substrates (carbohydrates, lipids, amino acids, water, electrolytes, vitamins and trace elements)
11. Two in One (TIO), an amino acid-glucose system
12. All-in-One (AIO), infusion contains all the required PN components,
13. AIO admixtures are safe, effective and low-risk formulations
14. AIO admixtures are sterile large volume parenteral infusions
15. Stable and sterile nutritional components
16. AIO admixtures can be manufactured in a serial industrial production as standard regimens
17. The limiting (quality) aspects of PN admixtures
18. The risk of instability is greatest when any PN admixture contains lipids, as the admixture is no longer a solution
19. Well-trained staff, under the supervision of a pharmacist, will have knowledge of the possible chemical/pharmaceutical interactions
20. Use of validated automated filling devices
21. For practical reasons some nutraceuticals or medications or proton pump inhibitors may be added to the admixture in order to
22. The recommendation is to prepare AIO admixtures under pharmaceutical supervision,
23. Inspection for signs of instability or incompatibility,

B

a) *allows the production of an increased quantity of PN admixtures at a decreased cost.*
b) *alternatively, special small diameter catheters my be introduced via a peripheral vein.*
c) *and as an alternative to central PN, avoiding the risks of central catheterisation.*
d) *and to follow precisely the management recommendations aimed at avoiding complications.*
e) *are amino acids, glucose, lipid, electrolytes, trace elements and vitamins.*
f) *are their physico-chemical compatibility and stability, and the risk of microbial contamination.*

g) *as an elective procedure in the operating theatre.*

h) *aseptically compounded for immediate use upon individual prescription.*

i) *between PN components thereby helping to resolve potential life-threatening stability problems prior to compounding.*

j) *but an emulsion that engenders additional issues associated with the stability of the final dispersion.*

k) *by which nutrients are provided intravenously.*

l) *following validated guidelines for types and amounts of macro- and micronutrients, under rigorously controlled order and conditions of mixing.*

m) *for practically all indications and applications.*

n) *in multi-compartment containers with extended expiry date, but not yet individually adapted and ready-to-use admixed.*

o) *in whom central catheterisation should be avoided for some period of time.*

p) *including lipids in the form of an emulsion.*

q) *is an aqueous formulation excluding lipid emulsion.*

r) *maintain effective drug concentration in the body, to decrease total volume of liquids, and to reduce the risk of contamination.*

s) *may be administered parenterally from: separate containers (multi-bottle system), or in a single container unit.*

t) *serious clinical problems during insertion, maintenance or after CVC removal.*

u) *such as precipitation, discolouration, gas formation, aggregation, creaming and coalescence, prior to and during administration is essential.*

v) *the catheter tip should be located under fluoroscopic guidance to lie in the superior vena cava just above the right atrium.*

w) *to treat or prevent malnutrition when oral/enteral nutrition is not possible.*

Exercise 2
Translate the expressions. Try to explain their meanings in English.

Peripheral parenteral nutrition, venous access, mandatory, alternative, avoiding the risks, rational method, central catheterisation, dilution, fat content, narrow cannula, follow precisely, management, recommendations, aimed at, duration and kind of therapy, access site, strict aseptic, elective procedure, operating theatre, comparable environment, jugular vein, subclavian vein, catheter tip, guidance, superior vena cava, right atrium, confirmed insertion, introduced, femoral vein, aftercare, removal, aetiology, prophylaxis, intravenous route, insufficient for, complete, partial, separate containers, admixture, single container unit, aqueous formulation, lipid emulsion, large volume, compounded, for immediate use, prescription, serial industrial production, multi-compartment containers, extended expiry date, subsequent microbial growth, solution, emulsion, final dispersion, supervision of a pharmacist, interactions, resolve problems, prior to, compounding conditions, validated, handling, laminar flow cabinets, implemented, automated filling devices, computer aided instrumentation, nutraceuticals, proton pump inhibitors, multiple running infusions, ingredients and additives, net effect, guidelines, rigorously controlled, precipitation, discolouration, gas formation, aggregation, creaming and coalescence, prior to, essential, safe and efficacious delivery.

Exercise 3
Prepare short talks and/or dialogues on these topics.

1. Parenteral nutrition
2. Peripheral parenteral nutrition
3. Central parenteral nutrition
4. Complications associated with central catheter insertion and care
5. Pharmaceutical aspects of parenteral nutrition support
6. Stability and compatibility of parenteral nutrition (PN) admixtures

Vocabulary 9

Fill in the meanings in your mother language:

adapt /ə'dæpt/
additive /'æd.ɪ.tɪv/
adipose /'æd.ɪ.pəʊz/
adverse /'æd.vɜːs/
aetiology /ˌiː.ti'ɒl.ə.dʒi/
aftercare /'ɑːftəˌkeə/
aggregation /ˌæg.rɪ'geɪ.ʃən/
aimed /eɪmd/ **at** /æt/
approximately /ə'prɒk.sɪ.mət.lɪ/
aqueous /'eɪ.kwi.əs/
aseptic /ˌeɪ'sep.tɪk/
atherogenic /ˌæθərəʊ'dʒɛnɪk/
atrium /'eɪ.tri.əm/ pl **atria**
automated /'ɔː.tə.meɪ.tɪd/
autopsy /'ɔː.tɒp.si/
aware /ə'weər/
awareness /ə'weə.nəs/
bariatric /bær.i'æt.rɪk/
bonding /'bɒn.dɪŋ/
baseline /'beɪsˌlaɪn/
bedside /'bedˌsaɪd/
beyond /bi'jɒnd/
bottle /'bɒt.lˌ/
broad /brɔːd/
cabinet /'kæb.ɪ.nət/
catabolic /kætə'bɒlɪc/
catabolism /kə'tæbəˌlɪzəm/
catheterisation /'kæθɪtəˌraɪ'zeɪ.ʃən/
chart /tʃɑːt/
coalescence /ˌkəʊə'lɛ.səns/
cognition /kɒg'nɪʃ.ən/
comparable /'kɒm.pər.ə.bəl/
compatibility /kəmˌpæt.ə'bɪl.ə.tɪ/
completion /kəm'pliːʃən/
complex /kɒm.pleks/
consensus /kən'sen.səs/
consequence /'kɒn.sɪ.kwəns/
considerable /kən'sɪd.ər.ə.bl̩/
container /kən'teɪ.nər/
contamination /kənˌtæm.ɪ'neɪ.ʃən/

costly /ˈkɒst.li/
cream /kriːm/
cut-off /kʌtˌɒf/ **value** /ˈvæljuː/
decline /dɪˈklaɪn/
deficiency /dɪˈfɪʃ.ənt .si/
define /dɪˈfaɪn/
depleted /dɪˈpliː.tɪd/
detrimental /ˌdet.rɪˈmen.təl/
diabetogenic /ˌdaɪəˈbet.əˈdʒen.ɪk/
diameter /daɪˈæm.ɪ.tər/
discolouration /dɪˌskʌl.əˈreɪ.ʃən/
dispersion /dɪˈspɜː.ʃən/
educated /ˈed.jʊ.keɪ.tɪd/
effect /ɪˈfekt/
efficacious /ˌefɪˈkeɪ.ʃəs/
efficiently /ɪˈfɪʃ.ənt.li/
elderly /ˈel.dəl.i/
engender /ɪnˈdʒen.də/
epidemiological /ˌep.ɪ.diː.
mi.əˈlɒdʒ.ɪ.kəl/
essential /ɪˈsen.tʃəl/
exceed /ɪkˈsiːd/
excess /ekˈses/
exclude /ɪkˈskluːd/
excrete /ɪkˈskriːt/
expiry /ɪkˈspaɪə.rɪ/ **date** /deɪt/
extended /ɪkˈsten.dɪd/
filling /ˈfɪl.ɪŋ/
flow /fləʊ/
fluoroscopic /ˌflʊər əˈskɒp ɪk/
formation /fɔːˈmeɪ.ʃən/
furthemore /ˈfɝː.ðɚ.mɔːr/
gas /gæs/
gastric /ˈgæs.trɪk/ **banding** /ˈbændɪŋ/
glucogenesis /ˌgluːkəˈdʒe.nɪ.sɪs/
handling /ˈhænd.lɪŋ/
history /ˈhɪs.tər.i/
imbalance /ˌɪmˈbæl.ənt s/
impaired /ɪmˈpeəd/
in order to /ˈɔː.dər/
incidence /ˈɪnt .sɪ.dənts/
include /ɪnˈkluːd/
individual /ˌɪn.dɪˈvɪd.ju.əl/
initial /ɪˈnɪʃ.əl/
instability /ˌɪn.stəˈbɪl.ɪ.ti/
isolator /ˈaɪ səˌleɪt.ər/
jugular vein /ˈdʒʌg.jʊ.ləˌveɪn/
laminar /ˈlæm.ə.nər/
laparoscopic /ˌlæp.ər.əsˈkɒp.ɪk/
lean /liːn/
limitation /ˌlɪm.ɪˈteɪ.ʃən/
link /lɪŋk/
lipid /ˈlɪp.ɪd/
majority /məˈdʒɒrɪtɪ/
mandatory /ˈmæn.də.tri/
manufacture /ˌmæn.jʊˈfæk.tʃər/
mood /muːd/
multiple /ˈmʌl.tɪ.pl̩/
muscle /mʌsəl/
nutraceutical /ˌnjuːtrəˈsjuːtɪkəl/
omeprazole /oʊˈmɛp rəˌzoʊl/
operating /ˈɒp.əˌreɪt.
ɪŋ/ **theatre** /ˈθɪə.tər/
osmolarity /ˌɒzməˈlær.ə.ti/
outcome /ˈaʊt.kʌm/
overfeeding /ˈəʊ.vərfiːdɪŋ/
overnutrition /ˈəʊ.vər.njuːˈtrɪʃ.ən/
partial /ˈpɑː.ʃəl/
perioperative /ˌper.ɪˈɒp.ər.ə.tɪv/
pharmacist /ˈfɑːmə.sɪst/
pharmacy /fɑːməsɪ/
polyurethane /ˌpɒlɪˈjʊərəˌθeɪn/
precipitation /prɪˌsɪpɪˈteɪ.ʃən/
precisely /prɪˈsaɪs.lɪ/
precursor /ˌpriːˈkɜː.sər/
predispose /ˌpriː.dɪˈspəʊz/
prescription /prɪˈskrɪp.ʃən/
preventive /prɪˈven.tɪv/
pro /prəʊ/ **-coagulatory** /
koʊˈæg jə ləˌtɔr i/
prophylaxis /ˌprɒf.ɪˈlæk.sɪs/
rational /ˈræʃ.ən.əl/
readily /ˈred.ɪ.li/
record /ˈrekɔːd/
refer /rɪˈfɜːr/
regimen /ˈredʒ.ɪ.mən/
removal /rɪˈmuː.vəl/
renal /ˈriː.nəl/ **clearance** /kliər.əns/
repair /rɪˈpeə/
resistance /rɪˈzɪs.tənts/

rigorously /'rɪg.ər.əs.lɪ/
running /'rʌn.ɪŋ/
sage /seɪdʒ/
separate /'sep.ər.ət/
serial /'sɪə.ri.əl/
serious /'sɪə.ri.əs/
setting /'setɪŋ/
shape /ʃeɪp/
single /'sɪŋgəl/
skeletal /'skel.ɪ.təl/
skilful /'skɪl.fəl/
solution /sə'lu:.ʃən/
spleen /spli:n/
stability /stə'bɪl.ɪ.ti/
storage /'stɔ:.rɪdʒ/
store /stɔ:r/
strict /strɪkt/
subclavian /sʌb'kleɪv.ɪ.ən/
artery /'ɑ:tərɪ/
summarize /'sʌm.ər.aɪz/
superior /su:'pɪə.ri.ər/ **vena cava** /ˌvi:.nə'keɪ.və/
supervision /ˌsu:.pə'vɪʒ.ən/
surplus /'sɜ:.pləs/
threshold /'θreʃ.h əʊld/
tissue /'tɪʃ.u:/
training /'treɪ.nɪŋ/
trend /trend/
triglyceride /traɪ.glɪs.ə.raɪd/
undergo /ˌʌn.də'gəʊ/ **(underwent, undergone)**
undesirable /ˌʌn.dɪ'zaɪə.rə.bl̩/
undiagnosed /ʌn'daɪ.əg.nəʊzd/
untreated /ʌn'tri:.tɪd/
validated /'væl.ɪˌdeɪ.tɪd/
vast /vɑ:st/
volunteer /ˌvɒl.ən'tɪər/
vulnerable /'vʌl.nər.ə.bl̩/
wasting /weɪst.ɪŋ/

Solution to Exercise 1
1k, 2c, 3o, 4d, 5g, 6v, 7b, 8t, 9w, 10s,11q, 12p, 13m, 14h, 15e, 16n, 17f, 18j, 19i, 20a, 21r, 22l, 23u

Unit 10 - Drugs and nutritional admixtures

To use AIO admix as a drug vehicle to patients with PN is attractive but problematic because of **complex nature of potential interactions** that may add substantially to the risks associated with PN. Specific emphasis is given concerning the properties of **AIO admixtures emulsions**, **chemical reactivity** of the components, **container** material and potential **adverse effects**. As a general rule, addition of drugs to AIO admixtures should be avoided. If it is inevitable for therapeutic and practical reasons a **strict GMP protocol** involving specific pharmaceutical expertise, including analytical assessment, is important in order to achieve **safe and effective** nutritional and drug therapy. Only selected drugs with acceptable extended **administration time**, a large therapeutic index, and appropriate physico-chemical properties are candidates for admixing. **Standardization** may help to facilitate institution-specific guidelines. An individual risk assessment must be documented to reflect the **responsibilities** of the (pharmaceutical) experts involved.

Composition of nutritional admixtures and formulas for parenteral nutrition

Parenteral nutrition (PN) can be divided into:

- **Total** parenteral nutrition (TPN) – all nutrient needs are provided **intravenously** without any significant oral or enteral intake
- **Supplementary parenteral nutrition** – a portion of the patient's nutrient needs is provided **via the gastrointestinal tract**, and the remainder is infused parenterally in sufficient amounts to meet optimal requirements.

The best approach to preparing parenteral feeding solution is to mix all nutrients **in one bag and to infuse them together**. All-in-one (AIO) bags may be filled from basic solutions and bulk additive sources, or appropriate **commercially produced two- or three-chamber bags** may be chosen as the basic solution and admixture source and are supplemented appropriately to **provide any lacking substances**. However, the clinical applicability of this approach may be limited by **stability problems** of some of the components and **incompatibilities** among some components. As parenterally fed patients must **metabolize or excrete all infused nutrients,** the **composition of nutritional formulas** should be adapted to nutritional **requirements**, metabolic **capacity**, metabolic **disturbances** and coexisting **deficiencies or overloading**. It is always necessary to understand the clinical situation comprehensively and to prescribe the formula most appropriate for a particular patient at all times during the course of their management.

Metabolic complications of parenteral nutrition

Metabolic complications of parenteral nutrition can be categorised as **deficiency states, acute metabolic complications** and **chronic** (long-term) metabolic complications.

Acute complications may occur during parenteral nutrition (PN) whenever the administered nutrient **formulations and/or dosages** do not take into account:

- detailed clinical **nutritional and biochemical assessment** of each patient
- proper evaluation of **nutrient requirements** and the need for **water** and **electrolyte** correction prior to PN initiation
- careful prescription appropriate to the patient's **metabolic state**

One must be aware that the practice of PN always requires biochemical assessment and correction of any electrolyte disorders **prior to the prescription** in order to avoid potentially **fatal acute** complications. **Chronic** complications of PN are more problematical. The aetiology of these **long-term side effects** is multiple and often not fully understood. Metabolic complications are more likely to occur in the absence of a nutrition support **team expert** in PN or when physicians do not perceive parenteral nutrition as useful adjunctive therapy and instead use it incautiously as urgent and lifesaving treatment. Patients with severe **malnutrition** and already existing **organ dysfunction** are at particular risk of the **refeeding syndrome** if PN is introduced too rapidly or aggressively. The risks of developing PN associated **liver disease** are increased, in **short bowel syndrome,** with small bowel less than 150cm, the **absence of a colon** in continuity, **the lack of** an adequate **bile circulation** (mostly due to resection of the terminal ileum or ileo-caecal valve), frequent (catheter) **infections, small bowel bacterial overgrowth**, the **lack of** any **enteral nutrition**, or **hypercaloric feeding**. The risks are even further increased in children, due to immaturity of the liver, especially in **premature** and dysmature **infants**. Parenteral nutrition can be complicated by many **metabolic problems**, which may arise from **inadequate or excessive** amounts of **nutrients** or from an inappropriate **composition** of parenteral nutrition formulations. Severe (long-term) complications comprise **cholestatic liver failure disease** and **bone demineralisation**. Patient-tailored monitoring of nutrient requirements and administration remains crucial to prevent complications.

Monitoring of nutritional support
Clinical monitoring

You need to develop a system, which suites your needs and circumstances, and to train your team so that **monitoring is undertaken and recorded** on a **regular and systematic** basis, so that each member of the team understands the purpose of this process and is able to participate in the interpretation of the recorded data. Use **serial data forms**, either paper or electronic, and place these on the patient's door or at the bottom of the bed, so that any member of the team can see not only **the current data**, but the **previous data** in a serial manner, so that any **change** can be perceived immediately and appropriate action taken. This saves an enormous amount of time sorting through the notes or a disorganised collection of data arranged in no proper order. The team soon get used to such a system and learn to **respond quickly when adverse trends are observed.** Such a system **coordinates** clinical, nutritional and laboratory **measurements**, allowing observation of changing patterns, thereby assisting interpretation. Careful, appropriate and systematic monitoring of clinical and laboratory parameters, combined with easily accessible serial data recording are mandatory for the optimal **management of nutritional support** by whatever route. Complications and outcomes should also be recorded to allow effective audit of the teams performance and to improve practice.

Some laboratory measures of response to nutrition

Malnutrition is responsible for increased morbidity and mortality and longer hospital stay with associated extra-costs. Optimal nutritional support may improve outcome. The **effectiveness** of this support should, therefore, be **tightly monitored**, including **mental and physical functions**. The nutritional support of malnourished patients is a primary therapy and as such its efficacy must be monitored. Most of the suitable parameters are different from those used to diagnose malnutrition because the latter are not sensitive enough. **Nitrogen balance, plasma transthyretin** and **urinary 3-methylhistidine** are useful but insufficiently used in daily practice, providing that people know the limit of specificity of these parameters and that **24 hour urine samples** (for N balance and 3-methylhistidine) are carefully collected. **Measurements** must be performed every 3 days or by 3-day periods (for urine parameters). In addition, CRP levels must be measured in order to interpret the results in the light of **variations** in **inflammatory status**. A **multi-disciplinary team** (biologist, physician, dietician) allows the best use of this monitoring.

Refeeding syndrome

The refeeding syndrome is a potentially **lethal** complication of refeeding in patients who are severely malnourished from whatever cause. It was first reported among those released from concentration camps following the Second World War. **Oral feeding** of these **grossly malnourished** individuals often resulted in fatality from **diarrhoea, heart failure** and **neurological complications**, including **coma** and **convulsions**. However, even at the present time the refeeding syndrome is not unusual complication of refeeding, with an incidence of 19 to 28%. The **incidence** of some form of the refeeding syndrome **in severely malnourished** patients started **on artificial feeding** is approximately 50%, with half of these developing the syndrome **within 3 days of starting** nutritional support. It occurs commonly with **enteral or parenteral realimentation** of malnourished patients. The refeeding syndrome is a complication of nutritional support in patients with **pathological weight loss, anorexia nervosa, cancer, postoperative phase, elderly, alcoholism**, etc. Its features are **salt and water retention** and **depletion of potassium, magnesium and phosphate** with a decrease in their **serum levels** during oral, enteral or parenteral realimentation. It can be associated with high mortality, especially when it is not diagnosed. Knowledge of the potential clinical symptoms like **tachypnoea, tachycardia and arrhythmia** is therefore essential for its **prevention, recognition, and treatment.**

Exercise 1
Match the column A with the column B. Try to learn the expressions and/or sentences by heart.

A

1. To use AIO admix as a drug vehicle to patients with PN
2. Specific emphasis is given concerning the properties of AIO
3. Addition of drugs to AIO admixtures should be avoided;
4. Only selected drugs with acceptable extended administration time, a large therapeutic index,
5. In total parenteral nutrition (TPN)
6. In supplementary parenteral nutrition a portion of the patient's nutrient needs
7. The best approach to preparing parenteral feeding solution
8. All-in-one (AIO) bags may be filled from basic solutions and bulk additive sources, or appropriate commercially produced two- or three-chamber bags may be chosen
9. As parenterally fed patients must metabolize or excrete all infused nutrients, the composition of nutritional formulas
10. Metabolic complications of parenteral nutrition can be categorised
11. The practice of PN always requires biochemical assessment and correction of any electrolyte disorders
12. Metabolic complications are more likely to occur when physicians do not perceive parenteral nutrition
13. Patients with severe malnutrition and already existing organ dysfunction
14. Parenteral nutrition can be complicated by metabolic problems, which may arise from
15. Severe (long-term) complications comprise
16. You need to train your team so that
17. Use serial data forms, so that any member of the team can see not only the current data,
18. The team soon get used to such a system and
19. Careful, appropriate and systematic monitoring of clinical and laboratory parameters,
20. The nutritional support of malnourished patients is a primary therapy
21. Nitrogen balance, plasma transthyretin and urinary 3-methylhistidine are useful, providing
22. The refeeding syndrome is a potentially lethal complication
23. Oral feeding of grossly malnourished individuals

24. The refeeding syndrome is a complication of nutritional support in patients
25. Its features are salt and water retention and depletion of potassium, magnesium and phosphate
26. Knowledge of the potential clinical symptoms like tachypnoea, tachycardia and arrhythmia

B

a) *admixtures emulsions, chemical reactivity of the components, container material and potential adverse effects.*

b) *all nutrient needs are provided intravenously without any significant oral or enteral intake.*

c) *and appropriate physico-chemical properties are candidates for admixing.*

d) *and as such its efficacy must be monitored.*

e) *are at particular risk of the refeeding syndrome if PN is introduced too rapidly or aggressively.*

f) *as deficiency states, acute metabolic complications and chronic (long-term) metabolic complications.*

g) *as the basic solution and admixture source and are supplemented appropriately to provide any lacking substances.*

h) *as useful adjunctive therapy and instead use it incautiously as urgent and lifesaving treatment.*

i) *but the previous data in a serial manner, so that any change can be perceived immediately and appropriate action taken.*

j) *cholestatic liver failure disease and bone demineralisation.*

k) *combined with easily accessible serial data recording are mandatory for the optimal management of nutritional support.*

l) *if it is inevitable, a strict GMP protocol including analytical assessment, is important.*

m) *inadequate or excessive amounts of nutrients or from an inappropriate composition of parenteral nutrition formulations.*

n) *is problematic because of complex nature of potential interactions.*

o) *is provided via the gastrointestinal tract, and the remainder is infused parenterally in sufficient amounts to meet optimal requirements.*

p) *is therefore essential for its prevention, recognition, and treatment.*

q) *is to mix all nutrients in one bag and to infuse them together.*

r) *learn to respond quickly when adverse trends are observed.*

s) *monitoring is undertaken and recorded on a regular and systematic basis.*

t) *of refeeding in patients who are severely malnourished from whatever cause.*

u) *often results in fatality from diarrhoea, heart failure and neurological complications, including coma and convulsions.*

v) *prior to the prescription in order to avoid potentially fatal acute complications.*

w) *should be adapted to nutritional requirements, metabolic capacity, metabolic disturbances and coexisting deficiencies or overloading.*

x) *that people know the limit of specificity of these parameters and that 24 hour urine samples are carefully collected.*

y) *with a decrease in their serum levels during oral, enteral or parenteral realimentation.*

z) *with pathological weight loss, anorexia nervosa, cancer, postoperative phase, elderly, alcoholism, etc.*

Exercise 2

Translate the expressions. Try to explain their meanings in English.

Admixtures, drug vehicle, complex nature, potential interactions, substantially, emphasis, adverse effects, as a general rule, inevitable, strict GMP protocol, expertise, assessment, achieve, administration time, facilitate, reflect, supplementary, provided, remainder, meet requirements, additive sources, commercially produced, lacking substances, applicability, adapted, metabolic disturbances, deficiencies or overloading, comprehensively, during the course, deficiency states, take into account, prescription, be aware, electrolyte disorders, prior to, perceive, adjunctive therapy, refeeding syndrome, short bowel syndrome, resection of the terminal ileum, ileo-caecal valve, premature infants, arise from, inadequate or excessive, inappropriate, comprise, cholestatic liver failure disease, crucial, suites your needs, understands the purpose, serial data forms, current data, previous action taken, proper order, get used to, adverse trends, observation, easily accessible, mandatory, performance, efficacy, sensitive, insufficiently used, inflammatory status, physician, grossly malnourished individuals, coma and convulsions, incidence, artificial feeding, realimentation, salt and water retention, depletion of potassium, magnesium and phosphate, serum levels, tachypnoea, tachycardia and arrhythmia recognition, treatment.

Exercise 3

Prepare short talks and/or dialogues on these topics.

1. Incompatibilities occurring upon admixing drugs to PN

2. Compounding nutritional formulas for parenteral nutrition
3. Clinical needs for all-in-one (AIO) compounding
4. Acute and long-term metabolic complications associated with parenteral nutrition
5. Monitoring support in normal clinical practice
6. Parameters suitable for monitoring the efficacy of nutrition support
7. Patients who are at risk of refeeding syndrome; the development of the refeeding syndrome

Vocabulary 10

Fill in the meanings in your mother language:

acceptable /ək'sept.ə.bl̩/
adjunctive /ə'dʒʌŋk.tɪv/
arrange /ə'reɪndʒ/
arrhythmia /ə'rɪð.mi.ə/
audit /'ɔːdɪt/
basis /'beɪ.sɪs/
bottom /'bɒt.əm/
carefully /'keə.fəl.i/
cholestatic /ˌkoʊ lə'stæt ɪk/
coexist /ˌkoʊ.ɪg'zɪst/
collect /kə'lekt/
commercially /kə'mɜː.ʃəl.i/
comprehensive /ˌkɒm.prɪ'hen.sɪv/
convulsion /kən'vʌl.ʃən/
correction /kə'rek.ʃən/
course /kɔːs/
data /'deɪ.tə/
demineralisation / diː'mɪnərəˌlaɪ.zeɪ.ʃən/
dysmature /dĭs'mət.jʊə/
emphasis /'em.fə.sɪs/
evaluation /ɪˌvæl.ju'eɪ.ʃən/
expert /'ek.spɜːt/
expertise /ˌek.spɜː'tiːz/
fatality /fə'tæl.ə.ti/
form /fɔːm/
grossly /'grəʊs.li/
heart /hɑːt/ **failure** /'feɪ.ljər/
ileo /'ɪlɪə/ **-caecal** /'si kəl/
ileum /'ɪl.i.əm/ pl **ilea**
immaturity /ˌɪm.ə'tʃʊə.rɪ.ti/
incautiously /ɪn'kɔːʃəs.lɪ/
index /'ɪn.deks/ pl **indices** /'ɪn.dɪ.siːz/
inevitable /ɪn'evɪt.ə.bəl/
initiation /ɪˌnɪʃ.i'eɪ.ʃən/
interpretation /ɪnˌtɜː.prɪ'teɪ.ʃən/
intravenously /ˌɪn.trə'viː.nəs.li/
manner /'mæn.ər/
methylhistidine /'mεθ əl'hɪstɪˌdiːn/
need /niːd/
overgrowth /ˌəʊ.və.grəʊθ/
overload /ˌəʊ.və'ləʊd/
participate /pɑː'tɪs.ɪ.peɪt/
pattern /'pæt.ən/
perceive /pə'siːv/
performance /pə'fɔː.məns/
portion /'pɔː.ʃən/
premature /'prem.ə.tʃər/
purpose /'pɜː.pəs/
reactivity /ˌri.æk'tɪv.ɪ.ţ i/
realimentation /riːˌæl.ɪ.men'teɪ.ʃən/
recognition /ˌrek.əg'nɪʃ.ən/
refeeding /riːˌfiːdɪŋ/
syndrome /'sɪn.drəʊm/
reflect /rɪ'flekt/
regular /'reg.jʊ.lər/
remainder /rɪ'meɪn.dər/
report /rə'poːt/
sensitive /'sent .sɪ.tɪv/
short /ʃɔːt/ **bowel** /'baʊ.əl/
syndrome /'sɪn.drəʊm/
small /smɔːl/ **bowel** /'baʊ.əl/
sorting /sɔːt.ɪŋ/
source /sɔːs/
specificity /ˌspes.ɪ'fɪs.ə.tɪ/

standardization /ˌstændədaɪˈzeɪʃən/
substantially /səbˈstænt.ʃəl.ɪ/
supplementary /ˌsʌp.lɪˈmen.tər.i/
tachycardia /ˌtæk.ɪˈkɑː.di.ə/
tachypnoea /ˌtæk.ɪp.ˈniː.ə/
tailored /ˈteɪl.əd/
take /ˈteɪk/ **action** /ˈæk.ʃən/
take /teɪk/ **into** /ɪntə/
account / əˈkaʊnt/
total /ˈtəʊtəl/
transthyretin /trænsˈθaɪ rɔ tən/
urgent /ˈɜː.dʒənt/
urinary /ˈjʊə.rɪ.nər.i/
valve /vælv/
vehicle /ˈviː.ɪ.klˌ/

Solution to Exercise 1
1n, 2a, 3l, 4c, 5b, 6o, 7q, 8g, 9w, 10f, 11v, 12h, 13e, 14m, 15j, 16s, 17i, 18r, 19k, 20d, 21x, 22t, 23u, 24z, 25y, 26p

Unit 11 - Nutritional support in different clinical situations 1

Nutritional support in severe malnutrition

Severe malnutrition is the result of **inadequate intake** of energy and other basic nutrients **in relation to expenditure**. It can also be due to losses of nutrients due to **poor intestinal absorption**. The rapidity of development of severe malnutrition depends on the degree of insufficient intake of nutrition as well as on the metabolic rate. During **simple (adapted) starvation** it develops relatively slowly over **a long period**. However, the **stress reaction and inflammation** can **accelerate** the progression of severe malnutrition. Then it can develop quickly; moreover malnutrition can be **concealed** by presence of **fat tissue**. Regardless of the aetiology, severe malnutrition is associated with **depletion of body protein, glycogen, potassium, phosphate, magnesium, trace elements and vitamins**. **Depletion of fat tissue** is dependent on the **rapidity** of malnutrition; chronic malnutrition is associated with severe loss of adipose tissue, while in stress malnutrition this is not the case. As malnutrition is commonly associated with an increased risk of **infection, delayed wound healing** and **surgical complications**, the severely malnourished subject must **receive nutritional support**, given preferably by the **oral or enteral** route. Only in the presence of **gastrointestinal dysfunction** is **parenteral** nutrition **indicated**.

- Severely malnourished patients need more **K, P, Mg, Zn, and vitamins** than well-nourished subjects.
- Final **energy and protein needs** are also higher and must be accommodated in order to accelerate repletion of deficits.
- If possible, oral and/or enteral nutrition is advocated for severely malnourished patients. The administration of standard **formulae for enteral nutrition** may be **supplemented** with parenteral **infusion of electrolytes, minerals and vitamins.**

- The early goal of feeding is improved function and accelerated **rehabilitation**. Restoration of lean mass is a longer term objective over weeks and months.

Preoperative nutrition

Most patients undergoing surgery can return to normal **oral feeding immediately**, or at any rate shortly after the operation. Several old traditional routines need to be changed. Proper anaesthetic techniques for **pain control** will help facilitate a return to the use of the oral route for feeding and **avoid postoperative ileus. Preoperative feeding** improves the outcome from surgery in patients with severe malnutrition and preoperative carbohydrates reduce postoperative insulin resistance and protein catabolism in elective surgery. **Postoperative enteral nutrition** reduces postoperative complications. There is some evidence of **benefit** from postoperative enteral and/or parenteral nutrition in previously malnourished patients, in those with postoperative complications and after **major trauma or burns**. So called **'immune- enhancing'** feeds have shown benefit in very severe trauma and in patients undergoing **major surgery** for upper gastrointestinal cancer. Feeding should be part of an integrated protocol of management throughout the patient's clinical course.

Nutritional support in critically ill and septic patients

The body **provides and diverts** energy and specific **substrates** to cover **energy** requirements as well as the needs of the body's **defences** and the **healing** process. **Gluconeogenesis** and increased **resistance to insulin** in **liver, muscle and adipose tissue** are integral parts of this reaction with the functions of improving **tissues growth and regeneration** as well as supplying metabolic pathways with reducing equivalents. These responses are **essential for survival** but occur at the expense of **loss of body proteins** (especially **muscle, skin,** and **gastrointestinal tissues**). It is even possible that **bone** contributes in some way to an adequate host response, because subacute as well as chronic inflammation leads to **osteoporosis**. This response of 'peripheral tissues' abates only when it is successful in **overcoming the primary disease**, including the reduction of infection, control of inflammation, heat loss etc. **Nutritional support** can **compensate** for negative energy and protein balance but it **cannot completely reverse catabolism** in peripheral tissues like muscle, skin and bone **until the convalescence** phase begins. The **catabolic response** to injury can be modified by treating and moderating its underlying cause but cannot be completely reversed by nutritional support.

Nutritional support can, however, **eliminate starvation** and **minimize tissue loss**, as well as assisting in the **maintenance of**

function and helping to **optimise recovery**. At least a part of the nutritional intake should be **enteral** because of its **beneficial effects** on gastrointestinal and **immune function**. This should be **started** as **early** as possible. Parenteral nutrition should be used in the presence of gastrointestinal dysfunction. Supplemental parenteral nutrition should be also given when enteral nutrition is insufficient in meeting requirements of nutrients. There is potential for harm if nutritional support is given without expert supervision and in the wrong dosage. Also it cannot compensate for inadequacies in the other aspects of care.

Nutritional support in trauma

Trauma is characterized by a combination of **cardiovascular**, **inflammatory** and **metabolic responses**. During the **cardiovascular** phase, priority is given to **resuscitation** and **maintenance of vital functions**. Nutritional support is useful during the **inflammatory and metabolic phase** and improves the patient's outcome. In trauma patients, **post-pyloric feeding** may be preferred to gastric feeding for the **first 3 to 4 days after trauma**. Immune-enhancing enteral diets may be useful in severely injured subjects. In **head-injured** patients, specific attention should be given to control of **intracranial pressure**. For this reason, overfeeding should be avoided.

Nutritional support in inflammatory bowel syndrome

The active phase of **inflammatory bowel disease** frequently leads to **protein- energy** malnutrition, which in children can lead to **growth retardation.** Furthermore, specific deficits of vitamins, especially **vitamin D, and of iron** and **calcium** have been described in some patients. Regular nutritional monitoring is, therefore, warranted in all patients with IBD. Nutritional support is indicated to **prevent and treat malnutrition**. Dietary **counselling** is usually insufficient, therefore **sip feeding** with standard polymeric diets or **tube feeding** are necessary. Tube feeding may be performed **overnight** to allow normal **oral nutrition by day.** Patients can either swallow a tube every evening, or may have a PEG tube safely inserted, even in Crohn's disease. Intravenous supplementation of vitamins, and iron may be necessary in patients with deficiencies due to reduced absorption or limited tolerance of oral supplements.

Adequate nutritional support **improves quality of life in IBD patients.** Enteral (and rarely parenteral) nutrition are also effective in treating active phases of **Crohn's disease** and are therefore **alternatives to medical treatment** in patients who are intolerant or unwilling to take steroids. In patients with chronic active CD sip feedings seems to allow reduction in steroid dosage and reduces disease activity. An elimination diet is difficult to construct but can be helpful in maintaining remission. The role of pharmaconutrients is still controversial.

Nutrition support in liver disease

Acute liver disease without fulminant hepatic failure induces the same **metabolic effects** as any disease associated with an acute phase response. The effect of nutritional **status** depends on the **duration** of the disease and the presence of any **underlying chronic liver disease** which may have already compromised the patients' nutritional status. Patients with **chronic liver disease** are at risk of malnutrition. Among patients with **advanced cirrhosis** there is a high prevalence of mixed protein energy malnutrition. These patients suffer from a significant **loss of total body protein** and a concomitant **loss of organ function**, such as **impaired skeletal muscle** or **immunological performance**.

Subjects at risk of malnutrition can **reliably** be **identified** by medical and nutritional **history** and **clinical examination** done in a **standardised** fashion, e.g. by **subjective global** assessment (SGA) or **anthropometry** (arm circumference, skinfold thickness). At the bedside, **bioimpendance analysis** can be used to quantitate the loss of body cell mass (phase angle). **Total body protein** is reduced to a greater degree in **cirrhosis of alcoholic origin** compared with other causes. With adequate nutrition body cell mass can be restored if metabolic conditions are stable. Protein-energy malnutrition is very common in **chronic liver disease** and negative nutrient balance due to inadequate intake is frequent. Thus, instead of imposing restrictive diets, which may be harmful, the goal of nutritional therapy is to ensure **sufficient provision of energy, nitrogen and micronutrients** to improve nutritional state.

Nutritional support in renal disease

The term protein-energy wasting in acute and chronic kidney disease (CKD) has been recently proposed by an expert panel for loss of body protein mass and fuel reserves. Protein-energy wasting should be diagnosed if three characteristics are present:

- **low serum levels** of **albumin, transthyretin** or **cholesterol**
- **reduced body mass** (low or reduced body mass or fat mass, or weight loss with reduced intake of protein and energy)
- **reduced muscle mass** (muscle wasting or sarcopenia, reduced circumference of mid-arm muscle)

The aetiology, diagnosis and nutritional treatment (as well as nutritional support) should be part of the **standard care** of patients with chronic and acute renal disease. The aims of nutritional support in patients with renal failure are dependent upon the **degree and character of kidney impairment**, degree of malnutrition, and associated disease. Patients with **chronic renal insufficiency** but without concurrent disease are at a high risk of malnutrition due to **uraemia-**associated factors, metabolic **acidosis**, impaired appetite and **oral intake** of food, and the gastrointestinal side effects of uraemia. The main purpose of nutritional management is to **prevent malnutrition**, to reduce or **control the accumulation of waste products**, and to **prevent bone and cardiovascular disease**.

Chronic renal **replacement therapy** leads to the **loss** of some nutritional substrates, such as **amino acids and water-soluble vitamins**, but also activation of **protein catabolism**. An adequate supply of energy, protein and vitamins must therefore be given to these patients. In **patients** with **renal insufficiency** complicated by **acute catabolic disease** and/or in patients with ARF, the stimulation of **immunocompetence**, **wound healing** and other reparative functions is the **principal goal** of nutritional therapy. In most situations, requirements exceed the minimal intake recommended for stable CRF patients or normal subjects. Intensive nutritional support must be provided to these patients and potential accumulation of waste and toxic products prevented by more intensive renal replacement therapy. **Renal failure** is a **pan-metabolic** and **pan-endocrine abnormality** affecting more or less **every metabolic pathway** in the body. In no other patient group is there such a narrow range between induction of **toxic effects** and the development of malnutrition. Nutritional assessment and intensive nutritional **education** are of great importance in all phases of renal transplantation, including the pre-transplant period. In cases of severe obesity, fat loss is recommended before surgery. During the first year, the major nutritional goal is to treat pre-existing malnutrition and **prevent excessive gain in weight.**

Exercise 1
Match the column A with the column B. Try to learn the expressions and/or sentences by heart.

A

1. The rapidity of development of severe malnutrition depends on the degree of insufficient intake of nutrition as well as on the metabolic rate
2. Severe malnutrition is associated with depletion of body protein, glycogen, potassium, phosphate, magnesium, trace elements and vitamins
3. Final energy and protein needs are also higher
4. The administration of standard formulae for enteral nutrition

5. Proper anaesthetic techniques for pain control will help facilitate
6. Preoperative feeding improves the outcome from surgery in patients with severe malnutrition
7. There is some evidence of benefit from postoperative enteral and/ or parenteral nutrition
8. The body provides and diverts energy and specific substrates
9. Nutritional support can compensate for negative energy and protein balance
10. Nutritional support can, however, eliminate starvation and minimize tissue loss,
11. In trauma patients, post-pyloric feeding
12. The active phase of inflammatory bowel disease
13. Dietary counselling is usually insufficient, therefore sip feeding with standard polymeric diets or tube feeding are necessary;
14. Enteral (and rarely parenteral) nutrition are also effective in treating active phases of Crohn's disease
15. Acute liver disease without fulminant hepatic failure
16. Among patients with advanced cirrhosis
17. These patients suffer from a significant loss of total body protein and a concomitant loss of organ function,
18. Subjects at risk of malnutrition can reliably be identified by medical and nutritional history and clinical examination done in a standardised fashion,
19. Total body protein is reduced to a greater degree in
20. Protein-energy malnutrition is very common in chronic liver disease
21. Protein-energy wasting in renal disease should be diagnosed if three characteristics are present:
22. The aims of nutritional support in patients with renal failure are
23. The main purpose of nutritional management is to prevent malnutrition,
24. Chronic renal replacement therapy leads to the loss of some nutritional substrates,
25. In patients with renal insufficiency complicated by acute catabolic disease and/ or in patients with ARF,
26. Nutritional assessment and intensive nutritional education are of great importance

B

a) a return to the use of the oral route for feeding and avoid postoperative ileus.

b) and are therefore alternatives to medical treatment in patients who are intolerant or unwilling to take steroids.

c) *and must be accommodated in order to accelerate repletion of deficits.*

d) *and negative nutrient balance due to inadequate intake is frequent.*

e) *and preoperative carbohydrates reduce postoperative insulin resistance and protein catabolism in elective surgery.*

f) *as well as assisting in the maintenance of function and helping to optimise recovery.*

g) *but it cannot completely reverse catabolism in peripheral tissues like muscle, skin and bone until the convalescence phase begins.*

h) *cirrhosis of alcoholic origin compared with other causes.*

i) *dependent upon the degree and character of kidney impairment, degree of malnutrition, and associated disease.*

j) *e.g. by subjective global assessment (SGA) or anthropometry (arm circumference, skinfold thickness).*

k) *frequently leads to protein-energy malnutrition, which in children can lead to growth retardation.*

l) *in all phases of renal transplantation, including the pre-transplant period.*

m) *in previously malnourished patients, in those with postoperative complications and after major trauma or burns.*

n) *induces the same metabolic effects as any disease associated with an acute phase response.*

o) *low serum levels of albumin, transthyretin or cholesterol, reduced body mass and reduced muscle mass.*

p) *may be preferred to gastric feeding for the first 3 to 4 days after trauma.*

q) *may be supplemented with parenteral infusion of electrolytes, minerals and vitamins.*

r) *patients can either swallow a tube every evening, or may have a PEG tube safely inserted, even in Crohn's disease.*

s) *severely malnourished patients need more K, P, Mg, Zn, and vitamins than well-nourished subjects.*

t) *such as amino acids and water-soluble vitamins, but also activation of protein catabolism.*

u) *such as impaired skeletal muscle or immunological performance.*

v) *the stimulation of immunocompetence, wound healing and other reparative functions is the principal goal of nutritional therapy.*

w) the stress reaction and inflammation can accelerate the progression of severe malnutrition.

x) there is a high prevalence of mixed protein energy malnutrition.

y) to cover energy requirements as well as the needs of the body's defences and the healing process.

z) to reduce or control the accumulation of waste products, and to prevent bone and cardiovascular disease.

Exercise 2
Translate the expressions. Try to explain their meanings in English.

Intestinal absorption, rapidity, insufficient intake, accelerate the progression, concealed, regardless of the aetiology, depletion, associated with, adipose tissue, delayed wound healing, surgical complications, repletion of deficits, is advocated, administration, improved function, a longer term objective, undergoing surgery, facilitate, evidence of benefit, major trauma or burns, integrated protocol of management, critically ill and septic patients, provides and diverts energy, cover requirements, defences, healing, tissues growth, regeneration, essential for survival, at the expense of, host response, overcoming the primary disease, compensate for, reverse catabolism, convalescence phase, treating and moderating, eliminate starvation, recovery, expert supervision, dosage, resuscitation, maintenance of vital functions, post-pyloric feeding, gastric feeding, intracranial pressure, inflammatory bowel syndrome, warranted, indicated, dietary counselling, sip feeding, tube feeding, swallow, inserted, limited tolerance, intolerant or unwilling, remission, fulminant hepatic failure, underlying disease, compromised status, advanced cirrhosis, high prevalence, reliably, be identified, arm circumference, skinfold thickness, bioimpendance analysis, be restored, imposing restrictive diets, harmful, improve nutritional state, protein-energy wasting, muscle wasting or sarcopenia, reduced circumference of mid-arm muscle, dependent upon, kidney impairment, renal insufficiency, concurrent disease, uraemia, metabolic acidosis, control the accumulation of waste products, renal replacement therapy, immunocompetence, wound healing reparative functions, principal goal, great importance, pre-transplant period.

Exercise 3
Prepare short talks and/or dialogues on these topics

1. Nutritional support in severely malnourished patients
2. The indications of preoperative and postoperative enteral or parenteral nutrition
3. Nutritional support in critically ill or septic patients

4. Nutritional support in trauma patients
5. Enteral and parenteral nutrition in patients with inflammatory bowel syndrome (IBS)
6. Nutritional therapy in acute liver disease and chronic liver diseases
7. Metabolic abnormalities in patients with renal disease

Vocabulary 11

Fill in the meanings in your mother language:

abate /ə'beɪt/
accelerate /æk'sel.əˌreɪt/
accommodate /ə'kɒm.ə.deɪt/
accumulation /əˌkjuː.mjʊ'leɪ.ʃən/
advocated /'æd.vəˌkeɪt.ɪd/
angle /'æŋ.gl̩/
anthropometry /ˌænθrə'pɒmɪtrɪ/
arm /ɑːm/
bioimpendance /'baɪəʊ/ɪm'piːdəns/
cause /kɔːz/
cholesterol /kə'les.tər.ɒl/
circumference /sə'kʌm.fər.əns/
compensate /'kɒm.pən.seɪt/
conceal /kən'siːl/
construct /kən'strʌkt/
counselling /'kaʊnt .səl.ɪŋ/
dosage /'dəʊ.sɪdʒ/
dysfunction /dɪs'fʌŋk.ʃən/
elimination /ɪˌlɪm.ɪ'neɪ.ʃən/
enhance /ɪn'hɑːns/
expense /ɪk'spens/
facilitate /fə'sɪl.ɪ.teɪt/
feed /fiːd/
fulminant /'fʊl.mɪ.nənt/
gain /geɪn/
global /'gləʊ.bəl/
gluconeogenesis /ˌglu koʊˌni ə'dʒɛn ə sɪs/
goal /gəʊl/
growth /grəʊθ/
harm /hɑːm/
healing /hiːlɪŋ/
host /həʊst/
ileus /'ɪl.i.əs/
immediately /ɪ'miː.di.ət.li/
immunocompetence /ˌɪm.jə.nəʊ.'kɒm.pɪ.təns/
impose /ɪm'pəʊz/
inadequacy /ɪ'næd.ɪ.kwə.sɪ/
inadequate /ɪ'næd.ɪ.kwət/
induce /ɪn'djuːs/
induction /ɪn'dʌk.ʃən/
intake /'ɪn.teɪk/
intolerant /ɪn'tɒlərənt/
intracranial /ˌɪn.trə'kraɪ.ni.əl/
maintenance /'meɪn.tɪ.nəns/
major /'meɪ.dʒər/
metabolic /ˌmet.ə'bɒl.ɪk/ **rate** /reɪt/
moderate /'mɒdəˌreɪt/
osteoporosis /ˌɒs.ti.əʊ.pə'rəʊ.sɪs/
overcome /ˌəʊ.və'kʌm/
overnight /ˌəʊ.və'naɪt/
pan- /pɑn/
panel /'pæn.əl/
post-pyloric /pəʊst.paɪ'lɔr ɪk/
postoperative /ˌpəʊst'ɒp.ər.ə.tɪv/
pre /priː/ **-transplant** /træn'splɑːnt/
pre-existing /ˌpriː.ɪg'zɪs.tɪŋ/
preferably /'pref.ər.ə.bli/
progression /prə'greʃ.ən/
provision /prə'vɪ.ʒən/
pyloric /paɪ'lɔr ɪk/
quantitate /'kwɒn tɪˌteɪt/
rapidity /rə'pɪd.ə.tɪ/
recovery /rɪ'kʌv.ər.i/
regardless /rɪ'gɑːd.ləs/
regeneration /rɪˌdʒenər'eɪʃən/
reliably /rɪ'laɪə.bli/
remission /rɪ'mɪʃ.ən/
renal /'riː.nəl/
reparative /rɪ'pær ə tɪv/

replacement /rɪˈpleɪs.mənt/
repletion /rɪˈpli ʃən/
retardation /ˌriː.tɑːˈdeɪ.ʃən/
sarcopenia /sɑːˈkəʊ.ˈpiː.ni.ə/
serum /ˈsɪə.rəm/ pl **sera**
significant /sɪgˈnɪf.ɪ.kənt/
skinfold /skɪn.fəʊld/
subacute /ˌsʌb.əˈkjuːt/
subjective /səbˈdʒek.tɪv/
suffer /ˈsʌf.ər/
sufficient /səˈfɪʃ.ənt/
therapy /ˈθer.ə.pi/
thickness /ˈθɪk.nəs/
trauma /ˈtrɔː.mə/
unwilling /ʌnˈwɪl.ɪŋ/
warrant /ˈwɒrənt/
waste /weɪst/
weight /weɪt/

Solution to Exercise 1
1w, 2s, 3c, 4q, 5a, 6e, 7m, 8y, 9g, 10f, 11p, 12k, 13r, 14b, 15n, 16x, 17u, 18j, 19h, 20d, 21o, 22i, 23z, 24t, 25v, 26l

Unit 12 - Nutritional support in different clinical situations 2

Nutrition in pulmonary and cardiac disease

Assessment for malnutrition is recommended in COPD patients because it is an indicator of poor prognosis. Recommendations suggest **supporting at-risk patients** but nutritional intervention alone rarely is of benefit without an integrated rehabilitation programme. **Modulation of dietary behaviour** is fundamental, with individualised **planned caloric intake** (with not too great an excess over energy requirements to avoid metabolic stress and excess CO_2 production) and **plurifractioning of meals during the day** to diminish postprandial dyspnoea and early satiety. Diets with high fat content have shown no benefit compared to standard or high carbohydrate formulations. In **acute exacerbations of COPD,** correct estimation of **caloric requirements** is best achieved by **indirect calorimetry** to **avoid metabolic overload and excessive CO_2 production.**

In mechanically ventilated patients, enteral formulae containing medium and long chain triglycerides and ω-3 fatty acids could be beneficial. Establishing the **presence of malnutrition** in CHF patients is important because it predicts a negative prognosis but its detection may be difficult because of the increase in extracellular fluids, therefore requiring adequate estimation of FFM. Nutritional intervention in CHF should be multidisciplinary because of the complex aetio-pathophysiology of cardiac cachexia but alone is rarely able to reverse malnutrition. Correct **counselling**, optimisation of **dietary patterns**, standard **oral supplements** or **tube feeding** when necessary, are currently recommended, while **caloric and protein requirements** then depend on **concomitant disease**/co-morbidity. **Amino acids** with anti-inflammatory and antioxidant properties appear promising future options.

Nutritional support in acute and chronic pancreatitis

The two major inflammatory diseases of the pancreas are **acute and chronic pancreatitis**. In both circumstances, **nutrient digestion and absorption** can be **impaired** in the short-term or definitely. Nutritional support is different in acute and chronic pancreatitis. In health, the pancreas plays an important part in the digestion and absorption of nutrients. Impaired pancreatic function has negative consequences for the host. Nutritional deficiencies can occur in acute and chronic pancreatitis.

Malnutrition in **acute pancreatitis** can be caused by the acute **catabolic stress** induced by the **systemic inflammatory response**, and in **chronic** pancreatitis due to **pain** and the **reduced digestion and absorption** of nutrients. Adequate administration of **fluid and food** can be a **major problem** in patients with acute pancreatitis. For many years, textbooks have advocated the **concept** that **oral or enteral feeding is harmful** in acute pancreatitis; such feeding was thought to stimulate **exocrine** pancreatic secretory **responses** and consequently **autodigestive processes**.

Conversely it is known that specific **nutritional deficiencies** can occur in patients with a **prolonged and complicated course** of **acute necrotising pancreatitis**. Also, it has been questioned **if early feeding changes the outcome** in uncomplicated, acute pancreatitis. During the evolution of **chronic** pancreatitis, **enzyme secretion** is gradually **decreased**. This results in **maldigestion** with **steatorrhoea** and **azotorrhea** when more than 90% of the pancreatic **tissue is destroyed**. In the late course of chronic pancreatitis, **diabetes** will develop due to the loss of insulin-producing beta cells in the pancreas. Up to 75-80% of patients with acute pancreatitis have **mild-to-moderate disease** and do not need specific nutritional support. **Early oral refeeding** can be started within a few days in patient who have no pain and disturbances within the gastrointestinal tract. Patients with **severe disease, complications,** or the **need for surgery** require early nutritional support.

In patients with **severe pancreatitis**, an **enteral jejunal approach** should be established, but parenteral nutrition is an alternative method **if enteral nutrition** is **insufficient**. For the future, several factors have to be clarified:

- the **optimal timing** of nutritional therapy
- the optimal **feeding type (oral, gastric, jejunal or TPN**);
- the optimal **nutrient formulation** (**semi-elemental** diet, **polymeric** diet, **immune-enhancing** diet, **prebiotics** or **probiotics**)

Future studies on clear stratification of patients according to nutritional status on hospital admission should be conducted.

Chronic pancreatitis

Abstinence from alcohol, **dietary modifications,** and **supplementation** of **pancreatic enzymes** are the cornerstones of nutritional management in patients with chronic pancreatitis. Clinical trials documenting a beneficial effect of enteral nutrition or parenteral nutrition in patients with chronic pancreatitis with severe maldigestion and malnutrition are lacking. **Enteral nutrition** can be useful if dietary recommendations fail, or **before and after pancreatic surgery. Jejunal** applications of **low-molecular diets** are well tolerated. The recommendations for enteral nutrition and parenteral nutrition are **empirical** because prospective **clinical trials** in patients with chronic pancreatitis using protocols for enteral nutrition or parenteral feeding **are lacking.**

Nutrition support in GI fistulas

Fistulas of the gastrointestinal (GI) tract can be divided generally into two groups:

- **internal**, consisting of an abnormal communication between **adjacent hollow viscera**
- **external** (enterocutaneous – EC) consisting of an abnormal communication between the **gastrointestinal tract** and the **surface** of the body

Additionally, more recently, wide **adoption of damage control surgery**, together with the open abdomen in trauma and emergency surgery, has confronted surgeons with an especially difficult adversary – the **exposed or entero-atmospheric fistula** (EAF). EC fistulas occur rarely, but they can present many medical and surgical problems.

The **therapeutic goals** in the management of **postoperative EC fistulas** are **closure** of the fistula and reestablishment of **intestinal continuit**y. Achieving of these goals is not easy, and often impossible, in the short term, in the malnourished patient who has been operated on a short period before the onset of fistula. **Treatment of fistulas** is complex and based on **bowel rest, enteral nutrition if possible**, but parenteral nutrition if not, pharmacological **suppression** of **secretion**, **suction drainage**, **physical rehabilitation** and careful **monitoring of all vital functions**. Whenever possible, some enteral nutrition should be introduced early, at least a part of nutritional support. Elective surgery should be considered if, after **3-5 weeks** of nutrition support, **spontaneous closure** has not occurred. Emergency surgery is indicated in patients who develop uncontrolled **sepsis**, or severe **haemorrhage**.

Nutritional support in extensive gut resection (short bowel syndrome)

The term short bowel syndrome (SBS) is used whenever **small bowel resection** leads to a situation in which the **uptake of nutrients and/or fluids** is **insufficient** for the maintenance of the **integrity and function** of the body. The **minimum length** of small bowel that is required for adequate absorption of nutrients varies depending on the **health** and **absorptive capacity of the remainder.** There is also a wide **variation between individuals** in the original length of the small intestine and it can be difficult to assess the length of the remaining bowel. Patients with short bowel syndrome inevitably have **intestinal failure,** but it should be noted that the functional nature of the best definitions of intestinal failure will mean that not all patients with intestinal failure have short bowel syndrome, since **major inflammatory or motility disorders** can **compromise** absorption **without** obligatory **loss of intestinal length.**

The clinical and metabolic status of a patient with short bowel syndrome depends on:

- the **extent and site of resection**
- the **presence or absence of the ileo-caecal valve**
- the function and **health** of **the remaining digestive tract** and associated organs
- the activity and course of the **underlying disease** leading to intestinal failure
- the process of **adaptation in the remaining intestine**
- the **age** of the patient
- the presence or absence of (a part of) the **colon** in continuity with the small bowel

The **minimum length** of small bowel ending in a jejunostomy needed to allow a patient to become independent from parenteral nutrition support is approximately **80 cm** for adults. With at least **half of the colon** remaining in **continuity** a patient may become **stable on intensive enteral nutrition** with as little as 50 cm of small bowel. Clinically, **SBS** is characterised by the presence of **diarrhoea, steatorrhoea, weight loss, dehydration, and malnutrition,** with **malabsorption** of **macronutrients, vitamins, fluid, electrolytes and trace elements** resulting in **hypovolaemia, hypoalbuminemia, and metabolic acidosis.**

After **resection of the jejunum,** the ileum is able to take over most absorptive functions, while **resection** of an equivalent length of the **ileum** is metabolically more **detrimental. Removal** of the **ileo-caecal valve decreases intestinal transit time** and contributes an increased risk of **retrograde bacterial colonisation** of the **small intestine.** Careful **fluid and electrolyte replacement** and **nutritional therapy** play a **critical**

role in the treatment of SBS. In most cases **parenteral nutrition** is **mandatory** in the early stages after resection, but, as soon as possible, enteral nutrition should be started and PN reduced as much as possible. **Enteral nutrition improves bowel function** as well as **facilitating intestinal adaptation**. In some patients long-term parenteral feeding, combined with oral or enteral nutrition, remains necessary. Such care can be provided in the home setting although the quality of life in these patients is a concern.

Nutritional consequences of bariatric surgery

Obesity can be understood as a state of current or past positive energy balance, resulting in **excessive accumulation of adipose tissue**. Although the status of non-energy nutritional sources is not relevant for diagnosis, it is presumed that obese subjects are globally very well nourished. This tenet has been shaken in some contexts, especially **after bariatric operations**. Such interventions were devised to create carefully dimensioned restrictive and/or malabsorptive mechanisms, **aiming to eliminate at least 50% of excess body weight**/EBW (difference between ideal and current weight), but not much more than 80%. Thus only a **minority of the subjects achieve ideal weight**, most remaining 20-25% above it. On the other hand only seldom do cases progress to being underweight.

Deficient nutrition should therefore be **extremely unusual** in bariatric populations. For more than two decades, especially once the **ill-conceived jejunoileal bypass of the 60s, 70s and early 80s** was abandoned in favour of **modern stomach-based operations**, this was universally accepted as true. The only precaution recommended by surgical societies was the daily ingestion of a multivitamin-multimineral supplement. **Recent experience** suggests otherwise, **namely** that this population should be considered at **risk for a long list of macro- and micronutrient deficiencies.** Interestingly even **before undergoing operation, iron-deficiency anaemia** and **low serum levels of vitamins A, D and B_{12}**, and of **folate, selenium and zinc** are now recognized **in morbidly obese** candidates. **Obesity** has always been classified as a **form of malnutrition**, but now it becomes clear that it is not incompatible with unquestionable undernutrition. **Bariatric therapy**, which was devised to cure severe obesity, is a highly commendable **surgical advance** which **removes comorbidities and prolongs life**, but it **may aggravate nutrient depletion**. A new profile is thus emerging, of the operated obese subject who may suffer from **multiple chronic deficits**, typically veiled and underdiagnosed. A deliberate and permanent effort is required to combat both dramatic **exacerbations** such as Wernicke's syndrome, and more subtle but relevant derangements including **anaemia and bone loss.**

Exercise 1
Match the column A with the column B. Try to learn the expressions and/or sentences by heart.

A

1. Assessment for malnutrition is recommended
2. Modulation of dietary behaviour is fundamental,
3. Diets with high fat content have shown no benefit
4. In acute exacerbations of COPD, correct estimation of caloric requirements is best achieved
5. Establishing the presence of malnutrition in CHF patients
6. Correct counselling, optimisation of dietary patterns, standard oral supplements or tube feeding when necessary,
7. The two major inflammatory diseases of the pancreas
8. Malnutrition in acute pancreatitis can be caused by the acute catabolic stress induced by the systemic inflammatory response,
9. Specific nutritional deficiencies can occur in patients
10. During the evolution of chronic pancreatitis, enzyme secretion is gradually decreased,
11. In the late course of chronic pancreatitis,
12. Early oral refeeding can be started within a few days in patient
13. In patients with severe pancreatitis, an enteral jejunal approach should be established,
14. Abstinence from alcohol, dietary modifications, and supplementation of pancreatic enzymes are the cornerstones
15. Fistulas of the gastrointestinal (GI) tract can be divided generally into two groups:
16. Treatment of fistulas is complex and based on bowel rest, enteral nutrition if possible, but parenteral nutrition if not,
17. Elective surgery should be considered if, after 3-5 weeks of nutrition support, spontaneous closure has not occurred;
18. The term short bowel syndrome (SBS) is used whenever small bowel resection leads to a situation in which
19. Not all patients with intestinal failure have short bowel syndrome,
20. The clinical and metabolic status of a patient depends on: the extent and site of resection, the presence or absence of the ileo-caecal valve,
21. Clinically, SBS is characterised by the presence of diarrhoea, steatorrhoea, weight loss, dehydration, and malnutrition,

22. After resection of the jejunum, the ileum is able to take over most absorptive functions,
23. Careful fluid and electrolyte replacement and nutritional therapy play a critical role in the treatment of SBS,
24. Obesity can be understood as a state of current or past positive energy balance, resulting in excessive accumulation of adipose tissue and bariatric operations
25. Recent experience suggests that this population should be considered at risk for macro- and micronutrient deficiencies, before undergoing operation,
26. Bariatric therapy, which was devised to cure severe obesity, is a highly commendable surgical advance

e) *by indirect calorimetry to avoid metabolic overload and excessive CO_2 production.*

f) *compared to standard or high carbohydrate formulations.*

g) *diabetes will develop due to the loss of insulin-producing beta cells in the pancreas.*

h) *emergency surgery is indicated in patients who develop uncontrolled sepsis, or severe haemorrhage.*

i) *enteral nutrition improves bowel function as well as facilitating intestinal adaptation.*

j) *in COPD patients because it is an indicator of poor prognosis.*

k) *internal, consisting of an abnormal communication between adjacent hollow viscera, and external consisting of an abnormal communication between the gastrointestinal tract and the surface of the body.*

l) *iron-deficiency anaemia and low serum levels of vitamins A, D and B_{12}, and of folate, selenium and zinc are now recognized in morbidly obese candidates.*

m) *is important because it predicts a negative prognosis.*

n) *of nutritional management in patients with chronic pancreatitis.*

B

a) *and in chronic pancreatitis due to pain and the reduced digestion and absorption of nutrients.*

b) *are acute and chronic pancreatitis.*

c) *are currently recommended, while caloric and protein requirements then depend on concomitant disease.*

d) *but parenteral nutrition is an alternative method if enteral nutrition is insufficient.*

o) *pharmacological suppression of secretion, suction drainage, physical rehabilitation and careful monitoring of all vital functions.*
p) *since major inflammatory or motility disorders can compromise absorption without obligatory loss of intestinal length.*
q) *the function and health of the remaining digestive tract, the course of the underlying disease and the adaptation in the remaining intestine.*
r) *the uptake of nutrients and/ or fluids is insufficient for the maintenance of the integrity and function of the body.*
s) *were devised to create carefully dimensioned restrictive and/or malabsorptive mechanisms, aiming to eliminate at least 50% of excess body weight, but not much more than 80%.*
t) *which removes comorbidities and prolongs life, but it may aggravate nutrient depletion.*
u) *which results in maldigestion with steatorrhoea and azotorrhea when more than 90% of the pancreatic tissue is destroyed.*
v) *while resection of an equivalent length of the ileum is metabolically more detrimental.*
w) *who have no pain and disturbances within the gastrointestinal tract.*
x) *with a prolonged and complicated course of acute necrotising pancreatitis.*
y) *with individualised planned caloric intake.*
z) *with malabsorption of macronutrients, vitamins, fluid, electrolytes and trace elements resulting in hypovolaemia, hypoalbuminemia, and metabolic acidosis.*

Exercise 2

Translate the expressions. Try to explain their meanings in English.

Nutritional intervention, of benefit, integrated, modulation of dietary behaviour, is fundamental, postprandial dyspnoea, early satiety, compared to, estimation of, metabolic overload, excessive CO_2 production, predicts detection, extracellular fluids, adequate estimation, correct counselling, dietary patterns, concomitant disease, promising future options, impaired pancreatic function, negative consequences, acute catabolic stress, systemic inflammatory response, administration of fluid and food, advocated the concept, exocrine responses, autodigestive processes, conversely, prolonged and complicated course, maldigestion, steatorrhoea, azotorrhea, mild-to-moderate disease, early oral refeeding, enteral jejunal approach, insufficient, timing, feeding type, nutrient formulation, stratification, hospital admission, clinical trials, dietary recommendations fail, jejunal applications, adjacent hollow viscera, onset, enterocutaneous, additionally, wide adoption, adversary surgical problems, bowel rest, suppression, suction drainage, introduced, spontaneous closure, extensive gut resection, uptake of nutrients, insufficient integrity, absorptive capacity, intestinal failure, inflammatory or motility disorders, compromise, extent and site, underlying disease, in continuity with, jejunostomy, independent from, approximately, hypovolaemia, hypoalbuminemia, metabolic acidosis, detrimental, ileo-caecal valve, retrograde, facilitating intestinal adaptation, home setting, current or past, excessive accumulation, presumed, devised, carefully dimensioned, aiming to eliminate, achieve ideal weight, abandoned, in favour of, precaution recommended, before undergoing operation, recognized derangements, abnormal findings, devised to cure, commendable surgical advance, aggravate nutrient depletion, deliberate and permanent effort, combat exacerbations.

Exercise 3
Prepare short talks and/or dialogues on these topics

1. Epidemiology of malnutrition and the importance of its correct detection in patients with cardiac and pulmonary disease
2. Physiology and patophysiology of pancreatic secretion and consequences for nutrient digestion
3. Benefits and limitation of early enteral or parenteral nutritional interventions in patients with acute pancreatitis
4. Nutritional recommendations in patients with chronic pancreatitis
5. Nutrition and metabolic care in the spontaneous healing of GI fistulas
6. The impact of extensive small bowel resection on digestion, absorption and metabolism
7. Nutritional consequences of bariatric surgery

Vocabulary 12

Fill in the meanings in your mother language:

absorptive /əbˈzɔːp.tɪv/
acidosis /ˌæs.ɪˈdəʊ.sɪs/
adjacent /əˈdʒeɪ.sənt/
adoption /əˈdɒp.ʃən/
advance /ədˈvɑːns/
adversary /ˈædvəsərɪ/
advocate /ˈæd.vəˌkeɪt/
aetio-pathophysiology / ˌiːtiəˌpæθ.əˌfɪz.iˈɒl.ə.dʒi/
aggravate /ˈæg.rə.veɪt/
autodigestive /ˈɔ toʊˈdʒɛstɪv/
azotorrhea /ˌæz.ə.təˈriːə/
bariatric /ˌbærɪˈætrɪk/
base /beɪs/
bypass /ˈbaɪ.pɑːs/

Chronic /ˈkrɒnɪk/ **Obstructive** /əbˈstrʌk.tɪv/ **Pulmonary** /ˈpʌl.mə.nər.i/ **Disease** /dɪˈziːz/ **COPD**
clarify /ˈklær.ɪ.faɪ/
closure /ˈkləʊ.ʒə/
colonisation /ˈkɒləˌnaɪz.eɪʃən/
combat /ˈkɒm.bæt/
commendable /kəˈmɛn.də.bəl/
communication /kəˌmjuːnɪˈkeɪʃən/
comorbidity /koʊ.mɔrˈbɪd ɪ ti/
compromise /ˈkɒmprəˌmaɪz/
concern /kənˈsɜːn/
consist /kənˈsɪst/
context /ˈkɒntɛkst/
contribute /kənˈtrɪb.juːt/
controversy /kənˈtrɒ.vɜː.sɪ/
cornerstone /ˈkɔːnəˌstəʊn/
cure /kjʊər/
current /ˈkʌr.ənt/
currently /ˈkʌr.ənt.li/
definitely /ˈdef.ɪ.nət.lɪ/
deliberate /dɪˈlɪb.ər.ət/
dimension /dɪˈmɛnʃən/
disease /dɪˈziːz/
disorder /dɪˈsɔː.dər/
drainage /ˈdreɪ.nɪdʒ/
dyspnoea /dɪs.pniː.ə/
emerge /ɪˈmɜːdʒ/
empirical emˈpɪrɪkə/
entero /ɛntərə/**-atmospheric** /æt.məsˈfɛr.ɪk/ **fistula** /ˈfɪs.tʃə.lə/
enterocutaneous /ɛntərə.kjuːˈteɪnɪəs/
estimation /ˌes.tɪˈmeɪ.ʃən/
exacerbation /ɪgˌzæs.əˈbeɪ.ʃən/
exhibit /ɪgˈzɪb.ɪt/
exocrine /ˈek.səʊ.kraɪn/
experience /ɪkˈspɪə.ri.ənt s/
exposed /ɪkˈspəʊzd/
external /ɪkˈstɜː.nəl/
extracellular /ˌek.strəˈsel.jə.lər/
fistula /ˈfɪs.tʃə.lə/ pl **fistulae**
gradually /ˈgrædʒ.ʊ.li/
gut /gʌt/
hollow /ˈhɒl.əʊ/
home /həʊm/ **setting** /ˈset.ɪŋ/
hypoalbuminemia /ˌhaɪ.poʊ.ælˌbjʊ.məˈni.mi.ə/
hypovolaemia /ˌhaɪ.pəʊ.vəˈliː.mɪ.ə/
ill-conceived /ˈɪl kənˈsivd/
in favour of /ˈfeɪ vər/
inevitably /ɪˈnev.ɪ.tə.bli/
integrity /ɪnˈteg.rə.ti/
jejunal /dʒɪˈdʒuːnəl/
jejunoileal /dʒɪ dʒuˈnɒ ˈɪlɪəl/
maldigestion /mæl.dɪˈdʒɛstʃən/
mechanical /məˈkæn.ɪ.kəl/
medium /miː.di.əm/
modification /ˌmɒd.ɪ.fɪˈkeɪ.ʃən/
modulation /ˌmɒd.jəˈleɪ.ʃən/
motility /ˌməʊ.ˈtil.i.ˈtiː/
namely /ˈneɪmlɪ/
necrotising /ˈnɛk rəˌtaɪz.ɪŋ/
obligatory /əˈblɪg əˌtɔr i/
optimal /ˈɒp.tɪ.məl/
optimisation /ˈɒp təˌmaɪ.zeɪ.ʃən/
otherwise /ˈʌð.ə.waɪz/
pancreatitis /ˌpæŋ.krɪ.əˈtaɪ.tɪs/
past /pɑːst/
plurifractioning /ˈplʊər ə ˈfrækʃən.ɪŋ/
precaution /prɪˈkɔː.ʃən/
predict /prɪˈdɪkt/
presume /prɪˈzjuːm/
relevant /ˈrel.ə.vənt/
respect /rɪˈspekt/
rest /rest/
restrictive /rɪˈstrɪk.tɪv/
retrograde /ˈrɛ.trə.greɪd/
secretory /ˈsek.rə.tər.i/
semi-elemental /ˈsɛmɪˌɛlɪˈmɛntəl/
shake /ʃeɪk/ **(shook, shaken)**
steatorrhoea /ˌstɪətəˈrɪə/
stratification /ˌstrætɪfɪˈkeɪʃən/
subtle /ˈsʌt.əl/
suction /ˈsʌk.ʃən/
suppression /səˈpreʃ.ən/
take /ˈteɪk/ **over** /ˈoʊ vər/
tenet /ˈten.ɪt/
timing /ˈtaɪ.mɪŋ/
tolerate /ˈtɒl.ər.eɪt/
transit /ˈtræn.sɪt/

underdiagnosed /ˈʌn
dərˈdaɪ əgˌnoʊzd/
underweight /ʌn.dərˈweɪt/
universal /ˌjuː.nɪˈvɜː.səl/
unquestionable /ʌnˈkwɛs.tʃə.nə.bəl/
veiled /veɪld/
ventilate /ˈven.tɪ.leɪt/
viscera /ˈvɪs.ər.ə/

Solution to Exercise 1
1j, 2y, 3f, 4e, 5m, 6c, 7b, 8a, 9x, 10u, 11g, 12w, 13d, 14n, 15k, 16o, 17h, 18r, 19p, 20q, 21z, 22v, 23i, 24s, 25l, 26t

Unit 13 - Nutritional support in different clinical situation 3

Nutrition in the elderly

The over 65 age group forms an ever **increasing proportion of the population,** particularly of Western countries. In the USA, for example, the fastest growing segment of the population is among those living 85 years and longer. The impact that these demographic changes have on the health care system is already being noticed in **acute**, **chronic** and **long-term care facilities**. Although European researches show a **low incidence** of undernutrition in the community among the **healthy elderly**, **protein energy malnutrition** (PEM) accompanied by micronutrient deficiencies is a major problem in the elderly suffering from **poor health**. Severe PEM has been found in 10-38% of older **out patients**, 5-12% of the **homebound**, 26-65% of elderly **hospital in-patients** and 5-85% of **institutionalised** individuals. In the developed world, malnutrition in the elderly occurs mainly in the context of disease. The elderly as a group are particularly susceptible to undernutrition especially when suffering from chronic mental or physical disease. Elderly patients should be screened for risk of undernutrition and have an appropriate **care plan**. Where significant undernutrition exists there is clear evidence of **benefit from nutrition support.** There is suggestive evidence that good nutrition and even the use of vitamin and mineral supplements may have an important **preventive role** in maintaining health and quality of life in the elderly. In making any care plan, ethical considerations are important, respecting the patient's autonomy, ensuring benefit and avoiding harm.

Nutritional support in burns patients

The incidence of **burn injuries** has decreased in Western countries, but they remain a challenge throughout the world. Overall, the metabolic responses of burns patients are similar to those of other trauma patients, but they are **more intense and prolonged.** A massive acute phase response is characteristic. Like other patients with severe trauma those with burns suffer **additional morbidity** from **shock, acute respiratory failure, sepsis** and **multiple organ dysfunction syndrome**. But burned patients benefit from management in specialised facilities due to some specific and additional medical characteristics.

- The **skin barrier** being destroyed, they present **cutaneous exudative fluid losses** containing large quantities of **proteins, minerals and micronutrients,** which cause acute **deficiency syndromes.**
- They are particularly prone to **infection** due **difficult venous access** and **destruction of the skin** (higher risk of catheter related infection)
- The **surface to repair** is extensive and explains the requirement for prolonged nutritional support.
- Burn patients stay for much longer periods in **intensive care units (ICU)** compared to those with other forms of trauma, and require more prolonged nutritional support.

The size of the burns will determine the responses to injury. Burns can be divided into **small**: 10-20% body surface area **(BSA)**; **large**: 20-40% BSA; **major**: 40-60%; and **massive**: if more than 60% BSA is involved. In the absence of inhalation injury which would make the patient dependent on intubation and mechanical ventilation and also nutritionally more vulnerable, patients with burns of **less than 20% BSA** can be managed **without artificial nutrition support**. Patients with major burns have increased nutritional requirements. **Energy expenditure varies over time** with the **largest increases** being observed during **the first weeks** after injury. **Enteral nutrition** is **the first choice,** parenteral nutrition being a second choice reserved for patients with gastrointestinal failure. Burns have large **trace element losses** with their **exudates** until wound closure; the **acute deficit** contributes to delay recovery; this can be reversed by early intravenous supplementation. Nutritional support includes **monitoring** daily weight changes and energy intakes.

Nutritional support in cancer patients

The rationale for using nutritional support in the cancer patient is the attempt to **reverse cancer cachexia**/ malnutrition and, consequently to **prevent complications** and the **mortality** associated with it. However, this goal is only partially attainable because cancer cachexia is not synonymous with undernutrition or starvation, but rather the result of **multiple metabolic aberrations.** This tenet, which has gained a worldwide acceptance following the discovery of many **mediators** which **interfere in the metabolism** of the cancer patients, are responsible for the **lean body mass erosion** and **fat depletion**, and cause a poor utilisation of the nutritive substrates, does not mean that adequate nutritional support is not important in these patients.

On the contrary, **nutritional support and anticachectic agents** are both **essential** in weight-losing patients, they are mutually interactive and their combination is the *conditio sine qua non* for a better nutritional and clinical outcome. Nutritional support is recommended in cancer patients in 3 main areas. In **perioperative conditions** artificial nutrition has proven to benefit malnourished patients and, thanks to the use of special immune nutrients, also in some patients who are not losing weight.

In oncological patients receiving **chemotherapy and/or radiation therapy**, nutritional support is recommended if **anorexia, nausea** and **vomiting**, or **mucositis** or progressive **weight loss** decrease the **compliance** with **cancer treatments**, cause progressive delays and ultimately reduce their efficacy. In some **incurable cancer patients** who are otherwise going to die from starvation, usually because of chronic malignant (sub)obstruction, rather than from tumour progression, PN is a **temporary lifesaving procedure.**

Cancer cachexia is a **frequent finding** with head-and-neck or upper gastrointestinal cancer and in all patients with **advanced stages** of disease. Cancer cachexia differs from simple starvation because it is due not only to **reduced nutrient intake** but is also associated with several **metabolic alterations** mediated by a **cascade of cytokines** and other **tumour-specific factors**. Weight loss, which is the characteristic feature of cachexia, has been widely recognised as an adverse prognostic and predictive factor.

Radiation enteropathy

Abdominal radiation therapy can result in significant **gastrointestinal, gynaecological, genitourinary and pelvic bone damage**. The incidence of radiation enteropathy **(RE)** has increased in recent years because of the use of radiation as a part of the multi-disciplinary **approach to cancer.** An accurate estimate of the prevalence of RE is difficult because the mildest types usually **escape clinical attention**, whereas the later and more severe types occur years after the end of the radiation therapy, and patients may then be admitted to other institutions or undergo **emergency surgery**. The prevalence of RE is **higher in elderly and slim patients**, and in subjects affected by **concurrent disease**, such as **hypertension** and **diabetes**. **Prior laparotomy** increases the risk of RE by a factor or 2, or by 3-7-fold in the case of major abdominal surgery. **Prior to concurrent chemotherapy** also increases the risk.

It has been estimated that **gastrointestinal complications** requiring **surgical intervention** develop in approximately 5-7% of patients who have undergone abdominal radiotherapy. **RE is not a uniform condition** that requires a standardised clinical approach. There is recent evidence that plasma citrulline may enable quantification and monitoring of epithelial radiation-induced small bowel damage, but this biochemical evaluation has not yet translated into the routine clinical approach. **Acute RE** is difficult to prevent, but frequently **reversible,** and patients should be treated conservatively, with **total bowel rest and TPN if necessary**. In **chronic RE**, PN may have a role if the RE involves **large parts of the small bowel** or if there is short bowel syndrome due to previous resectional surgery. In these patients **PN may be required** indefinitely. **In severe subacute RE,** not amendable to surgery because of multiple scattered lesions, **medium term PN**, in hospital or at home, is indicated and may allow resolution of intestinal obstruction and help to restore oral feeding.

Effect of anticachectic agents in cancer

It has been recognised for a long time in **catabolic states**, and in **cancer cachexia** in particular, that **artificial nutrition support** has a **limited impact**. The most favourable expected effect is a **prevention** of **further** nutritional **deterioration**. **Full replenishment** may sometimes occur, when malnutrition is primarily due to starvation rather than to multiple metabolic derangements, when **tumour growth is not rapid** and there is time and opportunity to reverse a state of depletion and, obviously when an **effective oncologic therapy** and nutritional support are associated in a combined modality approach. Since depletion **in most cancer patients** is not simply due to starvation but to **metabolic alterations**, recent research has focused, after the disappointing results of artificial nutrition, on the study of agents potentially able to interfere with some of the mediators of cachexia. It should be pointed out that these agents **cannot** be expected to **work alone,** but rather in the presence of an adequate **spontaneous food intake** or, in the case of hypophagia, in combination with **enteral or parenteral support**.

Nutritional support in AIDS

Although infection with HIV progresses **from acute to a chronic disease** treated by **multiple drug** therapy, nutritional status should not be forgotten. Until a cure for HIV is found, the patient should have access to **nutritional therapy** to maintain good nutritional status in order to **fight the infection** and maintain an effective function. Patients should be **monitored** for **obesity**, **cardiovascular diseases** and **diabetes** due to a low activity pattern and unbalanced intake of food. The goal is good nutritional status to facilitate compliance with drug therapy.

Exercise 1
Match the column A with the column B. Try to learn the expressions and/ or sentences by heart.

A

1. European researches show a low incidence

of undernutrition in the community among the healthy elderly,

2. There is suggestive evidence that good nutrition and even the use of vitamin and mineral supplements
3. The metabolic responses of burns patients are similar to those of other trauma patients,
4. Patients with burns suffer additional morbidity from
5. The skin barrier being destroyed, burns present cutaneous exudative fluid losses
6. Patients with burns are particularly prone to infection
7. The size of the burns will determine the responses to injury;
8. Energy expenditure varies over time with the largest increases
9. Burns have large trace element losses with their exudates until wound closure;
10. The rationale for using nutritional support in the cancer patient is the attempt to reverse cancer cachexia/malnutrition and,
11. Cancer cachexia is not synonymous with undernutrition or starvation,
12. Many mediators which interfere in the metabolism of the cancer patients, are responsible for
13. In perioperative conditions artificial nutrition has proven to benefit
14. In oncological patients receiving chemotherapy and/or radiation therapy, nutritional support is recommended if anorexia, nausea and vomiting, or
15. Cancer cachexia is a frequent finding with head-and-neck or upper gastrointestinal cancer
16. Abdominal radiation therapy can result in
17. The prevalence of RE is higher in elderly and slim patients,
18. Gastrointestinal complications requiring surgical intervention develop
19. Acute RE is difficult to prevent, but frequently reversible
20. In chronic RE, PN may have a role if the RE involves large parts of the small bowel
21. In severe subacute RE, not amendable to surgery because of multiple scattered lesions,
22. In catabolic states, and in cancer cachexia artificial nutrition support has a limited impact;
23. Full replenishment may sometimes occur, when malnutrition is primarily due to starvation rather than to multiple metabolic derangements, when tumour growth is not rapid

24. Although infection with HIV progresses from acute to a chronic disease treated by multiple drug therapy, the patient should have access to nutritional therapy

B

a) *and in all patients with advanced stages of disease.*
b) *and in subjects affected by concurrent disease, such as hypertension and diabetes.*
c) *and patients should be treated conservatively, with total bowel rest and TPN if necessary.*
d) *and there is time and opportunity to reverse a state of depletion and, obviously when an effective oncologic therapy and nutritional support are associated in a combined modality approach.*
e) *being observed during the first weeks after injury.*
f) *burns can be divided into small, large, major and massive.*
g) *but rather the result of multiple metabolic aberrations.*
h) *but they are more intense and prolonged.*
i) *consequently to prevent complications and the mortality associated with it.*
j) *containing large quantities of proteins, minerals and micronutrients, which cause acute deficiency syndromes.*
k) *due to difficult venous access and destruction of the skin.*
l) *in approximately 5-7% of patients who have undergone abdominal radiotherapy.*
m) *malnourished patients and, thanks to the use of special immune nutrients, also in some patients who are not losing weight.*
n) *may have an important preventive role in maintaining health and quality of life in the elderly.*
o) *medium term PN is indicated and may allow resolution of intestinal obstruction and help to restore oral feeding.*
p) *mucositis or progressive weight loss decrease the compliance with cancer treatments, cause progressive delays and ultimately reduce their efficacy.*
q) *or if there is short bowel syndrome due to previous resectional surgery.*
r) *protein energy malnutrition (PEM) accompanied by micronutrient deficiencies is a major problem in the elderly suffering from poor health.*
s) *shock, acute respiratory failure, sepsis and multiple organ dysfunction syndrome.*
t) *significant gastrointestinal, gynaecological,*

genitourinary and pelvic bone damage.

u) *the acute deficit contributes to delay recovery; this can be reversed by early intravenous supplementation.*

v) *the lean body mass erosion and fat depletion, and cause a poor utilisation of the nutritive substrates.*

w) *the most favourable expected effect is a prevention of further nutritional deterioration.*

x) *to maintain good nutritional status in order to fight the infection and maintain an effective function.*

Exercise 2

Translate the expressions. Try to explain their meanings in English.

Segment, impact, health care system, care facilities, incidence, accompanied by, suffering from, out patients, hospital in-patients, institutionalised individuals, particularly susceptible to, ethical considerations, ensuring benefit, avoiding harm, remain a challenge, acute respiratory failure, multiple organ dysfunction syndrome, cutaneous exudative fluid, acute deficiency syndromes, difficult venous access, intensive care units, determine the responses, inhalation injury, dependent on intubation, mechanical ventilation, vulnerable, gastrointestinal failure, trace element losses, delay recovery, reversed, attainable, multiple metabolic aberrations, worldwide acceptance, discovery, body mass erosion, fat depletion, utilisation, essential, mutually interactive, has proven to benefit, mucositis, compliance with treatments, reduce efficacy, incurable patients, temporary lifesaving procedure, frequent finding, advanced stages, metabolic alterations, adverse, predictive factor, genitourinary, pelvic bone damage, radiation enteropathy, accurate estimate, concurrent disease, major abdominal surgery, surgical intervention, recent evidence, radiation-induced small bowel damage, previous resectional surgery, not amendable to surgery, scattered lesions, resolution of obstruction, limited impact, deterioration, full replenishment, metabolic derangements, metabolic alterations, interfere with, pointed out to, facilitate compliance with drug therapy.

Exercise 3

Prepare short talks and/or dialogues on these topics

1. Protein-energy malnutrition (PEM) in the elderly
2. Patients with major burns and the advantages of enteral nutrition in burns patients
3. Indications for nutritional support in surgical and non-surgical cancer patients
4. Radiation enteropathy
5. Effect of anticachectic agents in cancer
6. Nutritional support for patients with AIDS

Vocabulary 13

Fill in the meanings in your mother language:

aberration /ˌæb.əˈreɪ.ʃən/
acceptance /əkˈsep.təns/
accurate /ˈæk.jʊ.rət/
acute /əˈkjuːt/
admit /ədˈmɪt/
agent /ˈeɪ dʒənt/
anticachectic /ˈæntɪ.kəˈkɛk tɪk/
attainable /əˈteɪ.nə.bəl/
cascade /kæsˈkeɪd/
citrulline /ˈsɪ trəˌlin/
concurrent /kənˈkʌr.ənt/
conditio /kənˈdɪʃ.ɪ.əʊ/ **sine qua non** /ˌsaɪni-kweɪ ˈnɒn/
conservative /kənˈsɜːvətɪv/
contrary /ˈkɒn.trə.ri/
damage /ˈdæm.ɪdʒ/
deterioration /dɪˌtɪə.ri.əˈreɪ.ʃən/
disappointing /ˌdɪsəˈpɔɪntɪŋ/
enteropathy /ˌɛn təˈrɒp ə θi/
escape /ɪˈskeɪp/
exudate /ˌek.sjuːˈdeɪt/
exudative /ɪgˈzu də tɪv/
factor /ˈfæk.tər/
favourable /ˈfeɪ.vər.ə.blˌ/
genitourinary /ˌdʒen.ɪ.təʊˈjʊə.rɪ.nər.i/
gynaecological /ˌgaɪ nɪˈkɒl ə dʒi.kəl/
homebound /ˈhoʊmˌbaʊnd/
hypertension /ˌhaɪ.pəˈten.tʃən/
hypophagia /ˌhaɪ.pəˈˈfeɪ.dʒə/
in particular /in.pəˈtɪk.jʊ.lər/
in-patient /ˈɪnˌpeɪ ʃənt/
incurable /ɪnˈkyʊər.ə.bəl/
institutionalise /ˌɪn stɪˈtu ʃə nlˌaɪz/
interfere /ˌɪn.təˈfɪər/
intestinal /ˌin.ˈtes.tin.əl/
investigation /ɪnˌves.tɪˈgeɪ.ʃən/
laparotomy /ˌlæp əˈrɒt ə mi/
lesion /ˈliː.ʒən/
lifesaving /ˈlaɪfˌseɪ.vɪŋ/
malignant /məˈlɪg.nənt/
massive /ˈmæsɪv/
mental /ˈmen.təl/
modality /məʊˈdæl.ə.ti/
morbidity /ˌmɔːˈbɪd.ɪ.ti/
mortality /mɔːˈtæl.ə.ti/
mucositis /ˈmyu kəs.aɪ.tɪs/
mutual /ˈmjuː.tʃu.əl/
notice /ˈnəʊ.tɪs/
obviously /ˈɒb.vi.əs.li/
out /aʊt/ **-patient** /ˈpeɪ.ʃənt/
pelvic /ˈpel.vɪk/
physical /ˈfɪz.ɪ.kəl/
point /ˈpɔɪnt/ **out** /aʊt/
potentially /pəˈten.ʃəl.i/
predictive /prɪˈdɪk.tɪv/
prone /prəʊn/
quantification /ˈkwɒn təˌfɪ.keɪ.ʃən/
randomise /ˈræn dəˌmaɪz/
recognise /ˈrɛk əgˌnaɪz/
replenishment /rɪˈplɛn.ɪʃ.mənt/
resectional /rɪˈsɛk ʃən.əl/
resolution /ˌrez.əˈluː.ʃən/
restore /rɪˈstɔːr/
reversible /rɪˈvɜː.sə.blˌ/
scattered /ˈskæt.əd/
screen /skriːn/
scrutiny /ˈskrut.n.i/
slim /slɪm/
suggestive /səˈdʒes.tɪv/
surgery /ˈsɜː.dʒər.i/
susceptible /səˈsep.tɪ.blˌ/
translate /trænsˈleɪt/
uniform /ˈjuː.nɪ.fɔːm/
venous /ˈviː.nəs/ **access** /ˈæk.ses/

Solution to Exercise 1

1r, 2n, 3h, 4s, 5j, 6k, 7f, 8e, 9u, 10i, 11g, 12v, 13m, 14p, 15a, 16t, 17b, 18l, 19c, 20q, 21o, 22w, 23d, 24x

Unit 14 - Nutritional support in different clinical situations 4

Nutritional support during pregnancy

In summary, pregnancy constitutes a special situation, in which adequate **nutrition is vital for both mother and child**. Delay in giving nutritional support to starving or semistarving pregnant women adversely affects the foetus and may result in increased foetal mortality and morbidity. Nutritional support should be implemented early in all such cases.

Nutritional support in neonatology

Although all **infants born before 37 weeks** gestation are '**premature**', this definition encompasses an extremely heterogeneous group of patients in terms of **prognosis**, **nutritional status** at birth, **concomitant disease** and nutritional **requirements**. Contrast, for example, the sick 600g infant born 15 weeks early and needing mechanical ventilation, inotropic support for hypotension, and fluid restriction, with a well, 35 week gestation infant, weighing 2.5 kg and nursed in a cot. The former has only a 50% chance of survival, is intolerant of even small volumes of milk feed and at high risk of necrotising enterocolitis (NEC). The latter has **immature suck** and **swallow** mechanisms, but **tolerates full milk feeds** within a few days of birth and has an excellent prognosis. **The most premature infants** and in particular those under 1.5 kg birth weight undoubtedly pose **the most difficult nutritional challenges**.

In the **newborn** infant with **gastrointestinal failure** as a consequence of **congenital or acquired bowel disease parenteral** nutrition is a life saving intervention. In the preterm infant immaturity of **gut function** also dictates that nutrients must initially be given parenterally if negative consequences of starvation are to be avoided. The premature newborn is **deprived acutely of nutrients** at the moment the **umbilical cord is cut** and it seems appropriate to **re-institute nutrient supply** as quickly as possible.

Current practice frequently errs on the side of over-caution, with delayed introduction and slow build up of nutrition, ensuring **over time a cumulative deficit** when **compared with in-utero nutrient** accretion rates. **Reducing this deficit** can be expected to lead to improvement in **growth** rates, although whether there will be a better **neurodevelopmental outcome** requires long term evaluation. The safety of a more 'aggressive' approach to early parenteral nutrition may not be fully established, but there is a strong a priori case for avoiding starvation and malnutrition. Full **enteral feeding** can be achieved over the **first one or two weeks** of life in many of the preterm infants who initially receive parenteral nutrition. Large clinical trials have indicated the superiority of preterm over term formula, and highlighted potential **advantages** of mother's **milk** despite its variable nutritional composition. The relative merits of supplemented mother's milk versus preterm formula needs further investigation.

Nutritional support in infants, children and adolescents

Provided they are carried out by experienced staff, the currently available methods of nutritional support including **EN and PN,** are **safe and effective** methods of treatment, improving the clinical condition, nutritional status, growth, and quality of life of many paediatric patients, as well as being life saving for a large number of infants and children. These patients, however, are particularly **susceptible** to severe **adverse effects** and complications of **errors in management**. Therefore meticulous care and an experienced paediatric team are essential to achieve the full benefits of nutritional support to paediatric patients.

Eating disorders – anorexia nervosa and bulimia nervosa

Eating disorders are classified within three categories (currently under revision): **Anorexia Nervosa (AN)**, **Bulimia Nervosa** and **Eating Disorders Non Otherwise Specified**. The common denominator for all of these forms of **obsessive engagement in body weigh**t and **eating patterns** associated with profound physical and psychological morbidity. The present lifetime prevalence of all eating disorders is 5%. **Anorexia nervosa** is characterised by extreme **low body weight and a fear of its increase.** The common symptoms of eating disorders fall under three headings: behavioural, psychopathological and physical symptoms. The **behavioural characteristics** are: cutting back on the **amount of food**, **strict rules** regarding food, **prolonged fasting** (more than 8 hours), **ritual behaviour** associated with purchase, preparation and consumption of food, **little variety** in foods, and **avoidance of social eating**. The **psychopathological features** are mainly those of **body image** disturbance; and the **physical symptoms** include: **weight loss** or **growth failure**, **menstrual impairment** and amenorrhoea, increased **sensitivity to low temperature**, **fatigue** and **weakness**. Anorexia nervosa is connected with **severe malnutrition**, which increases risk of malnutrition related complication development. Nutrition therapy is crucial but it can be **complicated** by **poor tolerance** and the onset of **refeeding syndrome**. Therefore careful feeding plan must be designed for each individual patient.

Nutrition therapy for neurological disorders

Nutritional issues associated with neurological diseases can be classified into two types. The **first** type arises from **nutritional deficiencies** (e.g. **Korsakov's** syndrome, **beriberi**), related to **alcoholism, malnutrition or malabsorption**. **Nutrient repletion** is required, although primary prevention is the cornerstone of their management. The **second** type is associated with severe **progressive** acute or chronic **degenerative disorders**, e.g. closed **head trauma**, **stroke**, **amyotrophic lateral** or **multiple sclerosis**, **Parkinson/Alzheimer's** disease, which **impair** the ability to **feed, chew, or swallow**. Nutritional therapies are valuable adjuncts to medical management of these conditions. All patients of the second type are at risk of malnutrition, and nutritional management is complex. Many have **dysphagia**, and the ability to **obtain, prepare and present food to the mouth** is often compromised. The pattern of dysfunction depends on the site and severity of the lesion(s). **Nutritional therapy** is an important part of treatment of these patients. The various methods of **dietary support** that are used in this group of patients (diet modifications, dietary supplements, enteral or even parenteral nutrition) are considered here.

Nutrition and wound healing

The **regeneration** of damaged tissue is a necessary condition for the survival from disease and injury connected with physical, chemical, infective or immune damage. It is a precisely regulated process controlled by **many humoral and cellular factors**. A **wound** is a **cutaneous** defect which is associated with a variable extent of **subcutaneous tissue damage**. Whereas in the early foetal period wounds heal without scarring, in later foetal phases and the postnatal period wound healing is not complete (ad integrum) and **scarring is the usual result**.

In the postnatal period **inflammation** plays a central role in wound healing and scarring is probably a consequence of this inflammation. Nutrition should be an indispensable part of the **complex care** of patients with large and non-healing wounds. The wound **healing process** is well orchestrated and composed from inflammation, proliferation and maturation. Local and systemic negative influences (including malnutrition) suppress this process. The resulting chronic wounds demand many resources in the clinical daily routine. Therefore, **local wound management** and the **treatment of systemic inflammation** and **nutrition support** are essential for successful wound healing and prevention of the development of chronic wounds. During the wound-healing process much energy is needed. Especially in malnourished subjects an in patients in catabolic phases of stress, the prompt assessment of nutritional status is necessary to **start supplementation** quickly, if applicable. **High protein** supplements with **essential micronutrients** seem to be especially beneficial.

Nutrition and pressure ulcers

A pressure ulcer is an area of localized **damage to the skin and underlying tissue** caused by **pressure, shear, friction** and or a combination of these. Pressure ulcers

(PU) remain a major healthcare problem throughout the world with prevalence rates ranging from 3 to 66% in health care organizations. Along with causing patients a great deal of discomfort, PU significantly increase the workload in all healthcare sectors and therefore are associated with high costs. **Frail, elderly and chronically ill** patients are particularly **vulnerable** in this connection. The problem of PU therefore is likely to increase as the **population ages** in most Western countries. **Protein** supplements can significantly reduce the development of pressure ulcers. Proper nutritional management is therefore a necessary **part of the complex care** of patients who are at risk of development of, or who already have developed, a pressure ulcer.

Nutritional support in the diabetic patient

The prevalence of diabetes mellitus is growing in developed countries and hence the **number of diabetic patients** who need enteral and parenteral nutrition support is rising. **Type 1 diabetes** is frequently encountered by those giving nutritional support, but due to the increasing prevalence of obesity in both developed and developing countries, **type 2 patient** numbers are increasing and form by far **the largest group** among diabetic patients requiring nutritional care. **During acute illness,** the **principles** of nutritional support of the diabetic are the **same** as those in the non-diabetic although there are **specific problems** particularly in **carbohydrate and fat** metabolism which may necessitate adjustments in **substrate administration** and **insulin** administration, especially since the **stress response** to injury causes **insulin resistance and hyperglycaemia.**

Insulin administration is frequently necessary during nutritional support of the diabetic as well as of some non-diabetic stressed patients. It should be administered according to changes and **trends in blood glucose level.** In the **unstable patient**, receiving nutritional support, insulin should be administered via **an i.v. pump** which allows **continuous delivery** and rapid **changes in dosage,** whereas in stable patients their normal subcutaneous insulin regime can be used and adjusted according to monitored blood glucose values.

Home artificial nutrition

Sometimes a person cannot obtain enough **nutrients from normal food** because of severe gastrointestinal disease impairing **nutritional intake or uptake by the gut**. If the loss of gastrointestinal function is permanent, life-long nutritional support will be necessary. This may be achieved by parenteral nutrition, in the case of **transient or permanent intestinal failure** or in the case of upper GI dysfunction (mainly **swallowing disorders**), or by long term enteral nutrition, provided in the home setting. **Home artificial**

nutrition (HAN) has become routine care in most developed countries allowing cost savings (less expensive, than in-hospital treatment), improved quality of life, proximity to family, and optimization of **normal social and professional life**. It has been proposed that nutritional support for acute or chronic GI dysfunction is the same in principle as dialysis for acute or chronic kidney failure and should be organized and funded in a comparable way.

Exercise 1
Match the column A with the column B. Try to learn the expressions and/or sentences by heart.

A

1. Delay in giving nutritional support to starving or semistarving pregnant women
2. Although all infants born before 37 weeks gestation are 'premature', this definition encompasses an extremely heterogeneous group of patients
3. In the newborn infant with gastrointestinal failure as a consequence of congenital or acquired bowel disease
4. In the preterm infant immaturity of gut function also dictates that nutrients
5. Full enteral feeding can be achieved over the first one or two weeks of life
6. Large clinical trials highlighted potential advantages of mother's milk
7. Paediatric patients are particularly susceptible
8. Eating disorders are classified within three categories:
9. Anorexia nervosa is characterised
10. The behavioural characteristics are: cutting back on the amount of food, strict rules regarding food, prolonged fasting (more than 8 hours),
11. The psychopathological features are mainly those of body image disturbance; and the physical symptoms include:
12. Nutrition therapy is crucial but it can be complicated by
13. Nutritional issues associated with neurological diseases can be classified into two types: the first type arises from nutritional deficiencies related to alcoholism, malnutrition or malabsorption;
14. Many patients have dysphagia, and the ability to obtain, prepare and present food to the mouth is often compromised;
15. The regeneration of damaged tissue is a necessary condition
16. A wound is a cutaneous defect which is associated

with a variable extent of subcutaneous tissue damage;

17. Inflammation plays a central role in wound healing
18. Local wound management and the treatment of systemic inflammation and nutrition support
19. A pressure ulcer is an area of localized damage to the skin and underlying tissue
20. Frail, elderly and chronically ill patients are particularly vulnerable;
21. The number of diabetic patients who need
22. Type 2 patient numbers are increasing and form by far
23. During acute illness, the principles of nutritional support of the diabetic are the same as those in the non-diabetic
24. In the unstable patient, receiving nutritional support,
25. Sometimes a person cannot obtain enough nutrients from normal food
26. Home artificial nutrition has become routine care allowing cost savings

B

a) *adversely affects the foetus and may result in increased foetal mortality and morbidity.*

b) *although there are specific problems, and insulin should be administered according to changes and trends in blood glucose level.*

c) *and scarring is probably a consequence of this inflammation.*

d) *Anorexia Nervosa (AN), Bulimia Nervosa and Eating Disorders Non Otherwise Specified.*

e) *are essential for successful wound healing and prevention of the development of chronic wounds.*

f) *because of severe gastrointestinal disease impairing nutritional intake or uptake by the gut.*

g) *by extreme low body weight and a fear of its increase.*

h) *caused by pressure, shear, friction and or a combination of these.*

i) *despite its variable nutritional composition.*

j) *enteral and parenteral nutrition support is rising.*

k) *for the survival from disease and injury connected with physical, chemical, infective or immune damage.*

l) *improved quality of life, proximity to family, and optimization of normal social and professional life.*

m) *in many of the preterm infants who initially receive parenteral nutrition.*

n) *in terms of prognosis, nutritional status at birth, concomitant disease and nutritional requirements.*

o) *insulin should be administered via an i.v. pump which allows continuous delivery and rapid changes in dosage.*

p) *must initially be given parenterally if negative consequences of starvation are to be avoided.*

q) *parenteral nutrition is a life saving intervention.*

r) *poor tolerance and the onset of refeeding syndrome.*

s) *protein supplements can significantly reduce the development of pressure ulcers.*

t) *ritual behaviour associated with purchase, preparation and consumption of food, little variety in foods, and avoidance of social eating.*

u) *the largest group among diabetic patients requiring nutritional care.*

v) *the second type is associated with severe progressive acute or chronic degenerative disorders, e.g. closed head trauma, stroke, amyotrophic lateral or multiple sclerosis, Parkinson/ Alzheimer's disease, which impair the ability to feed, chew, or swallow.*

w) *the wound healing process is composed from inflammation, proliferation and maturation.*

x) *to severe adverse effects and complications of errors in management.*

y) *various methods of dietary support that are used in this group of patients (diet modifications, dietary supplements, enteral or even parenteral nutrition) are considered here.*

z) *weight loss or growth failure, menstrual impairment and amenorrhoea, increased sensitivity to low temperature, fatigue and weakness.*

Exercise 2

Translate the expressions. Try to explain their meanings in English.

Semistarving pregnant women, foetal mortality and morbidity, implemented, premature, mechanical ventilation, inotropic support for hypotension, fluid restriction, milk feed, necrotising enterocolitis, suck and swallow mechanisms, congenital or acquired bowel disease, life saving intervention, negative consequences, deprived acutely of nutrient, umbilical cord is cut, current practice, over-caution, accumulative deficit, in-utero, nutrient accretion rates, formula, neurodevelopmental outcome, preterm infants, variable nutritional composition, carried out, currently available methods, susceptible, adverse effects, errors in management, meticulous care, common denominator, obsessive engagement in body weight, eating patterns, behavioural characteristics, strict rules, prolonged fasting, purchase, preparation and consumption, avoidance of social eating, amenorrhoea, fatigue, feeding plan, designed, nutrient repletion, progressive, degenerative disorders, stroke, amyotrophic lateral or multiple sclerosis, impair the ability to feed, chew, or swallow, dysphagia, regeneration, humoral and cellular factors, cutaneous defect, subcutaneous tissue damage, postnatal period, scarring, complex care, healing process, inflammation, proliferation, maturation, suppress, daily routine, prompt assessment, seem to be beneficial, pressure ulcers, great deal of discomfort, pressure, shear, friction, frail, elderly, chronically ill, complex care, requiring nutritional care, necessitate adjustments in substrate administration, stress response, insulin resistance, hyperglycaemia, changes and trends, unstable patient, continuous delivery, changes in dosage, adjusted, impairing, nutritional intake or uptake by the gut, transient or permanent, intestinal failure, home artificial nutrition, in principle.

Exercise 3
Prepare short talks and/or dialogues on these topics

1. The adverse effects of starvation on pregnancy and foetal outcome
2. The need for early nutritional support in the very low birth weight premature infant
3. Nutritional support in the premature newborn
4. Assessment of children and adolescents at risk of malnutrition
5. Treatment possibilities in anorexia and bulimia nervosa
6. The nutritional aspects of wound healing
7. The role of nutrition and nutrition supplements in pressure ulcer healing
8. Long-term dietary management of diabetic patients
9. Indications for home artificial nutrition

Vocabulary 14

a priori /ˌeɪ.praɪˈɔr.aɪ/
ability /əˈbɪl.ɪ.ti/
accretion /əˈkri ʃən/ **rate** /reɪt/
ad integrum /æd.ɪnˈtɛgrəm/
adjunct /ˈædʒ.ʌŋkt/
adjustment /əˈdʒʌst.mənt/
adversely /ˈæd.vɜː.sli/
Alzheimer's disease / ˈɔltsˌhaɪ.mərz.dɪˌziz/
amenorrhoea /ˌeɪ.men.əˈriː.ə/
applicable /əˈplɪk.ə.bl̩/
arise /əˈraɪz/
avoidance /əˈvɔɪ.dəns/
behaviour /bɪˈheɪ.vjə/
beriberi /ˌber.ɪˈber.i/
by /baɪ/ **far** /fɑː/
cellular /ˈsel.jʊ.lər/
chew /tʃuː/
clinical /ˈklɪn.ɪ.kəl/
compare /kəmˈpeər/
congenital /kənˈdʒen.ɪ.təl/
continuous /kənˈtɪn.ju.əs/
cot /kɒt/
cumulative /ˈkjuː.mjʊ.lə.tɪv/
cut /ˈkʌt/ **back** /bæk/ **on st**
degenerative /dɪˈdʒen.ər.ə.tɪv/

delivery /dɪˈlɪv.ər.i/
denominator /dɪˈnɒm.əˌneɪ.tər/
deprive /dɪˈpraɪv/
dietary /ˈdaɪ.ə.tər.i/
dysphagia /dɪsˈfeɪ.dʒi.ə/
eating /iː.tɪŋ/
encompass /ɪnˈkʌm.pəs/
encounter /ɪnˈkaʊn.tə/
engagement /ɛnˈgeɪ.dʒ.mənt/
err /ɜr/
experienced /ɪkˈspɪə.ri.ənst/
frail /freɪl/
friction /ˈfrɪk.ʃən/
fund /fʌnd/
gestation /dʒesˈteɪ.ʃən/
hence /hens/
heterogeneous /ˌhɛt.ər.əˈdʒi.ni.əs/
humoral /ˈhjuː.mər.əl/
image /ˈɪm.ɪdʒ/
immature /ˌɪm.əˈtʃʊər/
in utero /in.juːˈtər.əʊ/
initially /ɪˈnɪʃ.əl.i/
inotropic /ˌɪn.əˈtrəp.ɪk/
Korsakov 's syndrome /ˈsɪn droʊm/
lifetime /ˈlaɪfˌtaɪm/
localized /ˈləʊ.kəˌlaɪzd/
maturation /ˌmæt.jʊəˈreɪ.ʃən/
merit /ˈmɛr ɪt/
meticulous /məˈtɪk.jʊ.ləs/
multiple /ˈmʌl.tɪ.pl̩/
sclerosis /skləˈrəʊ.sɪs/
necrotising /ˈnɛk rəˌtaɪz.ɪŋ/
enterocolitis /ˌɛn.tə.roʊ.koʊˈlaɪ.tɪs/
neonatology /ˌni.oʊ.neɪˈtɒl.ə.dʒi/
neurodevelopmental /ˌnjʊə.
rəʊ.dɪˌvel.əpˈmen.təl/
nurse /nɜːs/
nutrition /njuːˈtrɪʃən/
obsessive /əbˈsesɪv/
orchestrate /ˈɔːkɪˌstreɪt/
over /ˈoʊ vər/ **-caution** /ˈkɔː.ʃən/
Parkinson's /ˈpɑː.kɪn.
sənz/ **disease** /dɪˈziːz/
particularly /pəˈtɪk.jʊ.lə.li/
postnatal /ˌpəʊstˈneɪ.təl/
promptly /ˈprɒmpt.li/
pump /pʌmp/
purchase /ˈpɜr tʃəs/
re /riː/ **-institute** /ˈɪn.stɪ.tjuːt/
regime /reɪˈʒiːm/
ritual /ˈrɪt.ju.əl/
scarring /skɑːr.ɪŋ/
severity /sɪˈver.ɪ.ti/
shear /ʃɪər/
site /saɪt/
solve /sɒlv/
subcutaneous /ˌsʌb.kjʊˈteɪ.ni.əs/
suck /sʌk/
superiority /səˌpɪər.iˈɔr.ɪ.ti/
term /tɜːm/
transient /ˈtræn.zi.ənt/
umbilical cord /ʌmˈbɪl.ɪ.kəlˌkɔːd/
unstable /ʌnˈsteɪ.bl̩/
uptake /ˈʌp.teɪk/
vital /ˈvaɪ.təl/
weakness /ˈwiːk.nəs/
workload /ˈwɜːk.ləʊd/

Solution to Exercise 1
1a, 2n, 3q, 4p, 5m, 6i, 7x, 8d, 9g, 10t, 11z, 12r, 13v, 14y, 15k, 16w, 17c, 18e, 19h, 20s, 21j, 22u, 23b, 24o, 25f, 26l

Bibliography

1. BASICS in clinical nutrition. Fourth Edition. Editor-in-chief Luboš Sobotka. Praha, Galén 2011. 724 p.
2. BAUMRUKOVÁ, Irena: English in Urgent Care Medicine. Exlibris 2015. 944 p.
3. COOPER, George: Be you own nutritionist. Rethink your relationship with food. Discover the True Art of healthy eating. Croydon, Short Books 2013. 277 p.
4. GOOD COOKING made easy. Compiled by Bridget Jones Twickenham, Hamlyn Publishing Bridgehouse 1986. 512 s.
5. MATĚJÍČKOVÁ, Radka, SOVJÁK, Richard: Human nutrition and prevention of food-borne diseases. Praha, Czech University of Agriculture 2009. 192 s.
6. PAYNE, Fiona: 101 Essential tips. Healthy Living. London, New York, Stuttgart, Moscow, Dorling Kindersley 1996. 72 p.
7. WEBSTER-GANDY, Joan: Understanding Food and Nutrition. Dorset, Family Doctor Publications Limited 2006. 164 p.

www.ingramcontent.com/pod-product-compliance
Lightning Source LLC
Chambersburg PA
CBHW020718180526
45163CB00001B/14
9781514493816